SpringerWienNewYork

Michael Hertl (ed.)

Autoimmune Diseases of the Skin

Pathogenesis, Diagnosis, Management

Third, Revised and Enlarged Edition

SpringerWienNewYork

Editor
Michael Hertl, MD
Professor and Chairman
Department of Dermatology and Allergology,
Philipps University,
Marburg,
Germany

Front Cover: Systemic lupus erythematosus (A) with subepidermal cytoid bodies and positive lupus band test in lesional skin (B), subacute lupus erythematosus (C) and livedo vasculopathy (D).

Printed with financial support of
Biotest AG
Dreieich, Germany

© 2001, 2005 and 2011 Springer-Verlag/Wien
Printed in Austria
SpringerWienNewYork is a part of Springer Science+Business Media
springer.at

The publisher and editor kindly wish to inform you that in some cases, despite their best efforts to do so, the obtaining of copyright permissions and usage of excerpts of text is not always successful.

© *Illustrations*: all illustrations with courtesy of the authors
Cover Design: WMXDesign GmbH, Heidelberg, Germany
Typesetting: le-tex publishing services GmbH, Leipzig, Germany
Printing and binding: Theiss GmbH, St. Stefan, Austria

Printed on acid-free and chlorine-free bleached paper
SPIN: 12550098
Library of Congress Control Number: 2010932332

With 95 colored figures

ISBN 978-3-211-99224-1   SpringerWienNewYork
ISBN 978-3-211-20686-8   2nd edition SpringerWienNewYork

Foreword

Based on recent advances in the understanding of the immunological pathogenesis of many chronic inflammatory disorders there is increasing evidence that several of them are characterized and potentially mediated by autoimmune phenomena. Classical examples are rheumatoid arthritis, myasthenia gravis, pemphigus vulgaris, lupus erythematosus and multiple sclerosis. Others, such as psoriasis vulgaris, some less well-characterized collagen vascular disorders, vasculitides and a subtype of chronic urticaria have a more or less pronounced autoimmune background that has to be considered in the overall management of these disorders. A significant portion of autoimmune diseases precipitate primarily or secondarily at the skin. Understanding the cutaneous symptoms may be therefore crucial for the diagnosis, classification and therapeutic management of organ-specific and systemic disorders that require special attention by the physician.

This book is set out to present the most recent scientific and clinically relevant state-of-the-art-knowledge on the broad spectrum of autoimmune disorders affecting the skin. It is meant to provide the most recent information on these disorders for clinicians as well as practicioners in dermatology, medicine, rheumatology, ENT, pediatrics, ophthalmology, orthopedics etc and for basic scientists interested in human autoimmunity. Each book chapter dealing with a distinct cutaneous autoimmmune disorder consists of an introduction focusing on the state of knowledge regarding pathogenesis and epidemiology followed by a practical guide how to identify and handle the particular disorder(s). Special attention is paid to genuine cutaneous autoimmune disorders such as autoimmune bullous skin disorders including pemphigus, pemphigoid and epidermolysis bullosa acquisita. These disorders can be considered as paradigms of organ-specific autoimmune disorders because autoantigens and autoantibody-mediated pathogenesis are well-characterized.

Major progress has been made in the diagnosis and classification of collagen vascular disorders such as systemic sclerosis, lupus erythematosus, dermatomyositis and overlap syndromes. These advances have provided the basis for more specific therapeutic interventions. Recent pathogenetic findings in psoriasis, lichen planus and chronic urticaria have led to novel therapeutic concepts that will replace the "classical" symptomatic treatments that have been established for decades. One striking example is the therapeutic effect of biologics in severe psoriasis vulgaris and psoriatic arthritis and the modulatory effect of high dose immunoglobulins in dermatomyositis and severe vasculitides. In addition to the book chapters on distinct clinical cutaneous disorders, the introductory chapter explains basic immunological principles leading to autoimmunity and the final chapter gives an overview of the mode of action of novel immunomodulatory drugs. The present book which is edited by my co-worker Dr. Michael Hertl is set out to combine major scientific advances in the understanding of autoimmunity with the clinical presentation and management of these disorders. I am convinced that the book constitutes a very successful effort to provide a handbook for those who are scientifically or clinically interested in autoimmune disorders of the skin. I wish the editor and the authors success with this endeavor.

Erlangen, July 2001   **Gerold Schuler**

Preface to the Third Edition

We are very grateful for the continuous positive reception of the book which led to the present, third completely revised and enlarged edition of Autoimmune Diseases of the Skin". The contents of the book reflect the rapid development of medical research and its impact on novel diagnostics and treatments in the field of autoimmune disorders.

The third edition of the book is dedicated to my father, Prof. Dr. Michael Hertl, who has been a devoted and most enthusiastic genuine clinician scientist all over his life. His never-ending broad interest to learn and extend his sight of the world has been the driving force for me to join the world of academic medicine.

Marburg, October 2010   **Michael Hertl**

Preface to the Second Edition

Thanks to the positive reception of the first edition of the book by the medical community both in Europe and in the USA, the present book has come to its second edition. All the chapters have been thoroughly revised and two new chapters on Vitiligo and Alopecia areata were included.

We hope that the present book will continue to provide state-of-the-art knowledge for those who are interested and clinically involved with autoimmune disorders of the skin.

The present edition of the book is dedicated to my clinical teacher, Professor Gerd-Klaus Steigleder, on the occasion of his 80th birthday.

Marburg, January 2005   **Michael Hertl**

Preface to the First Edition

Hundred years ago, Paul Ehrlich speculated whether an individual is able to produce toxic autoantibodies and about the implications of such antibodies for disease. The contention that an alteration of the body fluids causes disease followed the traditional teachings of Hipppocrates and Galen that disease results from dysfunction of the four humors. However, Ehrlich introduced the novel concept of antigen specificity that was based on his side chain theory of antibody formation: (1) antibodies are naturally occuring substances that serve as receptors on the cell surface; (2) the specificity of antibody for antigen is determined by a unique stereochemical configuration of atoms that permits the antibody to bind tightly and chemically to its appropriate antigen; (3) the number of different combining sites structures available is so great that each one differs from the others, with little or no cross reactivity among them; (4) and in order to induce active antibody formation, it is only necessary that appropriate receptors be present on the cells for antigen to interact with them and so stimulate their overproduction and liberation into the blood. According to this description by Paul Ehrlich, the antibody ap-peared to be a polymorphous cytoplasmic agent with a unique feature – a highly organized combining site (the haptophore group) that determined its unique antigen specificity.

It was Bordet who showed that anti-erythrocyte antibodies were capable of mediating immune hemolysis giving rise to the idea that self-produced hemolytic antibodies might assist in destroying autologous erythrocytes.

This and similar findings including the description of cytotoxic antibodies against a variety of other cell types prompted Ehrlich to say: "… the organism possesses certain contrivances by means of which the immunity reaction, so easily produced by all kinds of cells, is prevented from acting against the organism's own elements and so giving rise to autotoxins … so that we might be justified in speaking of a 'horror autotoxicus' of the organism. These contrivances are naturally of the highest importance for the individual" (P. Ehrlich and J. Morgenroth, Berlin. Klin. Wochenschr., 1901).

When Metalnikov was the first to demonstrate the generation of autoantibodies that were cytotoxic against spermatozoa in vitro, Ehrlich questioned that they were able to induce pathology *in vivo*.

It took, however, more than fourty years that some distinct organ-specific immune disorders were categorized as true autoimmune diseases. Among the first identified were autoimmune orchitis, allergic encephalomyelitis, autoimmune thyroiditis, pemphigus vulgaris and bullous pemphigoid. Noteworthy, some of these disorders are exclusively mediated by circulating autoantibodies such as the hemolytic anemias, thrombocytopenia, pemphigus, and pemphigoid while others, such as allergic autoimmune encephalomyelitis and autoimmune thyroiditis require the transfer of immunocompetent cells in addition to autoantibodies.

The existence of immunological tolerance was the logical consequence of Paul Ehrlich's postulate that there was a "horror autotoxicus" a mechanism that inhibited formation of potentially harmful autoantibodies to self *in vivo*. It was Owen to show that dizygotic calves whose circulation was connected *in utero* were unable to respond to each other's antigens after birth. Out of this and similar observations, the clonal deletion theory was invented by Burnet meaning that antigen present during embryonic life would somehow cause destruction of self-reactive clones. The observation that adult animals could be rendered unresponsive to foreign antigens by the administration of large doses of the antigen led to the notion that immunological tolerance could be also acquired.

The recognition of different central and peripheral immune mechanisms leading to immunological tolerance are all based on Ehrlich's concept of "horror autotoxicus", *i.e.* acquired or active immune regulation of unwanted immune responses against self. The finding that B lymphocytes generally require the help of T lymphocytes in their antibody response to a defined antigenic stimulus led to the discovery of distinct immune cell subsets including helper cells, cytotoxic cells and regulatory cells. The identification of the idiotypeanti idiotype network was born out of the discovery that the antigen binding site of the antibody itsself can act as an antigen for anti-idiotypic antibodies. Anti-idiotypic immune responses are part of the physiological immune surveillance aimed at limiting the extent of an immune response.

The identification of different lineages of antigen presenting cells has taken away much attention from T lymphocytes as the exclusive regulators of immune and autoimmune responses. Major interest has recently focused on dendritic cells, bone marrow-derived antigen presenting cells with potent capacity to induce primary T-cell-mediated immune responses. However, accumulating evidence has demonstrated that the dendritic cell system bears much more plasticity than originally thought. Dendritic cells can arise from several different types of progenitor cells and different functional types of dendritic cells can be generated from the same precursor. It thus appears that dendritic cells have the potential to modulate immune responses within the wide spectrum of immunity on the one hand and immunological tolerance on the other hand.

The rapid development of immunological research has also provided major insights in the pathogenesis of autoimmune disorders which has implications for classification, diagnosis and therapy of these disorders. Classical examples for well-characterized autoimmune disorders are myasthenia gravis, pemphigus vulgaris, and hemolytic anemia. Furthermore, the availability of recombinant forms of the major autoantigens of these disorders has provided critical tools to investigate autoimmunity versus immunological tolerance to these self proteins in affected patients and healthy individuals.

The increasing understanding of the mechanisms that lead to immunological tolerance to self and the role that HLA and non-HLA alleles play in antigen recognition by autoaggressive T cells may also lead to novel therapeutic strategies. Several clinical studies have sought to restore immunological tolerance to self by the administration of modified self peptides, such as the administration of altered peptide ligands of myelin proteins in multiple sclerosis. Immature dendritic cells hold great promise as highly efficient tools to induce immunological tolerance to defined self proteins or peptides as demonstrated in murine allograft rejection models. They may induce tolerance by inducing antigenspecific anergy of autoreactive T cells and/ or by the induction of regulatory T lymphocytes that inhibit the activation of autoaggressive T cells.

I am very grateful that internationally leading experts in the field of cutaneous autoimmune disorders spontaneously agreed to provide comprehensive and well-illustrated overviews of the major autoimmune disorders of the skin. It was truly fun to interact with all of them! In addition, I would like to acknowledge the support and efforts of Springer Verlag in making this kind of book possible. We hope that the concept of this book will indeed help to broaden the understanding of cutaneous autoimmune disorders for those working in the many clinical disciplines which are involved in the care of these patients. Finally, I thank my wife for her continous support and her help and criticism during the development of this book.

Erlangen, July 2001 **Michael Hertl**

Contents

List of Contributors

Tilo Biedermann, MD
Department of Dermatology
Eberhard Karls University Tübingen
Liebermeisterstr. 25
72076 Tübingen
Germany
Tel.: 0049 7071-2980836
Fax: 0049 7071-294117
e-mail: tilo.biedermann@med.uni-
tuebingen.de

Luca Borradori, MD
Department of Dermatology
Inselspital
University of Bern
Freiburgstrasse
3010 Bern
Switzerland
Tel. 0041 31 632 2288
Fax: 0041 31 632 8355
e-mail: luca.borradori@insel.ch

Caroline Bussmann, MD
Department of Dermatology and Allergy
University of Bonn
Sigmund-Freud-Str. 25
D-53127 Bonn
Tel. +49-228-287-15370
Fax. +49-228-287-14333

Jeffrey P. Callen, MD
Division of Dermatology
University of Louisville
310 East Broadway
Louisville, KY 40202
USA
Tel.: 001 502 583 1749
Fax: 001 502 583 3028
e-mail: Jefca@aol.com

Jan Dutz, MD
Division of Dermatology
Faculty of Medicine
University of British Columbia
835 West 10th Avenue
Vancouver BC
V5Z 4E8
Canada
Tel.: 001 604 875 4747
Fax: 001 604 8736 9919
e-mail: dutz@interchange.ubc.ca

Kevin McElwee, PhD
Department of Dermatology
and Skin Science
VGH Research Pavilion
828 West 10th Avenue, Room #467
Vancouver, BC V5Z 1L8
Tel: 001-604-875-4111 ext. 63908
Fax: 001-604-875-4376
e-mail: kmcelwee@interchange.ubc.ca

Rüdiger Eming, MD
Department of Dermatology
and Allergology
Philipp University Marburg
Deutschhausstraße 9
35037 Marburg
Germany
Tel.: 0049 6421 58 66280
Fax: 0049 6421 58 62902
e-mail: eming@med.uni-marburg.de

Robert I. Fox, MD, PhD
Allergy and Rheumatology Clinic
Scripps Memorial Hospital and Research
Foundation
9850 Genesee Ave, #860
La Jolla, CA 92037
USA
Tel.: 001 858 4572023
Fax: 001 858 457 2721
e-mail: robertfoxmd@mac.com

Camille Francès, MD
Service de Dermatologie-Allergologie
Hôpital Tenon
4, rue de la Chine
F-75020 Paris
France
Tel. +33 1 56 01 64 62
Fax +33 1 56 01 64 58
e-mail camille.frances@tnn.aphp.fr

Pia Freyschmidt-Paul, MD
Dermatology/Allergology
Schimmelpfengstraße 4
D-34613 Schwalmstadt
Germany
Tel.: 0049 6691 806 5112
Fax: 0049 6691 806 5129
e-mail: paul@hautarzt-hessen.de

Peter Fritsch, MD
Department of Dermatology
University of Innsbruck
Innrain 143
A-6020 Innsbruck
Austria
Tel.: 0043 650 790 35 55
Fax: 0043 512 9010 10 09
e-mail: peter.fritsch@i-med.ac.at

Clive Grattan, MD
Norfolk and Norwich University Hospitals
Colney Lane
Norwich
NR4 7UY
United Kingdom
Tel: 0044 1603 286 286
Fax: 0044 1603 287211
e-mail: clive.grattan@nnuh.nhs.uk

Wolfgang L. Gross, MD
Department of Rheumatology
University of Lübeck
Ratzeburger Allee 160
23538 Lübeck
Germany
Tel.: 0049 451 500 2368
Fax: 0049 451 500 3650
e-mail: wolfgang.gross@uk-sh.de

Michael Hertl, MD
Department of Dermatology and
Allergology
Philipp University Marburg
Deutschhausstraße 9
D-35037 Marburg
Germany
Tel.: 0049 6421 58 66280
Fax: 0049 6421 58 62902
e-mail: hertl@med.uni-marburg.de

Rolf Hofmann, MD
Dermaticum
Kaiser-Joseph-Straße 262
D-79098 Freiburg
Germany
Tel.: 0049 761 3837400
e-mail: rolf.hofmann@dermaticum.de

Nicolas Hunzelmann, MD
Department of Dermatology
University of Cologne
J.-Stelzmann-Str. 9
D-50924 Köln
Germany
Tel.: 0049 221 478 4517
Fax: 0049 221 478 4538
e-mail: Nico.Hunzelmann@uni-koeln.de

Arnd Jacobi, MD
Department of Dermatology and
Allergology
Philipp University Marburg
Deutschhausstraße 9
D-35037 Marburg
Germany
Tel.: 0049 6421 58 62944
Fax: 0049 6421 58 62902
e-mail: Arnd.Jacobi@med.uni-marburg.de

Reiji Kasukawa, MD
Institute of Rheumatic Diseases
Ohta General Hospital Foundation
5-25, Nakamachi, Koriyama
963-8004
Japan
Tel.: 0081 24 925 0088
Fax: 0081 24 931 1155
e-mail: ohta-found@ohta-hp.or.jp

Cristián Vera Kellet, MD
Centro Médico San Joaquín
Av. Vicuña Mackenna 4686
Macul
Chile
Tel.: 0056-2-552 1900
Fax: 0056-2-354 8620

Nicolas Kluger, MD
Service de Dermatologie
Université Montpellier I,
Hôpital Saint-Eloi,
CHU de Montpellier
80 avenue Augustin Fliche
F-34295 Montpellier cedex 5
France

Thomas Krieg, MD
Department of Dermatology and
Allergology
University of Köln
Kerpener Str. 62
D-50937 Köln
Germany
Tel: 0049 221 478 4500
Fax: 0049 221 478 4538
e-mail: thomas.krieg@uni-koeln.de

Emmanuel Laffitte, MD
FMH dermatologie et vénérologie
Hôpitaux Universitaires de Genève
rue Gabrielle-Perret-Gentil 4
CH-1211 Genève 14
Switzerland
Tel: 0041-022-372-94-30
Fax:: 0041-022-372-94-70221
e-mail:

Peter Lamprecht, MD
University of Lübeck
Department of Rheumatology
Vasculitis Center UKSH &
Clinical Center Bad Bramstedt
Ratzeburger Allee 160
D-23538 Lübeck
Germany
Tel.: 0049 451 500 2368
Fax: 0049 451 500 3650
e-mail: peter.lamprecht@uk-sh.de

Philipp von Landenberg, MD
Institut für Labormedizin (FfLM)
Solothurner Spitäler AG
CH-4600 Olten
Switzerland
Tel.: 0041 62 3115179
Fax: 0041 62 3115486
e-mail: Philipp.Landenberg@spital.so.ch

Natalija Novak, MD
Department of Dermatology and Allergy
University of Bonn
Sigmund-Freud-Str. 25
D-53127 Bonn
Tel. +49-228-287-15370
Fax. +49-228-287-14333
E-mail: Natalija.Novak@ukb.uni-bonn.de

Catherine Helene Orteu, MD
Department of Dermatology
The Royal Free Hospital
Pond Street
London NWS 2QG
United Kingdom
Tel.: 0044 20 7794 0500

Jörg Christoph Prinz, MD
Department of Dermatology and
Allergology
University of Munich (LMU)
Frauenlobstr. 9-11
D-80337 München
Germany
Tel.: 0049 89 5466 481
Fax: 0049 89 5160 6002
e-mail: Joerg.Prinz@med.uni-muenchen.de

Martin Röcken, MD
Department of Dermatology and
Allergology
University of Tübingen
Liebermeisterstraße 25
D-72076 Tübingen
Germany
Tel.: 0049 7071 29 84574
Fax: 0049 7071 29 5450
e-mail: Martin.Roecken@med.uni-
tuebingen.de

Karin Schallreuter, MD
Clinical and Experimental Dermatology
Department of Biomedical Sciences
University of Bradford
Richmond Road
Bradford/West Yorkshire BD7 1DP
United Kingdom
Tel.: 0044 1274 235 527
Fax: 0044 1274 235 290
e-mail: k.schallreuter@bradford.ac.uk

Dagmar Simon, MD
Department of Dermatology
University of Bern
Freiburgstrasse Eingang 14 A-D
CH-3010 Bern
Switzerland
Tel.: 0041 31 632 22 18
Fax: 0041 31 632 22 33
e-mail: e-mail: dagmar.simon@insel.ch

Hans-Uwe Simon, MD
Institute of Pharmacology
University of Bern
Friedbühlstrasse 49
CH-3010 Bern
Switzerland
Tel.: 0041 31 632 2530
Fax: 0041 31 632 49 92
hus@pki.unibe.ch

Miklòs Simon jr, MD
Department of Dermatology
University of Erlangen
Hartmannstr. 14
D-91052 Erlangen
Germany
Tel.: 0049 9131 853 2707
Fax: 0049 9131 853 3854
e-mail: miklos.simon@uk-erlangen.de

Christian Rose, MD
Department of Dermatology
University of Lübeck
Ratzeburger Allee 160
D-23538 Lübeck
Germany
Tel. 0049 451 50 270 50
Fax. 0049 451 50 270 55
e-mail: rose@dermatohistologie-luebeck.de

Richard D. Sontheimer, MD
John S. Strauss Endowed Chair in
Dermatology
Department of Dermatology
University of Iowa College of Medicine/
Health Care
200 Hawkins–Dr BT 2045-1
Iowa City, IA 52242-1090
USA
Tel.: 001 319 356 3609
Fax: 001 319 356 8317
e-mail: richard-sontheimer@uiowa.edu

Michael Sticherling, MD
Department of Dermatology
University of Erlangen
Hartmannstr. 14
D-91052 Erlangen
Germany
Tel.: 0049 9131 85 33851
Fax: 0049 9131 85 36175
Email: michael.sticherling@uk-erlangen.
de

Ingo H. Tarner, MD
Department of Rheumatology
Kerckhoff-Klinik
University of Giessen
Benekestr. 2-8
D-61231 Bad Nauheim
Tel.: 0049 6032/996 0
Fax: 0049 6032/996 2399
e-mail: Tarner@innere.med.uni-giessen.de

David Woodley, MD
Division of Dermatology
LAC and USC Medical Center
8th Floor General Hospital
1200 North State Street
Los Angeles, California, 90033
USA
Tel.: 001 213 717 2289 or
001-323 224 7056
Fax: 001 323 336 2654
e-mail: dwoodley@usc.edu

Giovanna Zambruno, MD
Laboratory of Molecular and Cell Biology
Istituto Dermopatico dell'Immacolata,
IRCCS
Via Monti di Creta 104
I-00167 Rome
Italy
Tel.: 0039 06 664 647 38
Fax: 0039 06 664 647 05
e-mail: g.zambruno@idi.it

Giovanni Di Zenzo, PhD
Laboratory of Molecular and Cell Biology
Istituto Dermopatico dell'Immacolata,
IRCCS
Via Monti di Creta 104
I-00167 Rome
Italy
Tel.: 0039 06 664 647 38
Fax: 0039 06 664 647 05
e-mail: g.dizenzo@idi.it

Detlef Zillikens, MD
Department of Dermatology
University of Lübeck
Ratzeburger Allee 160
D-23538 Lübeck
Germany
Tel.: 0049 451 500 2510
Fax: 0049 451 500 2981
e-mail: detlef.zillikens@derma.uni-
luebeck.de

Pathogenesis of Autoimmune Diseases

Martin Röcken and Tilo Biedermann

Autoimmunity and autoimmune disease

The term autoimmunity signifies the presence of specific memory-type immune reactions that are directed against one or more self-epitopes. Under most conditions, autoimmunity is determined in terms of immunoglobulins that react with either unknown or well-defined human antigens. Today it is supposed that the production of these autoantibodies requires prior activation of potentially autoreactive B cells by memory T cells. These T cells must not only recognize a closely related peptide structure. Importantly, these T cells can stimulate B cells only when primed by activated antigen presenting cells.

Autoimmunity is a relatively frequent event. Most likely, any individual raises immune reactions against numerous self antigens. This autoimmunity leads only very rarely to overt autoimmune disease. Therefore, the development of autoimmune disease requires trespassing of a large number of additional security levels, beyond autoimmune reactivity (Schwartz, 1998). This is illustrated by two frequent clinical phenomena: One of the best examples are antinuclear antibodies (ANA), which are found in even more than 50% of the female population older than 50 years. Compared to this frequency, ANA-associated autoimmune diseases are relatively rare and affect less than 2% (Rubin, 1997). The other is that only very few autoimmune diseases progress continuously. Most of them progress during short waves of disease activity and in between these waves have long periods of quiescence. Since autoreactive T and B cells do normally not disappear during these periods of quiescence, a series of control mechanisms protect from manifest autoimmune disease.

T and B cells

T cells are small lymphocytes that are characterized by their antigen recognition structure, the T cell receptor (TCR). According to the current state of knowledge, the TCR is only functional as a cell bound structure. Due to the low affinity for free peptide (Weber et al., 1992), the TCR recognizes only antigens that are presented by major histocompatibility complex

(MHC) molecules. The TCR acts in concert with an array of additional surface structures. The most important are the co-receptors, the CD4 and CD8 molecules. The CD8 molecule determines the interaction of the TCR with MHC class I and the CD4 molecule with MHC class II. Appropriate activation of T cells requires a series of additional events, such as adhesion molecules and costimulatory molecules (reviewed in Biedermann et al., 2004).

B cells are characterized by the production of antigen recognition structures, the B cell receptor and immunoglobulins. They produce immunoglobulins mainly when stimulated appropriately through T-B-cell interactions (Lanzavecchia, 1985). However, besides antigen specific signals, induction of immunoglobulin production by B cells requires CD40-CD40L interactions and cytokines (Banchereau et al., 1994). In contrast to the TCR, immunoglobulins may have a very high affinity for their specific antigen. They recognize free antigen and their major function seems to be the binding to either cell-bound or free antigens.

T cells develop in the thymus and B cells in the bone marrow. Importantly, the structure of the TCR is definitely determined in the thymus. Thus, the thymus constitutes an important site of education which ultimately determines the specificity of the ensuing T cells (Kisielow and von Boehmer, 1995). In contrast, the structure of the immunoglobulin recognition site is not terminally fixed when B cells leave the bone marrow and mature B cells undergo somatic mutation and the affinity of the antigen recognition site of secreted immunoglobulins can mature during the course of immune responses.

Thymic maturation and selection of T cells

Precursor T cells develop within the bone marrow and reach the thymus through the blood. These immature precursor cells undergo a series of activation and maturation events that ultimately result in a precursor population that expresses a TCR and both, CD4 and CD8 molecules. The TCR expresses two independent immunoglobulin-like chains, the α- and the β-chain. The β-chain is expressed together with a pre-α-chain; the definite TCR α-chain replaces the pre-α-chain prior to the development of the CD4+CD8+, double positive status. Normally, T cells express only one pair of TCR α/β-chains. This subsequent replacement of the pre-α-chain by a definite TCR-α-chain however, may lead to the occurrence of T cells which express two receptors, one single β-chain assorted with two different and independent α-chains. Thus, one T cell may have two, entirely independent specificities (Kretz-Rommel and Rubin, 2000; Stockinger, 1999).

Once the double positive status is achieved, T cells interact with thymic MHC molecules. This interaction of the double positive cells, which are highly sensitive to death signals, will decide their further outcome as most of the double positive cells die during this selection process. T cells with relatively high affinity for peptide loaded and possible also empty MHC molecules die through induction of apoptosis. T cells that express a TCR with an affinity that is too low for recognizing peptide loaded MHC molecules die from neglect. Only a small proportion of T cells, smaller than 10%, survives this selection and leaves the thymus as a single positive T cell, expressing either CD4 or CD8 and a TCR (Bouneaud et al., 2000; Kisielow et al., 1988; Rocha and von Boehmer, 1991). During thymic selec-

Fig. 1. Modes of intrathymic selection of T cells. T cells with a very high affinity T cell receptor (TCR) for self major histocompatibility complexes (MHC) die from active deletion, those with an intermediate affinity are positively selected and those with low affinity will die from neglect

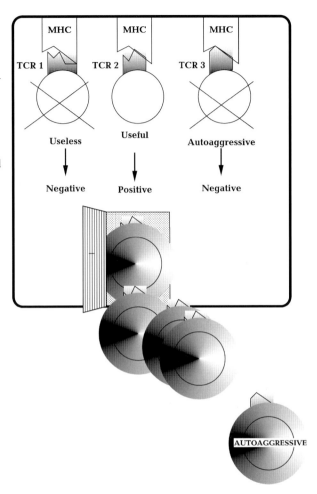

tion, TCR structures with high affinity for self may not only lead to deletion; another mode is temporary suppression of the TCR. If a T cell with two distinct TCR α-chains then receives at the same time a survival signal by the second receptor, this cell may become positively selected and result in a peripheral T cell population with two distinct TCR; one corresponding to an autoreative receptor (Fig. 1).

Tolerance of self-reactive T and B cells

Central tolerance and peripheral tolerance

The thymus and the apoptosis and paralysis occurring during the development of B cells recognizing abundant antigens in the periphery delete about 90% of self-reactive T and B cells. This phenomenon is termed as *central tolerance*. However, roughly 10% of these cells survive (Blackman et al., 1990; Kisielow et al., 1988). Moreover, not all antigens are presented in thymus, bone marrow or peripheral blood. In one individual, all cells express the same MHC class I and a large spectrum of common minor antigens. However, each cell also expresses its own set of antigens that is related to its function and localization. Thus, the mature immune system encounters a larger spectrum of antigens in the periphery than in the thymus. Tolerance against these antigens requires a multitude of mechanisms which are summarized under the term *peripheral tolerance* (Bonomo and Matzinger, 1993). While *central tolerance* is mainly based on deletion of potentially autoreactive T cells, a larger spectrum of mechanisms constitutes *peripheral tolerance* (Arnold et al., 1993; Rocken and Shevach, 1996).

Mechanisms of peripheral tolerance

One mechanism of peripheral tolerance may be deletion, too. Deletion is mainly associated with the sudden appearance of a large number of antigens. This mechanism has been demonstrated for antigens that were presented in large numbers, thus during infection or following injection of superantigens (Moskophidis et al., 1993; Webb et al., 1990). Whether this mechanism applies also under physiological conditions is not clear. But it may become relevant during tissue destruction, when large quantities of self-antigens are presented, thus in the case of skin burning, viral infections of skin, muscle or other organs or following a stroke. However, this phenomenon has not yet been analyzed in more detail.

Another mechanism is suppression of TCR expression. This has been shown with pregnant mice expressing a transgenic TCR that recognizes the foreign MHC class I molecule expressed by the father and the fetus. The level of this transgenic TCR is high before and after pregnancy, but low during pregnancy. These T cells are also functionally silenced. During pregnancy, pregnant female mice become even tolerant to otherwise highly immunogenic tumor cells expressing this same antigen (Alferink et al., 1998). Thus, suppression of a TCR expression is closely associated with the occurrence of peripheral tolerance and may contribute to it. These data, even though very elegant, do not exclude that other mechanisms significantly contribute to peripheral tolerance (Alferink et al., 1998; Schonrich et al., 1991).

One important example demonstrating the requirement for additional mechanisms was given by mice that simultaneously express a peptide antigen of the lymphocytic choriomeningitis virus (LCMV) by the endocrine pancreas and T cells with a TCR transgenic for the LCMV peptide (Ohashi et al., 1991; Oldstone et al., 1991). These animals have autoreactive CD8+ T cells that are functionally normal, express normal levels of the TCR and kill peptide loaded targets in vitro to the same extend as transgenic T cells from control animals. Nevertheless, these animals do not develop overt autoimmune disease, showing that, besides the target organ, the expression of an endogenous potentially immunogenic peptide and normal levels of TCR, other signals are required for the induction of autoimmune disease. Such a situation may be the consequence of 'ignorance' of the target structure by the autoreactive T cells (Ohashi et al., 1991). Ignorance may be the consequence of missing adhesion molecules or the absence of co-stimulatory signals (von Herrath et al., 1995).

However, it may also be due to expression of autoantigens at immunologically privileged sites, the expression of apoptosis inducing molecules capable of killing activated T cells or secondary to local silencing of activated T cells that recognize target tissues in the absence of co-stimulatory molecules.

Reactivity and mode of action are not only given by the TCR and the spectrum of co-stimulatory T cells expressed by T cells. Most importantly, T cell functions are determined by the cytokines they produce. Naive T cells produce only interleukin (IL-) 2 when stimulated by peptides and professional antigen presenting cells (APC; (Weinberg et al., 1990)). Subsequently, T cells develop towards memory cells that are theoretically capable of producing a large spectrum of cytokines. Today it is established that T cells normally do not secrete a random pattern of cytokines, but differentiate into phenotypes that produce distinct sets of cytokines associated with well defined functional phenotypes (Mosmann and Sad, 1996; Rocken et al., 1996; Rocken et al., 1992).

T cells that produce predominantly IL-2 and interferon-γ (IFN-γ) are associated with inflammatory, cell mediated immune responses. When expressing the CD4 molecule they are named Th1, when expressing the CD8 molecule, they are named Tc1 cells and induce 'type 1' immune responses. These types of immune responses are required for the control of infections with viruses, funghi or parasites. However, when directed against autoantigens, they may cause inflammatory autoimmune diseases (Adorini and Sinigaglia, 1997; Arnold et al., 1993; Katz et al., 1995; Kolb et al., 1995; Powrie, 1995; Racke et al., 1994; Rocken et al., 1996). These inflammatory autoimmune diseases are normally well localized to one single organ or a group of organs that share a common antigen. These T cells do not only induce direct tissue destruction, they also induce B cells to produce complement binding antibodies, which may enhance local inflammation and tissue destruction, as it is the case in patients with bullous pemphigoid (Budinger et al., 1998).

The most important counterpart of 'type 1' immune responses are 'type 2' responses. They are induced by CD4+ T cells capable of producing IL-4 and IL-13. These two cytokines seem to suppress multiple pro-inflammatory effector functions by macrophages, such as production of tumor necrosis factor (TNF). Th2 cells are primarily known by their capacity to switch the immunoglobulin isotype of human B cells towards IgE and probably also IgG4 (Mosmann and Coffman, 1989). Thus, Th2 cells do not generally extinct immune responses. They may even induce autoimmune responses and probably also autoimmune disease, such as pemphigus vulgaris, which is associated with autoantibodies of the IgG4 isotype and little local inflammation (Goldman et al., 1991; Hertl et al., 1998). However, when directed against epitopes that are associated with type 1-mediated inflammatory autoimmune disease, type 2 immune responses may exert anti-inflammatory, protective effects. Treating Th1 mediated diseases with Th2 cells or the cytokine IL-4 that most potently induces Th2 and suppresses Th1 has been demonstrated in animal models of organ specific autoimmune disease and skin inflammation (Racke et al., 1994; Rocken et al., 1996; Biedermann et al., 2001). Most importantly, however, this therapeutic strategy was also effective in humans suffering from psoriasis, a Th1 mediated autoimmune disease of the skin (Ghoreschi et al., 2003).

In recent years, additional subsets of Th cells and associated immune pathologies were identified. The best characterized of these subsets is the Th17 cells, defined by predominant production of IL-17. Subsequent to the description of Th17 cells, it was found that some of the autoimmune diseases that were believed to be 'type 1' mediated, in fact, are at least in part driven by Th17 cells. The best studied example is a model for multiple sclerosis, the experimental allergic encephalitis (EAE), for which it was shown that both Th1 and Th17 cells are capable to mediate autoimmune disease although with different strength and different pathology (Luger et al., 2008). Th17 mediated immune responses are often associated with infiltrates of polymorphonuclear Leukocytes (PMN). By morphology and involvement of effector immune cells and cytokines, inflammatory bowel diseases such as Crohn´s disease, rheumatoid arthritis, and psoriasis have often been compared to elucidate immune pathologies (Biedermann et al., 2000). Consequently, the association of Th17 responses to one was soon followed by well based characterizations of all these autoimmune diseases. Today Th17 cells are believed to mediate many of the hallmarks of psoriasis such as PMN infiltrates, acanthosis and papillomatosis (Nestle et al., 2009).

Another dimension of immune regualtion, probably increasingly important, are the different types of regulatory T cells that mediate immune tolerance and thus are counter regulators of autoimmunity. Cell mediated as well as cytokine mediated 'regulation' of immune responses by regulatory or Treg cells have been described. In contrast to all other phenotypes, these Treg cells seem to have the exquisite capacity of turning immune responses off. This regulatory effect may be of great importance in the treatment of autoimmune diseases, since Treg are obviously capable of silencing several types of immune responses including Th1, Th17, and Th2 dominated immune responses (Akdis et al., 2000; Groux et al., 1997). Referring to the historical attribution given to CD8+ T cells, suppressor T cells experience a time of renaissance. These CD4+ T cells are capable to suppress autoaggressive immune reactions and were found to express CD25, GITR, CTLA-4, and most importantly a specific transcription factor, forkhead box p3 (Foxp3) (Bluestone and Tang, 2004). Foxp3 is not only a marker for these Tr, it is of functional importance for the suppressive mode of action of Tr (Walker et al., 2003; Fontenot et al., 2003). As a consequence, patients deficient in the Foxp3 transcription factor develop a multiorgan autoimmune disease (Kriegel et al., 2004). Tr cells are very difficult to induce and grow to expand in vitro and probably also in vivo, but finding Foxp3 and increasingly elucidating the underlaying mechanisms of Tr development will help to answer the questions in regard to the significance these cells may play in the therapy of autoimmune disease.

Activation and differentiation of T cells

All organs are drained by dendritic APC (DC). These DC are normally considered as potent stimulators of T cells that prime primarily for interferon-γ (IFN-γ) producing CD4+ and CD8+ T cells (Banchereau and Steinman, 1998; Schuler and Steinman, 1997; Schuler et al., 1997). DC acquire this capacity following antigen uptake while they migrate to the draining lymph nodes. This capacity in activating and stimulating T cells to become efficient effector cells, capable of mediating inflammatory immune responses and of inducing immunoglobulin production by B cells, requires a certain activation status by these APC. Thus APC co-express adhesion molecules that permit adherence of naive and activated T cells. They express a panel of co-stimulatory molecules that are required for the activa-

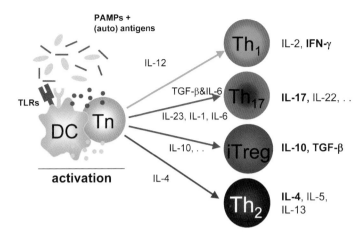

Fig. 2. Differentiation of T helper (Th) cells into either IFN-γ producing Th1, IL-17 producing Th17, IL-10 or TGF-β producing T reg or IL-4 producing Th2 cells. The differentiation into Th1, Th17, and Th2 cells is driven by the functional phenotype of the stimulating dendritic cells (DC), draining the site of inflammation. Innate immune sensing by DC is crucial for DC activation, maturation, and migration and also influences the phenotype of DC. PAMPs: Pathogen associated molecular pattern; TLRs: Toll-like-receptors; Tn: Naïve Th cell

tion of specifically binding T cells and, in addition, they produce cytokines. Both, the sum of cell bound signals and of APC derived cytokines results not only in the stimulation and maturation of the specific T cells but also determines their differentiation. Thus, the maturation process that APC and DC undergo during their migration from the periphery to the draining lymph node will ultimately determine, whether the primary activation of T cells may lead Th1, Th2, Th17, Th22 or inducible Treg cells (Kalinski et al., 1999; Moser and Murphy, 2000; Korn et al., 2009; Abraham et al., 2009) (Fig. 2).

When residing in peripheral organs, DC are continuously processing numerous antigens delivered by the local milieu. At this stage, DC have little migratory and antigen presenting capacity. Recent data suggest that the few immature and quiescent DC that migrate from peripheral organs to the draining lymph node are not capable of activating T cells to become autoaggressive. They seem either to contribute to the phenomenon of 'ignorance' or to promote the differentiation of naive but potentially autoreactive T cells towards an immunosuppressive Treg phenotype (Jonuleit et al., 2000). In sharp contrast, DC start to mature and to leave their residing site after an appropriate stimulus. Among those innate signals are highly conserved so called 'pathogen associated molecular pattern' (PAMP) derived from infectious agents, such as bacterial DNA, bind to Toll-like receptors (TLR) that are increasingly recognized as most relevant activators of DC. Obviously, this process is driven by more than just one such PAMP, but the impact of combinative innate immune sensing ist just beginning to be understood (Volz et al., 2010). These innate signals transform APC not only from an antigen processing towards an antigen presenting cell, capable of attracting naive and memory T cells into lymph nodes. These innate signals also determine the differentiation of APC towards different DC phenotypes that are capable to orchestrate Th1, Th2, Th17, Th22 or Treg cells. In consequence, DC and their capacity to di-

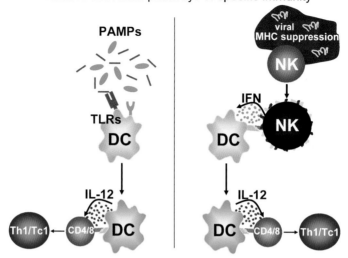

Fig. 3. PAMPs tend to induce IL-12 producing DC that control the development of IFN-γ producing Th1 or Tc1 cells. These type 1 immune responses are effective against microbes but may also be involved in tissue destruction during autoimmune diseases. Alternatively, DC with a similar phenotype may also be generated under the influence of activated natural killer (NK) cells and lead to Th1 or Tc1 cells

rect the functional phenotype of the future immune response, directed against either self or foreign antigens, is one central element of immune regulation (Banchereau and Steinman, 1998; Kalinski et al., 1999; Moser and Murphy, 2000). This concept was expanded by disclosing regulatory mechanisms underlaying DC induced immune responses. Thus, PAMPs present during the initial activation of DC generally instruct DC to produce IL-12 and PAMPs tend to promote Th1 development leading to a proper anti-infectious immunity (Figs. 2, 3). However, some PAMPs and other signals lead to an inappropriate Th2 immunity in response to microbes (Fig. 2). Interestingly, these Th2 reactions can be switched to effective Th1 reactions, a mechanism that may also regulate autoimmunity. Paradoxically, IL-4 is a potent factor driving this switch, because IL-4 instructs activated DC to produce IL-12 and promotes Th1 cell development (Biedermann et al., 2001). The paradox functional consequences achieved by IL-4 were investigated by the sequential analysis of immune responses. Immune responses in general develop via the consecutive activation of DC and then T cells. Thus, the contrasting effects of IL-4 on immune responses with opposing functional phenotypes are a result from IL-4 signaling in early DC activation leading to a Th1 phenotype and on IL-4 induced T cell differentiation inducing Th2 cells during a later stage. How exactly Th17 cells and Th2 cells are regulated and influence each other is a focus of ongoing research, but it seems as if Th2 cytokines modulate DC in a way that these DC are incapable to support Th17 differentiation and maintenance (Guenova et al. in preparation).

In addition to TLR signaling, there is a multitude of other recognition pathways that include the lectins and other cytosolic pathogen recognition receptors (PRR) such as the retinoic acid – inducible gene I (RIG-I) – like receptors (RLRs) and the nucleotide-binding domain and leucine-rich repeat – containing receptors (NLRs) (Iwasaki & Medzhitov, 2010; Volz et al., 2010). Other levels of innate recognition and regulation of inflammation include the inflammasome providing rapid IL-1 levels (Schroder & Tschopp, 2009) and recognition of apoptotic cell material (Nagata et al., 2010). In this context, it is interesting that complex cellular communication pathways support recognition and inflammation. Thus, activated NK cells can also prime DC to produce IL-12 and to induce CD8 T cell memory responses, a mechanism that may be also underlaying an activation of autoreactive lymphocytes (Mocikat et al., 2003) (Fig. 3).

Activation of self-reactive T and B cells

Autoimmune diseases require the presence of autoreactive T cells and, in the case of immunoglobulin mediated diseases, of autoreactive B cells. In view of the potent and large number of regulatory mechanisms that protect against autoimmune disease, activation of autoreactive T and B cells is thought to require a series of destabilizing events. One important aspect is the activation and reactivation of potentially autoreactive T cells (Rocken et al., 1992). However, induction of autoreative T cells or B cells alone does not induce or predispose for autoimmune diseases. For example, in individuals, which are genetically predisposed of developing autoimmune diabetes, the relative risk of becoming diabetes increases significantly if their T cells respond vigorously against endogenous antigens from pancreatic islet cells. In sharp contrast, individuals from the same population are largely protected against autoimmune diabetes, when they exert high immunoglobulin titers but weak T cell responses against the same antigens (Harrison et al., 1993). This further underlines that 'reactivity' does not equal autoimmune disease.

One of the fundamental questions that are still unanswered yields with the primary event leading to the induction of autoreactivity. Some data suggest that, in the presence of an appropriate genetic background, minimal events such as normal tissue necrosis may be sufficient for the induction of, perhaps even potentially harmful, autoreactivity (Albert et al., 1998; Matzinger and Anderson, 2001).

Most data suggest that a series of tolerance inducing mechanisms normally inhibits T and B cells to react against many autoantigens (Naucler et al., 1996). Therefore, stimuli that induce reactivity against these autoantigens have to overcome the diverse tolerance inducing barriers. Epidemiologic data suggest that the realization of autoimmune diseases is often preceded by infectious diseases and attention was given to the events by which infections may abolish the status of tolerance (Matzinger, 1994; Sinha et al., 1990). At least three mechanisms are thought to contribute to this phenomenon: reactivation of tolerant T and B cells, induction of autoreactive T cells by molecular mimicry and modification of the cytokine pattern during the course of infectious diseases.

Breaking T and B cell tolerance

Experiments with transgenic or non- transgenic mice animals have shown that, in principle, tolerant T and B cells can be reactivated by infectious agents. Infections are capable of restoring in silenced T cells the capacity to produce cytokines (Racke et al., 1994; Rocken et al., 1992). This phenomenon was extended to the situation of transplantation induced tolerance (Ehl et al., 1998). Similarly, reactivity and immunoglobulin production by B cells that were silenced either by exogenous or transgenic endogenous antigens can be restored with mitogens, including bacteria derived lipopolisacchrides (Goodnow et al., 1991; Louis et al., 1973). Even though these experiments have shown that infectious agents can abolish solid T and B cell tolerance there are little data showing that this reactivation of tolerant T and B cells can also lead to autoimmune disease. One first example suggesting such a situation is given by double transgenic mice that bear a TCR recognizing a transgenic self-antigen expressed by hepatocytes. Injection of bacterial DNA motifs that activate DC and promote DC-development also induced transient liver damage, as evidenced by an increase of transaminases. However, this phenomenon was short lived and no data are available proving that autoimmune disease can be the direct consequence of polyclonal T cell activation (Limmer et al., 1998). In small animal models, induction of autoimmune disease by bactrial DNA motifs or more complex bacterial lysates such as complete Freund's adjuvans required, in addition, always immunization with an antigen that mimics peptide motifs of the targeted self antigen (Bachmaier et al., 1999). Thus, in normal mice bacterial DNA motifs triggered the myocarditis only when co-administered with an altered self-peptide, derived from chlamydia.

These data suggest that immunization against antigens that are structurally related to self-antigens are essential for the induction of autoimmunity. This concept is further supported by functional and structural analysis of T cell eptipopes of infectious agents and potential self-antigens. Chlamydia peptides can share functional similarities with peptides expressed by mammalian heart muscle, while other infectious agents share important peptide sequences with potential self-antigens such as myelin basic protein. This aspect is especially significant since molecular mimicry does not require molecular identity. Studies with altered peptide ligands have shown that induction of cytokine production or T cell proliferation requires only poor structural relation as long as important anchor positions are conserved (Gautam et al., 1994; Wucherpfennig and Strominger, 1995). Various examples suggest that this may be of relevance for autoimmune diseases of the skin. Thus, the first eruption of the juvenile type of psoriasis is preceded by streptococcal infections in most patients (Prinz, 1999) and lichen planus is associated in a large number of patients with an acute or chronic liver disease (Chuang et al., 1999). In some patients lichen planus may even be provoked by active or even passive vaccination against hepatitis (Degitz and Röcken, 1997; Tessari et al., 1996).

Despite the experimental prove for both, re-activation of tolerant T cells and for molecular mimicry, the exact role of infections in the pathogenesis of autoimmune diseases remains open. One important alternative would be the direct infection and molecular alteration through infectious disease. One important example is chronic active hepatitis, where relatively weak immune responses follow the slowly progressing wave of infected hepato-

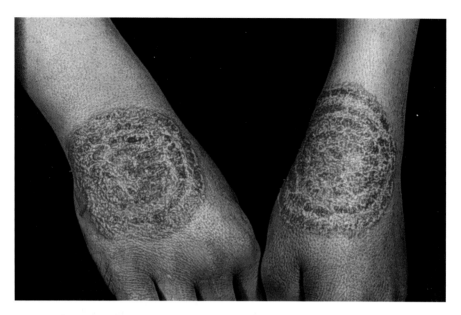

Fig. 4. Waves of inflammation as reflected by the migrating margins of eczema found during tinea infection

cytes and thus slowly destroy the liver. In this situation, activation of the T cell mediated immune responses, associated with a short aggravation of the hepatitis may lead to reduction and control of the viral load and cure from chronic progressive hepatitis (Berg et al., 1997; Gerlach et al., 1999; Moradpour and Blum, 1999). In the skin a very similar phenomenon is visible during fungal infections. The border, the clinically manifest eczema, reflects the immune reaction against a large burden of fungi. Inside the inflammatory margin, the eczema and the fungal load are significantly milder. In the case of fast growing fungi, the eczema may present as a policyclic disease (Fig. 4).

A third level where infections could directly interfere with autoreactive T cells is the pattern of cytokines that T cells produce. Thus, infection with the nematode nippostrongylus brasiliensis can not only restore reactivity in silenced CD4+ T cells but also induce IL-4 production by these silenced T cells (Rocken et al., 1996; Rocken et al., 1994; Rocken et al., 1992).

In conclusion, increasing understanding of the PRR-mediated activation if innate immune cells and their link to adaptive immunity has helped to create a concept that also applies to the activation of autoreactive T and B cells. Thus in a series of models, activating innate immunity has turned on or increased the adaptive immune response. These data emphasize the power of infectious diseases in mounting immune responses and in modulating the cytokine phenotype of established immune responses. PAMPs binding to TLR and other PRRs and regulating the transcription of pro-inflammatory genes through NFκB are the basis for this new understanding. Thus, PAMPs like immunostimulatory DNA binding TLR9, like lipopolysachharides binding TLR4 and others are capable of activating DC, B cells, and probably also T cells. Thus, instructing IL-12 producing DC via TLR9 can be achieved by injection of TLR9 ligands into mice. Using the model of progressive, Th2-mediated leishmaniasis infection in susceptible BALB/c mice, Zimmermann et al. showed that immunostimulatory DNA motifs are capable of reverting even fully established type 2 immune responses into IFN-γ dominated type 1 immune responses and DTHR (Zimmermann et al., 1998). Thus, injection of immunostimulatory DNA motifs and triggering TLR9 overcame the tolerance towards the parasite and restored control over *Leishmania major* in animals with a large parasite burden. In view of such a powerful Th1-inducing capacity, it was likely that similar immunostimulatory motifs are also capable of breaking self-tolerance and induce autoreactive Th1/Tc1 cells that cause inflammatory tissue destruction. Indeed, it was shown very recently that viruses provide TLR signals required for bypassing regulatory T cell-mediated tolerance (Yang et al., 2004). PAMPs may therefore be considered as the leading group of danger signals that nature provides and that may also lead to activation of autoreactive T and B cells.

In addition to PAMPs derived from microbes, there is increasing evidence suggesting that also endogenous ligands can trigger TLR and activate autoreactive lymphocytes (Ulevitch, 2004). Systemic lupus erythematosus is characterized by the production of autoantibodies against nucleic-acid-containing macromolecules such as chromatin or ribonucleoprotein particles. DC and B cells are effectively activated by immune complexes containing chromatin, a process that involves TLR9. This activation leads to proliferation of autoreactive T and B cells providing direct evidence for TLR promoted autoimmunity mediated by endogeneous ligands (Leadbetter et al., 2002; Boulé et al., 2004).

Autoimmune disease

Autoimmunity is a prerequisite for autoimmune disease. However, the events that lead from autoimmunity to an overt inflammatory disease are still unclear. Production and release of TNF seems to be important for this step, but the exact role of this cytokine is far from being elucidated (Green and Flavell, 2000). Without any doubt, autoreactive T cells are not only associated with autoimmune diseases but can directly cause the disease. Analysis from mice with non obese diabetes (NOD) revealed that both, CD4+ and CD8+ T cells are required for the induction of both, autoimmune inflammation and autoimmune disease (Bendelac et al., 1987). Similarly, transfer of MBP-reactive T cells (Mokhtarian et al., 1984) and even more precisely, MBP-reactive CD4+ T cells of the Th1 phenotype alone are capable of inducing severe autoimmune encephalitis, when transferred into naive mice (Racke et al., 1994).

T cells

A comparison of various models for organ-specific, inflammatory autoimmune disease unrevaled that organ specific inflammatory autoimmune diseases are primarily induced by T cells of the proinflammatory Th1 and Th17 phenotype. It is assumed that both, CD4+ and CD8+ T cells and also Th1 and Th17 cells are involved under most conditions, but the exact role of CD8+ T cells remains unclear. The best studied example investigating the exact role of Th1 and Th17 cells in autoimmunity is a model for multiple sclerosis, the experimental allergic encephalitis (EAE): In this model both Th1 and Th17 cells are capable to mediate autoimmune disease although with different strength and different pathology (Luger et al., 2008). These types of investigations and the functional characterization were performed in the past for Th1 cells for models of autoimmue diseases in small animals and for the analysis of autoimmune responses in humans with organ-specific autoimmune disease such as autoimmune diabetes (Kolb et al., 1995), multiple sclerosis (Martin et al., 1992; Zhang et al., 1998) or psoriasis (Austin et al., 1999; Vollmer et al., 1994). Analysis in regard to Th17 pathology are as performed for EAE (Luger et al., 2008) are still ongoing, but immune responses associated with infiltrates of polymorphonuclear Leukocytes (PMN) such as psoriasis seem to be mediated by Th17 (Nestle et al., 2009).

B cells and immunoglobulins

Probably the best example for an immunoglobulin-mediated disease is pemphigus vugaris. In patients, this disease is associated with little inflammation and seems to be directly mediated by the binding of autoreactive immunoglobulins to the desmogleins that guarantee the adherence between keratinocytes (Amagai et al., 1991). Indeed, transfer of patient sera and monoclonal antibodies directed against desmoglein III into the skin of new-born mice can directly induce acanthosis (Rock et al., 1989). This critical role for a direct binding of immunoglobulins to desmoglein structures is further supported by the observation that in patients with pemphigus vugaris the disease activity correlates closely with the serum levels of the autoantibodies (Hertl, 2006). Such a close association is unusual for other autoimmune diseases, including lupus erythematosus or bullous pemphigoid. For comparisons, bullous pemphigoid is of special interest. It is also an immunoglobulin mediated bullous skin disease. In sharp contrast to pemphigus vulgaris, the clinical manifestation of bullous pemphigoid does not only require deposition of autoantigens but also an inflammatory milieu that causes detachment of the basement membrane (Liu et al., 2000; Liu et al., 1998). Consequently, transfer of specific sera or immunoglobulins under the skin of new born nude mice alone is not sufficient for the induction of blisters. It requires, in addition, activation of the complement cascade and inflammation, involving the recruitment of granulocytes (Liu et al., 1995).

Tissue damage, Th1, and Th17 cells

Th1 and Th17 cells seem to be associated with two distinct types of tissue damage. One type of tissue damage is rather characterized by a sterile inflammation (Th1), the other with the strong accumulation of polymorphonuclear granulocytes (Th17).

Sterile Th1/Tc1 responses are found in lichen planus, most patients with multiple sclerosis or autoimmune diabetes. They are associated with activated macrophages, which seem

1

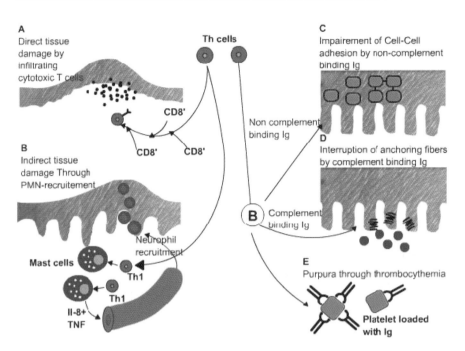

Fig. 5. Different types of inflammation induced by either IFNγ-producing Th1 and by IL-4-producing Th2 cells

to be the effector cells of these immune responses. Like macrophages that are stimulated in vitro in the presence of IFN-γ, they produce large amounts of TNF, oxygen radicals, NO and other mediators of inflammation (Stenger and Modlin, 1999). Activated CD8+ T cells (Tc1) with potent killer functions seem also to be involved (Zinkernagel, 1996). In concert, these mediators can cause severe tissue destruction that ultimately results in compensatory scar formation. Due to the capacity of the skin to regenerate even severe tissue damage, lichen planus heals under most conditions without scaring. However, persistent alopecia, onychodystrophy or even scars of the normal skin are potential complications (Fig. 5A).

Under other conditions, Th17 cells dominate autoimmune diseases, which are associated with a strong infiltrate of PMN. Such a constellation characterizes psoriasis, rheumatiod arthritis (RA) and most types of inflammatory bowel disease, especially Crohn's disease (Kron et al., 2009; Abraham et al., 2009). In addition, targeting the p40 subunit of both IL-12 and IL-23 also demonstrated to be an effective therapy for psoriasis indicating that induction of Th1 cells (IL-12) or induction and maintenance of Th17 cells (IL-23) together with some inherent effector functions of these two cytokines are crucial for the immune pathogenesis of psoriasis (Krueger GG et al., 2007). In this context, IL-17 and IL-17 induced cytokines regulate PMN infiltration and in addition, mast cells triggered by Th cells lead to strong PMN recruitment through their mediators: TNF, which induces the expression of intravascular adhesion molecules (Biedermann et al., 2000; Kneilling et al., 2009), and the IL-8, which is the most important chemokine attracting PMN (Biedermann et al., 2000). The communication pathways between Th1 and Th17 cells and mast cells still need to be characterized (Fig. 5B).

Interestingly, mast cells seem not only to recruit PMN during Th1/Th17 mediated immune responses. Activated mast cells are also abundant during immunoglobulin mediated destruction of the basement membrane in bullous pemphigoid. Adoptive transfer of bullous pemphigoid autoantibodies into the skin of newborn mice underlined that mast cells are required also for PMN recruitment in the pathogenesis of bullous pemphigoid (Chen et al., 2000).

Th2 T cells and T-B cell interactions (Fig. 2)

A large number of autoimmune diseases is immunoglobulin mediated. These 'humoral' diseases can roughly be divided into two major categories. Immunoglobulins can induce damage through direct binding of their target-antigen. This is the situation in most other bullous autoimmune diseases of the skin, especially pemphigus vulgaris. Alternatively immunoglobulins bind to circulating antigens and cause damage through deposition along basement membranes or in vessels. The former situation is given in the case of lupus (Rubin, 1997) the latter at sites of vasculitis.

Thus, immunoglobulins are responsible for all types of diseases caused by immunreaction type I, II and III according to the classification of Coombs & Gell. As the pattern of immune responses initiated by immunoglobulins strictly depends on the immunoglobuline isotype, the diseases caused by immunoglobulins depend not only on the antigen they recognize. The clinical spectrum of diseases initiated by autoantibodies ranges from urticaria, through cytopathic tissue damage leading to cytopenia, inflammatory tissue destruction following the deposition of immunoglobulins and complexes at membranes till to severe necrosis, as a consequence of acute vascular infarction.

Here again, T cells play a central regulatory role. Under most conditions, B cells start only to produce autoantibodies, when stimulated by antigen-specific T cells. During this stimulation, T cells release a distinct pattern of cytokines controlling the immunoglobulin switch in the responding B cells. Cytokines of the Th2-family, IL-4 and IL-13 induce the isotype switch towards IgE and isotypes that don't bind complement, IgG1 in the mouse and in humans probably IgG4. Th1 cells that are thought to organize the defense against intracellular pathogens and viruses induce preferentially complement-binding isotypes.

A well analyzed example is pemphigus vulgaris, where patients have frequently IgG4 antibodies against desmoglein 3 and predominant Th2 responses against this same autoantigen.

Therapeutic induction of functional tolerance

The therapeutic strategies available reflect a combination of corticosteroids and immunosuppressive agents, most of them acting on both T and B cells. Corticosteroids are used with the primary goal to reduce the acute inflammation and to limit tissue damage. They are also efficient in suppressing T and B cell responses, but long-term side effects are very important. Therefore, therapies normally combine corticosteroids with immunosuppressive agents in order to reduce immune responses to a level that optimally inhibits harmful immune reactions but still allows normal defense against infectious agents. Such therapies establish a fragile balance that is helpful in some but not all autoimmune diseases. Especially the late outcome is still poorly controlled and acute relapses and chronic infections may lead to new complications such as an increased frequency of atherosclerosis, at least in some groups of immunosuppressed individuals.

This led to the development of novel strategies. They are based on either of the three principles: efficient blockade of the effector functions of immune responses, absorbing harmful immunoglobulin fractions or correction of aberrant T cell responses.

The greatest progress is currently obtained by blocking immune functions with anti-TNF-antibodies. This seems to be more efficient and better tolerated than any of the previously described immmunosuppressive agents (Feldmann et al., 1996). However, therapies based on anti-TNF-antibodies inhibit any type of immuneresponse and therefore harbor a series of risks for patients with acute or chronic infections. Among autoimmune skin diseases psoriasis has been shown to improve under anti-TNF-therapies (Mease et al., 2000). This is an important prove of principle and we know today that this therapeutic approach can be very beneficial for our patients suffering from psoriasis, psoriasis arthritis, and acrodermatitis continua suppurativa of Hallopeau. In addition, neutralizing TNF may be a promising approach for acute diseases associated with inflammatory tissue destruction such as aphtous ulcers or pyoderma gangraenosum. In addition, antibodies to the p40 subunit of both IL-12 and IL-23 are now available (ustekinumab) and were successfully used in psoriasis (Krueger GG et al., 2007) possibly targeting Th1 and Th17 mediated autoimmune disease. However, we have to keep in mind that other highly effective, less invasive, and less expensive therapies are available for psoriasis.

Absorbency of harmful immunoglobulins is a logical approach that was developed from plasmapheresis. One problem is that it acts relatively late in the immune response and B cells continue to produce pathogenic immunoglobulins.

Large efforts were undertaken to develop T cell based immunotherapies. They may affect either antigen presenting cells, co-stimulation or the T cells directly. Today, strategies modulating the co-stimulation of T cells mediated through CD28/CTLA4 or LFA-2/LFA-3 seem to be one promising approach to alter autoreactive T cell responses (Abrams et al., 2000; Krueger and Ellis, 2003). One other possibility would be to correct harmful cytokine production by specific T cells. Three mechanisms are under study: induction of regulatory Tr cells capable of inhibiting immune responses in an antigen-specific fashion. The second would be the deviation of harmful Th1 or Th17 responses into a protective Th2 response or Treg responses. While tha latter seems to be difficult to achive, such an approach was followed up with Th2-responses. Th2 responses in contrast to Treg cells have a tendency to perpetuate and to establish an antiinflammatory Th2-memory, once they are initiated (Biedermann et al., 2001). Indeed, a first study performed with psoriasis patients demonstrated that IL-4 therapy is a highly effective treatment strategy for autoimmune diseases (Ghoreschi et al., 2003). The third reflects the opposite, the redirection of harmful Th2 responses into a Th1-phenotype or Th17 phenotype, an approach that may be of interest in IgE-mediated diseases.

These antigen-specific T cell based approaches are still at an early clinical experimental stage and even though not appropriate for acute interventions, the first studies demonstrated that it is a very promising approach (Ghoreschi et al., 2003). For future development, these vaccination approaches are of special interest as they circumvent a series of major problems associated with all other therapies. Two important aspects are: These therapies are highly specific for the targeted antigen structure and should therefore not interfere with the other physiologically required immune responses (Rocken et al., 1996). The other is that they target the site where T cell responses are translated from the innate to the adaptive immune response and they therefore should protection of long duration.

References

Abraham C. and Cho J. H. (2009). IL-23 and Autoimmunity: New Insights into the Pathogenesis of Inflammatory Bowel Disease. Annu. Rev. Med. *60*, 97–110

Abrams, J. R., Kelley, S. L., Hayes, E., Kikuchi, T., Brown, M. J., Kang, S., Lebwohl, M. G., Guzzo, C. A., Jegasothy, B. V., Linsley, P. S., and Krueger, J. G. (2000). Blockade of T lymphocyte costimulation with cytotoxic T lymphocyte-associated antigen 4-immunoglobulin (CTLA4Ig) reverses the cellular pathology of psoriatic plaques, including the activation of keratinocytes, dendritic cells, and endothelial cells. J. Exp. Med. *192*, 681–694

Adorini, L. and Sinigaglia, F. (1997). Pathogenesis and immunotherapy of autoimmune diseases. Immunol. Today *18*, 209–211

Akdis, C. A., Joss, A., Akdis, M., Faith, A., and Blaser, K. (2000). A molecular basis for T cell suppression by IL-10: CD28-associated IL-10 receptor inhibits CD28 tyrosine phosphorylation and phosphatidylinositol 3-kinase binding. Faseb J. *14*, 1666–1668

Albert, M. L., Sauter, B., and Bhardwaj, N. (1998). Dendritic cells acquire antigen from apoptotic cells and induce class I-restricted CTLs. Nature *392*, 86–89

Alferink, J., Tafuri, A., Vestweber, D., Hallmann, R., Hammerling, G. J., and Arnold, B. (1998). Control of neonatal tolerance to tissue antigens by peripheral T cell trafficking. Science *282*, 1338–1341

Amagai, M., Klaus-Kovtun, V., and Stanley, J. R. (1991). Autoantibodies against a novel epithelial cadherin in pemphigus vulgaris, a disease of cell adhesion. Cell *67*, 869–877

Arnold, B., Schonrich, G., and Hammerling, G. J. (1993). Multiple levels of peripheral tolerance. Immunol. Today *14*, 12–14

Austin, L. M., Ozawa, M., Kikuchi, T., Walters, I. B., and Krueger, J. G. (1999). The majority of epidermal T cells in Psoriasis vulgaris lesions can produce type 1 cytokines, interferon-gamma, interleukin-2, and tumor necrosis factor-alpha, defining TC1 (cytotoxic T lymphocyte) and TH1 effector populations: a type 1 differentiation bias is also measured in circulating blood T cells in psoriatic patients. J. Invest. Dermatol. *113*, 752–759

Bachmaier, K., Neu, N., de la Maza, L. M., Pal, S., Hessel, A., and Penninger, J. M. (1999). Chlamydia infections and heart disease linked through antigenic mimicry. Science *283*, 1335–1339

Banchereau, J., Bazan, F., Blanchard, D., Briere, F., Galizzi, J. P., van Kooten, C., Liu, Y. J., Rousset, F., and Saeland, S. (1994). The CD40 antigen and its ligand. Annu. Rev. Immunol. *12*, 881–922

Banchereau, J. and Steinman, R. M. (1998). Dendritic cells and the control of immunity. Nature *392*, 245–252

Bendelac, A., Carnaud, C., Boitard, C., and Bach, J. F. (1987). Syngeneic transfer of autoimmune diabetes from diabetic NOD mice to healthy neonates. Requirement for both L3T4+ and Lyt-2+ T cells. J. Exp. Med. *166*, 823–832

Berg, P. A., Klein, R., and Rocken, M. (1997). Cytokines in primary biliary cirrhosis. Semin. Liver Dis. *17*, 115–123

Biedermann, T., Kneilling, M., Mailhammer, R., Maier, K., Sander, C. A., Kollias, G., Kunkel, S. L., Hultner, L., and Rocken, M. (2000). Mast Cells Control Neutrophil Recruitment during T Cell-mediated Delayed-type Hypersensitivity Reactions through Tumor Necrosis Factor and Macrophage Inflammatory Protein 2. J. Exp. Med. *192*, 1441–1452

Biedermann, T., Mailhammer, R., Mai, A., Sander, C., Ogilvie, A., Brombacher, F., Maier, K., Levine, A. D., and Röcken M. (2001). Reversal of established delayed type hypersensitivity reactions following therapy with IL-4 or antigen-specific Th2 cells. Eur. J. Immunol. *31*, 1582–1591

Biedermann, T., Zimmermann, S., Himmelrich, H., Gumy, A., Egeter, O., Sakrauski, A. K., Seeg-muller, I., Voigt, H., Launois, P., Levine, A. D., Wagner, H., Heeg, K., Louis, J. A., and Röcken, M. (2001) IL-4 instructs TH1 responses and resistance to Leishmania major in susceptible BALB/c mice. Nat. Immunol. *2*, 1054–1060

Biedermann, T., Röcken, M., and Carballido, J. M. (2004). TH1 and TH2 lymphocyte development and regulation of TH cell-mediated immune responses of the skin. J. Investig. Dermatol. Symp. Proc. *9*, 5–14

Blackman, M., Kappler, J., and Marrack, P. (1990). The role of the T cell receptor in positive and negative selection of developing T cells. Science *248*, 1335–1341

Bluestone, J. A. and Tang, Q. (2004). Therapeutic vaccination using CD4+CD25+ antigen-specific regulatory T cells. Proc Natl Acad Sci U S A. www.pnas.org/cgi/doi/10.1073/pnas.0405234101

Bonomo, A. and Matzinger, P. (1993). Thymus epithelium induces tissue-specific tolerance. J. Exp. Med. *177*, 1153–1164

Boulé, M. W., Broughton, C., Mackay, F., Akira, S., Marshak-Rothstein, A., and Rifkin, I.R. (2004). Toll-like receptor 9-dependent and -independent dendritic cell activation by chromatin-immu-noglobulin G complexes. J. Exp. Med. *199*; 1631–1640

Bouneaud, C., Kourilsky, P., and Bousso, P. (2000). Impact of Negative Selection on the T Cell Rep-ertoire Reactive to a Self-Peptide. A Large Fraction of T Cell Clones Escapes Clonal Deletion. Immunity *13*, 829–840

Budinger, L., Borradori, L., Yee, C., Eming, R., Ferencik, S., Grosse-Wilde, H., Merk, H. F., Yancey, K., and Hertl, M. (1998). Identification and characterization of autoreactive T cell responses to bullous pemphigoid antigen 2 in patients and healthy controls. J. Clin. Invest. *102*, 2082–2089

Chen, R., Diaz, L., Giudice, G., and Liu, Z. (2000). The role of C5a in mast cell activation during subepidermal blistering in experimetnal bullous pemphigoid. J. Invest. Dermatol. *114 (A)*, 762

Chuang, T. Y., Stitle, L., Brashear, R., and Lewis, C. (1999). Hepatitis C virus and lichen planus: A case-control study of 340 patients. J. Am. Acad. Dermatol. *41*, 787–789

Degitz, K. and Röcken, M. (1997). Lichen ruber planus nach Hepatitis-B-Impfung. In Fortschritte der praktischen Dermatologie und Venerologie 1996, G. Plewig and B. Przybilla, eds. (Berlin Heidelberg New York: Springer), 426–427

Duhen, T., Geiger, R., Jarrossay, D., Lanzavecchia, A., and Sallusto, F. (2009). Production of in-terleukin 22 but not interleukin 17 by a subset of human skin-homing memory T cells. Nat. Immunol. *10*, 857–863

Ehl, S., Hombach, J., Aichele, P., Rulicke, T., Odermatt, B., Hengartner, H., Zinkernagel, R., and Pircher, H. (1998). Viral and bacterial infections interfere with peripheral tolerance induction and activate CD8+ T cells to cause immunopathology. J. Exp. Med. *187*, 763–774

Eyerich, S., Eyerich, K., Pennino, D., Carbone, T., Nasorri, F., Pallotta, S., Cianfarani, F., Odorisio, T., Traidl-Hoffmann, C., Behrendt, H., Durham, S. R., Schmidt-Weber, C. B., Cavani, A. (2009). Th22 cells represent a distinct human T cell subset involved in epidermal immunity and re-modeling. J Clin Invest. *119*, 3573–3585

Feldmann, M., Brennan, F. M., and Maini, R. N. (1996). Role of cytokines in rheumatoid arthritis. Annu. Rev. Immunol. *14*, 397–440

Fontenot, J. D., Gavin, M. A., and Rudensky, A. Y. (2003). Foxp3 programs the development and function of CD4+CD25+ regulatory T cells. Nat. Immunol. *4*, 330–336

Gautam, A. M., Lock, C. B., Smilek, D. E., Pearson, C. I., Steinman, L., and McDevitt, H. O. (1994). Minimum structural requirements for peptide presentation by major histocompatibility complex class II molecules: implications in induction of autoimmunity. Proc. Natl .Acad. Sci. U.S.A. *91*, 767–771

Gerlach, J. T., Diepolder, H. M., Jung, M. C., Gruener, N. H., Schraut, W. W., Zachoval, R., Hoffmann, R., Schirren, C. A., Santantonio, T., and Pape, G. R. (1999). Recurrence of hepatitis C virus after loss of virus-specific CD4(+) T-cell response in acute hepatitis C. Gastroenterology *117*, 933–941

Ghoreschi, K., Thomas, P., Breit, S., Dugas, M., Mailhammer, R., Van Eden, W., Van Der Zee, R., Biedermann, T., Prinz, J., Mack, M., Mrowietz, U., Christophers, E., Schlondorff, D., Plewig, G., Sander, C. A., and Röcken, M. (2003). Interleukin-4 therapy of psoriasis induces Th2 responses and improves human autoimmune disease. Nat. Med. *9*, 40–46

Goldman, M., Druet, P., and Gleichmann, E. (1991). TH2 cells in systemic autoimmunity: insights from allogeneic diseases and chemically-induced autoimmunity. Immunol. Today *12*, 223–227

Goodnow, C. C., Brink, R., and Adams, E. (1991). Breakdown of self-tolerance in anergic B lymphocytes. Nature *352*, 532–536

Green, E. A. and Flavell, R. A. (2000). The temporal importance of TNFalpha expression in the development of diabetes. Immunity *12*, 459–469

Groux, H., O'Garra, A., Bigler, M., Rouleau, M., Antonenko, S., de Vries, J. E., and Roncarolo, M. G. (1997). A CD4+ T-cell subset inhibits antigen-specific T-cell responses and prevents colitis. Nature *389*, 737–742

Harrison, L. C., Honeyman, M. C., DeAizpurua, H. J., Schmidli, R. S., Colman, P. G., Tait, B. D., and Cram, D. S. (1993). Inverse relation between humoral and cellular immunity to glutamic acid decarboxylase in subjects at risk of insulin-dependent diabetes. Lancet *341*, 1365–-1369

Hertl, M., Karr, R. W., Amagai, M., and Katz, S. I. (1998). Heterogeneous MHC II restriction pattern of autoreactive desmoglein 3 specific T cell responses in pemphigus vulgaris patients and normals. J. Invest. Dermatol. *110*, 388–392

Hertl M, Eming R, Veldman C. (2006) T cell control in autoimmune bullous skin disorders. J Clin Invest. 116:1159–66.

Iwasaki, A., Medzhitov, R. (2010). Regulation of Adaptive Immunity by the Innate Immune System. Science. *5963*, 291–295

Jonuleit, H., Schmitt, E., Schuler, G., Knop, J., and Enk, A. H. (2000). Induction of interleukin 10-producing, nonproliferating CD4(+) T cells with regulatory properties by repetitive stimulation with allogeneic immature human dendritic cells. J. Exp. Med. *192*, 1213–1222

Kalinski, P., Hilkens, C. M., Wierenga, E. A., and Kapsenberg, M. L. (1999). T-cell priming by type-1and type-2 polarized dendritic cells: the concept of a third signal. Immunol. Today *20*, 561–567

Katz, J. D., Benoist, C., and Mathis, D. (1995). T helper cell subsets in insulin-dependent diabetes. Science *268*, 1185–1188

Kisielow, P., Teh, H. S., Bluthmann, H., and von Boehmer, H. (1988). Positive selection of antigen-specific T cells in thymus by restricting MHC molecules. Nature *335*, 730–733

Kisielow, P. and von Boehmer, H. (1995). Development and selection of T cells: facts and puzzles. Adv. Immunol. *58*, 87–209

Kneilling, M., Mailhammer, R., Hültner, L., Schönberger, T., Fuchs, K., Schaller, M., Bukala, D., Massberg, S., Sander, C. A., Braumüller, H., Eichner, M., Maier, K. L., Hallmann, R., Pichler, B. J., Haubner, R., Gawaz, M., Pfeffer, K., Biedermann, T., Röcken, M. (2009). Direct crosstalk between mast cell-TNF and TNFR1-expressing endothelia mediates local tissue inflammation. Blood. *114*, 1696–706

Kolb, H., Kolb-Bachofen, V., and Roep, B. O. (1995). Autoimmune versus inflammatory type I diabetes: a controversy? Immunol. Today *16*, 170–172

Korn, T., Bettelli, E., Oukka, M., Kuchroo, V. K. (2009). IL-17 and Th17 Cells. Annu. Rev. Immunol. *27*, 485–517

Kretz-Rommel, A. and Rubin, R. L. (2000). Disruption of positive selection of thymocytes causes autoimmunity. Nat. Med. *6*, 298–305

Kriegel, M. A., Lohmann, T., Gabler, C., Blank, N., Kalden, J. R., and Lorenz, H. M. (2004). Defective suppressor function of human CD4+ CD25+ regulatory T cells in autoimmune polyglandular syndrome type II. J. Exp. Med. *199*, 1285–1291

Krueger, G. G , Ellis, C. N. (2003). Alefacept therapy produces remission for patients with chronic plaque psoriasis. Br. J. Dermatol. *148*,784–788

Krueger, G. G., Langley, R. G., Leonardi, C., Yeilding, N., Guzzo, C., Wang, Y., Dooley, L. T., Lebwohl, M.; CNTO 1275 Psoriasis Study Group. (2007). A human interleukin-12/23 monoclonal antibody for the treatment of psoriasis. N. Engl. J. Med. *356*, 580–592

Lanzavecchia, A. (1985). Antigen-specific interaction between T and B cells. Nature *314*, 537–539

Leadbetter, E. A., Rifkin, I. R., Hohlbaum, A. M., Beaudette, B.C., Shlomchik, M. J., and Marshak-Rothstein, A. (2002). Chromatin-IgG complexes activate B cells by dual engagement of IgM and Toll-like receptors. Nature *416*, 603–607

Limmer, A., Sacher, T., Alferink, J., Kretschmar, M., Schonrich, G., Nichterlein, T., Arnold, B., and Hammerling, G. J. (1998). Failure to induce organ-specific autoimmunity by breaking of tolerance: importance of the microenvironment. Eur. J. Immunol. *28*, 2395–2406

Liu, Z., Giudice, G. J., Swartz, S. J., Fairley, J. A., Till, G. O., Troy, J. L., and Diaz, L. A. (1995). The role of complement in experimental bullous pemphigoid. J. Clin. Invest. *95*, 1539–1544

Liu, Z., Shipley, J. M., Vu, T. H., Zhou, X., Diaz, L. A., Werb, Z., and Senior, R. M. (1998). Gelatinase B-deficient mice are resistant to experimental bullous pemphigoid. J. Exp. Med. *188*, 475–482

Liu, Z., Shapiro, S. D., Zhou, X., Twining, S. S., Senior, R. M., Giudice, G. J., Fairley, J. A., and Diaz, L. A. (2000). A critical role for neutrophil elastase in experimental bullous pemphigoid. J. Clin. Invest. *105*, 113–123

Louis, J. A., Chiller, J. M., and Weigle, W. O. (1973). The ability of bacterial lipopolysaccharide to modulate the induction of unresponsiveness to a state of immunity. Cellular parameters. J. Exp. Med. *138*, 1481–1495

Luger, D., Silver, P. B., Tang, J., Cua, D., Chen, Z., Iwakura, Y., Bowman, E. P., Sgambellone, N. M., Chan, C. C., Caspi, R. R. (2008). Either a Th17 or a Th1 effector response can drive autoimmunity: conditions of disease induction affect dominant effector category. J Exp Med. *205*, 799–810.

Martin, R., McFarland, H. F., and McFarlin, D. E. (1992). Immunological aspects of demyelinating diseases. Annu. Rev. Immunol. *10*, 153–187

Matzinger, P. (1994). Tolerance, danger, and the extended family. Annu. Rev. Immunol. *12*, 991–1045

Matzinger, P. and Anderson, C. C. (2001). Immunity or tolerance: Opposite outcomes of microchimerism from skin grafts. Nat. Med. *7*, 80–87

Mease, P. J., Goffe, B. S., Metz, J., VanderStoep, A., Finck, B., and Burge, D. J. (2000). Etanercept in the treatment of psoriatic arthritis and psoriasis: a randomised trial. Lancet *356*, 385–390

Mocikat, R., Braumüller, H., Gumy, A., Egeter, O., Ziegler, H., Reusch, U., Bubeck, A., Louis, J., Mailhammer, R., Riethmuller, G., Koszinowski, U., Röcken, M. (2003). Natural killer cells activated by MHC class I(low) targets prime dendritic cells to induce protective CD8 T cell responses. Immunity *19*, 561–569

Mokhtarian, F., McFarlin, D. E., and Raine, C. S. (1984). Adoptive transfer of myelin basic protein-sensitized T cells produces chronic relapsing demyelinating disease in mice. Nature *309*, 356–358

Moradpour, D. and Blum, H. E. (1999). Current and evolving therapies for hepatitis C. Eur. J. Gastroenterol. Hepatol *11*, 1199–1202

Moser, M. and Murphy, K. M. (2000). Dendritic cell regulation of TH1-TH2 development. Nat. Immunol. *1*, 199–205

Moskophidis, D., Lechner, F., Pircher, H., and Zinkernagel, R. M. (1993). Virus persistence in acutely infected immunocompetent mice by exhaustion of antiviral cytotoxic effector T cells. Nature *362*, 758–761

Mosmann, T. R. and Coffman, R. L. (1989). TH1 and TH2 cells: different patterns of lymphokine secretion lead to different functional properties. Annu. Rev. Immunol. *7*, 145–173

Mosmann, T. R. and Sad, S. (1996). The expanding universe of T-cell subsets: Th1, Th2 and more. Immunol. Today *17*, 138–146

Nagata, S., Hanayama, R., and Kawane, K. (2010). Autoimmunity and the clearance of dead cells. Cell. *140*, 619–630

Naucler, C. S., Larsson, S., and Moller, E. (1996). A novel mechanism for virus-induced autoimmunity in humans. Immunol. Rev. *152*, 175–192

Nestle, F. O., Kaplan, D. H., Barker, J. (2009). Psoriasis. N. Engl. J. Med. *361*, 496–509

Ohashi, P. S., Oehen, S., Buerki, K., Pircher, H., Ohashi, C. T., Odermatt, B., Malissen, B., Zinkernagel, R. M., and Hengartner, H. (1991). Ablation of "tolerance" and induction of diabetes by virus infection in viral antigen transgenic mice. Cell *65*, 305–317

Oldstone, M. B., Nerenberg, M., Southern, P., Price, J., and Lewicki, H. (1991). Virus infection triggers insulin-dependent diabetes mellitus in a transgenic model: role of anti-self (virus) immune response. Cell *65*, 319–331

Powrie, F. (1995). T cells in inflammatory bowel disease: protective and pathogenic roles. Immunity *3*, 171–174

Prinz, J. C. (1999). Which T cells cause psoriasis? Clin. Exp. Dermatol. *24*, 291–295

Racke, M. K., Bonomo, A., Scott, D. E., Cannella, B., Levine, A., Raine, C. S., Shevach, E. M., and Rocken, M. (1994). Cytokine-induced immune deviation as a therapy for inflammatory autoimmune disease. J. Exp. Med. *180*, 1961–1966

Rocha, B. and von Boehmer, H. (1991). Peripheral selection of the T cell repertoire. Science *251*, 1225–1228

Rock, B., Martins, C. R., Theofilopoulos, A. N., Balderas, R. S., Anhalt, G. J., Labib, R. S., Futamura, S., Rivitti, E. A., and Diaz, L. A. (1989). The pathogenic effect of IgG4 autoantibodies in endemic pemphigus foliaceus (fogo selvagem). N. Engl. J. Med. *320*, 1463–1469

Rocken, M., Urban, J. F., and Shevach, E. M. (1992). Infection breaks T-cell tolerance. Nature *359*, 79–82

Rocken, M., Saurat, J. H., and Hauser, C. (1992). A common precursor for CD4+ T cells producing IL-2 or IL-4. J. Immunol. *148*, 1031–1036

Rocken, M., Urban, J., and Shevach, E. M. (1994). Antigen-specific activation, tolerization, and reactivation of the interleukin 4 pathway in vivo. J. Exp. Med. *179*, 1885–1893

Rocken, M., Racke, M., and Shevach, E. M. (1996). IL-4-induced immune deviation as antigen-specific therapy for inflammatory autoimmune disease. Immunol. Today *17*, 225–231

Rocken, M. and Shevach, E. M. (1996). Immune deviation – the third dimension of nondeletional T cell tolerance. Immunol. Rev. *149*, 175–194

Rubin, R. L. (1997). Dubois Lupus Erythematosus, 5th Edition, D. J. Wallace and B. H. Hahn, eds. (Baltimore: Williams & Wilkens), 871–901

Schonrich, G., Kalinke, U., Momburg, F., Malissen, M., Schmitt-Verhulst, A. M., Malissen, B., Hammerling, G. J., and Arnold, B. (1991). Down-regulation of T cell receptors on self-reactive T cells as a novel mechanism for extrathymic tolerance induction. Cell *65*, 293–304

Schroder, K., Tschopp, J. (2009). The inflammasomes. Cell. *140*, 821–832

Schuler, G. and Steinman, R. M. (1997). Dendritic cells as adjuvants for immune-mediated resistance to tumors. J. Exp. Med. *186*, 1183–1187

Schuler, G., Thurner, B., and Romani, N. (1997). Dendritic cells: from ignored cells to major players in T-cell-mediated immunity. Int. Arch. Allergy Immunol. *112*, 317–322

Schwartz, R. H. (1998). Immunological tolerance. In Fundamental Immunology, 4th Edition, W. E. Paul, ed. (Philadelphia, New York: Lippincott-Raven), 701–740

Sinha, A. A., Lopez, M. T., and McDevitt, H. O. (1990). Autoimmune diseases: the failure of self tolerance. Science *248*, 1380–1388

Stenger, S. and Modlin, R. L. (1999). T cell mediated immunity to Mycobacterium tuberculosis. Curr. Opin. Microbiol. *2*, 89–93

Stockinger, B. (1999). T lymphocyte tolerance: from thymic deletion to peripheral control mechanisms. Adv. Immunol. *71*, 229–265

Strober, W. and Ehrhardt, R. O. (1993). Chronic intestinal inflammation: an unexpected outcome in cytokine or T cell receptor mutant mice. Cell *75*, 203–205

Tessari, G., Barba, A., and Schena, D. (1996). Lichen ruber planus following the administration of human anti-hepatitis B virus immunoglobulins [letter]. Acta Derm. Venereol. *76*, 154

Trifari, S., Kaplan, C. D., Tran, E. H., Crellin, N. K., Spits, H. (2009). Identification of a human helper T cell population that has abundant production of interleukin 22 and is distinct from T(H)-17, T(H)1 and T(H)2 cells. Nat. Immunol. *10*, 864–871

Ulevitch, R. J. (2004). Therapeutics targeting the innate immune system. Nat. Rev. Immunol. *4*, 512–520

Vollmer, S., Menssen, A., Trommler, P., Schendel, D., and Prinz, J. C. (1994). T lymphocytes derived from skin lesions of patients with psoriasis vulgaris express a novel cytokine pattern that is distinct from that of T helper type 1 and T helper type 2 cells. Eur. J. Immunol. *24*, 2377–2382

Volz, T., Nega, M., Buschmann, J., Kaesler, S., Guenova, E., Peschel, A., Röcken, M. Götz, F.*, Biedermann, T.* (2010). Natural Staphylococcus aureus-derived peptidoglycan fragments activate NOD2 and act as potent co-stimulator of the innate immune system exclusively in the presence of TLR signals. FASEB J 2010, in press. *Co-corresponding authors

von Herrath, M. G., Guerder, S., Lewicki, H., Flavell, R. A., and Oldstone, M. B. (1995). Coexpression of B7-1 and viral ("self") transgenes in pancreatic beta cells can break peripheral ignorance and lead to spontaneous autoimmune diabetes. Immunity *3*, 727–738

Walker, M. R., Kasprowicz, D. J., Gersuk, V. H., Benard, A., Van Landeghen, M., Buckner, J. H., and Ziegler, S. F. (2003). Induction of FoxP3 and acquisition of T regulatory activity by stimulated human CD4+CD25- T cells. J. Clin. Invest. *112*, 1437–1443

Webb, S., Morris, C., and Sprent, J. (1990). Extrathymic tolerance of mature T cells: clonal elimination as a consequence of immunity. Cell *63*, 1249–1256

Weber, S., Traunecker, A., Oliveri, F., Gerhard, W., and Karjalainen, K. (1992). Specific low-affinity recognition of major histocompatibility complex plus peptide by soluble T-cell receptor. Nature *356*, 793–796

Weinberg, A. D., English, M., and Swain, S. L. (1990). Distinct regulation of lymphokine production is found in fresh versus in vitro primed murine helper T cells. J. Immunol. *144*, 1800–1807

Wucherpfennig, K. W., and Strominger, J. L. (1995). Molecular mimicry in T cell-mediated autoimmunity: viral peptides activate human T cell clones specific for myelin basic protein. Cell *80*, 695–705

Yang, Y., Huang, C. T., Huang, X., and Pardoll, D. M. (2004). Persistent Toll-like receptor signals are required for reversal of regulatory T cell-mediated CD8 tolerance. Nat. Immunol. *5*, 508–515

Zhang, J., Hafler, D., Hohlfeld, R., and Miller, A., eds. (1998). Immunotherapy in neuroimmunologic diseases (London: Martin Dunitz Ltd)

Zimmermann, S., Egeter, O., Hausmann, S., Lipford, G. B., Rocken, M., Wagner, H., and Heeg, K. (1998). CpG oligodeoxynucleotides trigger protective and curative Th1 responses in lethal murine leishmaniasis. J. Immunol. *160*, 3627–3630

Zinkernagel, R. M. (1996). Immunology taught by viruses. Science *271*, 173–178

Autoantibody Detection Using Indirect Immunofluorescence on HEp-2 Cells

2

Philipp von Landenberg

Introduction

Non organ specific autoantibodies (AABs), are directed against highly conserved antigens of the body's own cells (Holborow et al., 1957). Diagnostically relevant target structures are predominantly located in the cell nucleus (antinuclear antibodies, ANA), but also in the cytoplasm. Screening for these AABs constitutes a major part of the diagnostic procedure for connective tissue and autoimmune liver diseases. Evidence is usually collected in a multistage diagnostic process in which initial screening is carried out using indirect immunofluorescence testing (IIF) on HEp-2 cells, an epithelial cell line derived from a human laryngeal carcinoma (Hahon et al., 1975). HEp-2 cells have replaced the frozen sections of organs, which were originally used as a substrate. Used in primary screening, the main advantage of IIF on HEp-2 cells is that it provides a good overview of most of the diagnostically relevant non-organ-specific AABs and their concentrations. Originally, immunological laboratories prepared their own HEp-2 cells, and diagnostic use of these cells was subject to great variability because of individual culture and fixation conditions. Nowadays preparations of acceptable quality are available from manufacturers of diagnostic equipment on standardized microscope slides as in vitro diagnostic material (EU Directive, 1998). The use of cells in IIF cannot be replaced by the use of lysed HEp-2 cells in enzyme immunoassays because only immunofluorescence can deliver information about all diagnostically relevant AABs. In spite of the now-acceptable quality of the available HEp-2 preparations for immunofluorescence, the results from different laboratories can differ considerably. This paper therefore aims to summarize current recommendations concerning IIF methodology and the interpretation of immunofluorescence patterns on HEp-2 cells. These recommendations will contribute to improve the comparability of diagnostic procedures and are intended to aid the interpretation of findings, independent of the laboratory in which the tests are performed. The recommendations were developed in close collaboration with clinical and laboratory scientists with the focus to improve diagnostic procedures for autoimmune diseases (Sack et al., 2007).

Reagents and Test Preparation

HEp-2 Cells

HEp-2 cells are available from numerous suppliers as a CE-certified and / or FDA approved diagnostic aid. They can also be obtained from cell banks (such as American Tissue and Cell Collection CCL-23; http://www.atcc.org) as a cell line for scientific investigations. The cells have been found to be heterogeneous in their morphology, antigen expression and cell division behavior. Modified HEp-2 cells also exist in which the expression of particular antigens, such as Ro60 has been increased by transfection. Certain criteria are important for the judgment of the cells' quality and can be heavily influenced in the production process by cell culture conditions, cell preparation, microscope slide preparation, fixation and the processing instructions given.

These criteria are:
1. cell density and distribution on the microscope slide,
2. number of mitoses (at least 3 to 5 mitoses per visual field at 200 × magnification),
3. expression of target antigens for relevant autoantibodies,
4. maintenance of morphology,
5. background fluorescence

Before it is used in the laboratory, the quality of each batch should be tested using defined monitoring procedures. There is so far no standardization of the preparation of HEp-2 cells or the composition of the test kits among manufacturers, although this would make it possible to ensure that differences in titer levels and fluorescence patterns detected on evaluation do not arise as a result of preparation procedures. Furthermore, only standardized procedures make possible longitudinal measurements and comparison of results from different laboratories. Batch monitoring requires the use of one negative serum and at least three positive serum samples with different fluorescence patterns resulting from defined antibody reactivity (e.g. centromeres, dsDNA, Ro/SS-A). These must be used in alternation each time the test is run.

Workplace

The preparation of IIF tests and subsequent evaluation by fluorescence microscopy are typically carried out in separate areas. In immunofluorescence laboratories it is especially important to ensure low levels of dust. The microscopy room must be large enough to allow two people to work simultaneously and must be adequately ventilated. Considerable amounts of heat can be produced, especially when microscopes with high-pressure mercury lamps are used. A network connection for laboratory computers simplifies working procedures and documentation.

Assay Procedure

All samples to be processed must be identifiable at all times with the help of the order specification and sample labelling.

Processing of Samples

Pre-analytic procedures are not critical for detection of autoantibodies. Hemolytic, lipemic, and icteric sera should be recorded in the protocol, as they may influence the test system. As a rule the reagents used have a CE certificate, so that analysis must be carried out according to the manufacturer's instructions. Deviations from incubation times, dilutions, or buffering systems can influence the test results when the microscope slides are evaluated and must therefore be validated in the laboratory. Samples are processed at room temperature (20 to 24 °C). When microscope slides from different manufacturers are used, it is necessary to ensure that the corresponding test components are used in each case. Buffer systems and conjugate concentrations, in particular, are usually adjusted for the relevant substrates on the microscope slides. It is also necessary to be aware of the expiry date and the correct storage method for each of the reagents used. With conjugate, in particular, a decrease in intensity is otherwise to be expected, which can lead to a lower titer of the autoantibody of interest. The volumes of serum and conjugate to be pipetted or dripped onto the appropriate application sites are often not clearly defined. Microscope slides frequently have application sites of different sizes. It is necessary to ensure that the whole application site is covered with serum / conjugate, but an application site should not be allowed to overflow because this immediately puts the next application site at risk of contamination. It is recommended that individual laboratories determine the optimal volumes for each microscope slide and include these in the corresponding internal instructions (Standard Operating Procedures, SOPs). The individual incubation stages should be carried out in a humidity chamber to prevent the sample from desiccation, which would significantly reduce the sample volume per application site. Easily cleanable flat plastic boxes are used for this purpose. The floor of the box is covered with a porous carrier material, such as cellulose, which is easy to moisten and should be renewed regularly. The microscope slides should not be placed directly on top of this material. The actual test starts when the serum, which has been diluted with the buffers supplied within the test kit (usually phosphate-buffered isotonic saline, PBS), is added to the HEp-2 cell monolayer. Under no circumstances should serum spill over onto adjacent fields. The incubation time is usually 30 min, normally followed by three 10-min washes in PBS. When cuvettes are used, the washing time is shortened to 3×2 to 5 min. The use of automatic washing equipment should be considered only after rigorous evaluation since it often gives unsatisfactory results because of increased background staining or cell detachments.

When washing the individual microscope slides, it is important first to remove all the serum or conjugate from each application site by briefly rinsing with washing buffer before placing the slides into the cuvette with washing buffer. This procedure is intended to pre-

Table 1. Typical Nuclear and Cytoplasmic Fluorescence Patterns of Anto-Antibodies

Patterns	HEp-2 Fluorescence	Common Antigens
nuclear patterns		
homogeneous	homogeneous or fine granular nuclear fluorescence, chromatin in metaphase positive	dsDNA, nucleosomes, histones
fine granular	fine/intermediate granular nuclear fluorescence, negative metaphase chromatin	Ro/SS-A, La/SS-B, Ku, Mi-2
coarse granular	coarse granular nuclear fluorescence with numerous condensations, excluding nucleoli	U1-RNP, Sm
nucleolar	nucleolar fluorescence Scl-70 (chromosomal association)	PM-Scl, Fibrillarin, Th/To
centromere	dot count according to interphase chromosome number AND mitosis chromatin	CENP-B
nuclear dots	multiple nuclear dots (commonly 13 to 25 per nucleus), negative metaphase chromatin	Sp100
pleomorphic	heterogeneous staining of interphase nuclei	PCNA
cytoplasmatic patterns		
homogeneous	cytoplasm homogeneous to fine granular	Rib-P (with positive nucleoli)
granular	fine to intermediate granular cytoplasm (or granular dots)	Jo-1
mitochondrial	fine-stitched cytoplasmatic fluorescence	AMA-M2
cytoskeletal	cytoskeleton associated fluorescence	Actin

vent high-titred and high avidity antibodies on other application sites from causing cross-contamination and false-positive results, even when incubation times are short. After addition of the fluorescent-labeled secondary antibody (conjugate) and an incubation period which normally lasts 30 minutes, the slide is washed again. The use of fluorescein isothiocyanate (FITC)-labeled secondary antibodies to human IgG is very common and, in our opinion, ideal. The value of additional use of secondary antibodies to other immunoglobulin classes needs to be investigated further. The FITC-labeled secondary antibodies are often treated with 0.01 g/1L Evans Blue to make the fluorescence signal easier to distinguish. To complete the test, the microscope slides are covered with a mounting medium containing glycerine (about 80% glycerine in PBS). This usually contains an antibleaching substance. The ideal quantity of mounting medium per microscope slide should be fixed for each laboratory individually. A large excess of mounting medium can lead to fogging and poor focus when slides are evaluated microscopically. Manufacturer-specific differences in mounting medium should be taken into consideration here. The practice of cleaning or drying around the application site with a paper towel or swab, which has become established at some laboratories, is unnecessary and causes errors by wiping substances into the cells and introducing dust and fibers. Gentle tapping of the microscope slide and drying on an absorbent surface are sufficient. After evaluation, the prepared slides can be kept in a refrigerator and analyzed for up to 24 h. However, after longer periods, reanalysis is difficult due to diffusion of the antibodies and bleaching-out of the fluorescent dyes, especially when the reactivity is weak. A prepared slide should therefore be hermetically shrink-wrapped and stored at − 20 °C, in case another analysis needs to be carried out later for monitoring or comparison purposes.

Serum Dilution

A serum dilution of 1:80 is used in screening for antibodies. The majority of test kits are designed so that 95% of sera from healthy control subjects show no staining, while sera with diagnostically relevant autoantibodies are detected. Reagents put together by individual laboratories (laboratory-made tests) must be adjusted during validation so that, at this dilution, negative sera from healthy blood donors are not recorded. The adjustments carried out by the manufacturer during batch monitoring must always be verified at the laboratory. It may be necessary to check whether changes of the testing procedure need to be made. However, these must also be validated.

The manufacturers should offer an adjustment here to accord with the consensus protocol. In the case of a positive result, the test is repeated using a geometric series of dilutions according to the strength of the primary fluorescence (1:160 to 1:5120). Titers of at least 1:160, are taken to be diagnostically relevant provided the test has been carried out and evaluated correctly (Kang et al., 2004). A titer of 1:80 can be seen as borderline because, in the majority of cases with this titer, no diagnostically relevant ANA specificities are found (Table 1).

Controls

In parallel to the sample processing, control tests with positive and negative samples must be run. For important patterns, sera containing disease-typical AABs should also be used at regular intervals (Fig. 1). Commercial control sera are available for this purpose, and positive probes defined by the laboratory itself can also be used. Ideally, defined control sera from commercial suppliers or the Center for Disease Control and Prevention (CDC) should be used. It is urgently recommended that laboratories take part in external quality assessments (http://www.ukneqas.org.uk) of independent suppliers in accordance with the national standards and guidelines.

2

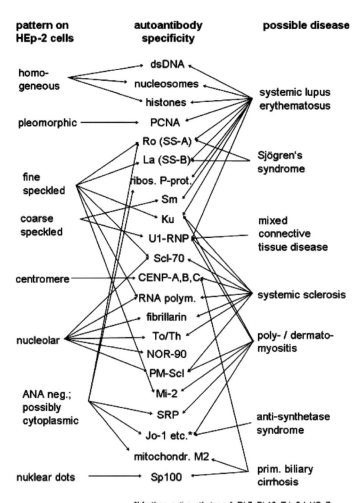

Fig. 1. Allocation of the HEp-2 cell immunofluorescence patterns listed in Table 1 to systemic inflammatory diseases that often underlie these patterns, or that are (with varying sensitivity and specificity) associated with them. The connecting lines indicate that, when the suspected diagnosis in the right-hand column and/or the fluorescence pattern in the left-hand column are present, the autoantibodies connected to them should be sought preferentially (*with permission modified from Sack et al., 2003*)

Microscopy

Precise pattern evaluation is carried out at $400 \times$ magnification (combination of $10 \times$ eyepiece and $40 \times$ objective). First the intensity of the fluorescence is judged. The evaluation must take into account several mitoses so that a clear decision on the presence or absence of fluorescence as well as a statement with regard to the basic pattern can be made (Table 1). The light intensity should not be less than that provided by a 50-watt mercury vapor lamp. Today, light emitting diodes (LEDs) are increasingly being used as a light source. Their constant brightness and long life (over 10,000 h of use) make them a real alternative to mercury vapor lamps (100 to 300 h of use depending on type; adjustment is necessary when bulbs are changed).

Efforts to standardize fluorescence intensity were not yet ultimately successful. Approaches such as the use of defined gray filters, standardized fluorescent beads (Kahn et al., 2006), or computer-assisted image analysis programs (Hiemann et al., 2007, 2009; Sack et al., 2003; Soda, 2007) are currently being evaluated.

Evaluation and Interpretation

HEp-2 cells contain a broad spectrum of detectable autoantigens. Primarily attention is directed toward nuclear patterns, but cytoplasmic patterns should also be considered. Mixed patterns are common. The individual patterns must be specified in the report, with details of different titers if appropriate. Certain patterns in IIF indicate disease-relevant AAB specificities and are an indication for using specific immunoassays. In an effective multistage diagnostic process it is therefore necessary to identify the autoantibodies that are typically responsible for a particular pattern. In the case of fluorescence patterns that cannot be characterized more closely, and whose clinical relevance is unknown, a note should at least be included to inform the clinician about the pattern so that future investigators can recognize it again (Fritzler, 2008). Antinuclear antibodies are subdivided into a few basic patterns. These patterns are often also present as mixed patterns. These can be differentiated by means of observation at different dilutions because, for example, a strong homogeneous fluorescence can mask other patterns at low serum dilutions and thus mask them. Depending on the suspected diagnosis it is useful to pay specific attention to the fluorescence patterns named in Fig. 1. The evaluation must be carried out by experienced workers who regularly undergo further training in autoimmune diagnostic procedures. Increasingly, attempts are being made to use computer-assisted interpretation aids; initial experiences in this area have recently been published (Kahn et al., 2006; Hiemann et al., 2007). Depending on the diagnostic questions posed and the fine characterization required for a differential diagnosis, screening should be followed by further diagnostic procedures based on specific immunoassays (radio, enzyme, or dot/line immunoassays) using highly purified (natural or recombinant) autoantigens. The diagnostic report must include the possible target antigens as well as a description of the fluorescence patterns found and their titers. Above all, the report needs to contain an assessment, f the findings in the light of the diagnostic, questions posed. The latter applies particularly for negative results. Because, in older patients, low-titred autoantibodies are often not an indication of illness, differential tests can be omitted if there is no clinical indication. It is not sufficient to report findings with the comment "positive ANA" without giving details of the pattern.

2

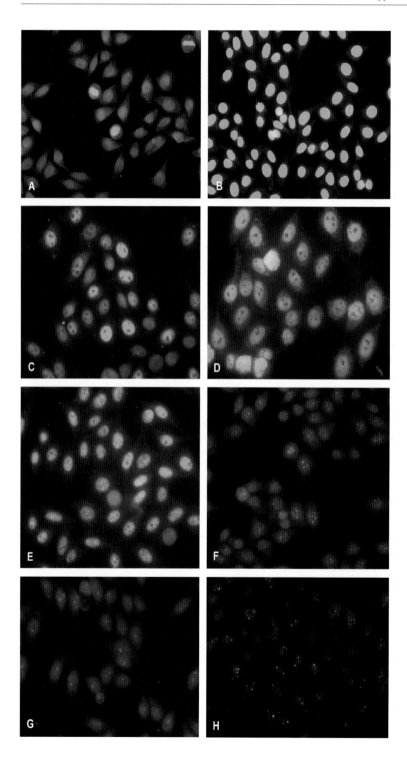

◄**Fig. 2.** Patterns of antinuclear autoantibodies on HEp-2 cells

A+B **Homogeneous pattern:** Homogeneous nucleoplasmic staining, strong homogenous chromosomal staining in mitotic cells.

C **Pleomorphic (PCNA):** Polymorphic nuclear staining, related to the cell cycle, from nuclear homogeneous to fine or coarse granular.

D **Fine speckled:** fine speckled nuclear in interphase cells, with no nucleolar decoration

E **Coarse speckled:** coarse speckled nucleoplasmic with no nucleolar decoration

F **Centromer:** discrete speckled nucleoplasmic staining in interphase cells, strong centromeric dots decorated in the metaphase plate

G **Nucleolar:** strong homogeneous nucleolar staining with usually weak homogenous nucleoplasmic staining

H **Nuclear dots:** nucleoplasmatic coarse speckled, antigen sp100.

magnification × 400

Summary

The detection of autoantibodies is an important element in the diagnosis and monitoring of disease progression in patients with autoimmune diseases. In laboratory diagnostic tests for connective tissue and autoimmune liver diseases, indirect immunofluorescence on HEp-2 cells plays a central role in a multistage diagnostic process. Despite the high quality of diagnostics, findings at different laboratories can differ considerably due to a lack of standardization, as well as subjective factors. This overview article formulates recommendations for the standardized processing and interpretation of the HEp-2 cell test for the detection of non-organ-specific (especially antinuclear) antibodies. It provides requirements regarding the diagnostic tests used, instructions for laboratory procedure and evaluation, and recommendations for interpretation. For an optimal laboratory diagnostic process, it is useful to have an informative, tentative clinical diagnosis and an experienced laboratory diagnostician. In addition, the following key elements are recommended: initial screening using indirect immunofluorescence on carefully chosen HEp-2 cells beginning with a serum dilution of 1:80 and evaluation under a microscope with powerful illumination; results from a titer of 1:160 and upwards being considered positive, internal laboratory quality control, and standardized interpretation.

References

Directive 98/79/EC of the European parliament and of the council of 27 October 1998 on invitro diagnostic medical devices. Official Journal of the European Communities L 331/1, 7.12.98, EN

Fritzler, M.J. (2008) Challenges to the use of autoantibodies as predictors of disease onset, diagnosis and outcomes. Autoimmun. Reviews 7:616–620

Hahon, N., H.L. Eckert & J. Stewart. (1975) Evaluation of cellular substrates for antinuclear antibody determinations. J. Clin. Microbiol. 2:42–5

Hiemann, R., N. Hilger, M. Weigert, et al. (2007) Image based description of immunofluorescence on, HEp-2 cells. Cytometry Part A 71:60

Hiemann, R., T. Büttner, T. Krieger, et al. (2009) Challenges of automated screening and differentiation of non-organ specific autoantibodies on HEp-2 cells. Autoimm. Rev. 9:17–22

Holborow, E.J., D.M.Weir & G.D. Johnson. (1957) A Serum Factor in Lupus Erythematosus with Affinity, for Tissue Nuclei. Br. Med. J. 2(5047):732–734

Kahn, E., A. Vejux, F. M´en´etrier, et al. (2006) Analysis, of CD36 expression on human monocytic cells, and atherosclerotic tissue sections with quantum dots: investigation by flow cytometry and spectral imaging microscopy. Anal. Quant. Cytol. Histol. 28:14–26

Kang, I., R. Siperstein, et al. (2004) Utility of age, gender, ANA titer and pattern as predictors of anti-, ENA and -dsDNA antibodies. Clin. Rheumatol. 23:,509–515

Sack, U., S. Knoechner, H. Warschkau, et al.,2003. Computer-assisted classification of HEp-2 immunofluorescence patterns in autoimmune diagnostics. Autoimmun. Rev. 2:298–304

Sack, U., K. Conrad, E. Csernok, et al. (2007) Standardization of Autoimmune Diagnostics in Germany: Activities of the German Group in the European Autoimmune Standardization Initiative. Ann., N. Y. Acad. Sci. 1109:31–36

Soda, P. (2007) Early Experiences in the Staining Pattern Classification of HEp-2 Slides. Proceedings of the Twentieth IEEE International Symposium on Computer-Based Medical Systems (CBMS'07):219–224

Michael Hertl and Rüdiger Eming

Introduction

Pemphigus vulgaris (derived from the Greek word "pemphix", meaning blister) belongs to the group of bullous autoimmune skin disorders. Clinically, the disorder is characterized by large, bullous, erosive defects on the skin and mucous membranes. This very rare disease usually occurs between the 4th and 6th decades of life and has an annual incidence of about $1-2/10^6$ (Europe and North America). Immunological studies typically show circulating autoantibodies to specific adhesion molecules in the epidermis. The binding of autoantibodies to desmosomal adhesion structures leads to functional loss of these autoantigens and thus to abnormal adhesion of epidermal keratinocytes corresponding to blisters or erosions. The strongest genetic association is with certain human leukocyte antigen (HLA) class II alleles (Lee et al., 2006).

In recent years desmoglein 3, a desmosomal adhesion protein, has been identified as an important autoantigen in pemphigus vulgaris and subsequently cloned (Amagai et al., 1991). In vivo and in vitro models have shown that desmoglein-3-reactive autoantibodies in the sera of pemphigus patients are the cause of pemphigus vulgaris (Amagai et al., 2000; Anhalt et al., 1982; Ishii et al., 2005; Kawasaki et al., 2006). The clinical manifestation of pemphigus vulgaris (mucosal or mucocutaneous type) correlates with the respective autoantibody profile. In patients with strictly mucosal involvement, only desmoglein-3-reactive autoantibodies are identified, while in patients with both mucosal and skin lesions both desmoglein-3 and desmoglein-1 autoantibodies are identified (Amagai et al., 1999). These new findings allow a classification of various pemphigus variants, not only by clinical phenotype, but also based on the specificity of the autoantibody profile.

Pathogenesis

Pemphigus vulgaris results from a loss of adhesion of epidermal keratinocytes due to binding of circulating autoantibodies to the desmosomal adhesion protein desmoglein 3 (Amagai et al., 1991; Hertl et al., 2006; Sitaru and Zillikens, 2005). Polyclonal autoantibodies can be identified in serum from affected patients; with regard to desmoglein-reactive immunoglobulins, during initial and acute stages of disease IgG4 isotypes predominate, while in chronic disease or during periods of remission IgG1 isotypes are present in greater numbers (Spaeth et al., 2001). The role of these autoantibodies in the pathogenesis of the disorder is further underscored by the following findings:

1. In the majority of patients, autoantibody titers correlate with the clinical activity of pemphigus;
2. newborns born to mothers with active disease can develop transitory blistering as a result of transplacental transfer of maternal autoantibodies; and
3. the injection of purified IgG from pemphigus serum leads to blistering of the skin in newborn mice, which histology shows to suprabasal acantholysis corresponding to pemphigus vulgaris (Amagai et al., 1998; Anhalt et al., 1982; Hertl et al., 2006).

Autoreactive CD4+ T cells appear to have an important function in autoantibody production. These are mainly helper T 2 (TH2) cells which regulate autoantibody production, especially of the TH2-dependent IgG4-subtype via secretion of interleukins 4, 5, and 13 (Hertl et al., 2006). The autoreactive T cells recognize portions (epitopes) of desmoglein 3, in association with certain HLA class II alleles (see Fig. 3). This is an interesting finding given that at this point the strongest genetic association in pemphigus vulgaris is with HLA class II alleles HLA-DRB1*0402 and HLADQB1* 0503 (Hertl et al., 2006; Lee et al., 2006). On the basis of binding algorithms, a limited number of T-cell epitopes of desmoglein 3 have been suggested that bind to the restricting HLA-DRB1*0402 allele (Wucherpfennig et al., 1995). This algorithm appears to be relevant since desmoglein-3-reactive T cells have been detected in peripheral blood of patients with pemphigus vulgaris which recognize the four or five proposed immunodominant epitopes of desmoglein 3 in association with the pemphigus-associated HLA class II alleles (Hertl et al., 2006). This discovery is very important for the development of T-cell-based specific immune therapies in pemphigus, especially for the induction of tolerance or an anergic state of autoaggressive desmoglein-3-specific T cells.

The fact that healthy carriers of the pemphigus-vulgaris-associated HLA class II haplotype also have autoreactive T cells suggests that the interaction between autoreactive T cells and B cells in pemphigus is controlled by other regulatory immune mechanisms as well. In a study conducted by our working group, we showed that desmoglein-3-specific, interleukin-10(IL-10)-producing, regulatory T cells are present in both pemphigus vulgaris patients and in healthy individuals with the respective HLA haplotypes (Hertl et al., 2006; Veldman et al., 2004). After stimulation with desmoglein 3 they are able to functionally inhibit pathogenic effector TH2 cells (Veldman et al., 2004) (see Fig. 3). The relevance of desmoglein-3-reactive, regulatory T cells in maintaining immunological tolerance is supported by the finding that these regulatory T cells occur in greater numbers in healthy individuals than in pemphigus patients.

Amagai and colleagues developed an animal model that is important in several ways for the pathogenesis of pemphigus. Desmoglein-3-reactive T and B lymphocytes from desmoglein-3-deficient mice immunized with desmoglein 3 were injected into immunodeficient mice with intact desmoglein-3 expression (Amagai et al., 2000). This led to induction of desmoglein-3-specific autoantibodies and development of erosions on the mucous membranes of the recipient mice similar to the clinical appearance of pemphigus vulgaris. Koch et al. produced a desmoglein- 3-deficient mouse (desmoglein-3 knockout mouse); due to abnormal intra-epidermal adhesion, the mouse developed erosions on the oral and nasal mucosa, but did not develop blisters on the skin (Koch et al., 1997). Eming et al. (2007) developed a humanized HLA class II transgenic mouse model for pemphigus in which the activation of desmoglein-3-reactive CD4+ T cells and subsequent production of pathogenic autoantibodies can be understood in vivo. This model demonstrates that the postulated immunodominant desmoglein-3 epitopes (which have already been identified in pemphigus vulgaris patients) are capable of inducing a specific autoantibody response.

Autoantibody profile and clinical appearance

The mucosal and mucocutaneous forms of pemphigus vulgaris are characterized by different autoantibody profiles. After lesions appear on the skin, there is nearly always simultaneous detection of IgG autoantibodies to desmoglein 1 and 3, two structurally similar desmosomal components. In pemphigus foliaceus, which is limited to the skin, antibodies are directed only at desmoglein 1 (Amagai et al., 1999).

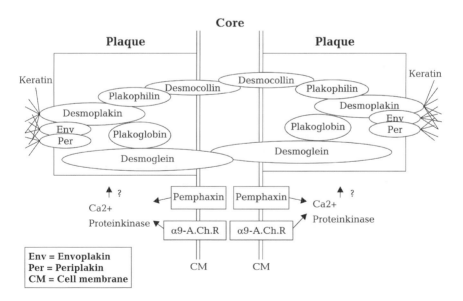

Fig. 1. Autoantigens of pemphigus. Schematic illustration of a desmosome, an adhesion complex between two epidermal keratinocytes with extra-cellular (nucleus) and intracellular (plaque) autoantigens in pemphigus.

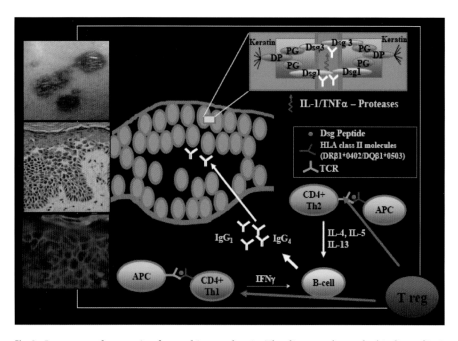

Fig. 2. Immunopathogenesis of pemphigus vulgaris. The diagram shows the binding of IgG autoantibodies to desmosomal adhesion molecules (desmogleins) in the epidermis; this causes loss of adhesion with subsequent blistering. The induction of autoantibody production by B cells is dependent on autoreactive desmoglein-specific CD4+ helper T cells, which recognize immunodominant regions (epitopes) of desmoglein. Regulatory, interleukin-10-secreting T cells (Treg) suppress the activation of autoreactive CD4+ T cells in vitro, either directly or indirectly via B cells and / or antigen-presenting cells (APC). Dsg: desmoglein; HLA: human leukocyte antigen;TH1 / TH2: CD4+ helper T cells, type 1 or 2; TCR: T-cell receptor.

A theory referred to as the "compensation theory" attempts to explain why pemphigus vulgaris and pemphigus foliaceus have differing clinical appearances based on the differences in expression of desmoglein 1 and 3 in the skin and mucous membranes (Mahoney et al., 1999) (Fig. 1). The mucous membranes consist of non-keratinized, stratified epithelium with relatively homogeneous expression of desmoglein 3 with only minimal expression of desmoglein 1. In the skin desmoglein 1 occurs mainly in the subcorneal epidermis, and less often in the suprabasal epidermis, while desmoglein 3 is expressed mainly in the basal and suprabasal layers. Thus, antibodies to desmoglein 3 in pemphigus vulgaris mainly cause suprabasal loss of adhesion of the non-keratinized mucosal epithelium. In pemphigus foliaceus, antibodies to desmoglein 1 cause a superficial, subcorneal blistering of the skin but not the mucous membranes (Fig. 1).

In addition, patients with pemphigus vulgaris occasionally have autoantibodies to other desmosomal adhesion molecules, e. g., to desmocollins (Fig. 2) (Hisamatsu et al., 2004). It is possible that in a significant portion of pemphigus patients serum testing would show

IgG reactivity with cholinergic receptors of epidermal keratinocytes; two acetylcholine receptors have been described as potential autoantigens in pemphigus: pemphaxin, an annexin homologue which binds acetylcholine, and alpha 9 acetylcholine receptor (Nguyen et al., 2000). The role of these autoantibodies in the pathogenesis of pemphigus vulgaris remains unclear.

The precise mechanism of loss of adhesion after binding of desmoglein-specific antibodies has not been completely elucidated (Amagai et al., 2006). In vitro tests show that binding of pemphigus antibodies to epidermal keratinocytes leads to rapid but transitory influx of Ca^2+ ions which probably disrupts signal transduction of the adhesion molecules. There may also be local activation of proteases such as plasminogen activator and phospholipase C, possibly leading to proteolytic cleavage of the extracellular portion of the desmoglein. In vitro and in vivo studies have shown that after pemphigus antibodies bind to epidermal keratinocytes, there is secretion of tumor necrosis factor alpha (TNF-α and interleukin 1. TNF-α seems to be involved in the pathogenesis of acantholysis, given that passive transfer of IgG antibodies from serum taken from mice with pemphigus who did not have TNF receptors less often leads to blistering than in normal control mice (Feliciani et al., 2000).

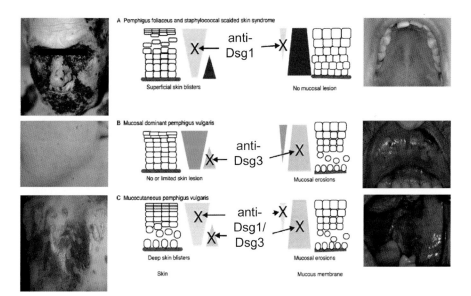

Fig. 3. Compensation theory of pemphigus. The effect of IgG antibodies to desmoglein 1 and 3 on epidermal adhesion is shown in the mucous membranes and skin (modified after Amagai, 2003). The isoforms of desmoglein, desmoglein 1 and 3, are expressed in different amounts in the basal and apical layers of the cutaneous and mucosal epidermis. Functionally, there may be desmoglein compensation that has not been inactivated by autoantibody binding. The clinical manifestation (pemphigus foliaceus, or cutaneous or mucocutaneous variants of pemphigus vulgaris) correlates with the autoantibody profile.

Table 1. Clinical classification of pemphigus

1.	**Pemphigus vulgaris**
1.1.	Pemphigus vegetans
1.1.1.	Type Neumann
1.1.2.	Type Hallopeau
1.2.	Pemphigus herpetiformis
2.	**Pemphigus foliaceus**
2.1.	Endemic forms (f.e. Fogo selvagem)
2.2.	Pemphigus erythematosus (Senear Usher)
2.3.	Pemphigus seborrhoicus
3.	**Paraneoplastic Pemphigus**
4.	**drug-induced Pemphigus**
5.	**IgA Pemphigus**
5.1.	Subcorneal pustular dermatosis type
5.2.	Intraepidermal neutrophilic dermatosis type

Clinical presentation

The different pemphigus variants may be distinguished based on their respective clinical features, the site of intra-epidermal blistering, and their characteristic antibody profiles (Tab. 1). Pemphigus vulgaris is the most common pemphigus variant with an incidence of 0.1 to 0.2 per 100 000; the prevalence is much higher among people of Jewish descent.

In about 80% of patients, pemphigus vulgaris initially presents with flaccid blisters or erosions on the mucous membranes, especially on the oral mucosa (Fig. 4). When there is involvement of the skin, fragile blisters are not always seen. Erosions are typically painful and have a shiny or crusty appearance. Nikolsky's signs I and II are positive in pemphigus vulgaris and can aid clinical diagnosis (Fig. 5, 6). Under tangential pressure to the apparently normal skin surrounding the lesion, the epidermis can be separated from the dermis (Nikolsky's sign I), while intact blisters may be pushed sideways (Nikolsky's sign II). Not only the oral mucosa, but also the nasal mucosa, the larynx, the pharynx, the anal and genital mucosa, and rarely the conjunctivae may also be affected (Fig. 4). A study by Hale and Bystryn reported that symptoms affecting the larynx or nasal mucosa were common complaints in patients with pemphigus vulgaris (Hale and Bystryn, 2001). Out of a total of 53 pemphigus vulgaris patients included in the study, 26 (49%) reported either laryngeal and/or nasal symptoms. Patients described pain in the pharynx, oropharyngeal dysphagia, and hoarseness or hemorrhagic crusts on the nasal mucosa, blood-tinged mucous, and nasal obstruction (Hale and Bystryn, 2001). A current study by Calka et al. (2006) points to the importance of a thorough gastrointestinal examination. In 12 out of

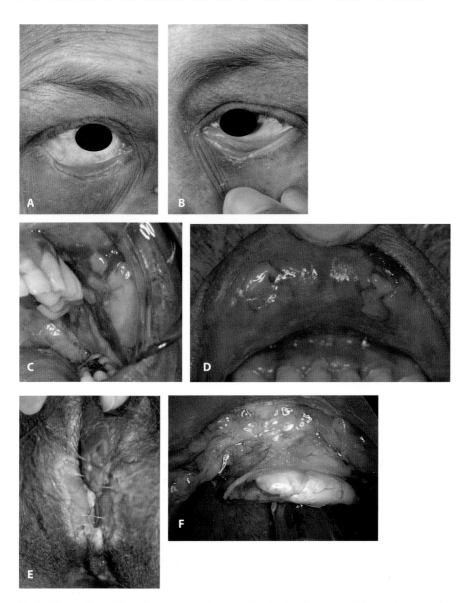

Fig. 4. Mucosal manifestations in pemphigus vulgaris. Involvement of the conjunctivae (a, b), buccal mucosa (c), upper lip (d), vulva (e), and larynx (f)

26 pemphigus vulgaris patients, endoscopic examination revealed erosive substance defects in the middle and distal thirds of the esophagus. Biopsies taken from the lesions show changes characteristic of pemphigus vulgaris on histology and under direct immunofluorescence (Calka et al., 2006). In addition, seven of the 12 patients had gastritis and

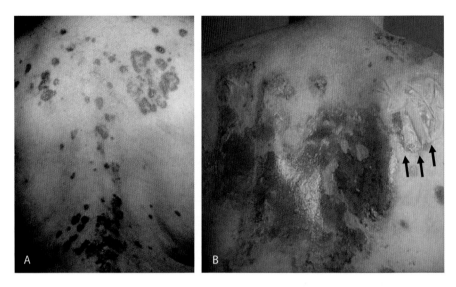

Fig. 5. Cutaneous manifestation in pemphigus vulgaris. Exanthematous appearance of flaccid blisters on the back (a) with subsequent development of large erosions (positive for Nikolsky's I sign) on clinically normal appearing skin (b, right shoulder)

one patient had duodenitis. In an Israeli study with 64 pemphigus patients, 14 (22%) had nail changes involving the fingernails, with clinical symptoms including paronychia, onycholysis, onychomadesis, dyschromasia, and subungual hemorrhage (Schlesinger et al., 2002). In general, nail involvement is rarely reported in pemphigus vulgaris. Before the advent of systemic immunosuppressant therapies, the mortality rate in pemphigus vulgaris was nearly 100% due to complications arising from the progressive skin and mucosal blistering and thus related dietary insufficiencies, secondary infections, protein loss, and increased catabolism.

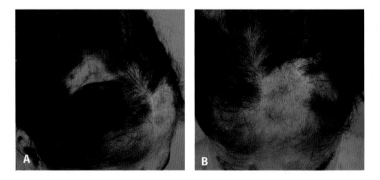

Fig. 6. Manifestation of pemphigus vulgaris on the skin and scalp. Crusty erosions and non-scarring alopecia on the scalp (a, b)

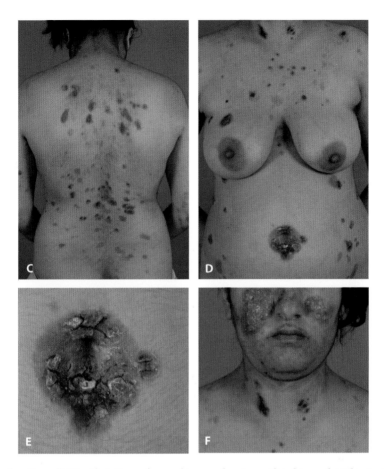

Fig. 6. (continued) **Manifestation of pemphigus vulgaris on the skin and scalp.** In sebor-rheic areas flaccid blisters (c, d) with centrifugal spread (e), extensive, plaque-like erosions on both cheeks (f)

Given that the majority of autoantibodies in pemphigus vulgaris are IgG4 antibodies, which can pass through the placenta, there is a risk the pregnant women with pemphigus vulgaris can pass autoantibodies on to the fetus. The resulting disorder, known as neonatal pemphigus, manifests clinically on newborn skin as exanthematous, crust-covered erosions that can persist for a few weeks (due to the half-life of maternal autoantibodies). Pemphigus vegetans is a variant of pemphigus vulgaris that occurs on intertriginous areas such as the axillae and the groin region; clinical presentation consists of blisters and secondary pustules that have a tendency to form verruciform or papillomatous vegetations (Fig. 7) (Ahmed and Blose, 1984). Mucosal involvement is relatively common, similar to pemphigus vulgaris. Neumann type is characteristically more aggressive than Hallopeau type disease. As in pemphigus vulgaris, both variants of pemphigus vegetans involve autoantibody activity against desmoglein 3 and desmoglein 1 (Tab. 2). Pemphigus herpe-

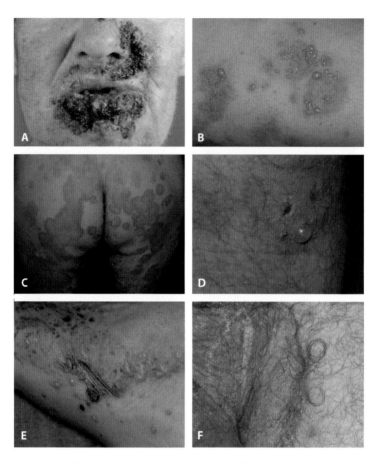

Fig. 7. Unusual manifestations of pemphigus vulgaris. Herpes simplex superinfection affecting the middle of the face in pemphigus vulgaris (a), pemphigus herpetiformis (b), eosinophilic spongiosis (c) with secondary blistering in pemphigus vulgaris (d), "Dyshidrosis" on the right plantar surface in pemphigus vulgaris (e), inguinal pemphigus vegetans (f)

Table 2. Autoantigens of pemphigus vulgaris

Pemphigus variant	Autoantigen	Characteristics*	Autoantibody isotype
Pemphigus vulgaris	**Desmoglein 3**	Initially (pathogen)	IgG
	Desmoglein 1	Common during disease development with the outcome of cutaneous involvement (pathogen)	IgG
	Acetylcholine receptor	Pathogenicity unclear	IgG
IgA Pemphigus	**Desmoglein 1**	Characteristic (IEN type)	IgA
	Desmoglein 3	Occasional (IEN type)	IgA
	Desmocollin 1-3	Characteristic (SPD type)	IgA

Table 2. (continued) Autoantigens of pemphigus vulgaris

Pemphigus variant	Autoantigen	Characteristics*	Autoantibody isotype
Pemphigus foliaceus	Desmoglein 1	Initially (pathogenic)	IgG
	Plakins	Rare (pathogenicity unclear)	IgG
Paraneoplastic Pemphigus	Desmoglein 3	Common (pathogenic)	IgG, IgA
	Desmoglein 1	Rare	IgG
	Plakins	(pathogenicity unclear)	IgG, IgA
	170 kD protein	Common (pathogenicity unclear)	IgG
	Desmocollin 1-3	Hallmark! (pathogenicity unclear) Rare (pathogenic in vitro)	
Drug-induced Pemphigus	Desmoglein 1	Common (pathogenicity unclear)	IgG
	Desmoglein 3	Less common (Pathogenicity unclear)	IgG
IgA Pemphigus	Desmoglein 1	Characteristic (IEN type)	IgA
	Desmoglein 3	Occasional (IEN type)	IgA
	Desmocollin 1-3	Characteristic (SPD type)	IgA

*IEN, intraepidermal neutrophilic dermatosis; SPD, subkorneale pustulöse Dermatose

tiformis is clinically characterized by herpetiform blisters, resembling dermatitis herpetiformis in appearance. Histological analysis shows eosinophilic spongiosis without marked acantholysis; circulating antibodies to desmoglein 1 and desmoglein 3 may be identified (Tab. 2, Fig. 7) (Ishii et al., 1998).

Differential diagnosis

Table 3 lists important differential diagnoses in pemphigus vulgaris. Along with infectious sources of blistering (e.g., bacterial or viral infection), immunological causes such as erythema exudativum multiforme, erosive lichen ruber of the mucous membranes, and bullous drug eruptions must be ruled out. Examples include bullous impetigo and staphylococcal scalded skin syndrome (SSSS), skin disorders that are caused directly by *Staphylococci* or indirectly by hematogenous spread of exotoxins. Stanley and Amagai reported that a staphylogenic exotoxin, as a serine protease, is able to proteolytically cleave the extracellular domains of desmoglein 1 (Stanley and Amagai, 2006). This leads to superficial loss of adhesion in the epidermis, with a clinical appearance resembling that of pemphigus foliaceus. Hereditary bullous skin disorders should also be considered which involve defects in cutaneous adhesion molecules which are also a target structure of circulating autoantibodies in acquired bullous autoimmune skin disorders (Tab. 3). First and foremost, however, differential diagnosis should rule out other pemphigus disorders.

Table 3. Differential Diagnosis of Pemphigus

	Disorder	Characteristics*
Epidermolysis bullosa	Epidermolysis bullosa simplex	Occurence at birth or early childhood; phenotype depends on mutated adhesion molecule; DIF and IIF negative
Autoimmune bullous disorders	Pemphigoid	DIF and IIF frequently positive (BMZ)
	Linear IgA bullous dermatosis	DIF and IIF frequently positive (BMZ)
	Epidermolysis bullosa acquisita	DIF and IIF frequently positive (BMZ)
	Dermatitis herpetiformis Duhring	DIF and IIF frequently positive (IgA)
Infectious diseases	Impetigo contagiosa	Microbiology, serological markers of inflammation; DIF and IIF negative
	Staphylococcal Scalded Skin Syndrome	Mainly limited epidermolysis, histopathology; DIF and IIF negative
	Herpes simplex Infection	Herpes simplex virus in blister fluid; DIF and IIF negative
	Varicella Zoster Infection	Clinics, general symptoms; DIF and IIF negative
Immunologic diseases	Bullous systemic lupus erythematosus	DIF and IIF positive (anti-collagen VII IgG), ANA positive; additional SLE criteria
	Erosive lichen planus	DIF: subepidermal *Cytoid bodies*, IIF negative; cutaneous involvement
	Erythema multiforme (EM)	History: DIF and IIF occasionally positive (majus form): ICS staining pattern (anti desmoplakin IgG)
	Bullous drug reaction (SJS, TEN)	EM-like phenotype or diffuse epidermolysis, histology; DIF and IIF negative
	Subcorneal pustular dermatosis (Sneddon Wilkinson disease)	Leukocytosis, serologic markers of inflammation, DIF and IIF negative
Other diseases	Porphyria cutanea tarda	Porphyrins in serum and urine; DIF and IIF negative; UV-exposed skin
	Bullosis diabeticorum	Serum/ urine glucose, DIF and IIF negative
	Traumatic/toxic blisters	History, DIF and IIF negative

*   ANA: antinuclear antibodies, BMZ: basement membrane zone; DIF: direct immunofluorescence microscopy; EM: erythema multiforme; ICS: intercellular staining pattern; IIF: indirect immunofluorescence microscopy; SJS: Stevens Johnson syndrome; SLE: systemic lupus erythematosus; TEN: toxic epidermal necrolysis.

Pemphigus foliaceus

Pemphigus foliaceus mainly occurs on seborrheic areas of the body (face, scalp, and the area between the shoulder blades) (Fig. 8, 9), affecting the skin only, with painful, crust-covered erosions. In chronic disease, the erosions may spread, covering large areas and contributing via secondary pyoderma and catabolic metabolism to the morbidity and mortality associated with the disease. Clues to diagnosis include IgG antibodies to desmoglein 1. In rare cases there are also autoantibodies to intracellular, desmosomal plaque proteins (see Tab. 2). In endemic variants in Brazil, Tunisia, and other regions in northern Africa, patients also have IgG autoantibodies to desmoglein 1 (Warren et al., 2000).

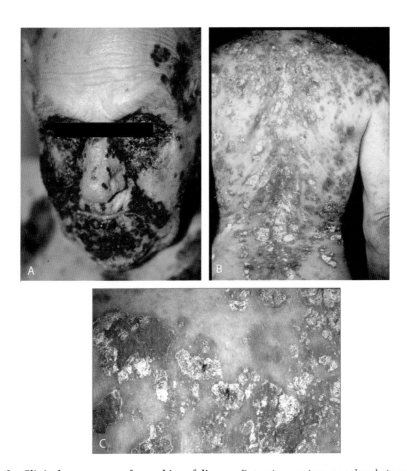

Fig. 8. Clinical appearance of pemphigus foliaceus. Extensive erosions on seborrheic areas of the face (a), leaf-like (Lat. folium: leaf) flaky crusts on seborrheic areas of the back (b), Close-up of the scaly crust–covered erosions (c)

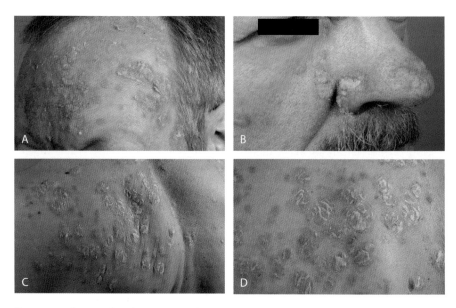

Fig. 9. Pemphigus seborrhoicus. Pemphigus seborrhoicus is a special form of pemphigus foliaceus; superficial, crusty erosions presenting as seborrheic eczema (a, b), on the shoulder blades of the same patient one sees scaly, partly erosive erythematous papules and plaques (c, d)

A rare clinical variant of pemphigus foliaceus is pemphigus erythematosus (Senear-Usher syndrome). The superficial erosions and accompanying erythema and hyperkeratosis mainly affect the trunk and sun-exposed areas of the skin, sometimes resembling cutaneous lupus erythematosus (Gomi et al., 1999; Senear and Usher, 1926). Antibodies to desmoglein 1 and possibly other desmosomal antigens may be identified; often there are also antinuclear antibodies (Gomi et al., 1999).

Pemphigus seborrheicus is a very superficial variant of pemphigus foliaceus with extensive erythematous plaques and erosions on seborrheic areas (Fig. 9).

Paraneoplastic pemphigus

Paraneoplastic pemphigus (PNP) is usually characterized by painful, extensive mucosal erosions and lichenoid papules on the palms of the hands and soles of the feet (Fig. 10). The clinical appearance, usually polymorphous with flaccid or taut blisters on the upper trunk or with multiforme-like, extensive erythema with epidermolysis, can sometimes resemble toxic-epidermal necrolysis (Lyell syndrome). This relatively rare disease is often as-

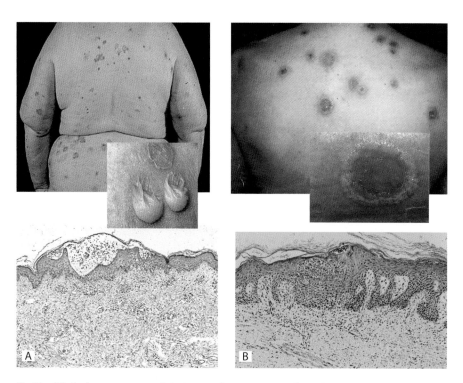

Fig. 10. Clinical appearance of IgA pemphigus. Intraepidermal, neutrophilic dermatosis with flaccid pustules covering the entire trunk (a), subcorneal pustulosis with an anular arrangement of erythematous plaques on the back (b) with corresponding histopathological correlates

sociated with B-cell lymphoma or other malignant hematological disorders and may precede clinical manifestation of cancer. PNP may also be associated with benign tumors, e. g., thymomas or Castleman disease (a benign angioproliferative lymph node hyperplasia that usually begins retroperitoneally). Unlike other pemphigus disorders, loss of adhesion of the lung epithelium can also occur (obliterating bronchiolitis); on endobronchial biopsy typical intraepidermal acantholysis of the bronchial epithelium is seen. This complication is fatal in 30% of patients due to intrapulmonary hemorrhage. PNP is primarily associated with antibodies against multiple proteins in the plakin family such as desmosomal plaque proteins desmoplakin I, II, envoplakin, periplakin and against hemidesmosomal adhesion molecules such as plektin and BP230 or against other, unidentified autoantigens (Amagai et al., 1998; Anhalt et al., 1990; Hashimoto et al., 1995; Kazerounian et al., 2000). IgG antibodies to a 170 kD antigen which was recently been identified as the protease inhibitor alpha-2 macro-globuline-like-1 (Schepens et al, 2010) have a high diagnostic value in confirming clinical diagnosis. IgG antibodies to desmoglein 3 and 1 are identified in the majority of patients with PNP and presumably also play a role the pathogenesis of disease (Amagai et al., 1998) (see Tab. 2).

3

Drug-induced pemphigus

Drug-induced pemphigus is normally caused or triggered by drugs that contain thiol or sulfur groups (which are then metabolized to thiols). These include D-penicillamine, captopril, propranolol, indomethacin, phenylbutazone, pyridinol, pyroxicam, and antitubercular drugs (Korman et al., 1991). Clinical appearances usually correspond to pemphigus foliaceus. In rare instances erosions on the oral mucosa may also occur as seen in pemphigus vulgaris. Antibodies are usually identified against desmoglein 1 and less often against desmoglein 3 (see Tab. 2).

IgA pemphigus

IgA pemphigus is characterized clinically by pustules that have a tendency to coalesce, forming anular lesions that are more strongly pronounced at the periphery (Fig. 11). Mucosal involvement is rare. IgA pemphigus is also associated with benign and malignant monoclonal IgA gammopathies and gastrointestinal disorders. Direct immunofluorescence studies show intercellular IgA deposits in the epidermis, but no IgG deposits. In-

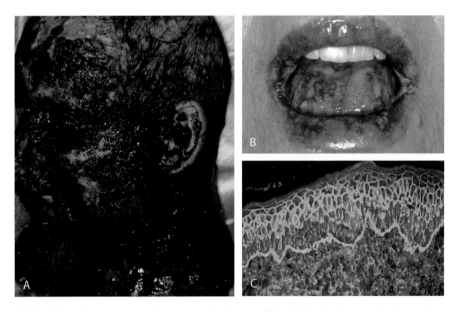

Fig. 11. Clinical appearance of paraneoplastic pemphigus. Massive, hemorrhagic erosions on the skin of the face (a), erosive stomatitis with fibrin coating (b), IgG and / or IgA deposits intercellularly in the epidermis and at the dermoepidermal junction zone (c)

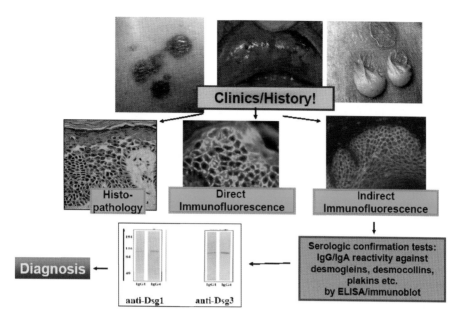

Fig. 12. Algorithm for diagnosing pemphigus. Beginning with clinical appearance, in addition to guiding histology, direct and indirect immunofluorescence studies also play a key role in diagnosis; immunoserological testing can be used to confirm the diagnosis or for preliminary diagnosis of disease course

direct immunofluorescence studies show circulating IgA antibodies in about 50% of patients. There are two immunopathological sub-forms: intraepidermal neutrophilic disease which is generally associated with IgA antibodies to desmoglein 1 or 3 (Fig. 11) and the subcorneal pustular sub-type which is associated with IgA antibodies to desmocollin 1 (Hashimoto et al., 1997; Karpati et al., 2000;Yasuda et al., 2000) (Fig. 11, see Tab. 2). Clinically, both variants are characterized by fragile blisters or pustules on an erythematous, scaly background.

Diagnosis

Diagnosis of pemphigus vulgaris is based on clinical presentation, histology, and direct and indirect immunofluorescence (Fig. 12). It is advisable to select recent, intact blisters for performing a biopsy, ensuring that surrounding perilesional tissue is also included. The tissue is fixed in formalin for histological analysis, while for immunofluorescence the plain specimen is frozen (e.g., in liquid nitrogen (N2)) or placed in Michel's medium (Morrison, 2001).

Histological analysis

Histological analysis of lesional skin serves as only a rough guide in diagnosing pemphigus because it does not always enable classification of specific variants. The primary function of histology is to identify the level at which blistering is taking place and thus to classify the disorder as belonging to the pemphigus group – or distinguish it from subepidermal blistering.

Histologically, pemphigus vulgaris is characterized by intraepidermal loss of keratinocyte adhesion, known as acantholysis. Typically, in the basement membrane zone there are basal keratinocytes attached to the floor of the blister. Occasionally an inflammatory infiltrate is also seen which mainly consists of eosinophils forming clusters of infiltrates in the epidermis. This is referred to as eosinophilic spongiosis.

While suprabasal blistering is typical of pemphigus vulgaris, in pemphigus foliaceus blistering is more superficial, with subcorneal blistering (Fig. 13). Characteristic histopathological changes in PNP are interface dermatitis with vacuolization of the basal cells and lichenoid infiltrate at the junction zone. There is also keratinocyte necrosis with mild acantholysis. Both clinical variants of IgA pemphigus have subcorneal or intraepidermal neutrophil infiltrates, but classic signs of acantholysis are generally absent.

Direct and indirect immunofluorescence studies

In all pemphigus disorders, direct immunofluorescence studies of perilesional skin show an intercellular, reticular (desmosomal) pattern of fluorescence of tissue-bound IgG autoantibodies (or IgA in IgA pemphigus) in the epidermis. There may also be ipsi loco deposits of complement factor. In PNP there are also band-like IgG (and C3) deposits at the dermoepidermal junction zone. Indirect immunofluorescence studies may be used to identify circulating autoantibodies in patient serum. In routine diagnostic testing, monkey esophagus is often used as a tissue substrate. Typically, there is a reticular pattern of intercellular reactivity of IgG antibodies with epithelial or epidermal cells (Fig. 13). Sera from patients with PNP have a typical intercellular staining pattern not only with the above-named substrates, but also in plakin-rich substrates such as guinea pig esophagus and rat or epithelium from monkey bladder (Fig. 13); normal pemphigus sera generally do not react to the latter substrate.

Immunoserological diagnosis with autoantigens

The availability of extracts from the epidermis or cultured keratinocytes as well as recombinant epidermal and dermal adhesion and structural proteins has considerably improved the sensitivity and specificity of diagnosis. In addition, serological diagnosis of pemphi-

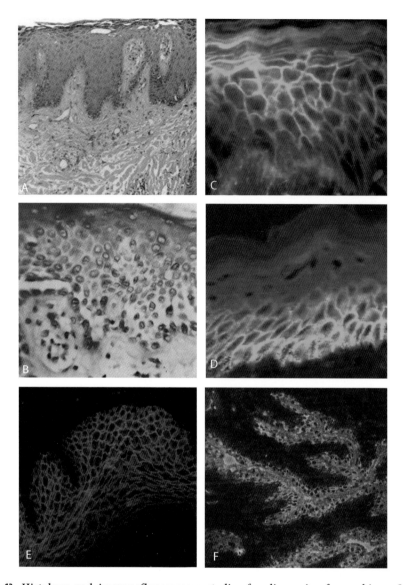

Fig. 13. Histology and immunofluorescence studies for diagnosis of pemphigus. Sub-corneal blistering (a) with IgG precipitates ipsi loco (b) in pemphigus foliaceus; suprabasal loss of adhesion with acantholysis (c) and detection of IgG precipitates ipsi loco (d) in pemphigus vulgaris; typical reticular fluorescence pattern of pemphigus sera on indirect immunofluorescence studies on monkey esophagus (e), reticular fluorescence pattern of sera using rat bladder epithelium in paraneoplastic pemphigus (f).

gus diseases has been significantly improved by the availability of commercial test systems. ELISA tests (MBL, Japan) are available for detecting autoantibodies to desmoglein 1 and 3. Generally speaking, autoantibody titers correlate with the clinical activity of pemphigus (Amagai et al., 2000). Immunoblot studies with recombinant desmoglein 3 have shown that in active disease IgG4 autoantibodies dominate, while IgG1 and IgG4 antibodies are detectable in chronic disease in equal amounts (Spaeth et al., 2001). With keratinocyte extracts, the sera from patients with PNP demonstrate typical IgG reactivity on immunoprecipitation with a complex of proteins containing various plakins (e.g., envoplakin, periplakin, desmoplakin 1/2), bullous pemphigoid antigen, BPAG 1 or BP230, desmogleins and a 170 kD protein (Amagai et al., 1998; Anhalt et al., 1990; Hashimoto et al., 1995; Kazerounian et al., 2000). This test is only available at specialized laboratories.

Parameters for assessment of clinical course

As yet there are no universally agreed-upon parameters for evaluating the clinical course of pemphigus. There have been various initiatives to define treatment targets more clearly, as partial and complete clinical remission, relapse, etc. (Murrell et al., 2008). There are currently two international projects underway to define the degree of mucosal and skin involvement using quantitative and qualitative parameters. One is the Autoimmune Bullous Skin Disorder Score (ABSIS) (Pfutze et al., 2007) which assesses the percentage of skin and mucosal involvement as well as qualitative changes in lesional skin. The acuteness and extent of skin lesions are weighted (Fig. 14). For example: blisters or acute oozing erosions would be weighted by a factor of 1.5, signs of initial re-epithelization by a factor of 1, and re-epithelization by a factor of 0.5 (Fig. 14). In addition to counting the number of mucosal lesions affecting specifically defined areas of the oral cavity, the ABSIS score also includes subjective impairment experienced by the patient, especially as it affects eating and drinking. The Pemphigus Disease Area Intensity Score (PDAI), developed by a working group in the United States, examines skin and mucosal changes as well as residual post-inflammatory lesions. Prospective studies are currently underway to compare the value of this score with the ABSIS score (Rosenbach et al., 2009). Increasingly, quality of life parameters are being included when evaluating the treatment response (Mayrshofer et al., 2005).

Therapy

The advent of systemic immunosuppressants has significantly improved the prognosis for patients with pemphigus vulgaris and other bullous autoimmune skin disorders. The goal of therapy is to achieve complete remission irrespective of whether the lesions are restricted to the mucosa or whether there is mucocutaneous involvement. Administration of high-dose systemic corticosteroids, initially in combination with other immunosuppressants, has been shown over the years to more quickly reduce the necessary dose and duration of systemic steroid use (Bystryn and Steinman, 1996; Hofmann et al., 2009; Martin et al., 2009). Prednisolone and methylprednisolone are the most frequently used sys-

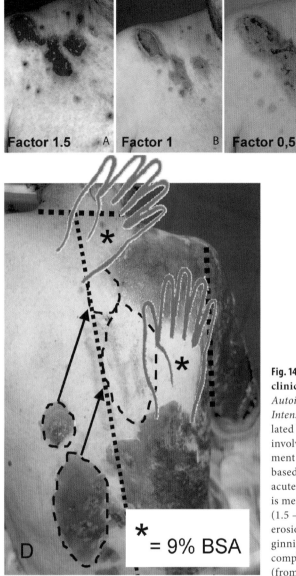

Fig. 14. Parameters for evaluating clinical course of pemphigus. The *Autoimmune Bullous Skin Disorder Intensity Score* (ABSIS) is calculated based on the extent of skin involvement (percentage involvement of the body surface area based on the "rule of nines") and acuteness of the skin lesions which is measured with a weighted score (1.5 – acute blisters and/or oozing erosions (a); 1 – dry erosions/beginning re-epithelization (b); 0.5 – complete re-epithelization (c)) (from Pfütze et al., 2007).

temic corticosteroids. In terms of potency, methylprednisolone is thought to be about 20% more potent than prednisolone. The notion of "dose-equivalence" should nevertheless not be taken at face value given that there are significant clinically relevant differences in the pharmacokinetics and pharmacodynamics between the two substances (Barth et al., 1994). For instance, it is much easier to control and predict the therapeutic effects of methylprednisolone (Barth et al., 1994). If therapy is absolutely imperative during the first trimester of pregnancy, animal studies have shown that the teratogenic potential associated with methylprednisolone is lower (Pfeiffer, 2001). In German-speaking countries, the most commonly used adjuvant immunosuppressants are azathioprine and mycophenolate mofetil, along with chlorambucil, cyclophosphamide, methotrexate, and cyclosporine A (Hofmann et al., 2009; Martin et al., 2009) (Tab. 4). Clinical experience regarding their effectiveness is discussed briefly in the following.

Table 4. Treatment of pemphigus

Drug	PV[§]	PF[§]	PNP[§]	IgA-P[§]	Evidence Level[#]	Dose[*]	Most common side effects[+]
Systemic glucocorticoids (Prednisolone)	+	+	+	(+)	I	Initially 1–2 mg/kg/d p.o.	Ulcus ventriculi et duodeni, diabetes mellitus, hypertension, osteoporosis, aseptic bone necrosis, opportunistic infections, Cushing's syndrome, glaucoma, cataract
Azathioprine	+	+	(+)	(+)	I	1–2.5 mg/kg/d p.o.	Caveat: Thiopurine methyl transferase activity! pancytopenia, hepatopathy, nephropathy, nausea
Mycophenolate Mofetil	+	+	+	(+)	I	1–3 g/d p.o.	pancytopenia, hepatopathy, nausea, gastrointestinal symptoms
Cyclophosphamide	+	+	+	(+)	I-II	100–200 mg/d p.o. or i.v.-Pulse Therapy (750 mg/m² BSA)	Pancytopenia, hemorrhagic cystitis, hepatopathy, stomatitis, nausea, alopecia, infertility, increased incidence of cancer; teratogenicity
Chlorambucil	+	+	+	–	IV	0.1–0.2 mg/kg/d p.o.	Pancytopenia, seizures, neuropathy, hepatopathy, exanthems, infertility, diarrhea
Methotrexate	+	+	–	–	IV	10–20 mg/Woche p.o. oder s.c.	Pancytopenia, hepatopathy, stomatitis, nephropathy, nausea, infertility, alopecia, teratogenicity
Ciclosporin A	(+)	(+)	–	–	I-II	2.5–5 mg/kg/d p.o.	hypertension, nephrotoxicity; increased incidence of cancer

Table 4. (continued) Treatment of pemphigus

Drug	PV[§]	PF[§]	PNP[§]	IgA-P[§]	Evidence Level[#]	Dose*	Most common side effects[+]
Diaminodi-phenyl Sulfone (DADPS)	+	+	–	+	I,IV	1–2 mg/kg/d p.o.	Caveat: Glucose-6-phosphate acitivity, methemoglobinemia, hemolytic anemia, agranulocytosis, hepatopathy
Retinoids (Acit-retin)	–	–	–	+	IV	Initial: 0.5–1.0 mg/kg/d p.o.; Maintenance dose: 0.5 mg/kg/d p.o.	Exfoliative dermatitis; alopecia, hyperlipi-demia, teratogenic-ity!, no concomitant treatment with methotrexate or tetra-cyclines
Immunoad-sorption	+	+	(+)	–	III-IV	3–4×/Week in 3–4 week intervals	Anaphylactic reac-tions, hypogamma-globulinemia
Intravenous Immunglobulin (IVIG)	+	+	(+)	(+)	I-II	2 g/kg/month i.v. (cycle)	Caveat: selective IgA deficiency, anaphylax-ia, nephropathy, head ache, nausea, fever
Rituximab (anti CD20)	+	+	+	+	III-IV	2 × 1 g i.v. (days 1 and 15) or 375 mg/m² BSA (days 1,8,15,22)	Anaphylaxia, severe infections, cardiac insufficiency, rarely: progressive multifocal leukencephalopathy (PML)

§   PV, Pemphigus vulgaris; PF, Pemphigus foliaceus, PNP, paraneoplastic Pemphigus; IgA-P, IgA-Pemphigus.

$ +, effective; (+) questionable efficacy fraglich wirksam, – not effective, data missing

Evidence levels relate to clinical trials in Pemphigus vulgaris or pemphigus foliaceus: I – prospective, randomized study, II – non-randomized, case-control study, III – case series or descriptive case reports, IV – single case reports/expert opinions

*   Initial treatment dose

+   Most relevant side effects

Given that there are only few controlled, prospective studies on the efficacy of specific immunosuppressants and immunomodulators in the treatment of bullous autoimmune skin disorders, the efficacy profiles of the drugs in this review are mostly based on ob-servational studies with smaller numbers of patients. These have been published in a cur-rent Cochrane meta-analysis (Martin et al., 2009). In addition, three new treatment procedures are proposed and discussed for treatment-refractory pemphigus: immunoadsorption, high-dose immunoglobulin therapy, and the anti-CD20 antibody, rituximab.

In pemphigus vulgaris, high-dose (1–2 mg/kg/day of prednisolone equivalent) systemic corticosteroids are initially given, and, depending on clinical response are then tapered over the course of several months based on a logarithm. Adverse effects, such as arterial hypertension, diabetes mellitus, osteoporosis, increased susceptibility to infection, gastrointestinal ulcers, and aseptic bone necrosis, continue to cause significant morbidity and mortality in pemphigus vulgaris and appropriate accompanying preventive therapies must be given (Bystryn and Steinman, 1996) (Tab. 4). Lever et al. have used intermittent pulse therapy (500–1000 mg methylprednisolone or 200 mg dexamethasone), which is given, e. g., in monthly cycles. A working group in India reported positive results with five years of corticosteroid pulse therapy (Pasricha et al., 1988).

Before initiating immunosuppressant therapy, florid / chronic infections (e. g., Tbc, HIV, hepatitis B / C) and cancer must be excluded. Women of childbearing age should be advised to use contraception. Before beginning alkylating agents (cyclophosphamide, chlorambucil), patients must be informed about the mutagenic and carcinogenic effects of these cytotoxic immunosuppressants and their suppression of spermiogenesis and oogenesis.

Azathioprine has been used for years and is considered the immunosuppressant therapy of choice (Aberer et al., 1987; Martin et al., 2009) (Tab. 4). Combining systemic corticosteroids with azathioprine allows the cumulative steroid dose to be significantly reduced. The lag time of two to three months until the immunosuppressant effect takes place must be taken into consideration. A prospective, randomized multicenter study has shown that azathioprine has a steroid-sparing effect and achieves clinical remission more quickly than corticosteroid monotherapy (Chams-Davatchi et al., 2007). Before beginning azathioprine therapy, it is important to assess the activity of thiopurine-S methyltransferase (TPMT) in order to identify lacking or deficient levels of TMPT, as standard dosages could lead to toxic myelosuppression (Deufel et al., 2004). TPMT activity can be measured in erythrocytes (phenotyping) or using mutation analysis (genotyping). Either method can be used alternatively, taking into consideration respective limitations (e. g., for phenotyping, contamination with foreign erythrocytes following blood transfusion must be recalled) (Deufel et al., 2004). Azathioprine should not be given in combination with allopurinol which slows the metabolism of azathioprine causing significantly elevated serum levels of the drug.

Mycophenolate mofetil has a similar efficacy profile to that of azathioprine. In a controlled prospective therapy study on pemphigus vulgaris and pemphigus foliaceus, mycophenolate mofetil 2 g/day in combination with prednisolone had a significant steroid-sparing effect compared with monotherapy with systemic corticosteroids (Mimouni et al., 2003). A prospective multicenter randomized study with 39 pemphigus patients showed that mycophenolate mofetil (2 g/day) and azathioprine (2 mg/kg/day) each in combination with methylprednisolone (initially 2 mg/kg/day) were similar in terms of clinical effectiveness and steroid-sparing effect (Beissert et al., 2006). In this study, there were no significant differences between the two substances in regard to serious (WHO grade 3) or life-threatening (WHO grade 4) side effects (Beissert et al., 2006). Gastrointestinal complaints are the most commonly reported side effect of mycophenolate mofetil therapy. Studies on kidney transplant patients have suggested that gastro-resistant administration of mycophenolic acid in the form of mycophenolate sodium, which leads to delayed release of the drug in the small intestine, can improve gastrointestinal tolerance without compromising immunosuppressive effectiveness (Chan et al., 2006).

Cyclophosphamide has also been used to treat refractory pemphigus, usually administered as pulse therapy (500–750 mg / m2 i. v.) (Ahmed and Hombal, 1987; Bystryn and Steinman, 1996; Martin et al., 2009; Pasricha et al., 1988). In a larger, prospective multicenter study on pemphigus, patients demonstrated a similar efficacy profile to azathioprine and mycophenolate mofetil (Chams-Davatchi et al., 2007). Potential adverse effects are more commonly seen in cyclophosphamide than azathioprine or mycophenolate mofetil, and include nausea, diarrhea, alopecia, bone marrow suppression with pancytopenia, hemorrhagic cystitis, and sterility (Chams-Davatchi et al., 2007) (see Tab. 4). Younger patients in particular must be informed of potential teratogenic and carcinogenic effects. Chlorambucil has been used successfully in severe pemphigus with an initial dose of 0.1 mg / kg / day which is then reduced after six weeks to a total daily dose of 2 mg. Under longer-term chlorambucil use, about 30% of patients have reversible thrombocytopenia. The increased risk of developing a hematological disorder as a result of the cumulative chlorambucil dose has led to decreased used of this immunosuppressant.

In a limited number of pemphigus patients with involvement of the oral mucosa, cyclosporine A has been used for systemic therapy or given as a topical treatment (Martin et al., 2009). However, a single randomized, controlled study with 33 patients reported that there was no advantage of combination therapy with prednisolone (1 mg / kg / day) and cyclosporine A (5 mg / kg / day) over monotherapy with methylprednisolone (initially 1 mg / kg / day) (Ioannides et al., 2000).

Methotrexate has also occasionally been used successfully in pemphigus vulgaris and may be given orally or subcutaneously at a dose of 10–15 mg / per week (Bystryn and Steinman, 1996).

In our experience, diaminodiphenyl sulfone (DADPS) can be used as an effective adjuvant therapy in pemphigus foliaceus and IgA pemphigus. Potentially severe side effects include hemolysis, hepatopathy, and agranulocytosis (see Tab. 4). Before beginning therapy, glucose-6-phosphate dehydrogenase activity should be assessed. A current multicenter randomized, double-blind, placebo-controlled study by Werth et al. has investigated the efficacy of dapsone as a steroid-sparing adjuvant therapy in pemphigus vulgaris (Werth et al., 2008). Nineteen pemphigus vulgaris patients were included whose disease activity could be controlled with systemic corticosteroids and / or other immunosuppressant drugs, but who experienced exacerbations repeatedly after reducing steroids. The target criterion of the study was a reduction to 7.5 mg / day or less (prednisolone equivalent) within one year. Study participants were given dapsone at a dosage of 200 mg / day or placebo as adjuvant therapy along with immunosuppressant therapy. In three out of ten patients in the placebo group therapy was successful while five out of nine of the dapsone patients achieved the primary goal. These results show only a tendency toward a steroid-sparing effect of dapsone, given that the results were not statistically significant, although this may also be a result of the small number of patients included (Werth et al., 2008). In IgA pemphigus, the therapies of choice are DADPS, systemic retinoids (acitretin, etretinate), and psoralen plus UVA (PUVA) (Bystryn and Steinman, 1996) (see Tab. 4).

An important adjuvant immunomodulatory therapy in treatment-refractory pemphigus is high-dose, intravenous immunoglobulin therapy (Amagai et al., 2009; Enk, 2009;

Enk et al., 2003; Jolles, 2001). Given as monotherapy, studies on a limited number of patients have shown that two to four monthly treatment cycles of high-dose immunoglobulins (2 g/kg/month for two to five days) brought about a significant decline in disease activity and an improved response to subsequent immunosuppressant drugs such as rituximab (Ahmed et al., 2006; Enk et al., 2003). Amagai and colleagues also showed in a multicenter, controlled study that one-time administration of i.v. immunoglobulins in steroid-resistant pemphigus was very effective (Amagai et al., 2009).

Additional treatment strategies in difficult cases of pemphigus have targeted rapidly reducing circulating IgG autoantibodies; plasmapheresis has been used successfully, especially in the United States (Bystryn, 1988). Recently, more selective immunoadsorption techniques with protein A or analogous surfaces have been used to target circulating IgG as selectively as possible and thus also remove IgG autoantibodies. Several case studies have reported that the combination of adjuvant immunoadsorption and immunosuppressant therapy is a treatment alternative that can more quickly control the activity of refractory pemphigus (Eming and Hertl, 2006; Zillikens et al., 2007).

Based on a recently published consensus paper written by German-speaking dermatologists, adjuvant immunoadsorption therapy is indicated in pemphigus when
1. there is involvement of more than 30% of body surface area,
2. there is involvement of more than 25% of the oral or genital mucosa,
3. one or both conjunctivae are affected, or
4. there is involvement of the esophageal mucosa (Zillikens et al., 2007).

Treatment is also indicated when there is
1. more than three-months-long, treatment-refractory disease and/or
2. at least one immunosuppressant therapy (systemic corticosteroids in combination with an immunosuppressant agent, e.g., azathioprine or mycophenolate mofetil) has been unsuccessful (Zillikens et al., 2007).

In Germany, a nationwide multicenter therapy study to evaluate the effect of adjuvant immunophoresis in active pemphigus is currently in the planning.

Another important improvement in therapy of pemphigus is rituximab, a monoclonal antibody to the CD20 molecule which is expressed on B cells. There are now two prospective studies and a number of case studies reporting the successful use of rituximab in severe pemphigus (Ahmed et al., 2006; Arin et al., 2005; Joly et al., 2007). Rituximab is given four times in weekly intervals at a dose of $375 \, mg/m^2$ i. v. (oncological protocol) or in two doses of 1 g i.v. given 14 days apart (rheumatologic protocol). Studies report complete and long-term B-cell depletion under therapy which was maintained for six to twelve months in peripheral blood.

Based on a recently published recommendation by German-speaking dermatologists, the indications for rituximab therapy are analogous to those for adjuvant immunoadsorption (Hertl et al., 2008). Rituximab therapy is also indicated in PNP. The drug should not be given to women who are pregnant or nursing, to patients under 18 years of age, or to those with sensitivity to murine proteins, active hepatitis B/C, HIV infection, or another uncontrollable infection (Hertl et al., 2008) (see Tab. 4). Potential adverse effects related to infusion include fever, chills, headache, urticarial exanthems, and angioedema. Severe bacterial or viral infections can also occur. Isolated reports of progressive, multifocal leukoencephalopathy have also been reported under adjuvant rituximab therapy in systemic lupus erythematosus and vasculitis (Hertl et al., 2008).

In everyday clinical practice an easily overlooked complication in pemphigus are secondary herpes simplex infections of lesional or perilesional skin (see Fig. 7). Clinical symptoms of secondary infection generally occur as disseminated herpetiform blisters or punctate erosions with a punched-out appearance. The possibility of herpes simplex superinfection should also be recalled in sudden clinical "recurrence" of disease affecting the face or intertriginous areas. After confirming diagnosis, e.g., identification under direct immunofluorescence of herpes simplex virus in a bladder smear, the therapy of choice is systemic acyclovir.

Summary

Autoimmune bullous disorders of the pemphigus group present a major clinical challenge based on their severe clinical course and limited therapeutic options. Making the diagnosis of pemphigus requires histology,direct and indirect immunofluorescence and eventually, serological analyses with recombinant autoantigens. Currently, there is no consensus on generally accepted clinical partameters that help to measure disease activity and clinical responses or relapses. The therapeutic standard of pemphigus consists of a "global" nonspecific immunosuppression with systemic glucocorticoids and immunosuppressive adjuvants causing severe side-effects and comorbidity. Due to the relative rareness of pemphigus, only few evidence-based controlled therapeutic trials have been performed. In light of limited approved immunosuppressive in the treatment of pemphigus, the "off-label-use" of potent immunosuppressive drugs is daily routine. Novel treatments, such as immunadsorption, rituximab and intravenous immunoglobulins bear the potential to induce clinical remissions in refractory pemphigus cases. The use of these drugs in pemphigus is described in recently published therapeutic guidelines

References

Aberer W, Wolff-Schreiner EC, Stingl G, Wolff K (1987) Azathioprine in the treatment of pemphigus vulgaris. A long-term follow-up. J Am Acad Dermatol 16:527–533

Ahmed AR, Blose DA (1984) Pemphigus vegetans. Neumann type and Hallopeau type. Int J Dermatol 23:135–141

Ahmed AR, Hombal S (1987) Use of cyclophosphamide in azathioprine failures in pemphigus. J Am Acad Dermatol 17:437–442

Ahmed AR, Spigelman Z, Cavacini LA, Posner MR (2006) Treatment of pemphigus vulgaris with rituximab and intravenous immune globulin. N Engl J Med 355:1772–1779

Amagai M, Klaus-Kovtun V, Stanley JR (1991) Autoantibodies against a novel epithelial cadherin in pemphigus vulgaris, a disease of cell adhesion. Cell 67:869–877

Amagai M, Nishikawa T, Nousari HC, Anhalt GJ, Hashimoto T (1998) Antibodies against desmoglein 3 (pemphigus vulgaris antigen) are present in sera from patients with paraneoplastic pemphigus and cause acantholysis in vivo in neonatal mice. J Clin Invest 102:775–782

Amagai M, Tsunoda K, Zillikens D, Nagai T, Nishikawa T (1999) The clinical phenotype of pemphigus is defined by the anti-desmoglein autoantibody profile. J Am Acad Dermatol 40:167–170

Amagai M, Tsunoda K, Suzuki H, Nishifuji K, Koyasu S, Nishikawa T (2000) Use of autoantigen-knockout mice in developing an active autoimmune disease model for pemphigus. J Clin Invest 105:625–631

Amagai M, Ahmed AR, Kitajima Y, Bystryn JC, Milner Y, Gniadecki R, Hertl M, Pincelli C, Kurzen H, Fridkis-Hareli M, Aoyama Y, Frusic-Zlotkin M, Muller E, David M, Mimouni D, Vind-Kezunovic D, Michel B, Mahoney M, Grando S (2006) Are desmoglein autoantibodies essential for the immunopathogenesis of pemphigus vulgaris, or just "witnesses of disease"? Exp Dermatol 15:815–831

Amagai M, Ikeda S, Shimizu H, Iizuka H, Hanada K, Aiba S, Kaneko F, Izaki S, Tamaki K, Ikezawa Z, Takigawa M, Seishima M, Tanaka T, Miyachi Y, Katayama I, Horiguchi Y, Miyagawa S, Furukawa F, Iwatsuki K, Hide M, Tokura Y, Furue M, Hashimoto T, Ihn H, Fujiwara S, Nishikawa T, Ogawa H, Kitajima Y, Hashimoto K (2009) A randomized double-blind trial of intravenous immunoglobulin for pemphigus. J Am Acad Dermatol 60:595–603

Anhalt GJ, Kim SC, Stanley JR, Korman NJ, Jabs DA, Kory M, Izumi H, Ratrie H, 3rd, Mutasim D, Ariss-Abdo L, et al. (1990) Paraneoplastic pemphigus. An autoimmune mucocutaneous disease associated with neoplasia. N Engl J Med 323:1729–1735

Anhalt GJ, Labib RS, Voorhees JJ, Beals TF, Diaz LA (1982) Induction of pemphigus in neonatal mice by passive transfer of IgG from patients with the disease. N Engl J Med 306:1189–1196

Arin MJ, Engert A, Krieg T, Hunzelmann N (2005) Anti-CD20 monoclonal antibody (rituximab) in the treatment of pemphigus. Br J Dermatol 153:620–625

Beissert S, Werfel T, Frieling U, Bohm M, Sticherling M, Stadler R, Zillikens D, Rzany B, Hunzelmann N, Meurer M, Gollnick H, Ruzicka T, Pillekamp H, Junghans V, Luger TA (2006) A comparison of oral methylprednisolone plus azathioprine or mycophenolate mofetil for the treatment of pemphigus. Arch Dermatol 142:1447–1454

Bystryn JC (1988) Plasmapheresis therapy of pemphigus. Arch Dermatol 124:1702–1704

Bystryn JC, Steinman NM (1996) The adjuvant therapy of pemphigus. An update. Arch Dermatol 132:203–212

Calka O, Akdeniz N, Tuncer I, Metin A, Cesur RS (2006) Oesophageal involvement during attacks in pemphigus vulgaris patients. Clin Exp Dermatol 31:515–519

Chams-Davatchi C, Esmaili N, Daneshpazhooh M, Valikhani M, Balighi K, Hallaji Z, Barzegari M, Akhyani M, Ghodsi SZ, Seirafi H, Nazemi MJ, Mortazavi H, Mirshams-Shahshahani M (2007) Randomized controlled open-label trial of four treatment regimens for pemphigus vulgaris. J Am Acad Dermatol 57:622–628

Chan L, Mulgaonkar S, Walker R, Arns W, Ambuhl P, Schiavelli R (2006) Patient-reported gastro-intestinal symptom burden and health-related quality of life following conversion from mycophenolate mofetil to enteric-coated mycophenolate sodium. Transplantation 81:1290–1297

Deufel T, Geßner R, Lackner KL, Schwab M, Steimer W, Steiner M, von Ahsen N, M. K (2004) Guidelines fort the laboratory management of thiopurine drug therapy. J Lab Med 28:477–482

Eming R, Hertl M (2006) Immunoadsorption in pemphigus. Autoimmunity 39:609–616

Eming R, Schmidt J, Schwietzke S, Podstawa E, Muller R, Sonderstrup G, Hertl M (2007) HLA class II-restricted autoaggressive T cells shape the autoantibody response against desmoglein 3 (dsg3) in an HLA-transgenic mouse model of pemphigus vulgaris (PV). Exp Dermatol 16:218A

Enk A (2009) Guidelines on the use of high-dose intravenous immunoglobulin in dermatology. Eur J Dermatol 19:90–98

Enk A, Hertl M, Messer G, Meurer M, Rentz E, Zillikens D (2003) [The use of high dose intravenous immunoglobulins in dermatology]. J Dtsch Dermatol Ges 1:183–190

Feliciani C, Toto P, Amerio P, Pour SM, Coscione G, Shivji G, Wang B, Sauder DN (2000) In vitro and in vivo expression of interleukin-1alpha and tumor necrosis factor-alpha mRNA in pemphigus vulgaris: interleukin-1alpha and tumor necrosis factor-alpha are involved in acantholysis. J Invest Dermatol 114:71–77

Gomi H, Kawada A, Amagai M, Matsuo I (1999) Pemphigus erythematosus: detection of anti-desmoglein-1 antibodies by ELISA. Dermatology 199:188–189

Hale EK, Bystryn JC (2001) Laryngeal and nasal involvement in pemphigus vulgaris. J Am Acad Dermatol 44:609–611

Hashimoto T, Amagai M, Watanabe K, Chorzelski TP, Bhogal BS, Black MM, Stevens HP, Boorsma DM, Korman NJ, Gamou S, et al. (1995) Characterization of paraneoplastic pemphigus autoantigens by immunoblot analysis. J Invest Dermatol 104:829–834

Hashimoto T, Kiyokawa C, Mori O, Miyasato M, Chidgey MA, Garrod DR, Kobayashi Y, Komori K, Ishii K, Amagai M, Nishikawa T (1997) Human desmocollin 1 (Dsc1) is an autoantigen for the subcorneal pustular dermatosis type of IgA pemphigus. J Invest Dermatol 109:127–131

Hertl M, Eming R, Veldman C (2006) T cell control in autoimmune bullous skin disorders. J Clin Invest 116:1159–1166

Hertl M, Zillikens D, Borradori L, Bruckner-Tuderman L, Burckhard H, Eming R, Engert A, Goebeler M, Hofmann S, Hunzelmann N, Karlhofer F, Kautz O, Lippert U, Niedermeier A, Nitschke M, Pfutze M, Reiser M, Rose C, Schmidt E, Shimanovich I, Sticherling M, Wolff-Franke S (2008) Recommendations for the use of rituximab (anti-CD20 antibody) in the treatment of autoimmune bullous skin diseases. J Dtsch Dermatol Ges 6:366–373

Hisamatsu Y, Amagai M, Garrod DR, Kanzaki T, Hashimoto T (2004) The detection of IgG and IgA autoantibodies to desmocollins 1-3 by enzyme-linked immunosorbent assays using baculovirus-expressed proteins, in atypical pemphigus but not in typical pemphigus. Br J Dermatol 151:73–83

Hofmann SC, Kautz O, Hertl M, Sticherling M, Zillikens D, Bruckner-Tuderman L (2009) Results of a survey of German dermatologists on the therapeutic approaches to pemphigus and bullous pemphigoid. J Dtsch Dermatol Ges 7:227–233

Ioannides D, Chrysomallis F, Bystryn JC (2000) Ineffectiveness of cyclosporine as an adjuvant to corticosteroids in the treatment of pemphigus. Arch Dermatol 136:868–872

Ishii K, Amagai M, Komai A, Ebharas T, Chorzelski TP, Nishikawa T, Hashimoto T (1998) Desmoglein 1 and desmoglein 3as autoimmune target of herpetiform pemphigus. J Invest Dermatol 110:510A

Ishii K, Harada R, Matsuo I, Shirakata Y, Hashimoto K, Amagai M (2005) In vitro keratinocyte dissociation assay for evaluation of the pathogenicity of anti-desmoglein 3 IgG autoantibodies in pemphigus vulgaris. J Invest Dermatol 124:939–946

Jolles S (2001) A review of high-dose intravenous immunoglobulin (hdIVIg) in the treatment of the autoimmune blistering disorders. Clin Exp Dermatol 26:127–131

Joly P, Mouquet H, Roujeau JC, D'Incan M, Gilbert D, Jacquot S, Gougeon ML, Bedane C, Muller R, Dreno B, Doutre MS, Delaporte E, Pauwels C, Franck N, Caux F, Picard C, Tancrede-Bohin E, Bernard P, Tron F, Hertl M, Musette P (2007) A single cycle of rituximab for the treatment of severe pemphigus. N Engl J Med 357:545–552

Karpati S, Amagai M, Liu WL, Dmochowski M, Hashimoto T, Horvath A (2000) Identification of desmoglein 1 as autoantigen in a patient with intraepidermal neutrophilic IgA dermatosis type of IgA pemphigus. Exp Dermatol 9:224–228

Kawasaki H, Tsunoda K, Hata T, Ishii K, Yamada T, Amagai M (2006) Synergistic pathogenic effects of combined mouse monoclonal anti-desmoglein 3 IgG antibodies on pemphigus vulgaris blister formation. J Invest Dermatol 126:2621–2630

Kazerounian S, Mahoney MG, Uitto J, Aho S (2000) Envoplakin and periplakin, the paraneoplastic pemphigus antigens, are also recognized by pemphigus foliaceus autoantibodies. J Invest Dermatol 115:505–507

Koch PJ, Mahoney MG, Ishikawa H, Pulkkinen L, Uitto J, Shultz L, Murphy GF, Whitaker-Menezes D, Stanley JR (1997) Targeted disruption of the pemphigus vulgaris antigen (desmoglein 3) gene in mice causes loss of keratinocyte cell adhesion with a phenotype similar to pemphigus vulgaris. J Cell Biol 137:1091–1102

Korman NJ, Eyre RW, Zone J, Stanley JR (1991) Drug-induced pemphigus: autoantibodies directed against the pemphigus antigen complexes are present in penicillamine and captopril-induced pemphigus. J Invest Dermatol 96:273–276

Lee E, Lendas KA, Chow S, Pirani Y, Gordon D, Dionisio R, Nguyen D, Spizuoco A, Fotino M, Zhang Y, Sinha AA (2006) Disease relevant HLA class II alleles isolated by genotypic, haplotypic, and sequence analysis in North American Caucasians with pemphigus vulgaris. Hum Immunol 67:125–139

Lever WF (1953) Pemphigus. Medicine. 32(1):1–123

Mahoney MG, Wang Z, Rothenberger K, Koch PJ, Amagai M, Stanley JR (1999) Explanations for the clinical and microscopic localization of lesions in pemphigus foliaceus and vulgaris. J Clin Invest 103:461–468

Martin LK, Werth V, Villanueva E, Segall J, Murrell DF (2009) Interventions for pemphigus vulgaris and pemphigus foliaceus. Cochrane Database Syst Rev:CD006263

Mayrshofer F, Hertl M, Sinkgraven R, Sticherling M, Pfeiffer C, Zillikens D, Messer G, Rzany Fur Die Deutschebsd-Studiengruppe B (2005) [Significant decrease in quality of life in patients with pemphigus vulgaris. Results from the German Bullous Skin Disease (BSD) Study Group]. J Dtsch Dermatol Ges 3:431–435

Mimouni D, Anhalt GJ, Cummins DL, Kouba DJ, Thorne JE, Nousari HC (2003) Treatment of pemphigus vulgaris and pemphigus foliaceus with mycophenolate mofetil. Arch Dermatol 139:739–742

Morrison LH (2001) Direct immunofluorescence microscopy in the diagnosis of autoimmune bullous dermatoses. Clin Dermatol 19:607–613

Murrell DF, Dick S, Ahmed AR, Amagai M, Barnadas MA, Borradori L, Bystryn JC, Cianchini G, Diaz L, Fivenson D, Hall R, Harman KE, Hashimoto T, Hertl M, Hunzelmann N, Iranzo P, Joly P, Jonkman MF, Kitajima Y, Korman NJ, Martin LK, Mimouni D, Pandya AG, Payne AS, Rubenstein D, Shimizu H, Sinha AA, Sirois D, Zillikens D, Werth VP (2008) Consensus statement on definitions of disease, end points, and therapeutic response for pemphigus. J Am Acad Dermatol 58:1043–1046

Nguyen VT, Ndoye A, Shultz LD, Pittelkow MR, Grando SA (2000) Antibodies against keratinocyte antigens other than desmogleins 1 and 3 can induce pemphigus vulgaris-like lesions. J Clin Invest 106:1467–1479

Pasricha JS, Thanzama J, Khan UK (1988) Intermittent high-dose dexamethasone-cyclophosphamide therapy for pemphigus. Br J Dermatol 119:73–77

Pfutze M, Niedermeier A, Hertl M, Eming R (2007) Introducing a novel Autoimmune Bullous Skin Disorder Intensity Score (ABSIS) in pemphigus. Eur J Dermatol 17:4–11

Rosenbach M, Murrell DF, Bystryn JC, Dulay S, Dick S, Fakharzadeh S, Hall R, Korman NJ, Lin J, Okawa J, Pandya AG, Payne AS, Rose M, Rubenstein D, Woodley D, Vittoria C, Werth BB, Williams EA, Taylor L, Troxel AB, Werth VP (2009) Reliability and Convergent Validity of Two Outcome Instruments for Pemphigus. J Invest Dermatol

Schepens I, Jannin F, Begre N, Läderach U, Marcus K, Hashimoto T, Favre B, Borradori L (2010) The protease inhibitor alpha-2-macroglobuline-like-1 is the p170 antigen recognized by paraneoplastic pemphigus autoantibodies in human. PLOS ONE 5(8):1–8

Schlesinger N, Katz M, Ingber A (2002) Nail involvement in pemphigus vulgaris. Br J Dermatol 146:836–839

Senear F, Usher B (1926) An unusual type of pemphigus: combining features of lupus erythematosus. Arch Derm Syphilol 13:761–781

Sitaru C, Zillikens D (2005) Mechanisms of blister induction by autoantibodies. Exp Dermatol 14:861–875

Spaeth S, Riechers R, Borradori L, Zillikens D, Budinger L, Hertl M (2001) IgG, IgA and IgE autoantibodies against the ectodomain of desmoglein 3 in active pemphigus vulgaris. Br J Dermatol 144:1183–1188

Stanley JR, Amagai M (2006) Pemphigus, bullous impetigo, and the staphylococcal scalded-skin syndrome. N Engl J Med 355:1800–1810

Veldman C, Hohne A, Dieckmann D, Schuler G, Hertl M (2004) Type I regulatory T cells specific for desmoglein 3 are more frequently detected in healthy individuals than in patients with pemphigus vulgaris. J Immunol 172:6468–6475

Warren SJ, Lin MS, Giudice GJ, Hoffmann RG, Hans-Filho G, Aoki V, Rivitti EA, Santos V, Diaz LA (2000) The prevalence of antibodies against desmoglein 1 in endemic pemphigus foliaceus in Brazil. Cooperative Group on Fogo Selvagem Research. N Engl J Med 343:23–30

Werth VP, Fivenson D, Pandya AG, Chen D, Rico MJ, Albrecht J, Jacobus D (2008) Multicenter randomized, double-blind, placebo-controlled, clinical trial of dapsone as a glucocorticoid-sparing agent in maintenance-phase pemphigus vulgaris. Arch Dermatol 144:25–32

Wucherpfennig KW, Yu B, Bhol K, Monos DS, Argyris E, Karr RW, Ahmed AR, Strominger JL (1995) Structural basis for major histocompatibility complex (MHC)-linked susceptibility to autoimmunity: charged residues of a single MHC binding pocket confer selective presentation of self-peptides in pemphigus vulgaris. Proc Natl Acad Sci U S A 92:11935–11939

Yasuda H, Kobayashi H, Hashimoto T, Itoh K, Yamane M, Nakamura J (2000) Subcorneal pustular dermatosis type of IgA pemphigus: demonstration of autoantibodies to desmocollin-1 and clinical review. Br J Dermatol 143:144–148

Zillikens D, Derfler K, Eming R, Fierlbeck G, Goebeler M, Hertl M, Hofmann SC, Karlhofer F, Kautz O, Nitschke M, Opitz A, Quist S, Rose C, Schanz S, Schmidt E, Shimanovich I, Michael M, Ziller F (2007) Recommendations for the use of immunoapheresis in the treatment of autoimmune bullous diseases. J Dtsch Dermatol Ges 5:881–887

Introduction

It is almost 60 years since Lever (1953), on the basis of specific clinical and histological features, recognized bullous pemphigoid (BP) as a distinct disorder within the large group of blistering disorders, including the pemphigus group. One milestone in the evolution of our understanding of BP was the demonstration by Jordon et al. (Jordon et al., 1967) that the disease was associated with *in vivo* bound and circulating autoantibodies directed against proteins of the basement membrane zone of stratified epithelia. Complementary DNAs for the two targeted autoantigens bullous pemphigoid antigen 230 (BP230, BPAG1-e) and bullous pemphigoid antigen 180 (BP180, BPAG2 or type XVII collagen) were subsequently isolated independently by various groups (Stanley et al., 1988, Diaz et al., 1990, Sawamura et al., 1991; Li et al., 1992; Giudice et al., 1992; Hopkinson et al., 1992). Today, BP has emerged as an example of organ-specific autoimmune disease and it represents the most frequent autoimmune blistering disorder.

In this review, we will discuss the clinical and immunopathological features of BP, its differential diagnosis and therapeutic options. We will also focus on recent progress in our understanding of the pathophysiology of this disorder and on the role of targeted autoantigens in the maintenance of epithelial-stromal adhesion.

Clinical features

In the **prodromal, non-bullous phase** manifestations of BP are frequently nonspecific and, thus, misleading. Patients complain of severe itch accompanied or not by excoriated, eczematous, papular and or urticated lesions that may persist for several weeks or months, or even remain the only signs of the disease.

In the **bullous stage** vesicles and bullae develop on apparently normal or erythematous skin together with urticated and infiltrated plaques that have occasionally an an-

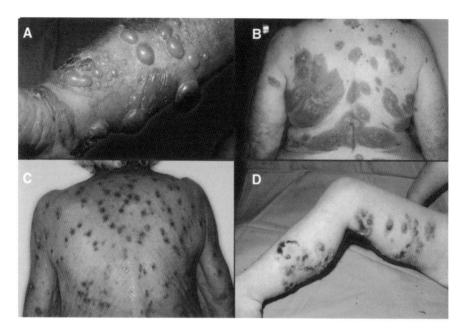

Fig. 1. Bullous pemphigoid. **Panel A**: bullous lesions on the forearms; **Panel B**: widespread urticated papules and plaques on the trunk distributed in a figurate pattern; **Panel C**: prurigo nodularis-like presentation with generalized papular and excoriated lesions; **Panel D**: childhood form of bullous pemphigoid with vesicular and bullous lesions arranged in jewel-like clusters. The patient had IgA autoantibodies targeting BP180.

nular or figurate pattern. The blisters are tense, with a clear exudate, and may persist for several days, leaving eroded and crusted areas (Fig. 1). The lesions are frequently distributed symmetrically and predominate on the flexural aspects of the limbs, and abdomen. In the intertriginous spaces, vegetating plaques can be seen. Involvement of the oral cavity is observed in 10–30% of cases. The mucosae of eyes, nose, pharynx, esophagus and ano-genital areas are more rarely affected (reviewed in Lever, 1953; Liu et al., 1986; Korman, 1987).

Several **clinical variants** of BP have been described (reviewed in Liu et al., 1986; Korman, 1987). Lesions remain occasionally localized, such as on the pretibial area ("pretibial pemphigoid"), around stomas, on the vulvar region ("vulvar pemphigoid"), on irradiated areas or confined to a paralyzed limb. Palmo-plantar involvement mimicking dyshidrosiform eczema ("dyshidrosiform pemphigoid") can also be observed. Several other variants, such as a prurigo nodularis-like ("pemphigoid nodularis"), erythroderma-like form, intertrigo-like variants or forms mimicking severe bullous drug eruption have been described. These variants have all been reported with various terms: only dermatologists can afford to have so different names for the same condition!

A peculiar form of BP typically associated with pregnancy, for which a separate term appears justified, is **gestational pemphigoid** (also called "pemphigoid gestationis" or "herpes gestationis") (reviewed in Shornick, 1993; Jenkins et al., 1993). This disease is also rarely

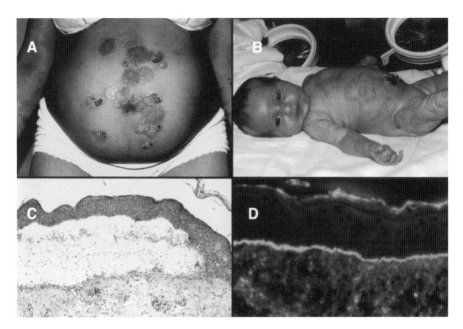

Fig. 2. Panel A: pemphigoid gestationis: infiltrated plaques, vesicles and bullae in the periumbelical area and abdomen; **Panel B**: transplacentar passage of autoantibodies from a mother with gestational pemphigoid: neonate with a generalized eruption consisting of erythematous plaques with a figurate configuration and blisters; **Panel C**: bullous pemphigoid: light microscopy study shows a subepidermal blister with an inflammatory infiltrate in the blister cavity and in the upper dermis consisting predominantly of eosinophils and neutrophils; **Panel D**: bullous pemphigoid: direct immunofluorescence microscopy depicting linear IgG deposits at the epidermal basement membrane.

found with either a choriocarcinoma or a hydatiform mole. Gestational pemphigoid, the estimated frequency of which is of one case in 10'000 to 40'000 pregnancies, starts during the second or third trimester of pregnancy or, more rarely, after delivery. In the early phase, itchy papular and urticated lesions are observed, with later on development of vesicles and bullae (Fig. 2). The eruption begins on the periumbilical and abdominal area and can generalize. Relapses are frequently observed during subsequent pregnancies and they might also be triggered by either menstruation or intake of oral contraceptives.

Presentation and clinical Setting

BP typically affects the elderly, with onset after 60 years of age. Its incidence has been estimated between 6.1 and 40 new cases per million per year. In a recent prospective study encompassing the entire Swiss population, the incidence was found to be of 12.7 new cases per million per year (Bernard et al., 1995; Jung et al., 1999; Marazza et al., 2009). It rapidly increases with aging and the relative risk for patients older than 90 years has been estimated to be approximately 300 fold higher than for subjects of 60 years of age or younger. In contrast to most autoimmune diseases, men have a higher risk of suffering from BP than women (Jung et al., 1999). Although BP is usually a disease of the elderly, it may be not as rare as commonly stated in children (Nemeth et al., 1991, Trueb et al., 1999, Waisbourd-Zinman et al., 2008).

Increasing evidence indicates that certain HLA class II alleles, that are prevalent in BP, play an important role in restricting autoreactive T cell responses to the BP target antigens (see below) and may thus be critical in the pathogenesis of the disease (Büdinger et al., 1998). A predominance of the class II HLA allele DQβ1*0301 has been found in Caucasian patients with BP and other variants, such as gestational pemphigoid and cicatricial pemphigoid (Delgado et al., 1996). However, the association of HLA class II alleles is most likely more polymorphic. In one report, the restriction with the allele DQβ1*0301 has been found to apply to men only (Banfield et al., 1998), while in a Japanese study BP was associated with the alleles DRβ1*04, DRβ1*1101 and DQβ1*0302 (Okazaki et al., 2000).

The potential occurrence of malignant diseases in patients with BP is most likely related to the old age of the patients. Some reports have suggested an increased frequency of certain cancers (such as of digestive tract, urinary bladder, and lung) and lymphoproliferative disorders. However, in two case-control studies, this excess of malignancy in BP was not significant (Venning et al., 1990; Lindelöf et al., 1990).

BP has been also described in patients with other autoimmune disorders, such as rheumatoid arthritis, Hashimoto's thyroiditis, dermatomyositis, lupus erythematosus, and autoimmune thrombocytopenia. Although a case-control study did not find any increased risk for autoimmune disorders in BP (Taylor et al., 1993), it is likely that these associations are not fortuitous, but reflect a genetically determined susceptibility to develop autoimmune diseases.

In some cases BP has been thought to be induced by trauma, burns, radiotherapy, UV radiation and, more significantly, drug intake (reviewed in Vassileva, 1998). With regard to the latter, diuretics (such as furosemide), non-steroidal anti-inflammatories, D-penicillamine, antibiotics (ampicillin and ciprofloxacin), iodine, and captopril are the most frequently implicated drugs. In a case-control study, an association was found with aldosterone antagonists and neuroleptics (Bastuji-Garin et al., 1996). It is not clear yet by which mechanisms drugs affect the development of BP, but it is likely that these patients have an underlying susceptibility to the disease and the drugs act as triggers. BP has also been found in association with certain dermatoses, such as psoriasis and lichen planus. In these conditions, it has been speculated that the inflammatory process at the dermo-epidermal junction is responsible for the exposure of antigens to autoreactive T lymphocytes leading to a secondary immune response (reviewed in Chan et al., 1998). Finally, BP has been described in patients presenting with neurological disorders, such as multiple sclerosis, Shy-Dragger syndrome, or amyotrophic lateral sclerosis (Masouyé et al., 1989; Chosidow et al., 2000). While the significance of these associations is unclear, it is intriguing to note that one of the two autoantigens of BP, the BP antigen 230 (BP230) (see below), has several isoforms (such as BPAG1-a) that are expressed in the central and peripheral nervous system and in muscles (Leung et al., 2001, Steiner-Champliaud et al., 2010) The possibility that in certain cases autoantibodies to BP230 might cross react with these isoforms and contribute to the neurological manifestations remains to be evaluated (Laffitte et al., 2005).

Diagnosis

Because of the clinical and immunopathological overlap with other autoimmune subepidermal blistering disorders, diagnosis of BP relies on the characterization of the targeted antigens. However, immunofluorescence microscopy studies are very useful for an initial classification. Although the validity of the approach needs confirmation, we frequently perform a work-up including IF microscopy studies in elderly patients with itch with or without skin manifestations to exclude a prodromal, non-bullous phase of BP.

1. *Light microscopy studies* of an early bulla show a subepidermal blister with a dermal inflammatory infiltrate composed predominantly of eosinophils and neutrophils (**Fig. 2**). In early non-bullous phases, subepidermal clefts and eosinophilic spongiosis can be found. Nevertheless, in the early phase of the disease or in atypical cases of BP histological features are either not diagnostic or not specific enough to allow distinction from other subepidermal autoimmune blistering diseases.
2. *Direct immunofluorescence microscopy studies* characteristically show linear deposits of IgG and or C3, and more rarely, of other Ig classes along the epidermal basement membrane (Fig. 2). Testing of autologous patient's skin after treatment with 1 M NaCl can allow the distinction of patients with BP (deposits on the epidermal side of the split or on both side of the split) from those with epidermolysis bullosa acquisita or anti-epiligrin mucous membrane pemphigoid (deposits on the dermal side) (Gammon et al., 1990).
3. *Indirect immunofluorescence studies* demonstrate the presence of circulating IgG autoantibodies in 60 to 80% of patients, that typically bind to the epidermal side of saline separated normal human skin (Gammon et al., 1984a). The latter substrate has been found to be superior than intact skin and other substrates such as monkey esophagus. In gestational pemphigoid, patients have IgG1 and IgG3 complement-fixing antibodies which are best detectable by a complement-binding indirect method.
4. *Enzyme linked immunosorbent assays (ELISA)* utilizing recombinant proteins encompassing various portions of BP180 (such as the NC16A domain, the COOH-terminal portion or its entire ectodomain) have been found to be highly specific and sensitive (Table 1). Antigens are tested under native conditions and, by this mean, reactivities against conformational antigens are not missed. (Giudice et al., 1994, Ide et al., 1995; Zillikens et al., 1997a and 1997b; Nakatani et al., 1998; Haase et al., 1998; Hofmann et al., 2002; Mariotti et al., 2004; Sakuma-Oyama et al., 2004; Thoma-Uszynski et al., 2004, Tsuji-Abe et al., 2005; 2006; Sitaru et al., 2007). ELISAs using BP230 recombinant proteins have been so far less sensitive and specific compared to BP180-ELISAs but have confirmatory diagnostic value (Table 1) (Kromminga et al., 2004; Thoma-Uszynski et al., 2004; Yoshida et al., 2006, Tampoia et al., 2009). In contrast to previous published

Table 1. A survey of published ELISA studies in bullous pemphigoid.

Study	BP sera	Control sera	IIF[1] (%)	Anti-gen	Recombinant protein[2]	Se[4] (%)	Sp (%)
Zillikens D. et al., 1997	50	107	84	BP180	P-NC16A (AA 490-562)	94.0	100
Nakatani C. et al., 1998	110	50	89	BP180	P-NC16A (AA 507-548)	96.0	100
					P-C-terminus (AA 1365-1413)	38.0	100
Husz S et al., 2000	43	60	NK	BP180 BP230	Combination of 3 peptides (BP180: AA 507-528; BP230: AA 1814-1834, AA 1793-1813)	91.0	88.0
Hata Y. et al 2000	83	40	100	BP180	E-ectodomain (AA 490-1497)	66.3	95.0
					P-NC16A (AA 490-566)	70	92.5
Kobayashi M. et al., 2002	64	538	100	BP180	P-NC16A (AA 490-566)	84.4	98.9
Hofmann SC. et al., 2002	116	100	100	BP180	E-NC16A+ Col 15 (AA 490-811)	80.0	99.0
					E-C-terminus (AA 1351-1497)	47.0	97.0
Sakuma-Oyama Y. et al., 2004	102	94	100	BP180	NC16A (commercial kit)[3]	89.0	97.9
Mariotti F. et al., 2004	78	107	100	BP180	P-NC16A (AA 490-562)	82.0	100
					Combination of 2 P-fragments (AA 1080-1107, AA 1331-1404)	41.0	99.1
Thoma-Uszynski S. et al., 2004	127	51	NK	BP180	E-ectodomain (AA 485-1497)	95.3	94.0
				BP230	Combination of 3 eukaryotic fragments (N: AA 1 1307; C1: AA 1881-2649; C2: AA 2077-2649;)	81.5	64.8
Kromminga A. et al., 2004	56	76	100	BP230	Combination of 5 E-fragments (N1: AA 1-671; N2: AA 607-1073; N3: AA 1014-1758; C1 AA 1710-2189; C2: AA 2137-2649)	62.5	93.4
Tsuji-Abe Y. et al., 2005	14	447	100	BP180	NC16A (commercial kit)[3]	78.6	98.9
Yoshida M. et al., 2006	239	430	100	BP180	NC16A (commercial kit)[3]	69.9	98.8
		109		BP230	Combination of 2 P-fragments (N: AA 1-979; C: AA 1870-2650)	72.4	99.5

3

Table 1. (*continued*) A survey of published ELISA studies in bullous pemphigoid.

Study	BP sera	Control sera	IIF[1] (%)	Anti-gen	Recombinant protein[2]	Se[4] (%)	Sp (%)
Sitaru et al., 2007	118	107	94	BP180	Tetramers of NC16A	89.8	87.8
Di Zenzo et al., 2008	49	80	96	BP180+ BP230	Combination of 1P and 2 E-fragments BP180-NC16A/ BP180-ECD/ BP230-NH2term	100	82
Feng et al., 2008	42	24	100	BP180	NC16A (commercial kit)[3]	97.6	96
Tampoia et al., 2009	20	82	100	BP180	NC16A (commercial kit)[3]	90	97.6
				BP230	BP230 (commercial kit)[3]	60	97.6

[1] Percentage of positivity by indirect immunofluorescence microscopy. [2]Recombinant proteins used as substrate. P- for prokaryotic or E- for eukaryotic expressed protein. [3]A commercially available ELISA kit (MBL, Naka-ku, Nagoya, Japan). Se: Sensitivity; Sp: specificity; NK: not known; AA: amino acid. [4]Noteworthy, in most studies, sensitivity is largely overestimated, since selected serum samples from BP patients with positive indirect IF studies were used.

claims, clinical experience indicates that the sensitivity of the commercially available BP180-ELISAs (70%–97.6%) is not superior to indirect immunofluorescence microscopy studies using salt-split normal skin when unselected BP sera are tested. However, the sensitivity can be increased up to 100% (Di Zenzo et al., 2008) when various ELISAs using the NC16A domain and other extracellular portions of BP180 or of BP230 are used in combination (Nakatani et al., 1998; Hofmann et al., 2002; Mariotti et al., 2004; Thoma-Uszynski et al., 2006; Yoshida et al., 2006; Di Zenzo et al., 2008). These ELISAs have several advantages over traditional diagnostic approaches: they allow multiple sample testing, are rapid and easy to perform, and can be better standardized (Fig. 3). Finally, although not yet demonstrated in controlled studies, they probably are of diagnostic help in patients suspected of having BP when, for various reasons, direct immunofluorescence studies cannot be performed. ELISAs have nowadays largely replaced immunoblot and immunoprecipitation techniques, which are technically much more demanding.

5. *Immunoblot and immunoprecipitation studies* of keratinocyte extracts show in 60% to 100% of patients' sera the presence of autoantibodies binding to BP180 and / or BP230 (Stanley et al., 1981; Labib et al., 1986; Mueller et al., 1989; Bernard et al., 1989). Recombinant forms of BP180 and BP230 expressed in prokaryotic or eukaryotic systems (such as baculoviruses, epithelial cell lines, and yeast) have also been used to facilitate the detection of auto-antibodies (Tanaka et al., 1991, Giudice, 1993, Haase et al., 1998). In gestational pemphigoid, patients' autoantibodies predominantly recognize BP180 (Morrison et al., 1988). These technical approaches are currently only performed in particular cases, such as for ELISA-negative serum samples or in investigative studies.

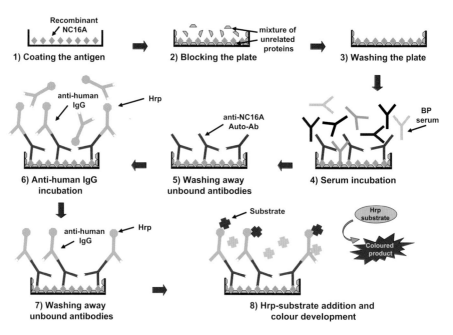

Fig. 3. Principle of BP180-NC16A ELISA. The ELISA based on the use of a recombinant protein corresponding to NC16A domain is highly sensitive and specific. The ELISA procedure involves (1) coating of antigen; (2) blocking of the nonspecific binding sites with a mixture of unrelated proteins; (3) washing the plate; (4) incubation of coated antigen with BP sera and controls; (5) washing to remove unbound autoantibodies (Auto-Ab); (6) incubation with anti-human IgG antibody conjugated with horseradish peroxidise (Hrp); (7) washing to remove unbound autoantibodies; (8) addition of peroxidise substrate and stopping the reaction that produces coloured products and reading of optical density (OD) at 450 nm with a microplate reader.

Differential diagnosis

Manifestations of BP might resemble those of a variety of dermatoses, including drug reactions, contact dermatitis, prurigo, fixed urticaria, vasculitis, arthropod reaction and scabies. Clinical history, pathologic features and negative immunofluorescence microscopy findings are essential to distinguish these disorders from BP. Diseases within the pemphigus group can be easily differentiated on the basis of distinctive immunopathological features. In dermatitis herpetiformis IF microscopy findings, the clinical setting with associated (clinical or subclinical) coeliac disease and the serological profile (see **Dermatitis herpetiformis chapter**) are peculiar. In contrast, the distinction of BP from certain autoimmune blistering disorders is difficult. However, a recent study has found that in patients with a blistering disorder associated with linear deposits of IgG or C3 in the epidermal basement membrane the presence of certain clinical criteria (that is, absence of skin atrophy, absence of mucosal involvement, absence of head and neck involvement and age greater than 70 years) indicates to a diagnosis of BP with high sensitivity and specificity (Vaillant et al., 1998, Joly et al., 2004). Paraneoplastic pemphigus, an autoimmune blistering disorder with potential multiorgan involvement associated with a neoplasia, might present with clinical features reminiscent of BP. However, its immunopathological features are peculiar enough to allow its differentiation from BP. The distinction of the following subepidermal blistering disorders may be challenging:

1. **Epidermolysis bullosa acquisita (EBA)** shows a wide spectrum of presentations (Gammon, 1984b; Briggaman et al., 1985; Gammon and Briggaman, 1993) (**see EBA chapter**). The *classical "non-inflammatory" form* includes skin fragility, blistering, erosions, with milia formation, skin atrophy and scarring that typically develop over trauma-exposed sites, such as arms, elbows, hands and feet. Occasionally, nail dystrophy and scarring alopecia are observed. While the features of this classical form are suggestive, a substantial number of patients have *an "inflammatory" form* of EBA mimicking BP, characterized by a widespread eruption with blisters involving intertriginous and flexural areas that heal without milia or atrophic scars. In addition, in the course of the disease, a mixture of inflammatory and non inflammatory features may be observed. Mucosal involvement can occur and potentially results in significant morbidity. Diagnosis of EBA relies on the detection of autoantibodies that bind to the dermal side of 1 M NaCl separated skin and specifically react with type VII collagen, the major component of anchoring fibrils (Briggaman et al., 1985; Woodley et al., 1984). Correct diagnosis of EBA is important for at least two reasons: the disease might be associated with other conditions, such as Crohn's disease, rheumatoid arthritis, and systemic lupus erythematosus, and second, EBA is thought to be more resistant to treatment than BP.

2. **Linear IgA bullous dermatosis** (LABD) was originally considered a distinct entity defined on the basis of the immunopathological finding of linear IgA deposits in the cutaneous BMZ (Chorzelski et al., 1979; Wojnarowska et al., 1988). The condition, thought to represent the most common autoimmune blistering disorder of childhood, is associated with urticated, annular and or polycyclic lesions, with development of vesicles and bullae. The latter might be distributed in "jewel-like" clusters or "string of pearls" patterns. Involvement of mucosae is not unusual. Childhood features of LABD are often peculiar, with involvement of the genital area or around the mouth, whereas adulthood LABD is more polymorphic. The autoantigens of LABD are heterogeneous. The two most characteristic target antigens are a protein of 97 kDa and a 120 kDa protein, termed the LABD antigen 1 (LABD97) and LAD-1 respectively. These two molecules correspond to the cleaved, shedded ectodomain of BP180 (Zone et al., 1998; Pas et al., 1997; Hirako et al., 1998 and 2003; Schäcke et al., 1998). It is thought that extracellular processing of BP180, which is catalyzed by members of the ADAMs family (A Disintegrin And Metalloprotease) (Franzke et al., 2004), results in the formation of neoepitopes which are specifically targeted by patients' IgA and, occasionally IgG, autoantibodies. Nevertheless, some patients with *bona fide* LABD have been found to possess IgA (and IgG) autoantibodies that recognize BP180 and BP230 (Ghohestani et al., 1997), type VII collagen (Hashimoto et al., 1996) or other, as yet uncharacterized antigens (Wojnarowska et al., 1991). Some of these LABD patients therefore fulfill the diagnostic criteria for BP or EBA. In summary, LABD most likely comprises a group of subepidermal blistering disorders rather than a single nosologic entity.

3. **Anti-p200 pemphigoid**, a recently identified entity within the group of autoimmune subepidermal blistering diseases. Clinical features are identical to those observed in BP, that is, vesicles and tense blisters together with eczematous and urticarial papules and plaques. Rarely, patients have a dermatitis herpetiformis-like grouped papulovesicles and oral and / or mucosal lesions can occur. Immunologically, these patients can be differentiated from BP based on the detection of circulating autoantibodies that bind the dermal side of NaCl-separated human skin. Patients' autoantibodies specifically recognize a 200 kDa protein of the dermo-epidermal junction, the laminin gamma 1 chain (Dilling et al., 2007; Dainichi et al., 2009).

4. **Mucous membrane pemphigoid** (MMP) includes a heterogeneous group of blistering diseases, which have in common the predominant involvement of the mucosae and a chronic course. Scarring is typical except for a subset of patients with disease restricted to the oral mucosa (Mutasim et al., 1993; Chan et al., 1993; Chan et al., 2002). In contrast to BP, MMP skin lesions generally involve the scalp, head, and the upper trunk, and they are found in up to 25% of patients. The oral mucosa and the conjunctiva, and, less frequently, nose, esophagus, larynx and genitals are affected. Subsets of patients with either pure ocular involvement, predominant oral mucosal involvement without cutaneous lesions, or with both oral and cutaneous lesions have been identified (Chan et al., 1993). Erosions and scarring of the mucosae might result in significant morbidity. Ocular disease can lead to symblepharon formation, entropion, and trichiasis. In addition, stenoses of the nasopharynx, larynx, esophagus and urethra are observed. Patients with a MMP phenotype might exhibit IgG and / or IgA autoantibodies of different specificity, that recognize BP180 and BP230 (Bernard et al., 1990a; Calabresi et al., 2007), the 97 / 120 kDa LABD antigen, laminin-332 (laminin-5) and laminin-311 (laminin-6) (Domloge-Hultsch et al., 1992; Chan et al., 1997), type VII collagen (Luke et al., 1999) or the β4 integrin subunit (Tyagi et al., 1996). Importantly, in the so called anti-epiligrin mucous membrane pemphigoid associated with anti-laminin-332 autoantibodies an increased relative risk for solid cancer (adenocarcinomas), especially in the first year after blister onset, has been reported (Egan et al., 2003). The latter observation probably accounts for the high incidence of mortality observed among these patients.

Therapy and Prognosis

BP is a chronic disease showing spontaneous exacerbations and remissions, that is associated with potential significant morbidity and has a serious impact on the quality of life (severe itch, bullous and eroded lesions, impetiginization…). Although the majority of patients go into remission under treatment, the mortality rate, estimated between 12 to 40% in the first year, is considerable (Roujeau et al., 1998, Colbert et al., 2004). It is likely that practice patterns (e. g., use systemic corticotherapy or immunosuppressive drugs) critically affect overall morbidity (Roujeau et al., 1998). Older age, low general condition (Karnovsky index of ≤ 40) and use of high doses of oral corticosteroids, but not the extent of the disease, are the most important prognostic factor affecting mortality rate (Rzany et al., 2002; Joly et al., 2005).

The treatment of BP is still based more on clinical experience rather than on evidence. However, results of controlled studies have recently started to change the practices and the therapeutic algorithm followed by dermatologists (Korman, 2000, Laffitte and Borradori, 2001). As a matter of fact, potent topical corticosteroids (such as clobetasol proprionate), have been demonstrated in a large multicenter study to constitute a more effective therapy for BP when compared to oral corticosteroids in terms of control of the disease, side effect profile and overall survival (Joly et al., 2002). Furthermore, a mild regimen with clobetasol propionate cream 10–30 g per day tapering over 4 months is not inferior than the original treatment protocol (clobetasol propionate cream, 40 g per day initially, with tapering over 12 months). This mild regimen allows a 70% reduction of the cumulative doses of corticosteroids, and, in patients with moderate disease, it reduces the risk of death and further improves the side effect profile (Joly et al., 2009). Systemic corticosteroids have been widely utilized in clinical practice and their efficacy have been confirmed in uncontrolled and controlled studies (Morel et al., 1984; Dreno et al., 1993, Joly et al., 2002). However, their use is associated with significant side effects (Roujeau et al., 1998, Joly et al., 2002). For patients with extensive disease, oral prednisone at the dosage of 0.5 to 1 mg per kg per day usually controls the disease within three weeks. This dose is then progressively tapered over a period of 6 to 9 months. The concomitant use of immunosuppressive drugs, such as azathioprine (Burton et al., 1978; Guillaume et al., 1993), mycophenolate mofetil, methotrexate, and less frequently, chlorambucil and cyclophosphamide, is a matter of debate. Some clinicians prefer to introduce them only when corticosteroids alone fail to control the disease, or if the latter are contraindicated. The only controlled study available so far failed to prove an advantage of using a combination of prednisone and azathioprine *versus* prednisone alone, since more complications were observed in the azathioprine group. However, in the latter study, the dose of azathioprine used was not adjusted based on TPMT levels. The choice of a immunosuppressive drug depends on the profile of its side effects, patients' overall condition, the experience of the physician with the molecule, and finally, cost issues. For example, although mycophenolate mofetil is likely to have less hepatic side effects compared to azathioprine, the latter is much cheaper and may show a more rapid onset of action with a better corticosteroid sparing effect (Beissert et al., 2007). Dapsone (Venning et al., 1989) and the association of nicotinamide and minocycline or tetracycline (Fivenson et al., 1994) have also been tried alone or as adjuvant with some success and may be helpful in mild disease. In certain treatment-resistant cases, pulse corticosteroid therapy, intravenous immunoglobulins, plasmapheresis and photophoresis have been utilized. The experience with biologicals, such as rituximab, in BP is still anecdotal (Reguiaï et al., 2009). Finally, in all BP patients, it is important to undertake all measures aimed at preventing the complications of both the cutaneous lesions and of the treatment.

Disease activity and relapse markers

In preliminary studies encompassing almost invariably retrospective cohorts with a limited number of patients, evidence has been provided indicating that IgG ELISA-BP180 NC16A values parallel disease severity and or activity (Haase et al., 1998, Schmidt et al., 2000a). Nevertheless, data from larger prospective studies are required to draw more substantiated conclusions. One has to keep in mind that up to 20–30% of unselected BP serum samples lack reactivity against the NC16A domain. A recent prospective study on BP patients after cessation of corticosteroid treatment has indicated that, besides greater age (> 80 years), the detection of a high-titer ELISA-BP180 (NC16A) score (3 x higher than the cutoff) and, to a lesser degree, of a positive direct immunofluorescence at the moment of therapy stopping are good indicators for an increased relapse risk (Bernard et al., 2009).

The phenotype of the disease seems to relate to the autoantibody profile. For example, reactivity with both the NH_2- and COOH-terminal region of the ectodomain of BP180 was found to be more frequently detected by ELISA in patients with mucosal lesions (Balding et al., 1996; Hofmann et al., 2002).

Challenging situations

An unresolved issue is how to deal with elderly patients with an itchy skin eruption who have circulating antibodies to the BM and show reactivity with BP180 and BP230, but without evidence for deposits of immunoreactants in the skin as assessed by IF microscopy and with unspecific histologic findings (Rieckhoff-Cantoni et al., 1992; Hashisuka et al., 1996). It is likely that in these cases the use of a more sensitive technique such as immunoelectron microscopy would disclose immune deposits in the skin at an earlier stage. Classification of this relatively large group of patients remains problematic in the absence of a consensus statement on definition of diagnostic criteria for definite and probable or early BP. As a matter of fact, some of these patients with initially negative direct immunofluorescence findings, but with circulating anti-basement membrane antibodies, develop BP later on.

Pathogenesis

BP180 and BP230 are components of hemidesmosomes, junctional adhesion complexes

Recent cell biological studies have specified the role of BP180 and BP230 in maintenance of dermo-epidermal adhesion (Borradori and Sonnenberg, 1999). These two proteins are components of hemidesmosomes (HD), junctional complexes promoting adhesion of epithelial cells to the underlying BM in stratified and other complex epithelia, such as skin and mucous membranes (**Fig. 4**).

BP180 is a transmembrane molecule with a large collagenous extracellular domain (ECD) serving as cell adhesion molecule (Giudice et al., 1991; Hopkinson et al., 1992) (**Fig. 5**). The idea that this protein is important for cell attachment is further supported by the observation that mutations in the gene encoding BP180 underly a form of non-lethal junctional epidermolysis bullosa characterized by skin blistering and fragility, alopecia, dental and nail abnormalities (Jonkmann et al., 1995, McGrath et al., 1995). In contrast, BP230 is a cytoplasmic component belonging to the plakin family of proteins (Stan-

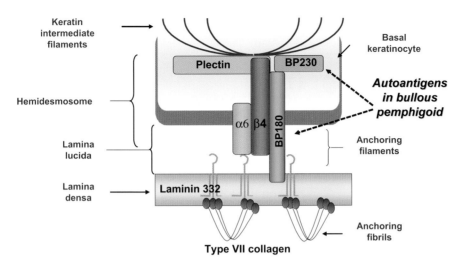

Fig. 4. Schematic representation of a hemidesmosome at the ventral side of a basal keratino-cyte depicting some major structural components. The two intracellular hemidesmosomal components BP230 (BPAG1-e) and plectin are implicated in the attachment of the keratin intermediate filament network and interact with the cytoplasmic domain of the transmembrane components BP180 (also called BPAG2, type XVII collagen) and integrin α6β4. The latter, by means of their extracellular domain, are able to interact with extracellular matrix proteins within the basement membrane, such as laminin-332, that is in turn connected with type VII collagen, the major component of anchoring fibrils in the upper dermis. Lamina densa, lamina lucida, anchoring filaments and anchoring fibrils are structures within the basement membrane zone that can be visualized by electron microscopy studies.

ley et al., 1988; Sawamura et al., 1991; Green et al., 1992) that consist of a central coiled-coil region flanked by two globular end domains (**Fig. 5**). The recent description of a mild form epidermolysis bullosa simplex due to mutations in the dystonin gene, encoding the coiled-coil domain of the epithelial isoform of BP230 (BPAG1-e), illustrates the role of BP230 in maintenance of cytoarchitecure and cell resilience (Groves et al., 2010).

These two antigens by means of interactions with each other and with the other components of HD, including the α6β4 integrin and plectin, contribute to the assembly and stabilization of HD, and, therefore, to the maintenance of cell-substrate adhesion (Hopkinson et al., 1995, Borradori et al., 1997, Koster et al., 2003). Specifically, BP230 and plectin (Guo et al., 1995, Andrä et al., 1997; Fontao et al., 2003) connect the keratin filaments to the basal plasma membrane, while the transmembrane hemidesmosomal proteins BP180 and the α6β4 integrin act as cell surface receptors for extracellular matrix proteins, including laminin-332. The latter interacts with type VII collagen, the major component of anchoring fibrils in the dermis. Because of their close structural organization and functional synergy, it is not unexpected that abnormalities of different structural components of HD (e.g. due to either autontibodies or a gene mutation) might result in a similar clinical phenotype.

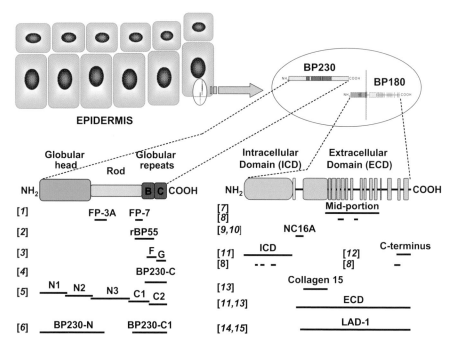

Fig. 5. Structural and domain organization of the bullous pemphigoid antigen 230 (BP230) and the bullous pemphigoid antigen 180 (BP180). BP230 is predicted to contain a central coil-coiled domain flanked by two globular domains, while BP180 is a type II transmembrane protein with a large extracellular collagenous domain. LAD-1 corresponds to a 120 kDa molecule generated by physiologic processing of BP180. The identified antigenic sites on the various portions of both antigens are depicted and the corresponding original studies are cited: [1] Miller et al., 1993; [2] Gaucherand et al., 1995; [3] Skaria et al., 2000; [4] Hamada et al., 2001; [5] Kromminga et al., 2004; [6] Thoma-Uszynski et al., 2004; [7] Egan et al., 2001; [8] Di Zenzo et al., 2004; [9] Zillikens et al., 1997; [10] Zimina et al., 2008; [11] Perriard et al., 1999; [12] Murakami et al., 1998; [13] Schumann et al., 2000; [14] Chritophoridis et al., 2000; [15] Di Zenzo et al., 2008.

BP, an example of organ-specific autoimmune disease

The autoimmune etiology of BP appears now clearly established: 1) patients have autoantibodies and autoreactive T cells to well characterized self-antigens; 2) tissue injury occurs where antibody-antigen complexes are found; 3) *in vitro* models with human skin and *in vivo* animal models of the disease have provided unequivocal evidence for the pathogenic role of autoantibodies; specifically, mice that lack mouse BP180, but express human BP180 have been generated. In these "humanized" mice, passively transferred, maternally-transferred or actively produced BP autoantibodies react to human BP180 molecules expressed in the skin and induce BP-like skin lesions in the neonates or adult mice; 4) in gestational pemphigoid, the transplacentar transfer of anti-BP180 autoantibodies from the mother into the neonate can cause a transient bullous eruption; 5) the levels of IgG and IgE autoantibodies directed against the immunodominant region of BP180 autoantibodies parallel disease activity; 6) the disease occurs in association with distinct HLA genotypes and responds to immunosuppressive therapy.

Humoral immune response

Almost all BP patients have autoantibodies binding to an immunodominant region of BP180, the NC16A domain, which is located extracellularly close to its transmembrane domain. Memory B cells specific for the NC16A domain, which can be induced in vitro to synthesize autoantibodies have been identified (Leyendeckers et al., 2003). Nevertheless, additional antigenic sites exist on both the extracellular and intracellular domain of BP180, which is recognized by up to 96% of the BP sera (Diaz et al., 1990; Giudice et al., 1993; Giudice et al., 1994; Zillikens et al., 1997; Perriard et al., 1999; Nakatani et al., 1998; Nie and Hashimoto, 1999; Egan et al.1999; Schumann et al., 2000; Egan et al., 2001; Hofmann et al., 2002; Di Zenzo et al., 2004; Mariotti et al., 2004; Thoma-Uszynski et al., 2006; Di Zenzo et al., 2008) (**Fig. 5**). Interestingly, there is a subgroup of patients who react with different BP180 extracellular epitopes, but not with the NC16A domain suggesting a possible role of non-NC16A epitopes in the pathogenesis of disease (Mariotti et al., 2004 and unpublished observations). Recently, it has also been reported that autoantibodies preferentially recognize the phosphorylated BP180 ectodomain (Zimina et al., 2007 and 2008).

BP patients also exhibit significant reactivity with BP230. In an initial study, 38% of BP sera recognized synthetic peptides representing sequences in the COOH-terminal region of BP230 by immunoblot (Rico et al., 1990). Subsequent studies showed that approximately 60% of BP sera have IgG autoantibodies that recognize the COOH-terminal domain of BP230. Specifically, immunodominant antigenic sites have been mapped within a region encompassing the B and C subdomains of BP230 (Skaria et al., 2000; Hamada et al., 2001). Nevertheless, IgG autoantibodies binding to the N-terminal and the central α-helical coiled-coil domain are also found (Skaria et al., 2000; Tanaka et al., 1991; Miller et al., 1993; Ide et al., 1995; Gaucherand et al., 1995; Thoma-Uszynski et al., 2004) (**Fig. 5**).

The presence of several antigenic sites throughout BP230 and BP180 most likely results from an "epitope spreading" (ES) phenomenon. This term describes the observation that in the course of an autoimmune disease, both B and T cell responses (see below) are not restricted to an unique "immunodominant" epitope, but they spread involving additional "secondary" epitopes within the same protein or on distinct molecules, that may play a key role for the progression of the disease (Vanderlugt and Miller, 1996; Chan et al., 1998). This phenomenon may explain the occasional finding that BP sera contain autoantibodies targeting other components of the hemidesmosomal adhesion complex, such as plectin and laminin-332 (Kawahara et al., 1998; Laffitte et al., 2001). Analysis of the epitope pattern in the disease course indicated that patients with either BP or gestational pemphigoid exhibit a specific reactivity profile and that binding to intracellular epitopes are detectable at an early stage of the disease (Di Zenzo et al., 2004; Di Zenzo et al., 2007). We have recently assessed the dynamics of the humoral response to human BP180 in mice grafted with skin obtained from transgenic mice expressing human BP180. The results showed that antibodies develop first against epitopes on the extracellular domain of BP180, and later on against intracellular epitopes (Di Zenzo et al., 2010). Recently, evidence for ES phenomena produced by autoaggressive B (and T) cells has been found. Most ES events occurred intramolecularly involving IgG response against BP180. Of note, in some patients IgG reactivity targeted first BP180 and then spread to BP230 epitopes. Noteworthy, IgG reactivity against the intracytoplasmic BP230 never preceded that recognizing the transmembrane BP180 protein (own unpublished observations). Altogether these findings are in keeping with the current model of autoimmune disease that predicts an initial involvement of an extracellular immunodominant epitope (BP180 ECD) triggering an inflammatory cascade with tissue damage leading subsequently to exposure with recognition of antigenic reactive sites on the intracellular domain of BP180 and BP230.

In addition to the IgG isotype, patients with BP have frequently IgE and IgA autoantibodies binding to both BP180 and BP230. IgE autoantibodies have been found to bind to the NC16A domain, other sites of the BP180 ectodomain and intracellular domain as well as to BP230 (Ghohestani et al., 1998; Fairley et al., 2005; Christophoridis et al., 2000; Messingham et al., 2009; Dresow et al., 2009). It should be noted that normal healthy subjects may possess IgG autoantibodies to basement membrane proteins as assessed by indirect immunofluorescence studies, immunoblot and ELISA, but usually at low titers (Desai et al., 2008; Wieland et al., 2010). Positive BP180 and BP230 ELISA values are also found in elderly patients with various pruritic skin disorders (Hofmann et al., 2003, 2009; Jedlickova et al., 2008 Feliciani et al., 2009). Nevertheless, based on the low incidence of BP, even in the elderly, the number of prospectively followed patients is insufficient to draw any conclusion about the predictive positive value of positive ELISAs results to identify elderly subjects who later on will develop BP.

Cellular immune response and inflammatory cascade

Only a limited number of studies have thus far addressed the role of autoreactive T cells in the pathogenesis of BP and related disorders. Some studies have assessed autoreactive T cell responses to the ectodomain of BP180 in patients with BP, gestational pemphigoid and in healthy individuals (Büdinger et al., 1998, Lin et al., 1999). Autoreactive T cells react with the same regions of BP180 and BP230 that are recognized by IgG autoantibodies (Thoma-Uszynski et al., 2006). Strikingly, epitope recognition appeared to be restricted by certain HLA class II alleles, such as the HLA-DQβ1*0301 allele, that are prevalent in BP (Delgado et al., 1996). CD4 T cell lines and clones derived from BP patients were shown to produce both Th1 and Th2 cytokines (Büdinger et al., 1998).

Since Th1 cytokines (such as IFNγ) are able to induce the secretion of IgG1 and IgG2, while Th2 cytokines (such as IL-4, IL-5, and IL-13) have been shown to regulate the secretion of IgG4 and IgE (reviewed in Romagnani, 1992), the detection of anti-BP180 and anti-BP230 antibodies of the IgG1, IgG4 and IgE isotype (Bernard et al., 1990b; Fairley et al., 2005) in BP patients suggest that both autoreactive Th1 and Th2 cells are involved in the regulation of the response to the BP target antigens. This idea is further supported by the analysis of the cytokine expression profile in both patients lesional tissue and sera, that shows an increase in most cytokines with significant correlations betweeen their level and skin lesions number (D'Auria et al., 1999). The relative low concentrations of IFNγ and IL-2 compared to those of IL-4, IL-5 and IL-10 suggests a predominance of a Th2 response (D'Auria et al., 1999). In line with this data, blister fluid and serum of patients with BP are extremely rich in CCL18 a chemokine frequently associated with inflammatory Th2-type responses. Specifically, Langerhans cells, antigen-presenting cells of the dermis and eosinophils have been identified as producers of CCL18, levels of which seem to parallel the disease course in most cases (Günther et al., 2009). Recently, grafts of human BPAG2 (BP180) transgenic skin placed on syngeneic wild type mice elicited IgG that bound human BP180 in the skin. Of note, MHC II-/- mice grafted with BPAG2 transgenic skin did not develop anti-BP180 IgG indicating that MHC II:CD4 + T cell interactions were crucial for these responses. Transgenic skin grafts on wild type mice developed neutrophil-rich infiltrates, dermal edema, subepidermal blisters, and deposits of immunoreactants in epidermal BM (Olasz et al., 2007). Recently, an active stable BP animal model has been established by transferring splenocytes from wild-type mice, that had been immunized by grafting of human BPAG2(BP180)-transgenic mouse skin, into mice generated by crossing Rag-2⁻/⁻ with BP180-humanized mice. The recipient mice continuously produced anti-human BP180 IgG Abs in vivo and developed blisters and erosions with BP-like features (Ujiie et al., 2010).

A recent analysis of cell subsets with immunoregulatory functions in untreated BP patients has shown that while CD4 + CD25 + FOXP3 + Treg, NKT and NK cell present normal frequency and function in BP patients, γδT cells were reduced (Rensing-Ehl et al., 2007; Oswald et al., 2009).

Liu and coworkers have generated a humanized mouse strain, in which the murine BPAG2(BP180)NC14A is replaced with the homologous human BPAG2(BP180)NC16A epitope. When pretreated with mast cell activation blocker or depleted of complement or neutrophils, these BP180 humanized mice become resistant to BP development following passive transfer of human BP autoantibodies (Liu et al., 2008). Thus, a growing body of evidence suggests that, besides autoantibodies, also T cell and other innate immune system players are important in the induction and progression of tissue damage and thus BP pathogenesis.

Pathogenic mechanism of blister formation

Animal models of disease based on the passive transfer of antibodies have been extensively used to dissect the functional pathways contributing to tissue injury in BP (Liu et al., 1993, 1995, 1997, 1998, 2000a, 2000b, 2005; 2008 Yamamoto et al., 2002; Nishie et al., 2007 and 2009). The transferred antibodies were either raised against the murine homologue of the human BP180NC16A domain or obtained and purified from BP patients and subsequently injected into hamster, neonatal wild-type and / or "humanized" mice expressing human BP180. Most of the data obtained in these models are in agreement with findings in BP patients. Overall, they show that the mechanisms by which IgG autoantibodies are pathogenic include complement activation, recruitment of inflammatory cells and liberation of proteases, such as matrix metalloproteinase (MMP)-9 and neutrophil elastase, which are detected in patient lesional skin and blister fluid (Gammon et al., 1984b; Stahle-Bäckdahl et al., 1994; Verraes et al., 2001; Shimanovich et al., 2004; Nelson et al., 2006;) (**Fig. 6**).

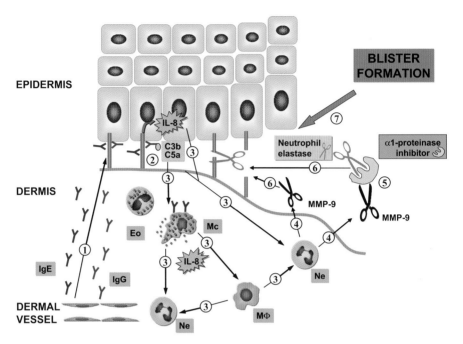

Fig. 6. Mechanisms of blister formation in bullous pemphigoid. Binding of autoantibodies to the target antigens results in an inflammatory response with complement activation, accumulation of neutrophils and eosinophils and liberation of proteolytic enzymes. The following steps are shown: (1) IgG and IgE autoantibodies bind to BP180 (and BP230); (2) The complement system is activated, while basal keratinocytes produce interleukin-8 (IL-8); (3) Macrophages (MΦ), neutrophils (Ne), mast cells (Mc) and eosinophils (Eo) are recruited and activated, specifically during the acute inflammatory process. Mast cells bind IgE antigen-specific autoantibodies and release the content of their granules; (4) Neutrophils secrete various proteases; (5) Matrix metalloproteinase 9 (MMP-9) inactivates the α1-proteinase inhibitor of neutrophil elastase; (6) Neutrophil-derived MMP-9 and neutrophil elastase cleave the extracellular domain of BP180 and various extracellular matrix proteins and cause dermo–epidermal dysadhesion with basal keratinocytes detachment and blister formation.

Specifically, these proteinases, which are strongly expressed by neutrophils and eosinophils, are thought to proteolytically degrade various extracellular matrix proteins as well as the extracellular domain of BP180 (Stahle-Bäckdahl et al., 1994; Verraes et al., 2001; Chen et al., 2001, 2002; Sitaru et al., 2002; Zhao et al., 2006).

Besides IgG, also IgE anti-BP180 autoantibodies also contribute to lesion development by stimulating degranulation of basophils and / or mast cells (Dimson et al., 2003). Recently, IgE purified from patients with BP injected into human skin grafted onto nude mice were able to induce histological separation of the epidermis from the dermis and inflammatory skin changes reminiscent of those observed in BP (Fairley et al., 2007). In addition, eosinophils appear to play an important role in mediating inflammatory process and tissue injury (Zone et al., 2007) (**Fig. 6**). While IL-5 promotes growth and activation of eosinophils, eotaxin is an eosinophil-specific chemokine, produced by fibroblasts and probably keratinocytes, regulating eosinophil migration (Wakugawa et al., 2000). High levels of IL-5 and eotaxin have been recently detected in blister fluid of BP patients. Keratinocytes are also likely to contribute to the local inflammation by releasing both pro-inflammatory cytokines as well as proteases. Recently, autoantibodies to BP180 have been shown to directly modulate the expression of IL-6 and IL-8 as well as tissue-type plasminogen activator by cultured keratinocytes (Schmidt et al., 2000b and 2004). Finally, a new study shows that anti-BP180 IgG autoantibodies reduce hemidesmosomal BP180 content, potentially weakening by this means dermo-epidermal cohesion (Iwata et al., 2009).

The pathogenic relevance of autoantibodies to the cytoplasmic protein BP230 has received less attention than given to BP180 autoantibodies. Although reactivity against this antigen often has been considered an epiphenomenon, several observations suggest its contribution to the pathogenesis of BP: 1. Immunization of rabbits with BP230-derived peptides seemed to increase the local inflammatory response following epidermal damage (Hall et al., 1993); 2. The passive transfer in neonatal mice of antibodies against BP230-derived peptides has been claimed to induce a dermal inflammatory reaction with subepidermal microdetachments (Kiss et al., 2005); 3. BP230-specific autoantibodies are readily detectable in the majority of BP patients, even after a relatively short duration of disease (Thoma-Uszynski et al., 2004; Di Zenzo et al., 2008).

Unresolved issues and perspectives

The etiologic factors underlying the initiation of the BP remain unclear. One of the major challenges will be the elucidation of the predisposing factors, including genetic polymorphism, leading to a break of autotolerance. It is important to better characterize the humoral and cellular immune response in the various phases of the disease and to further verify to which extent findings obtained from mouse models of BP can be applied to the situation in humans. Spontaneous animal models of BP in cats, horses, and minipigs (Olivry et al., 1999, 2000a, 2000b) could provide important tools for gaining further insight into the pathophysiology of the disease. This insight will not only further our understanding of autoimmune diseases in general, but, hopefully, also facilitate the development of diagnostic tools for the identification of patients at risk for BP. Better knowledge of the autoimmune response in BP is a crucial step towards the design of novel immunomodulatory approaches devoid of the severe side effects of current immunosuppressive treatments. For example, preliminary observations indicate that the new biological therapies using monoclonal antibodies able to modulate immune respose (by targeting for example B and / or T cells) may be useful in controlling BP (Szalbocs et al., 2002). Finally, it would not be surprising that better knowledge of the pathophysiology of BP and other blistering disorders will lead to a revision of their classification based on the targeted antigens. It is likely that additional factors, such as genes regulating the inflammatory and tissue repair response, critically affect clinical features and final outcome.

Summary

Our understanding of BP, a blistering disorder of the skin and mucosae, has greatly improved. BP has emerged as a paradigm of organ-specific autoimmune disease. Patients' autoantibodies are directed against BP180 and BP230. These two autoantigens are components of hemidesmosomes, adhesion complexes in human skin that promote dermo-epidermal cohesion. Animal models have provided unequivocal evidence for the pathogenic significance of these autoantibodies as well as novel insights into the cascade of events leading to subepidermal separation. Improved knowledge of the pathophysiology of BP will hopefully allow the development of new immunomodulatory treatments for this potentially devastating disease.

References

Andrä K, Lassmann H, Bittner R, Shorny S, Fässler R, Propst F, Wiche G (1997) Targeted inactivation of plectin reveals essential function in maintaining the integrity of skin, muscle, and heart cytoarchitecture. Gen Develop 11:3143–3156

Balding SD, Prost C, Diaz LA, Bernard P, Bedane C, Aberdam D, Giudice GJ (1996) Cicatricial pemphigoid autoantibodies react with multiple sites on the BP180 extracellular domain. J Invest Dermatol 106:141–146.

Banfield CC, Wojnarowska F, Allen J, George S, Venning VA, Welsh KI (1998) The association of HLA-DQ7 with bullous pemphigoid is restricted to men. Br J Dermatol 138:1085–1090.

Bastuji-Garin S, Joly P, Picard-Dahan C, Bernard P, Vaillant L, Pauwels C, Salagnac V, Lok C, Roujeau JC (1996) Drugs associated with bullous pemphigoid. A case-control study. Arch Dermatol 132:272–276

Beissert S, Werfel T, Frieling U, Böhm M, Sticherling M, Stadler R, Zillikens D, Rzany B, Hunzelmann N, Meurer M, Gollnick H, Ruzicka T, Pillekamp H, Junghans V, Bonsmann G, Luger TA (2007) A comparison of oral methylprednisolone plus azathioprine or mycophenolate mofetil for the treatment of bullous pemphigoid. Arch Dermatol 143:1536–42

Bernard P, Didierjean L, Denis F, Saurat JH, Bonnetblanc JM (1989) Heterogeneous bullous pemphigoid antibodies: detection and characterization by immunoblotting when absent by indirect immunofluorescence. J Invest Dermatol 92:171–174.

Bernard P, Prost C, Lecerf V, Intrator L, Combemale P, Bedane C, Roujeau JC, Revuz J, Bonnetblanc JM, Dubertret L (1990a) Studies of cicatricial pemphigoid autoantibodies using direct immunelectron microscopy and immunoblot analysis. J Invest Dermatol 94:630–635

Bernard P, Aucouturier P, Denis F, Bonnetblanc JM (1990b) Immunoblot analysis of IgG subclass of circulating antibodies in bullous pemphigoid. Clin Immunol Immunopath 54:484–494

Bernard P, Vaillant L, Labeille B, Bedane C, Arbeille B, Denoeux JP, Lorette G, Bonnetblanc JM, Prost C (1995) Incidence and distribution of subepidermal autoimmune bullous skin diseases in three French regions. Bullous diseases French study group. Arch Dermatol 131:48–52

Bernard P, Reguiai Z, Tancrède-Bohin E, Cordel N, Plantin P, Pauwels C, Vaillant L, Grange F, Richard-Lallemand MA, Sassolas B, Roujeau JC, Lok C, Picard-Dahan C, Chosidow O, Vitry F, Joly P (2009) Risk factors for relapse in patients with bullous pemphigoid in clinical remission: a multicenter, prospective, cohort study. Arch Dermatol 145:537–42

Borradori L, Koch PJ, Niessen CM, Erkeland S, van Leusden M, Sonnenberg A (1997) The localization of bullous pemphigoid antigen 180 (BP180) in hemidesmosomes is mediated by its cytoplasmic domain and seems to be regulated by the b4 integrin subunit. J Cell Biol 136:1333–1347.

Borradori L, Sonnenberg A (1999) Structure and function of hemidesmosomes: more than simple adhesion complexes. J Invest Dermatol 112:411–418.

Briggaman RA, Gammon WR, Woodley DT (1985) Epidermolysis bullosa acquisita of the immunopathological type (dermolytic pemphigoid). J Invest Dermatol 85:79s–84s

Büdinger L, Borradori L, Yee C, Eming R, Ferencik S, Grosse-Wilde H, Merk HF, Yancey K, Hertl M (1998) Identification and characterization of autoreactive T cell responses to bullous pemphigoid antigen 2 in patients and healthy controls. J Clin Invest 102:2082–2089

Burton JL, Harman RM, Peachey RD, Warin RP (1978) A controlled trial of azathioprine in the treatment of pemphigoid. Br J Dermatol 99:14

Calabresi V, Carrozzo M, Cozzani E, Arduino P, Bertolusso G, Tirone F, Parodi A, Zambruno G, Di Zenzo G (2007) Oral pemphigoid autoantibodies preferentially target BP180 ectodomain. Clin Immunol 122:207–213

Chan LS, Yancey KB, Hammerberger C, Soong HK, Regezi JA, Johnson K, Cooper KD (1993) Immune-mediated subepithelial blistering diseases of mucous membranes. Arch Dermatol 129:448–455

Chan LS, Majmudar AA, Tran HH, Meier F, Schaumburg -Lever G, Chen M, Woodley DT, Marinkovich PM (1997) Laminin-6 and laminin-5 are recognized by autoantibodies in a subset of cicatricial pemphigoid. J Invest Dermatol 108:848–853

Chan LS, Vanderlugt CJ, Hashimoto T, Nishikawa T, Zone JJ, Black MM Wojnarowska F, Stevens SR, Chen M, Fairley JA, Woodley DT, Miller SD, Gordon KB (1998) Epitope spreading: lessons from autoimmune skin diseases. J Invest Dermatol 110:103–109

Chan LS, Ahmed AR, Anhalt GJ, Bernauer W, Cooper KD, Elder MJ, Fine JD, Foster CS, Ghohestani R, Hashimoto T, Hoang-Xuan T, Kirtschig G, Korman NJ, Lightman S, Lozada-Nur F, Marinkovich MP, Mondino BJ, Prost-Squarcioni C, Rogers RS 3rd, Setterfield JF, West DP, Wojnarowska F, Woodley DT, Yancey KB, Zillikens D, Zone JJ (2002) The first international consensus on mucous membrane pemphigoid: definition, diagnostic criteria, pathogenic factors, medical treatment, and prognostic indicators. Arch Dermatol 138:370–9

Chen R, Ning G, Zhao ML, Fleming MG, Diaz LA, Werb Z, Liu Z (2001) Mast cells play a key role in neutrophil recruitment in experimental bullous pemphigoid. J Clin Invest 108:1151–8.

Chen R, Fairley JA, Zhao ML, Giudice GJ, Zillikens D, Diaz LA, Liu Z (2002) Macrophages, but not T and B lymphocytes, are critical for subepidermal blister formation in experimental bullous pemphigoid: macrophage-mediated neutrophilinfiltration depends on mast cell activation. J Immunol 169:3987–92.

Chorzelski TP, Jablonska S, Beutner EH, Bean SF, Furey NL (1979) Linear IgA bullous dermatosis. In: Immunopathology and the Skin (Beutner EH, Chorzelski TP, Bean SF, eds). New York, NY: John Wiley & Sons Inc:315–323

Chosidow O, Doppler V, Bensimon G, Joly P, Salachas F, Lacomblez L, Prost C, Camu W, Frances C, Herson S, Meininger V (2000) Bullous pemphigoid and myotrophic lateral sclerosis: a new clue for understanding the bullous disease ? Arch Dermatol 136:521–524.

Christophoridis S, Budinger L, Borradori L, Hunziker T, Merk HF, Hertl M (2000) IgG, IgA and IgE antibodies against the ectodomain of BP180 in patients with bullous and cicatricial pemphigoid and linear IgA bullous dermatosis. Br J Dermatol 143:349–55

Colbert RL, Allen DM, Eastwood D, Fairley JA (2004) Mortality rate of bullous pemphigoid in a US medical center. J Invest Dermatol 122:1091–5

Dainichi T, Kurono S, Ohyama B Ishii N, Sanzen N, Hayashi M, Shimono C, Taniguchi Y, Koga H, Karashima T, Yasumoto S, Zillikens D, Sekiguchi K, Hashimoto T (2009) Anti-laminin gamma-1 pemphigoid. Proc Natl Acad Sci U S A. 106:2800–5.

D'Auria L, Cordiali Fei P, Ameglio F (1999) Cytokines and bullous pemphigoid. Eur Cytokine Netw 10:123–134

Delgado JC, Turbay D, Yunis EJ, Yunis JJ, Morton ED, Bhol K, Norman R, Alper CA, Good RA, Ahmed R (1996) A common major histocompatibility complex class II allele HLA-DQB1* 0301 is present in clinical variants of pemphigoid. Proc Natl Acad Sci 93:8569–8571

Desai N, Allen J, Ali I, Venning V, Wojnarowska F (2008) Autoantibodies to basement membrane proteins BP180 and BP230 are commonly detected in normal subjects by immunoblotting. Australas J Dermatol 49:137–41

Diaz LA, Ratrie H, Saunders WS, Futamura S, Squiquera HL, Anhalt GJ, Giudice GK (1990) Isolation of a human epidermal cDNA corresponding to the 180-kDa autoantigen recognized by bullous pemphigoid and herpes gestationis sera. J Clin Invest 86:1088–1094.

Dilling A, Rose C, Hashimoto T, Zillikens D, Shimanovich I (2007) Anti-p200 pemphigoid: a novel autoimmune subepidermal blistering disease. J Dermatol 34:1–8

Dimson OG, Giudice GJ, Fu CL, Van den Bergh F, Warren SJ, Janson MM, Fairley JA (2003) Identification of a potential effector function for IgE autoantibodies in the organ-specific autoimmune disease bullous pemphigoid. J Invest Dermatol 120:784–8.

Di Zenzo G, Grosso F, Terracina M, Mariotti F, De Pita O, Owaribe K, Mastrogiacomo A, Sera F, Borradori L, Zambruno G (2004) Characterization of the anti-BP180 autoantibody reactivity profile and epitope mapping in bullous pemphigoid patients. J Invest Dermatol 122:103–10

Di Zenzo G, Calabresi V, Grosso F, Caproni M, Ruffelli M, Zambruno G (2007) The intracellular and extracellular domains of BP180 antigen comprise novel epitopes targeted by pemphigoid gestationis autoantibodies. J Invest Dermatol 127:864–73

Di Zenzo G, Thoma-Uszynski S, Fontao L, Calabresi V, Hofmann S C., Hellmark T, Sebbag N, Pedicelli C, Sera F, Lacour JP, Wieslander J, Bruckner-Tuderman L, Borradori L, Zambruno G, Hertl M (2008) Multicenter prospective study of the humoral autoimmune response in bullous pemphigoid. Clin Immunol 128:415–426.

Di Zenzo G, Calabresi V, Olasz EB, Zambruno G, Yancey KB (2010) Sequential intramolecular epitope spreading of humoral responses to human BPAG2 in a transgenic model. J Invest Dermatol 130:1040–1047.

Domolge-Hultsch N, Gammon WR, Briggaman RA, Gil SG, Carter WG, Yancey KB (1992) Epiligrin, the major human keratinocyte ligand, is a target in both an acquired autoimmune and in inherited subepidermal blistering skin disease. J Clin Invest 90:1628–1633

Dreno B, Sassolas B, Lacour P, Montpoint S, Lota I, Giordano F, Royer P (1993) Methylprednisolone versus prednisolone methylsulfobenzoate in pemphigoid: a comparative multicenter study. Ann Dermatol Venereol 120:518–21.

Dresow SK, Sitaru C, Recke A, Oostingh GJ, Zillikens D, Gibbs BF (2009) IgE autoantibodies against the intracellular domain of BP180. Br J Dermatol 160:429–32

Egan CA, Taylor TB, Meyer LJ, Petersen MJ, Zone JJ (1999) Bullous pemphigoid sera that contain antibodies to BPAg2 also contain antibodies to LABD97 that recognize epitopes distal to the NC16A domain. J Invest Dermatol 112:148–52

Egan CA, Reddy D, Nie Z, Taylor TB, Schmidt LA, Meyer LJ, Petersen MJ, Hashimoto T, Marinkovich MP, Zone JJ (2001) IgG anti-LABD97 antibodies in bullous pemphigoid patients' sera react with the mid-portion of the BPAg2 ectodomain. J Invest Dermatol 116:348–50

Egan CA, Lazarova Z, Darling TN, Yee C, Yancey KB (2003) Anti-epiligrin cicatricial pemphigoid: clinical findings, immunopathogenesis, and significant associations. Medicine 82:177–86.

Fairley JA, Fu CL, Giudice GJ (2005) Mapping the binding sites of anti-BP180 immunoglobulin E autoantibodies in bullous pemphigoid. J Invest Dermatol 125:467–72

Fairley JA, Burnett CT, Fu CL, Larson DL, Fleming MG, Giudice GJ (2007) A pathogenic role for IgE in autoimmunity: bullous pemphigoid IgE reproduces the early phase of lesion development in human skin grafted to nu / nu mice. J Invest Dermatol 127:2605–11

Feliciani C, Caldarola G, Kneisel A, Podstawa E, Pfütze M, Pfützner W, Hertl M (2009) IgG autoantibody reactivity against bullous pemphigoid (BP) 180 and BP230 in elderly patients with
pruritic dermatoses. Br J Dermatol 161:306–312

Feng S, Lin L, Jin P, Wu Q, Zhou W, Sang H, Shao C (2008) Role of BP180NC16a-enzyme-linked
immunosorbent assay (ELISA) in the diagnosis of bullous pemphigoid in China. Int J Dermatol
47:24–8

Fivenson DP; Breneman DL; Rosen GB; Hersh CS; Cardone S; Mutasim (1994) Nicotinamide and
tetracycline therapy of bullous pemphigoid. Arch Dermatol 6:753–758

Fontao L, Favre B, Riou S, Geerts D, Jaunin F, Saurat JH, Green KJ, Sonnenberg A, Borradori L
(2003) Interaction of the bullous pemphigoid antigen 1 (BP230) and desmoplakin with intermediate filaments is mediated by distinct sequences within their COOH terminus. Mol Biol
Cell 14:1978–92.

Franzke CW, Tasanen K, Borradori L, Huotari V, Bruckner-Tuderman L (2004) Shedding of
collagen XVII / BP180: Structural motifs influence cleavage from cell surface. J Biol Chem
279:24521–24529.

Gammon WR, Briggaman RA, Inman AO III, Queen LL, Wheeler CE (1984a) Differentiating anti-
lamina lucida and anti-sublamina densa anti-BMZ antibodies by indirect immunofluorescence
on 1.0 M sodium chloride-separated skin. J Invest Dermatol 82:139–144.

Gammon WR, Inman AO III, Wheeler CE Jr. (1984b) Differences in complement-dependent
chemotactic activity generated by bullous pemphigoid and epidermolysis bullosa acquisita immune complexes: demonstration by leukocytic attachment and organ culture methods. J Invest
Dermatol 83:57–61

Gammon WR, Kowalewski C, Chorzelski TP, Kumar V, Briggaman RA, Beutner EH (1990) Direct
immunofluorescence studies of sodium chloride-separated skin in the differential diagnosis of
bullous pemphigoid and epidermolysis bullosa acquisita. J Am Acad Dermatol 22:664–670

Gammon WR, Briggaman RA (1993) Epidermolysis bullosa acquisita and bullous systemic lupus
erythematosus. Dermat Clin 11:535–547

Gaucherand M, Nicolas JF, Paranhos Baccala G, Rouault JP, Réano A, Magaud JP, Thivolet J, Jolivet
M, Schmitt D (1995) Major antigenic epitopes of bullous pemphigoid 230 kDa antigen map
within the C-terminal end of the protein. Evidence using a 55 kDa recombinant protein. Br J
Dermatol 132:190–6

Ghohestani RF, Nicolas JF, Kanitakis J, Claudy A (1997) Linear IgA bullous dermatosis with IgA
antibod ies exclusively directed against the 180- and 230-kDa epidermal antigens J Invest Dermatol 108:854–858

Ghohestani RF, Cozzani E, Delaporte E, Nicolas JF, Parodi A, Claudy A (1998) IgE antibodies in
sera from patients with bullous pemphigoid are autoantibodies preferentially directed against
the 230-kDa epidermal antigen (BP230). J Clin Immunol 18:202–9

Giudice GJ, Squiquera HL, Elias PM, Diaz LA (1991) Identification of two collagen domains within
the bullous pemphigoid autoantigen, BP180. J Clin Invest 87:734–738

Giudice GJ, Emery DJ, Diaz LA (1992) Cloning and primary structural analysis of the bullous
pemphigoid autoantigen BP180. J Invest Dermatol 99:243–250.

Giudice GJ, Emery DJ, Zelickson BD, Anhalt GJ, Liu Z , Diaz LA (1993) Bullous pemphigoid and
herpes gestationis autoantibodies recognize a common non-collagenous site on the BP180 ectodomain. J Immunol 151:5742–5750

Giudice GJ, Wilske KC, Anhalt GJ, Fairley JA, Taylor AF, Emery DJ, Hofman RG, Diaz LA (1994)
Development of an ELISA to detect anti-BP180 autoantibodies in bullous pemphigoid and herpes gestationis. J Invest Dermatol 102:878–881

Green KJ, Virata MLA, Elgart GW, Stanley JR, Parry DAD (1992) Comparative structural analysis
of desmoplakin, bullous pemphigoid antigen and plectin: members of a new gene family involved in organization of intermediate filaments. Int J Biol Macromol 14:145–153

Groves RW, Liu L, Dopping-Hepenstal PJ, Markus HS, Lovell PA, Ozoemena L, Lai-Cheong JE, Gawler J, Owaribe K, Hashimoto T, Mellerio JE, Mee JB, McGrath JA (2010) A homozygous nonsense mutation within the dystonin gene coding for the coiled-coil domain of the epithelial isoform of BPAG1 underlies a new subtype of autosomal recessive epidermolysis bullosa simplex. J Invest Dermatol, e-pub Feb 18

Guillaume JC, Vaillant L, Bernard P, Picard C, Prost C, Labeille B, Guillot B, Foldes-Pauwels C, Prigent F, Joly P (1993) Controlled trial of azathioprine and plasma exchange in addition to prednisolone in the treatment of bullous pemphigoid. Arch Dermatol 129:49–53

Günther C, Carballido-Perrig N, Kopp T, Carballido JM, Pfeiffer C (2009) CCL18 is expressed in patients with bullous pemphigoid and parallels disease course. Br J Dermatol 160:747–55

Guo L, Degenstein L, Dowling J-C, Yu QC, Wollmann R, Perman B, Fuchs E (1995) Gene targeting of BPAG1: abnormalities in mechanical strength and cell migration in stratified epithelia and neurologic degeneration. Cell 81:233–243

Haase C, Büdinger L, Borradori L, Yee C, Merk HF, Yancey KB, Hertl M (1998) Detection of IgG autoantibodies in the sera of patients with bullous and gestational pemphigoid: ELISA studies utilizing a baculovirus-encoded form of bullous pemphigoid antigen 2. J Invest Dermatol 110:282–286

Hachisuka H, Kurose K, Karashima T, Mori O, Maeyama Y (1996) Serum from elderly individuals contains anti-basement membrane zone antibodies. Arch Dermatol 132:1201–1205

Hall RP 3rd, Murray JC, McCord MM, Rico JM, Streilein RD (1993) Rabbits immunized with a peptide encoded for by the 230-kd bullous pemphigoid antigen cDNA develop an enhanced inflammatory response to UVB irradiation: a potential animal model for bullous pemphigoid. J Invest Dermatol 101:9–14.

Hamada T, Nagata Y, Tomita M, Salmhofer W, Hashimoto T (2001) Bullous pemphigoid sera react specifically with various domains of BP230, most frequently with C-terminal domain, by immunoblot analyses using bacterial recombinant proteins covering the entire molecule. Exp Dermatol 10:256–63

Hashimoto T, Ishiko, A, Shimizu H, Tanaka T, Dodd HJ, Bhogal BS, Black MM, Nishikava T (1996) A case of linear IgA bullous dermatosis with IgA anti-type VII collagen autoantiboies. Br J Dermatol 134:336–339

Hata Y, Fujii Y, Tsunoda K, Amagai M (2000) Production of the entire extracellular domain of BP180 (type XVII collagen) by baculovirus expression. J Dermatol Sci 23:183–90

Hirako Y, Usukura J, Uematsu J, Hashimoto T, Kitajima Y, Owaribe K (1998) Cleavage of BP180, a 180-kDa bullous pemphigoid antigen, yields a 120-kDa collagenous extracellular polypeptide. J Biol Chem 273:9711–9717

Hirako Y, Nishizawa Y, Sitaru C, Opitz A, Marcus K, Meyer HE, Butt E, Owaribe K, Zillikens D (2003) The 97-kDa (LABD97) and 120-kDa (LAD-1) fragments of bullous pemphigoid antigen 180 / type XVII collagen have different N-termini. J Invest Dermatol 121:1554–6.

Hofmann S, Thoma-Uszynski S, Hunziker T, Bernard P, Koebnick C, Stauber A, Schuler G, Borradori L, Hertl M (2002) Severity and phenotype of bullous pemphigoid relate to autoantibody profile against the NH2- and COOH-terminal regions of the BP180 ectodomain. J Invest Dermatol 119:1065–73.

Hofmann SC, Tamm K, Hertl M, Borradori L (2003) Diagnostic value of an enzyme-linked immunosorbent assay using BP180 recombinant proteins in elderly patients with pruritic skin disorders. Br J Dermatol 149:910–12

Hofmann SC, Otto C, Bruckner-Tuderman L, Borradori L (2009) Isolated NC16a-ELISA testing is of little value to identify bullous pemphigoid in elderly patients with chronic pruritus. Eur J Dermatol 19:634–5

Hopkinson SB, Riddelle KS, Jones JCR (1992) Cytoplasmic domain of the 180-kD bullous pemphigoid antigen, a hemidesmosomal component: molecular and cell biologic characterization. J Invest Dermatol 99:264–270.

Hopkinson SB, Baker SE, Jones JCR (1995) Molecular genetic studies of a human epidermal autoantigen (the 180-kD bullous pemphigoid antigen / BP180): identification of functionally important sequences within the BP180 molecule and evidence for an interaction between BP180 and α6 integrin. J Cell Biol 130:117–125

Husz S, Kiss M, Molnar K, Marczinovits I, Molnár J, Tóth GK, Dobozy A (2000) Development of a system for detection of circulating antibodies against hemdesmosomal proteins in patients with bullous pemphigoid. Arch Dermatol Res 292:217–24

Ide A, Hashimoto T, Amagai M, Tanaka M, Nishikawa T (1995) Detection of autoantibodies against the bullous pemphigoid and pemphigus antigens by an enzyme-linked immunosorbent assay using the bacterial recombinant proteins. Exp Dermatol 5:112–116

Iwata H, Kamio N, Aoyama Y, Yamamoto Y, Hirako Y, Owaribe K, Kitajima Y (2009) IgG from patients with bullous pemphigoid depletes cultured keratinocytes of the 180-kDa bullous pemphigoid antigen (type XVII collagen) and weakens cell attachment. J Invest Dermatol 129:919–26

Jedlickova H, Racovska J, Niedermeier A, Feit J, Hertl M (2008) Anti-basement membrane zone antibodies in elderly patients with pruritic disorders and diabetes mellitus. Eur J Dermatol 18:534–8.

Jenkins RE, Shornick JK, Black MM (1993) Pemphigoid gestationis. J Eur Acad Dermatol 2:163–173

Joly P, Roujeau JC, Benichou J, Picard C, Dreno B, Delaporte E, Vaillant L, D'Incan M, Plantin P, Bedane C, Young P, Bernard P, Bullous Diseases French Study Group (2002) A comparison of oral and topical corticosteroids in patients with bullous pemphigoid. N Engl J Med; 346:321–7

Joly P, Courville P, Lok C, Bernard P, Saiag P, Dreno B, Delaporte E, Bedane C, Picard C, Sassolas B, Plantin P, D'Incan M, Chosidow O, Pauwels C, Lambert D, Loche F, Prost C, Tancrede-Bohin E, Guillaume JC, Roujeau JC, Gilbert D, Tron F, Vaillant L, French Bullous Study Group (2004) Clinical criteria for the diagnosis of bullous pemphigoid: a reevaluation according to immunoblot analysis of patient sera. Dermatology 208:16–20

Joly P, Benichou J, Lok C, Hellot MF, Saiag P, Tancrede-Bohin E, Sassolas B, Labeille B, Doutre MS, Gorin I, Pauwels C, Chosidow O, Caux F, Estève E, Dutronc Y, Sigal M, Prost C, Maillard H, Guillaume JC, Roujeau JC (2005) Prediction of survival for patients with bullous pemphigoid: a prospective study.Arch Dermatol 141:691–8

Joly P, Roujeau JC, Benichou J, Delaporte E, D'Incan M, Dreno B, Bedane C, Sparsa A, Gorin I, Picard C, Tancrede-Bohin E, Sassolas B, Lok C, Guillaume JC, Doutre MS, Richard MA, Caux F, Prost C, Plantin P, Chosidow O, Pauwels C, Maillard H, Saiag P, Descamps V, Chevrant-Breton J, Dereure O, Hellot MF, Esteve E, Bernard P (2009) A comparison of two regimens of topical corticosteroids in the treatment of patients with bullous pemphigoid: a multicenter randomized study. J Invest Dermatol 129:1681–7

Jonkman MF, de Jong MC, Heeres K, Pas HH, van der Meer JB, Owaribe K, Martinez de Velasco AM, Niessen CM, Sonnenberg A (1995) 180-kD bullous pemphigoid antigen (BP180) is deficient in generalized atrophic benign epidermolysis bullosa. J Clin Invest 95:1345–1352.

Jordon RE, Beutner EH, Witebsky E, Blumental G, Hale WC, Lever WC (1967) Basement zone antibodies in bullous pemphigoid. J Am Med Assoc 200:751–756

Jung M, Kippes W, Messer G, Zillikens D, Rzany B (1999) Increased risk of bullous pemphigoid in male and very old patients: a population based study on incidence. J Am Acad Dermatol 41:266–268

Kawahara Y, Amagai M, Ohata Y, Ishii K, Hasegawa Y, Hsu R, Yee C, Yancey KB, Nishikawa T (1998) A case of cicatricial pemphigoid with simultaneous IgG autoantibodies against the 180 kd bullous pemphigoid antigen and laminin 5. J Am Acad Dermatol 38:624–627

Kiss M, Husz S, Janossy T, Marczinovits I, Molnár J, Korom I, Dobozy A (2005) Experimental bullous pemphigoid generated in mice with an antigenic epitope of the human hemidesmosomal protein BP230. J Autoimmun 24:1–10

3

Kobayashi M, Amagai M, Kuroda-Kinoshita K, Hashimoto T, Shirakata Y, Hashimoto K, Nishikawa T (2002) BP180 ELISA using bacterial recombinant NC16a protein as a diagnostic and monitoring tool for bullous pemphigoid. J Dermatol Sci 30:224–32

Koster J, Geerts D, Favre B, Borradori L, Sonnenberg A (2003) Analysis of the interactions between BP180, BP230, plectin and the integrin alpha6beta4 important for hemidesmosome assembly. J Cell Sci; 116:387–99

Korman NJ (1987) Bullous pemphigoid. J Am Acad Dermatol 16:907–24

Korman NJ (2000) New and emerging therapies in the treatment of blistering diseases. Dermatol Clin 18:127–137

Kromminga A, Sitaru C, Hagel C, Herzog S, Zillikens D (2004) Development of an ELISA for the detection of autoantibodies to BP230. Cli Immunol 111:146–52

Labib RS, Anhalt GJ, Patel HP, Mutasim DF, Diaz LA (1986) Molecular heterogeneity of the bullous pemphigoid antigens as detected by immunoblotting. J Immunol 136:1231–1235.

Laffitte E, Borradori L (2001) Fiche thérapeutique: prise en charge de la pemphigoïde bulleuse. Ann Dermatol Venerol 128:677–80

Laffitte E, Favre B, Fontao L, Riou S, Jaunin F, Tamm K, Saurat J-H, Borradori L (2001) Plectin, an unusual target in bullous pemphigoid. Br J Dermatol 44:136–8

Laffitte E, Burkhard PR, Fontao L, Jaunin F, Saurat JH, Chofflon M, Borradori L (2005) Bullous pemphigoid antigen 1 isoforms: potential new target auto-antigens in multiple sclerosis? Br J Dermatol 152:537–54.

Leung CL, Zheng M, Prater SM, Liem RK (2001) The BPAG1 locus: Alternative splicing produces multiple isoforms with distinct cytoskeletal linker domains, including predominant isoforms in neurons and muscles. J Cell Biol 20 154:691–7.

Lever WF (1953) Pemphigus. Medicine 32:1–123

Leyendeckers H, Tasanen K, Bruckner-Tuderman L, Zillikens D, Sitaru C, Schmitz J, Hunzelmann N (2003) Memory B cells specific for the NC16A domain of the 180 kDa bullous pemphigoid autoantigen can be detected in peripheral blood of bullous pemphigoid patientsand induced in vitro to synthesize autoantibodies. J Invest Dermatol 120(3):372–8

Li K, Guidice GJ, Tamai K, Do HC, Sawamura D, Diaz LA, Uitto J (1992) Cloning of partial cDNA for mouse 180-kDa bullous pemphigoid antigen (BPAG2), a highly conserved collagenous protein of the cutaneous basement membrane zone. J Invest Dermatol 99:258–63.

Lin MS, Gharia MA, Swartz SJ, Diaz LA, Giudice GJ (1999) Identification and characterization of epitopes recognized by T lymphocytes and autoantibodies from patients with herpes gestationis J Immunol 162:4999–4997

Lindelöf B, Islam N, Eklund G, Arfors L (1990) Pemphigoid and cancer. Arch Dermatol 126:66–68

Liu HH, Su DWP, Rogers RS III (1986) Clinical variants of pemphigoid. Int J Dermatol 25:17–27

Liu Z, Diaz LA, Troy JL, Taylor AF, Emery DJ, Fairley JA, Giudice GJ (1993) A passive transfer model of the organ-specific autoimmune disease, bullous pemphigoid, using antibodies generated against the hemidesmosomal antigen, BP180. J Clin Invest 92:2480–2488

Liu Z, Giudice GJ, Swartz SJ, Fairley JA, Till GO, Troy JL, Diaz LA (1995) The role of complement in experimental bullous pemphigoid. J Clin Invest 95:1539–44

Liu Z, Giudice GJ, Zhou X, Swartz SJ, Troy JL, Fairley JA, Till GO, Diaz LA (1997) A major role for neutrophils in experimental bullous pemphigoid. J Clin Invest 100:1256–63

Liu Z, Shipley JM, Vu TH, Zhou X, Diaz LA, Werb Z, Senior RM (1998) Gelatinase B-deficient mice are resistant to experimental bullous pemphigoid. J Exp Med 188:475–82

Liu Z, Shapiro SD, Zhou X, Twining SS, Senior RM, Giudice GJ, Fairley JA, Diaz LA (2000a) A critical role for neutrophil elastase in experimental bullous pemphigoid. J Clin Invest 105:113–123

Liu Z, Zhou X, Shapiro SD, Shipley JM, Twining SS, Diaz LA, Senior RM, Werb Z (2000b) The serpin alpha1-proteinase inhibitor is a critical substrate for gelatinase B/MMP-9 in vivo. Cell 102:647–55

Liu Z, Li N, Diaz LA, Shipley M, Senior RM, Werb Z (2005) Synergy between a plasminogen cascade and MMP-9 in autoimmune disease. J Clin Invest 115:879–87

Liu Z, Sui W, Zhao M, Li Z, Li N, Thresher R, Giudice GJ, Fairley JA, Sitaru C, Zillikens D, Ning G, Marinkovich MP, Diaz LA (2008) Subepidermal blistering induced by human autoantibodies to BP180 requires innate immune players in a humanized bullous pemphigoid mouse model. J Autoimmun 31:331–8

Luke MC, Darling TN, Hsu R, Summers RM, Smith JA, Solomon BI, Thomas GR, Yancey KB (1999) Mucosal morbidity in patients with epidermolysis bullosa acquisita. Arch Dermatol 135:954–95.9

Marazza G, Pham HC, Schärer L, Pedrazzetti PP, Hunziker T, Trüeb RM, Hohl D, Itin P, Lautenschlager S, Naldi L, Borradori L, Autoimmune bullous disease Swiss study group (2009) Incidence of bullous pemphigoid and pemphigus in Switzerland: a 2-year prospective study. Br J Dermatol 161:861–8.

Mariotti F, Grosso F, Terracina M, Ruffelli M, Cordiali-Fei P, Sera F, Zambruno G, Mastrogiacomo A, Di Zenzo G (2004) Development of a novel ELISA system for detection of anti-BP180 IgG and characterization of autoantibody profile in bullous pemphigoid patients. Br J Dermatol 151:1004–10

Masouyé I, Schmid E, Didierjean L, Abba Z, Saurat JH (1989) Bullous pemphigid and multiple sclerosis: more than a coincidence? Report of three cases. J Am cad Dermatol 21:63–68

McGrath JA, Gatalica B, Christiano AM, Li K, Owaribe K, McMillan JR, Eady RA, Uitto J (1995) Mutations in the 180-kD bullous pemphigoid antigen (BPAG2), a hemidesmosomal transmembrane collagen (COL17A1), in generalized atrophic benign epidermolysis bullosa. Nature Genet 11:83–86

Messingham KA, Noe MH, Chapman MA, Giudice GJ, Fairley JA (2009) A novel ELISA reveals high frequencies of BP180-specific IgE production in bullous pemphigoid. J Immunol Methods 346:18–25

Miller JE, Rico JM, Hall RP (1993) IgG antibodies from patients with bullous pemphigoid bind to fusion proteins encoded by BPAg1 cDNA. J Invest Dermatol 101:779–782.

Morel P, Guillaume JC (1984) Treatment of bullous pemphigoid with prednisolone only: 0.75 mg/kg/day versus 1.25 mg/kg/day. A multicenter randomized study Ann Dermatol Venereol 111:925–928

Morrison LH, Labib RS, Zone JJ, Diaz LA, Anhalt GJ (1988) Herpes gestationis autoantibodies recognize a 180-kD human epidermal antigen. J Clin Invest 8:2023–2026.

Mueller S, Klaus-Kovtun V, Stanley JR (1989) A 230 kD basic protein is the major bullous pemphigoid antigen. J Invest Dermatol 92:32–38.

Murakami H, Nishioka S, Setterfield J, Bhogal BS, Black MM, Zillikens D, Yancey KB, Balding SD, Giudice GJ, Diaz LA, Nishikawa T, Kiyokawa C, Hashimoto T (1998) Analysis of antigens targeted by circulating IgG and IgA autoantibodies in 50 patients with cicatricial pemphigoid. J Dermatol Sci 17:39–44

Mutasim DF, Pelc NJ, Anhalt GJ (1993) Cicatricial pemphigoid. Dermatol Clin 11:499–510

Nakatani C, Muramatsu T, Shirai T (1998) Immunoreactivity of bullous pemphigoid (BP) autantibodies against the NC16A and C-terminal domains of the 180 kDa BP antigen (BP180): immunoblot analysis and enzyme-linked immunosorbent assay using BP180 recombinant proteins. Br J Dermatol 139:365–70

Nelson KC, Zhao M, Schroeder PR, Li N, Wetsel RA, Diaz LA, Liu Z (2006) Role of different pathways of the complement cascade in experimental bullous pemphigoid. J Clin Invest 116:2892–900

Nemeth AJ, Klein AD, Gould EW, Schachner LA (1991) Childhood bullous pemphigoid. Clinical and immunologic features, treatment, and prognosis. Arch Dermatol 127:378–386

Nie Z, Hashimoto T (1999) IgA antibodies of cicatricial pemphigoid sera specifically react with C-terminus of BP180. J Invest Dermatol 112:254–5.

Nishie W, Sawamura D, Goto M, Ito K, Shibaki A, McMillan JR, Sakai K, Nakamura H, Olasz E, Yancey KB, Akiyama M, Shimizu H (2007) Humanization of autoantigen. Nat Med 13:378–83.

Nishie W, Sawamura D, Natsuga K, Shinkuma S, Goto M, Shibaki A, Ujiie H, Olasz E, Yancey KB, Shimizu H (2009) A novel humanized neonatal autoimmune blistering skin disease model induced by maternally transferred antibodies. J Immunol 183:4088–93.

Olasz EB, Roh J, Yee CL, Arita K, Akiyama M, Shimizu H, Vogel JC, Yancey KB (2007) Human bullous pemphigoid antigen 2 transgenic skin elicits specific IgG in wild-type mice. J Invest Dermatol 127:2807–17.

Olivry T, Chan LS, Xu L, Chace P, Dunston SM, Fahey M, Marinkovich MP (1999) Novel feline autoimmune blistering disease resembling bullous pemphigoid in humans: IgG autoantibodies target the NC16A ectodomain of type XVII collagen (BP180/BPAG2). Vet Pathol 36:328–35

Olivry T, Borrillo AK, Xu L, Dunston SM, Slovis NM, Affolter VK, Demanuelle TC, Chan LS (2000a) Equine bullous pemphigoid IgG autoantibodies target linear epitopes in the NC16A ectodomain of collagen XVII (BP180, BPAG2). Vet Immunol Immunopathol 73:45–52

Olivry T, Mirsky ML, Singleton W, Dunston SM, Borillo AK, Xu L, Traczyk T, Rosolia DL, Chan LS (2000b) A spontaneously rising porcine model of bullous pemphigoid. Arch Dermatol Res 292:37–45

Okazaki A, Miyagawa S, Yamashina Y, Kitamura W, Shirai T (2000) Polymorphisms of HLA-DR and -DQ genes in Japanese patients with bullous pemphigoid. J Dermatol 27:149–156

Oswald E, Fisch P, Jakob T, Bruckner-Tuderman L, Martin SF, Rensing-Ehl A (2009) Reduced numbers of circulating gammadelta T cells in patients with bullous pemphigoid. Exp Dermatol 18:991–3

Pas HH, Kloosterhuis GJ, Heeres K, van der Meer JB, Jonkman MF (1997) Bullous pemphigoid and linear IgA dermatosis sera recognize a similar 120-kDa keratinocyte collagenous glycoprotein with antigenic cross-reactivity to BP180. J Invest Dermatol 108:423–429

Perriard J, Jaunin F, Favre B, Büdinger L, Hertl M, Saurat J-H, Borradori L (1999) IgG autoantibodies from bullous pemphigoid (BP) patients bind antigenic sites on both the extracellular and the intracellular domain of the BP antigen 180. J Invest Dermatol 112:141–147.

Reguiaï Z, Tchen T, Perceau G, Bernard P (2009) Efficacy of rituximab in a case of refractory bullous pemphigoid. Ann Dermatol Venereol 136:431–4

Rensing-Ehl A, Gaus B, Bruckner-Tuderman L, Martin SF (2007) Frequency, function and CLA expression of CD4 + CD25 + FOXP3 + regulatory T cells in bullous pemphigoid. Exp Dermatol 16:13–21

Rico MJ, Korman NJ, Stanley JR, Tanaka T, Hall RP (1990) IgG antibodies from patients with bullous pemphigoid bind to localized epitopes on synthetic peptides encoded bullous pemphigoid antigen cDNA. J Immunol 145:3728–3733.

Rieckhoff-Cantoni L, Bernard P, Didierjean L, Imhof K, Kinloch-de-Loes S, Saurat JH (1992) Frequency of bullous pemphigoid-like antibodies as detected by Western immunoblot analysis in pruritic dermatoses. Arch Dermatol 128:791–794

Romagnani S (1992) Human Th1 and Th2 subsets: regulation of differentiation and role in protection and immunopathology. Int Arch Allergy Appl Immunol 98:279–285.

Roujeau JC, Lok C, Bastuji-Garin S, Mhalla S, Enginger V, Bernard P (1998) High risk of death in elderly patients with extensive bullous pemphigoid. Arch Dermatol 134:465–469

Rzany B, Partscht K, Jung M, Kippes W, Mecking D, Baima B, Prudlo C, Pawelczyk B, Messmer EM, Schuhmann M, Sinkgraven R, Büchner L, Büdinger L, Pfeiffer C, Sticherling M, Hertl M, Kaiser HW, Meurer M, Zillikens D, Messer G (2002) Risk factors for lethal outcome in patients with bullous pemphigoid: low serum albumin level, high dosage of glucocorticosteroids, and old age. Arch Dermatol 138:903–8

Sakuma-Oyama Y, Powell AM, Oyama N, Albert S, Bhogal BS, Black MM (2004) Evaluation of a BP180-NC16a enzymelinked immunosorbent assay in the initial diagnosis of bullous pemphigoid. Br J Dermatol 151:126–31

Sawamura D, Li K, Chu ML, Uitto J (1991) Human bullous pemphigoid antigen (BPAG1). Amino acid sequences deduced from cloned cDNAs predict biologically important peptide segments and protein domains. J Biol Chem 266:17784–17790.

Schäcke H, Schumann H, Hammami-Hauasli N, Raghunath M, Bruckner-Tuderman L (1998) Two forms of collagen XVII in keratinocytes. A full-length transmembrane protein and a soluble ectodomain. J Biol Chem 273:25937–25943

Schmidt E, Obe K, Brocker EB, Zillikens D (2000a) Serum levels of autoantibdies to BP180 correlate with disease activity in patients with bullous pemphigoid. Arch Dermatol 136:174–178

Schmidt E, Reimer S, Kruse N, Jainta S, Brocker EB, Marinkovich MP, Giudice GJ, Zillikens D (2000b) Autoantibodies to BP180 associated with bullous pemphigoid release interleukin-6 and interleukin-8 from cultured human keratinocytes. J Invest Dermatol 115:842–848

Schmidt E, Wehr B, Tabengwa EM, Reimer S, Brocker EB, Zillikens D (2004) Elevated expression and release of tissue-type, but not urokinase-type, plasminogen activator after binding of autoantibodies to bullous pemphigoid antigen 180 incultured human keratinocytes. Clin Exp Immunol 135:497–504

Schumann H, Baetge J, Tasanen K, Wojnarowska F, Schäcke H, Zillikens D, Bruckner-Tuderman L (2000) The shed ectodomain of collagen XVII / BP180 is targeted by autoantibodies in different blistering skin diseases. Am J Pathol 156:685–95

Shimanovich I, Mihai S, Oostingh GJ, Ilenchuk TT, Bröcker EB, Opdenakker G, Zillikens D, Sitaru C (2004) Granulocyte-derived elastase and gelatinase B are required for dermal-epidermal separation induced by autoantibodies from patients with epidermolysis bullosa acquisita and bullous pemphigoid. J Pathol 204:519–27

Shornick JK (1993) Herpes gestationis. Dermatol Clin 11:527–533

Sitaru C, Schmidt E, Petermann S, Munteanu LS, Bröcker EB, Zillikens D (2002) Autoantibodies to bullous pemphigoid antigen 180 induce dermal-epidermal separation in cryosections of human skin. J Invest Dermatol 118:664–71

Sitaru C, Dähnrich C, Probst C, Komorowski L, Blöcker I, Schmidt E, Schlumberger W, Rose C, Stöcker W, Zillikens D (2007) Enzyme-linked immunosorbent assay using multimers of the 16th non-collagenous domain of the BP180 antigen for sensitive and specific detection of pemphigoid autoantibodies. Exp Dermatol 16:770–7

Skaria M, Jaunin F, Hunziker T, Riou S, Schumann H, Bruckner-Tuderman L, Hertl M, Bernard P, Saurat JH, Favre B, Borradori L (2000) IgG autoantibodies from bullous pemphigoid patients recognize multiple antigenic reactive sites located predominantly within the B and C subdomain of the COOH-terminus of BP230. J Invest Dermatol 114:998–1004

Stahle-Bäckdahl M, Inoue M, Giudice GJ, Parks WC (1994) 92-kD gelatinase is produced by eosinophils at the site of blister formation in bullous pemphigoid and cleaves the extracellular domain of recombinant 180 kD in bullous pemphigoid autoantigen. J Clin Invest 93:2022–2230

Stanley JR, Hawley-Nelson P, Yuspa SH, Shevach EM, Katz SI (1981) Characterization of bullous pemphigoid antigen: a unique basement membrane protein of stratified squamous epithelia. Cell 24:897–903

Stanley JR, Tanaka T, Mueller S, Klaus-Kovtun V, Roop D (1988) Isolation of complementary DNA for bullous pemphigoid antigen by use of patients' autoantibodies. J Clin Invest 82:1864–1870

Steiner-Champliaud MF, Schneider Y, Favre B, Paulhe F, Praetzel-Wunder S, Faulkner G, Konieczny P, Raith M, Wiche G, Adebola A, Liem RK, Langbein L, Sonnenberg A, Fontao L, Borradori L (2010) BPAG1 isoform-b: complex distribution pattern in striated and heart muscle and association with plectin and alpha-actinin. Exp Cell Res 316:297–313

Szabolcs P, Reese M, Yancey KB, Hall RP, Kurtzberg J (2002) Combination treatment of bullous pemphigoid with anti-CD20 and anti-CD25 antibodies in a patient with chronic graft-versus-host disease. Bone Marrow Transplant 30:327–9

Tampoia M, Lattanzi V, Zucano A, Villalta D, Filotico R, Fontana A, Vena GA, Di Serio F (2009) Evaluation of a new ELISA assay for detection of BP230 autoantibodies in bullous pemphigoid. Ann N Y Acad Sci 1173:15–20

Tanaka M, Hashimoto T, Amagai M, Shimizu N, Ikeguchi N, Tsubata T, Hasegawa A, Miki K, Nishikawa T (1991) Characterization of bullous pemphigoid antibodies by use of recombinant bullous pemphigoid antigen proteins. J Invest Dermatol 97:725–728.

Taylor G, Venning V, Wojnarowska F, Welch K (1993) Bullous pemphigoid and autoimmunity. J Am Acad Dermatol 29:181–184

Thoma-Uszynski S, Uter W, Schwietzke S, Hofmann SC, Hunziker T, Bernard P, Treudler R, Zouboulis CC, Schuler G, Borradori L, Hertl M (2004) BP230- and BP180 specific autoantibodies in bullous pemphigoid. J Invest Dermatol 122:1413–1422

Thoma-Uszynski S, Uter W, Schwietzke S, Schuler G, Borradori L, Hertl M (2006) Auto-reactive T and B cells from bullous pemphigoid (BP) patients recognize similar antigenic regions of BP180 and BP230. J Immunol 176:2015–23

Trüeb RM, Didierjean L, Fellas A, Avraam E, Borradori L (1999) Childhood bullous pemphigoid. Report of a case with characterization of the targeted antigens. J Am Acad Dermatol 40:338–344

Tsuji-Abe Y, Akiyama M, Yamanaka Y, Kikuchi T, Sato-Matsumura KC, Shimizu H (2005) Correlation of clinical severity and ELISA indices for the NC16A domain of BP180 measured using BP180 ELISA kit in bullous pemphigoid. J Dermatol Sci 37:145–9

Tyagi S, Bhol K, Natarajan K, Livir-Rallatos C, Foster CS, Ahmed AR (1996) Ocular cicatricial pemphigoid antigen: partial sequence and biochemical characterization. Proc Natl Acad Sci USA 93:14714–14719

Ujiie H, Shibaki A, Nishie W, Sawamura D, Wang G, Tateishi Y, Li Q, Moriuchi R, Qiao H, Nakamura H, Akiyama M, Shimizu H (2010) A novel active mouse model for bullous pemphigoid targeting humanized pathogenic antigen. J Immunol 184:2166–74

Vaillant L, Bernard P, Joly P, Labeille B, Bedane C, Arbeille B, Thomine B, Bertrand B, Lok C, Roujeau JC (1998) Evaluation of clinical criteria for diagnosis of bullous pemphigoid. French bullous study group. Arch Dermatol 134:1075–1080

Vanderlugt CJ, Miller SD (1996) Epitope spreading. Curr Opin Immunol 8:831–836

Vassileva S (1998) Drug-induced pemphigoid: bullous and cicatricial. Clin Dermatol 16:379–387

Venning VA, Millard PR, Wojnarowska F (1989) Dapsone as first line therapy for bullous pemphigoid. Br J Dermato 120:83–92

Venning VA, Wojnarowska F (1990) The association of bullous pemphigoid and malignant disease: a case control study. Br J Dermatol 123:439–445

Verraes S, Hornebeck W, Polette M, Borradori L, Bernard P (2001) Respective contribution of neutrophil elastase and matrix metalloproteinase 9 in the degradation of BP180 (type XVII collagen) in human bullous pemphigoid. J Invest Dermatol 117:1091–6

Waisbourd-Zinman O, Ben-Amitai D, Cohen AD, Feinmesser M, Mimouni D, Adir-Shani A, Zlotkin M, Zvulunov A (2008) Bullous pemphigoid in infancy: Clinical and epidemiologic characteristics. J Am Acad Dermatol 58:41–8

Wakugawa M, Nakamura K, Hino H, Toyama K, Hattori N, Okochi H, Yamada H, Hirai K, Tamaki K, Furue M (2000) Elevated levels of eotaxin and interleukin-5 in blister fluid of bullous pemphigoid: correlation with tissue eosinophilia. Br J Dermatol 143:112–116

Wieland CN, Comfere NI, Gibson LE, Weaver AL, Krause PK, Murray JA (2010) Anti-bullous pemphigoid 180 and 230 antibodies in a sample of unaffected subjects. Arch Dermatol 146:21–5

Wojnarowska F, Marsden RA, Bhogal B, Black MM (1988) Chronic bullous disease of childhood, childhood cicatricial pemphigoid, and linear IgA disease of adults. A comparative study demonstrating clinical and immunological overlap. J Am Acad Dermatol 19:792–805

Wojnarowska F, Whitehead P, Leigh IM, Bhogal BS, Black MM (1991) Identification of the target antigen in chronic bullous disease of childhood and linear IgA disease of adults. Br J Dermatol 124:157–162

Woodley DT, Briggaman RA, O'Keefe EJ, Inman AO, Queen LL, Gammon WR (1984) Identification of the skin basement-membrane autoantigen in epidermolysis bullosa acquisita. N Engl J Med 310:1007–1013

Zhao M, Trimbeger ME, Li N, Diaz LA, Shapiro SD, Liu Z (2006) Role of FcRs in animal model of autoimmune bullous pemphigoid. J Immunol 177:3398–405

Zillikens D, Mascaro JM, Rose PA, Liu Z, Ewing SM, Caux F, Hoffmann RG, Diaz LA, Giudice GJ (1997a) A highly sensistive enzyme-linked immunosorbent assay for the detection of circulating autoantibodies in patients with bullous pemphigoid. J Invest Dermatol 109:679–683.

Zillikens D, Rose PA, Balding SD, Liu Z, Olague-Marchan M, Diaz LA, Giudice GJ (1997b) Tight clustering of extracellular BP180 epitopes recognized by bullous pemphigoid autoantibodies. J Invest Dermatol 109:573–579

Zimina EP, Fritsch A, Schermer B, Bakulina AY, Bashkurov M, Benzing T, Bruckner-Tuderman L (2007) Extracellular phosphorylation of collagen XVII by ecto-casein kinase 2 inhibits ectodomain shedding. J Biol Chem 282:22737–46.

Zimina EP, Hofmann SC, Fritsch A, Kern JS, Sitaru C, Bruckner-Tuderman L (2008) Bullous pemphigoid autoantibodies preferentially recognize phosphoepitopes in collagen XVII. J Invest Dermatol 128:2736–9

Zone JJ, Taylor TB, Meyer LJ, Petersen MJ (1998) The 97-kDa linear IgA bullous disease antigen is identical to a portion of the extracellular domain of the 180-kDa bullous pemphigoid antigen, BPAG2. J Invest Dermatol 110:207–210

Zone JJ, Taylor T, Hull C, Schmidt L, Meyer L (2007) IgE basement membrane zone antibodies induce eosinophil infiltration and histological blisters in engrafted human skin on SCID mice. J Invest Dermatol 127:1167–74

Yamamoto K, Inoue N, Masuda R, Fujimori A, Saito T, Imajoh-Ohmi S, Shinkai H, Sakiyama H (2002) Cloning of hamster type XVII collagen cDNA, and pathogenesis of anti-type XVII collagen antibody and complement in hamster bullous pemphigoid. J Invest Dermatol 118:485–92

Yoshida M, Hamada T, Amagai M, Hashimoto K, Uehara R, Yamaguchi K, Imamura K, Okamoto E, Yasumoto S, Hashimoto T (2006) Enzyme-linked immunosorbent assay using bacterial recombinant proteins of human BP230 as a diagnostic tool for bullous pemphigoid. J Dermatol Sci 41:21–30

Autoimmune Bullous Skin Disorders

3.3 Dermatitis Herpetiformis Duhring

3

Christian Rose and Detlef Zillikens

Introduction

Dermatitis herpetiformis is an intensely pruritic, chronic autoimmune blistering skin disease characterized by granular IgA deposits along the dermal-epidermal junction and an association with celiac disease. The term dermatitis herpetiformis (DH) was first proposed by Louis Duhring (1884). He described a chronic disorder characterized by intense pruritus and pleomorphic skin lesions. Table 1 summarizes a selection of historical milestones in our understanding of DH. Marks et al. (1966) first described small-bowel changes in 9 of 12 patients with DH. Subsequently, both diseases were found to be associated with certain HLA haplotypes (Sachs et al., 1996). Almost all patients express HLA-DQ2 or HLA-DQ8. Another major advance was the finding of Cormane (1967), who described immunoglobulins to be deposited at the dermal-epidermal junction in patients with DH. Two years later, van der Meer (1969) identified this immunoglobulin as IgA. Subsequently, Chorzelski and

Table 1. Milestones in Studies on Dermatitis herpetiformis (DH)

Clinical description and introduction of the designation DH	Duhring, 1884
First use of sulphonamides for the treatment	Costello, 1940
Association of DH and small bowel disease	Marks et al., 1966
In-situ deposits of immunglobulin at the DEJ*	Cormane, 1967
Granular in-situ deposits of IgA at the DEJ	van der Meer, 1969
Differentiation of linear IgA disease from DH	Chorzelski et al., 1979
Detection of IgA anti-endomysium antibodies	Chorzelski et al., 1983
Characterization of tissue transglutaminase as the autoantigen of anti-endomysium antibodies	Dieterich et al., 1997
Identification of epidermal transglutaminase as an autoantigen	Sárdy et al., 2002

*DEJ; Dermal-epidermal junction

coworkers (1979) separated linear IgA disease from DH on the basis of different findings by immunofluorescence microscopy. Whereas in DH, granular IgA deposits are found, linear IgA disease is characterized by linear IgA deposits at the dermal-epidermal junction. Later, it became evident that the two diseases have a different immunogenetic background and that linear IgA disease is not associated with gastrointestinal changes.

Clinical Appearance / Classification

DH most commonly manifests in adult life, but is also found in childhood or elderly patients. The average age of over 40 years was observed in various large studies (Alonso-Llamazares et al., 2007; Rose et al., 2010) A slight male predominance with the ratio of 1.5:1 has been noted (Fry, 2002). Typically, patients with DH present with an intense pruritic eruption of erythematous papules or vesicles. The lesions are distributed symmetrically on the extensor surfaces. Areas of predilection include scalp, elbows, knees, sacrum and buttocks (Fig. 1A–C). The symmetrical distribution of the lesions on the buttocks has led to the coining of the descriptive phrase "gluteal butterfly". The primary lesion of DH is a small tense blister and rarely, tiny blisters are grouped; this rare appearance led to the designation dermatitis herpetiformis. Sometimes larger blisters are found. Severe pruritus, which is often described as burning or stinging, is a hallmark of DH and may precede the cutaneous eruption. Frequently, only crusted or eroded lesions are present. Occasionally, DH manifests with urticarial plaques or haemorrhagic maculae on the palms and soles (Kárpáti et al., 1986; Hofmann et al., 2009) (Fig. 1D). Oral involvement is very rare (Fraser et al., 1973). Earlier reports of a more frequent oral involvement in DH may have included patients with linear IgA bullous dermatosis where oral lesions are more common. The differential diagnosis of DH includes scabies, eczema and subacute or chronic prurigo. If blisters are encountered, other autoimmune blistering diseases have to be considered.

It is now well-accepted that all DH patients have celiac disease (CD), although most patients have no overt gastrointestinal symptoms. Marks et al. (1966) first reported abnormalities of the jejunal mucosa in patients with DH. Subsequently, it was recognized that the gastrointestinal abnormalities in DH are the same as in CD (Fry et al., 1967). Confusion concerning the incidence of the enteropathy in patients with DH is derived mainly from two aspects: Firstly from the inadequate criteria for the diagnosis of CD and secondly from confusing DH and linear IgA disease. Before differentiating the two diseases, some patients with linear IgA disease may have been considered to suffer from DH without bowel disease. Essentially all DH patients have histologic changes of CD that vary from mononuclear infiltrates in the lamina propria and minimal villous atrophy to complete flattening of the small intestinal mucosa (Fig. 2). The typical histological changes are not always found when a single jejunal biopsy specimen is taken and multiple biopsies from the jejunal mucosa increase the frequency to detect the abnormalities by light microscopy (Brow et al., 1971). Today, CD is considered as the result of a complex interplay of intrinsic and extrinsic factors. The spectrum of clinical manifestations ranges from oligosymptomatic and silent diseases to severe malabsorption. Gluten peptides are presented by antigen-

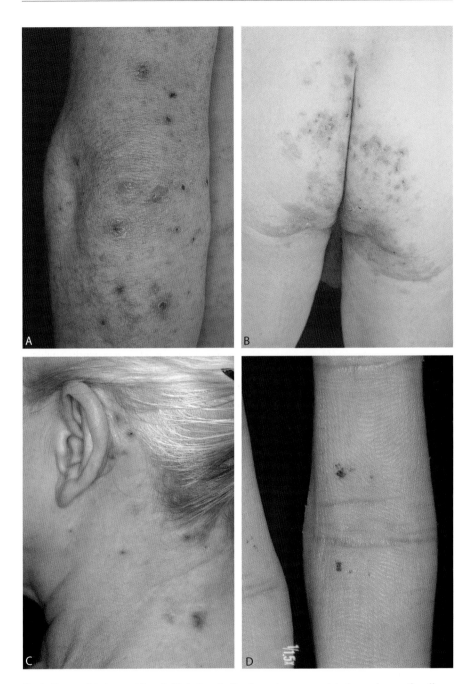

Fig. 1. Dermatitis herpetiformis Duhring **A.** Erythematous, excoriated papules on the elbow. **B.** Excoriated papules and plaques in a nearly symmetrical distribution on the buttocks ("gluteal butterfly"). **C.** Excoriated papules behind the ear and on the neck. **D.** Petechial lesions on the volar aspects of fingers.

3

A

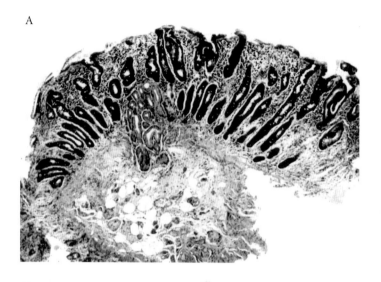

B

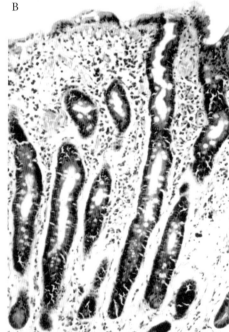

Fig. 2. A. Histopathologic examination of a small bowel biopsy from a patient with dermatitis herpetiformis demonstrating a virtually complete loss of villi (low magnification). **B.** The crypts are elongated and hyperplastic and an inflammatory infiltrate is present in the lamina propria (high magnification)

presenting cells and drive the immune response leading to an inflammatory reaction in the connective tissue of the lamina propria of the small bowel (Green and Cellier, 2007).

DH and CD are mainly found in Europe, but can be seen in other populations with European ancestry. In Scandinavia, Ireland, and Great Britain, DH is found more frequently than in other parts of Europe. Children appear to be more commonly affected in Italy and Hungary (Ermacora et al., 1986; Kárpáti et al., 1996). In the Anglo-Saxon and Scandinavian population, the prevalence of DH ranges from 10 to 39 per 100,000 inhabitants (Mobacken et al., 1984; Smith et al., 1992). The disease is rare in Afro-Caribbeans, Asians and Orientals. The varying frequency among different ethnical populations is most probably related to the different genetic background. HLA studies in patients with DH and CD led to identical findings. Both diseases are strongly associated with HLA DQ2 (in 90% of patients), compared with only 20% in normal controls. The remaining 10% of patients of both diseases carry the HLA DQ8 haplotyp. The presence of either of both alleles provides a sensitivity of close to 100% for CD and DH. In individuals lacking these alleles, CD and DH is virtually excluded. Thus, HLA analysis for the relevant DQ alleles can be a useful exclusion test when the diagnosis of DH and CD based on other tests is not possible (Caproni et al., 2009).

DH and CD may be associated with various autoimmune disorders, including autoimmune thyroiditis, type I diabetes, lupus erythematosus, Sjogren's disease, vitiligo, and others. DH is associated with an additional autoimmune disorder in approximately 10% of patients (Reunala and Collin, 1997). These associations have been thought to be a consequence of a common genetic background. In CD, it was demonstrated that the likelihood of an associated autoimmune disease is related to the duration of exposure to gluten and is higher in patients with CD diagnosed at a later stage (Ventura et al., 1999). In the majority of cases, the associated autoimmune disorder appeared before a gluten-free diet had been initiated, suggesting that long-standing untreated CD predisposes to the occurrence of other autoimmune disorders in the same patient. In addition, long-standing CD is associated with increased frequency of lymphomas of the gut (Collin et al., 1994). Whether patients with DH share the same risks of developing lymphoma is not known. A recent cohort study including 846 DH patients found no increased risk of malignancy or mortality in DH patients compared to controls (Lewis et al., 2008).

Diagnosis

Direct Immunofluorescence Microscopy

The diagnosis of DH is based on the finding of granular IgA deposits at the epidermaldermal junction by direct immunofluorescence microscopy. Without this finding, the diagnosis of DH should be questioned (Fry, 2002). Direct immunofluorescence microscopy is performed on a biopsy taken from clinically uninvolved perilesional skin. Lesional skin may be devoid of IgA, most likely due to degradation of the cutaneous IgA by enzymes released by neutrophils. If no IgA is found on the first section, serial sections of the biopsy should be studied. In skin areas that have never been affected by the disease, IgA has been found to be scant or absent (Zone et al., 1996). This may explain occasional reports where direct immunofluorescence microscopy findings were negative (Beutner et al., 2000). IgA deposition is found in two patterns. In addition to focal granular deposits localized in the tips of the papillary dermis (Fig. 3), IgA can be deposited continuously in the upper dermis beneath the basement membrane. In a recent study, we observed continuous deposits somewhat more frequently than focal dermal papillae deposits (Rose et al., 2010). There is

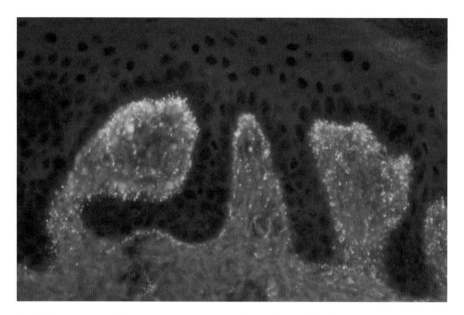

Fig. 3. Direct immunofluorescence microscopy of a perilesional skin biopsy showing granular deposits of IgA at the dermal-epidermal junction

no correlation between the direct immunofluorescence microscopy pattern and the clinical presentation of the disease (Beutner EH et al., 1992). Occasionally, granular IgM, IgG, and C3 deposits may also be seen in the upper dermis. It is essential to distinguish the continuous granular pattern of IgA deposits from the homogeneous linear IgA deposition which is characteristic for linear IgA disease. The granular IgA staining in the skin ultrastructurally corresponds to IgA-positive amorphous grains. They are of different size and are scattered throughout the papillary dermis and represent IgA and immune complexes (Kárpáti et al., 1990). Sárdy et al. (2002) identified epidermal transglutaminase (eTG) as the autoantigen in DH. It was demonstrated that eTG is colocalized with IgA deposits in the papillary dermis in DH patients. These results lead to the hypothesis that in DH patients, circulating immune complexes containing IgA and eTG may be trapped in the skin.

Histopathology

As skin lesions are severely pruritic they often become excoriated and the histological findings in these lesions may be nonspecific. A recent histopathological study of patients with DH showed that in nearly 40% of the biopsies, only a lymphocytic infiltrate with fibrosis and ectatic capillaries were seen (Warren and Cockerell, 2002). Therefore, biopsies for histopathologic examination should be taken from an early papule, papulovesicle, or a small blister with healthy appearing skin immediately adjacent to it. Typical histological

A

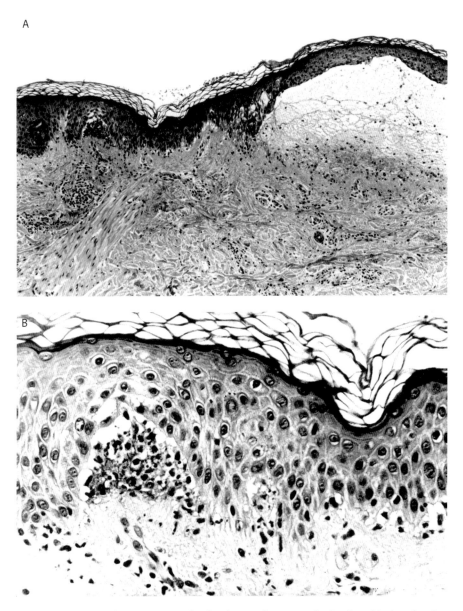

Fig. 4. A. Histological examination of a skin biopsy from a newly developed lesion showing a subepidermal blister and a sparse superficial inflammatory infiltrate (low magnification). **B.** Next to the blister, neutrophils are found along the dermal-epidermal junction and clustered in a dermal papilla (high magnification)

changes are best seen in the vicinity of early blisters (Fig. 4). The initial inflammatory event is variable edema in the papillary dermis with discrete subepidermal vacuolar alteration and neutrophils along the dermal-epidermal junction. As the lesion develops, neutrophils, to a lesser extent eosinophils, and fibrin accumulate within the dermal papillae and form microabscesses. These become confluent resulting in a subepidermal blister. It has been demonstrated that split formation occurs within the lamina lucida of the basement membrane zone (Smith et al., 1992). The IgA deposits have been shown to act as a chemoattractant for neutropils (Hendrix et al., 1990). In addition, interleukin 8, which is another chemoattractant for neutrophils, is strongly expressed by basal keratinocytes in lesional skin of DH patients (Graeber et al., 1993). In early stages of the disease, the inflammatory infiltrate contains mostly neutrophils, but in later stages, variable numbers of eosinophils can be present. In rare cases eosinophils can dominate and flame figures can be found (Rose et al., 2003). Histological changes in DH are indistinguishable from those in linear IgA disease. Other autoimmune subepidermal blistering diseases may also show an inflammatory infiltrate mainly composed of neutrophils and eosinophils and may mimic DH histopathologically, including epidermolysis bullosa acquisita, mucous membrane pemphigoid, bullous pemphigoid, and anti-laminin γ1 pemphigoid (Rose et al., 2004). Since histopathologic studies may not reliably differentiate between DH and these diseases, immunofluorescence microscopy is mandatory to establish the correct diagnosis. Analyses by immunoblotting and enzyme-linked immunosorbent assay aid in further characterizing the specificity of the autoantibodies. In addition, in bullous systemic lupus erythematosus, neutrophils and nuclear dust are found in the upper dermis and along the dermal-epidermal junction but in contrast to DH, mucin is commonly found in the reticular dermis. Rarely, a bullous drug eruption or an arthropod bite can mimic DH histopathologically (Ackerman et al., 1997, Rose et al., 2003). Since DH patients invariably also suffer from CD, one can question the necessity for a small intestinal biopsy to document the bowel disease if the diagnosis of DH is already established (Caproni et al., 2009).

Serological Findings

Chorzelski et al. (1983) first reported that sera from patients with DH and CD show IgA autoantibodies to endomysium, a specialized structure of connective tissue (Fig. 5). These IgA anti-endomysium autoantibodies allow a screening for CD with an almost 100% sensitivity and specificity (Corrao et al., 1994). As in DH patients associated CD is often mild, detection of these autoantibodies is lower ranging from 52% to 90% (Caproni et al., 2009). Dieterich et al. (1997) identified tissue transglutaminase (tTG) as the autoantigen of anti-endomysium antibodies. Detection of IgA autoantibodies to tTG by enzyme-linked immunosorbent assays (ELISA) using human recombinant tTG is a sensitive and specific test for the diagnosis of both treated and untreated patients with CD and DH (Dieterich et al., 1998; Sulkanen et al., 1998; Dieterich et al., 1999). Furthermore, our own studies showed that levels of IgA anti-tTG antibodies reflect the extent of histological changes in the gut of patients with DH. These antibodies were not detected in patients with linear IgA disease or other subepidermal autoimmune bullous diseases (Rose et al., 1999). Therefore, the determination of serum levels of antibodies to tTG should be routinely used for the diagnosis of DH (Caproni et al., 2009).

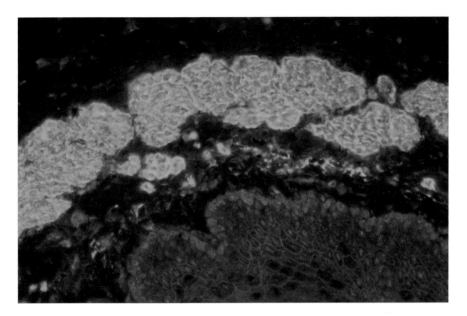

Fig. 5. IgA anti-endomysium antibodies on monkey esophagus by indirect immunfluorescence microscopy. These antibodies are found in the serum of patients with dermatitis herpetiformis and celiac disease and are directed to tissue transglutaminase

Recently, it has been shown that determination of highly specific antibodies against deamidated gliadin peptides (IgA and IgG) may be considered as the most reliable serological test to identify CD in DH patients (Sugai et al., 2006; Sugai et al., 2009). This new ELISA has a high diagnostic accuracy and in children, the combined investigation of antibodies against deamidated gliadin peptides and anti-tTG increased the diagnostic sensitivity to detect CD (Prause et al., 2009). The presence of IgA antibodies against endomysium, tTG and deamidated gliadin peptides in DH patients reflect their bowel disease. Indirect immunofluorescence microscopy, however, has failed to identify any antibody in DH sera reactive with normal human skin (Kadunce et al., 1989).

In 2002, Sárdy and colleagues reported a serological difference between DH and CD. Patients with DH produce two IgA antibody populations against eTG. The first one binds exclusively eTG, whereas the second one cross-reacts with tTG. The tTG cross-reactive eTG-specific antibodies may also be found in CD without DH but show a lower avidity for eTG than in patients with DH. Antibodies against eTG can be detected by ELISA; they are not seen by indirect immunofluorescence microscopy. In a recent study on 52 DH-patients, we demonstrated that IgA antibodies against eTG (95%) were more commonly detected than those against tTG (79%). Under a gluten-free diet, IgA reactivities to eTG and tTG decreased similarly. Interestingly, in rare DH patients, where pruritic cutaneous lesions persisted despite a gluten-free diet, antibodies against eTG remained detectable. The production of antibodies against eTG, independent of a gluten-free diet, may explain the persistence of cutaneous disease in these patients (Rose et al., 2009).

Therapy

Treatment of DH should consider changes in both the skin and the gut. Dapsone usually controls the skin eruption within days and this rapid response helped to support the clinical diagnosis of DH in the past. Dapsone is most commonly used in the treatment of skin lesions of DH and is normally well-tolerated by this patient group (Buckley et al., 1983; Rose et al., 2009). Although there are no controlled clinical trials, dapsone is considered to be more effective than sulfonamides such as sulphapyridine and sulphamethoxypyridazine. The initial dose of dapsone is around 1.5 mg / kg daily and if no control of symptoms is achieved, the dose is usually increased by 50 mg daily every 2 weeks leading to a maximum dose of 400 mg daily (Fry, 1988). If the skin rash has cleared, the dose should be tapered to the minimal dose required to suppress the symptoms. After a daily dose of 50 mg is achieved, the time interval between each dose should be increased before the drug is discontinued completely. When treating children, the recommended dose of dapsone is 2 mg / kg per day (Prendiville and Esterly, 1991). Side effects of dapsone include hemolytic anemia, methemoglobinemia and rarely agranulocytosis. Hemolysis occurs early in the treatment and a complete blood count is therefore checked two and four weeks after starting dapsone. Patients of Mediterranean ancestry should be screened for glucose-6-phosphate dehydrogenase deficiency prior to treatment. In these patients, use of dapsone can lead to severe hemolysis. Methemoglobinemia reaches a steady state about two weeks after initiation of dapsone and may cause cyanosis, shortness of breath and angina. Other side effects of dapsone include hepatitis, hypoalbuminemia, headache, lethargy, peripheral neuropathy, and the dapsone syndrome (lymphadenopathy and hepatitis). Most side effects related to the use of dapsone occur within the first three months of its use.

Sulphapyridine and sulphamethoxypyridazine are alternatives in patients who do not tolerate dapsone (Fry, 1988; McFadden et al., 1989). The initial dose of sulphapyridine is 2.0 g daily and the maximum dose should not exceed 4.0 g per day. Most patients require 0.5 to 2.0 g sulphapyridine daily to control the rash. The initial dose of the long-acting sulphonamide sulphamethoxypyridazine is 1 g daily. This may be increased to a daily maximum of 1.5 g, but in many patients symptoms are controlled with 0.5 g daily. Side effects of both sulphonamides include nausea, lethargy and drug rash. Rarely, agranulocytosis may occur. In addition, side-effects of sulphapyridine are bone marrow depression, hemolytic anemia, and nephrolithiasis. There is a considerable variation between patients regarding the dose of the three drugs (dapsone, sulphapyridine and sulphamethoxypyridazine) that is required to control the rash. A combination of two of the drugs can be used to reduce side-effects. None of the three sulphonamides affects the deposition of IgA in the skin, serum levels of IgA anti-endomysium antibodies, or the associated intestinal disease.

Alternative therapies for DH patients who do not tolerate sulphonamides include cholestyramine, sodium cromoglycate, cyclosporin, heparin, colchicine and a combination of tetracycline and nicotinamide (Silvers et al., 1980; Zemstov and Neldner, 1993; Shah and Ormerod, 2000). Intensive heparinization resulted in rapid improvement of DH in a few days. After withdrawal of heparin, skin lesion recurred within one week (Alexander, 1963; Tan et al., 1996). The mode of action of heparin in DH is unclear. Interestingly, both dapsone and heparin are able to inhibit proteolytic enzymes which are released in skin lesions of DH (Olkarinen et al., 1986).

The treatment of CD and DH should always include a gluten-free diet. Since most patients with DH do not suffer from gastrointestinal symptoms and skin lesions can be controlled by dapsone, it is important to carefully inform the patient of the necessity to maintain a gluten-free diet for a lifetime. Since such a diet is difficult to maintain, patients need to be motivated and carefully educated, and the support of a dietitian is essential. In addition, in many countries, self-supportive groups have been established that aid the patient in dealing with the diet. Gluten is present in most common grains (wheat, rye, barley) but not in rice and corn. It was thought that oats also contain gluten and play a role in inducing DH, but recently oats have been shown to be devoid of toxicity in DH patients (Hardman et al., 1997; Reunala et al., 1998). Patients benefit from a gluten-free diet in different aspects. Though only 5–10% of DH patients have gastrointestinal symptoms such as diarrhea, bloating and abdominal pain, these improve under a gluten free diet. In addition, iron or folate deficiency, which also is found in some DH patients, will ameliorate. Under a strict diet, most patients are able to reduce the dose of dapsone required to control their skin disease and in some patients, dapsone can be discontinued completely after two–three years. However, it may take months and even years until an effect of the diet can be appreciated by the patient (Garioch et al., 1994).

IgA deposits are slowly cleared from the skin once gluten is removed from the diet (Fry et al., 1973). After an average of 12 years of avoiding gluten, no IgA was found in the skin of three of 12 patients studied. When these three patients were re-challenged with gluten, it induced new IgA deposits in their skin and two patients also developed cutaneous lesions (Fry et al., 1982; Leonard et al., 1983). In two studies, after 5–10 years of a strict gluten-free diet, the risk to develop lymphoma in DH-patients decreases (Collin et al., 1996; Lewis et al., 1996). Furthermore, a gluten-free diet may be helpful in preventing the occurrence of additional autoimmune diseases in DH and CD patients. Interestingly, two studies have shown that patients with DH have an increased life expectancy. This finding resulted from a reduction in ischemic heart disease and was independent of a gluten-free diet (Swerdlow et al., 1993; Lear et al., 1997).

Summary

Dermatits herpetiformis (DH) is a pruritic autoimmune subepidermal bullous disease and is considered as a specific cutaneous manifestation of celiac disease (CD). The diagnosis of DH is based on the detection of granular IgA deposits in biopsies of normal-appearing perilesional skin. CD and DH patients have the same genetic predisposition and demonstrate IgA anti-endomysium antibodies in their sera. These antibodies are directed against tissue transglutaminase. Serum levels of IgA antibodies to tissue transglutaminase reflect the extent of histopathologic changes of the small bowel and are routinely assessed in patients with DH and CD. The autoantigen of DH is epidermal transglutaminase which is found in the skin of DH-patients at the same site as the granular IgA deposits. Detection of anti-IgA antibodies against epidermal transglutaminase is a sensitive serological test in the diagnosis of DH. Skin lesions can be controlled by dapsone, but the drug does not affect the small bowel disease. For CD, the treatment of choice is a gluten-free diet that should be maintained for a lifetime. In most patients, the diet eventually results in remission of the skin lesions, a clearance of IgA deposits from the skin and an improvement of the bowel disease. The question why some patients with mild CD produce antibodies against epidermal transglutaminase and develop DH still remains to be elucidated.

References

Ackerman AB, Chongchitnant N, Sanchez J, Guo Y, Bennin B, Reichel M, Randall MB (1997) Histologic diagnosis of inflammatory skin diseases, 2nd ed. Williams & Wilkins, Baltimore, pp 271–278

Alexander O´D (1963) The treatment of dermatitis herpetiformis with heparin. Br J Dermatol 75:289–293

Alonso-Llamazares J, Gibson LE, Rogers III RS (2007) Clinical, pathologic, and immunopathologic features of dermatitis herpetiformis: review of the Mayo clinic experience. Int J Dermatol 46:910–919

Beutner EH, Chorzelski TP, Reunala TL, Kumar V (1992) Immunopathology of dermatitis herpetiformis. Clin Dermatol 9:295–311

Beutner EH, Baughman RD, Austin BM, Plunkett RW, Binder WL (2000) A case of dermatitis herpetiformis with IgA endomysial antibodies but negative direct immunofluorescent findings. J Am Acad Dermatol 43:329–332

Brow J, Parker F, Weinstein W, Rubin CE (1971) The small intestinal mucosa in dermatitis herpetiformis: severity and distribution of the small intestinal lesion and associated malabsorption. Gastroenterology 60:355–361

Buckley DB, English J, Molloy W, Doyle CT, Welton MJ (1983) Dermatitis herpetiformis: a review of 119 cases. Clin Exp Dermatol 8:477–487

Caproni M, Antiga E, Melani L, Fabbri P, The Italian Group of Cutaneous Immunopathology (2009) Guidelines for the diagnosis and treatment of dermatitis herpetiformis. JEADV 23:633–638

Collin P, Pukkala E, Reunala T (1996) Malignancy and survival in dermatitis herpetiformis: a comparison with coeliac disease. Gut 38:528–530

Cormane RH (1967) Immunofluorescent studies of the skin in lupus erythematosus and other diseases. Pathologica Eur 2:170–180

Corrao G, Corazza GR, Andreani ML, Torchio P, Valentini RA, Galatola G, Quaglino D, Gasbarrini G, di Orio F (1994) Serological screening of coeliac disease: choosing the optimal procedure according to various prevalence values. Gut 35:771–775

Costello M (1940) Dermatitis herpetiformis treated with sulfapyridine. Arch Dermatol Syphilol 41:134

Chorzelski TP, Jablonska S, Beutner EH, Bear SF, Furey NL (1979) Linear IgA bullous dermatosis. In: Beutner EH, Chorzelski TP, Bear SF (eds) Immunopathology of the skin. 2nd ed. John Wiley & Sons; New York, pp 315–323

Chorzelski TP, Sulej J, Tchorzewska H, Jablonska S, Beutner EH, Kumar V (1983) IgA class endomysium antibodies in dermatitis herpetiformis and coeliac disease. Ann N Y Acad Sci 4:325–334

Dieterich W, Ehnis T, Bauer M, Donner P, Volta U, Riecken EO, Schuppan D (1997) Identification of tissue transglutaminase as the autoantigen of celiac disease. Nature Med 3:797–801

Dieterich W, Laag E, Schöpper H, Volta U, Ferguson A, Gillett H, Riecken EO, Schuppan D (1998) Autoantibodies to tissue transglutaminase as predictors of celiac disease. Gastroenterology 115:1317–1321

Dieterich W, Laag E, Bruckner-Tuderman L, Reunala T, Kárpáti S, Zágoni T, Riecken EO, Schuppan D (1999) Antibodies to tissue transglutaminase as serologic markers in patients with dermatitis herpetiformis. J Invest Dermatol 113:133–136

Duhring LA (1884) Dermatitis herpetiformis. JAMA 3:225–229

Ermacora E, Prampolini L, Tribbia G, Pezzoli G, Gelmetti C, Cucchi G, Tettamanti A, Giunta A, Gianotti F (1986) Long-term follow-up of dermatitis herpetiformis in children. J Am Acad Dermatol 15:23–30

Fraser NG, Kerr NW, Donald D (1973) Oral lesions in dermatitis herpetiformis. Br J Dermatol 89:439–450

Fry L, Keir P, McMinn RMH, Cowan JD, Hoffbrand AV (1967) Small-intestinal structure and function and haematological changes in dermatitis herpetiformis. Lancet II:729–734

Fry L, Seah PP, Riches DJ, Hoffbrand AV (1973) Clearance of skin lesions in dermatitis herpetiformis after gluten withdrawal. Lancet I:288–291

Fry L, Leonard JN, Swain F, Tucker WFG, Haffenden G, Ring N, McMinn RMH (1982) Long-term follow-up of dermatitis herpetiformis with and without dietary gluten withdrawal. Br J Dermatol 107:631–640

Fry L (1988) Fine points in the management of dermatitis herpetiformis. Semin Dermatol 7:206–211

Fry L (2002) Dermatitis herpetiformis: problems, progress and prospect. Eur J Dermatol 12:523–531

Garioch JJ, Lewis HM, Sargent SA, Leonard JN, Fry L (1994) 25 years´ experience of gluten-free diet in the treatment of dermatitis herpetiformis. Br J Dermatol 131:541–545

Graeber M, Baker BS, Garioch JJ (1993) The role of cytokines in the generation of skin lesions in dermatitis herpetiformis. Br J Dermatol 129:530–532

Green PHR, Cellier C (2007) Celiac disease. N Engl J Med 357:1731–1743

Hardman CM, Garioch JJ, Leonard JN, Thomas HJ, Walker MM, Lortan JE, Lister A, Fry L (1997) Absence of toxicity of oats in patients with dermatitis herpetiformis. N Engl J Med 337:1884–1887

Hendrix JD, Karen L, Mangum MT, Zone JJ, Gammon WR (1990) Cutaneous IgA deposits in bullous diseases function as ligands to mediate adherence of activated neutrophils. J Invest Dermatol 94:667–672

Hofmann SC, Nashan D, Bruckner-Tuderman L (2009) Petechiae on the fingertips as presenting symptom of dermatitis herpetiformis Duhring. JEADV 23:732–733

Kadunce DP, Meyer LJ, Zone JJ (1989) IgA class antibodies in dermatitis herpetiformis: reaction with tissue antigens. J Invest Dermatol 93:253–258

Kárpáti S, Torok E, Kosnai I (1986) Discrete palmar and plantar symptoms in children with dermatitis herpetiformis Duhring. Cutis 3:184–187

Kárpáti S, Meurer M, Stolz W, Schrallhammer K, Krieg T, Braun-Falco O (1990) Dermatitis herpetiformis bodies. Arch Dermatol 126:1469–1474

Lear JT, Neary RH, Jones P, Fitzgerald DA, English JS (1997) Risk factors for ischaemic heart disease in patients with dermatitis herpetiformis. J R Soc Med 90:247–249

Leonard J, Haffenden G, Tucker W, Unsworth J, Swain F, McMinn R, Holborow J, Fry L (1983) Gluten challenge in dermatitis herpetiformis. N Engl J Med 308:816–819

Lewis HM, Reunala TL, Garioch JJ, Leonard JN, Fry JS, Collin P, Evans D, Fry L (1996) Protective effect of gluten-free diet against development of lymphoma in dermatitis herpetiformis. Br J Dermatol 135:363–367

Lewis NR, Logan RFA, Hubbard RB, West J (2008) No increase in risk of fracture, malignancy or mortality in dermatitis herpetiformis: a cohort study. Aliment Pharmacol Ther 27:1140–1147

Olkarinen AL, Reunala T, Zone JJ, Kilstala U, Uitto J (1986) Proteolytic enzymes in blister fluids from patients with dermatitis herpetiformis. Br J Dermatol 114:295–302

Marks J, Shuster S, Watson AJ (1966) Small bowel changes in dermatitis herpetiformis. Lancet II:1280–1282

McFadden JP, Leonard JN, Powles AV, Rutman AJ, Fry L (1989) Sulphamethoxypyridazine for dermatitis herpetiformis, linear IgA disease and cicatricial pemphigoid. Br J Dermatol 121:759–762

Mobacken H, Kastrup W, Nilsson L. (1984) Incidence and prevalence of dermatitis herpetiformis in Western Sweden. Acta Derm Venereol 64:400–404

Prendiville JS, Esterly NB (1991) Childhood dermatits herpetiformis. Clin Dermatol 9:375–381

Reunala T, Collin P (1997) Diseases associated with dermatitis herpetiformis. Br J Dermatol 136:315–318

Reunala T, Collin P, Holm K, Pikkarainen P, Miettinen A, Vuolteenaho N, Maki M (1998) Tolerance to oats in dermatitis herpetiformis. Gut 43:490–493

Prause C, Richter T, Koletzko S, Uhlig HH, Hauer AC, Stern M, Zimmer KP, Laass MW, Probst C, Schlumberger W, Mothes T (2009) New developments in serodiagnosis of childhood celiac disease: assay of antibodies against deamidated gliadin. Ann N Y Acad Sci 1173:28–35

Rose C, Dieterich W, Bröcker EB, Schuppan D, Zillikens D (1999) Circulating autoantibodies to tissue transglutaminase differentiate patients with dermatitis herpetiformis from those with linear IgA disease. J Am Acad Dermatol 61:39–43

Rose C, Bröcker EB, Krahl D (2003) Dermatitis herpetiformis with flame figures mimicking an arthropod bite. Am J Dermatopathol 25:277–278

Rose C, Bröcker EB, Zillikens D (2004) Relevance of histological examination in the diagnosis of autoimmune bullous dermatoses. J Dtsch Dermatol Ges 2:96–104

Rose C, Armbruster FP, Ruppert J, Igl BW, Zillikens D, Shimanovich I (2009) Autoantibodies against epidermal transglutaminase are a sensitive diagnostic marker in patients with dermatitis herpetiformis on a normal or gluten-free diet. J Am Acad Dermatol 41:957–961

Rose C, Bröcker EB, Zillikens D (2010) Clinical, histological and immunpathological findings in 32 patients with dermatitis herpetiformis Duhring. J Dtsch Dermatol Ges 8:265–271

Sachs JA, Awad J, McCloskey D, Navarrete C, Festenstein H, Elliot E, Walker-Smith JA, Griffiths CE, Leonard JN, Fry L (1986) Different HLA associated gene combinations contribute to susceptibility for coeliac disease and dermatitis herpetiformis. Gut 27:515–520

Sárdy M, Odenthal U, Kárpáti S, Paulsson M, Smyth N (1999) Recombinat human tissue transglutaminase ELISA for the diagnosis of gluten-sensitive enteropathy. Clin Chem 45:2142–2149

Sárdy M, Kárpáti S, Merkl B, Paulsson M, Smyth N (2002) Epidermal transglutaminase (TGase 3) is the autoantigen of dermatitis herpetiformis. J Exp Med 195:747–757

Seissler J, Borns S, Wohlrab U, Morgenthaler NG, Mothes T, Boehm BO, Scherbaum WA (1999) Antibodies to human tissue transglutaminase measured by radioligand assay: evidence for high diagnostic sensitivity for celiac disease. Horm Metab Res 31:375–379

Silvers DN, Juhlin EA, Berczeller PH, McSorley J (1980) Treatment of dermatitis herpetiformis with colchicine. Arch Dermatol 116:1373–1374

Shah SAA, Ormerod AD (2000) Dermatitis herpetiformis effectively treated with heparin, tetracycline and nicotinamide. Clin Exp Dermatol 25:204–205

Smith JB, Tulloch JE, Meyer LJ, Zone JJ (1992) The incidence and prevalence of dermatitis herpetiformis in Utah. Arch Dermatol 128:1608–1610

Smith JB, Taylor TB, Zone JJ (1992) The site of blister formation in dermatitis herpetiformis is within the lamina lucida. J Am Acad Dermatol 27:209–213

Sulkanen S, Halttunen T, Laurila K, Kolho KL, Korponay-Szabo IR, Sarnesto A, Savilahti E, Collin P, Mäki M (1998) Tissue transglutaminase autoantibody enzyme-linked immunosorbent assay in detecting celiac disease. Gastroenterology 115:1322–1328

Sugai E, Hwang HJ, Vázquez H, Smecuol E, Niveloni S, Mazure R, Mauriño E, Aeschlimann P, Binder W, Aeschlimann D, Bai JC (2010) New serology assays can detect gluten sensitivity among enteropathy patients seronegative for anti-tissue transglutaminase. Clin Chem 56:661–665

Sugai E, Smecuol E, Niveloni S, Vázquez H, Label M, Mazure R, Czech A, Kogan Z, Mauriño E, Bai JC (2006) Celiac disease serology in dermatitis herpetiformis. Which is the best option for detecting gluten sensitivity? Acta Gastroenterol Latinoam 36:197–201

Swerdlow AJ, Whittaker S, Carpenter LM, English JSC (1993) Mortality and cancer incidence in patients with dermatitis herpetiformis: a cohort study. Br J Dermatol 129:140–144

Tan CC, Sale JE, Brammer C, Irons RP, Freeman JG (1996) A rare case of dermatitis herpetiformis requiring parenteral heparin for long-term control. Dermatology 192:185–186

Van der Meer JB (1969) Granular deposits of immunoglobulins in the skin of patients with dermatitis herpetiformis. Br J Dermatol 81:493–503

Ventura A, Magazzu G, Greco L for the SIGEP study group for autoimmune disorders in celiac disease (1999) Duration of exposure to gluten and risk for autoimmune disorders in patients with celiac disease. Gastroenterology 117:297–303

Warren SJP, Cockerell CJ (2002) Characterization of a subgroup of patients with dermatitis herpetiformis with nonclassical histologic features. Am J Dermatopathol 24:305–308

Zemtsov A, Neldner K (1993) Successful treatment of dermatitis herpetiformis with tetracycline and nicotinamide in a patient unable to tolerate dapsone. J Am Acad Dermatol 28:505–506

Zillikens D, Kawahara Y, Ishiko A, Shimizu H, Mayer J, Rank CV, Liu Z, Giudice GJ, Tran HH, Marinkovich MP, Bröcker EB, Hashimoto T (1996) A novel subepidermal blistering disease with autoantibodies to a 200-kDa antigen of the basement membrane zone. J Invest Dermatol 106:1333–1336

Zone JJ, Laurence JM, Peterson MJ (1996) Deposition of granular IgA relative to clinical lesions in dermatitis herpetiformis. Arch Dermatol 132:912–918

Gene Kim, Mei Chen, Dafna Hallel-Halevy, and David T. Woodley

Introduction

Epidermolysis bullosa acquisita (EBA) was first described before the turn of the century and was designated as an acquired form of epidermolysis bullosa (EB) because the clinical features were so reminiscent of children who were born with genetic forms of dystrophic EB (Elliott, 1985). EBA is an acquired, subepidermal bullous disease and is classified as one of the "primary" bullous diseases of the skin. In its classical form, it is a mechanobullous disease with skin fragility and trauma-induced blisters that have minimal inflammation and heal with scarring and milia – features that are highly reminiscent of hereditary dystrophic forms of epidermolysis bullosa (DEB). In DEB, there is a hereditary defect in the gene that encodes for type VII (anchoring fibril) collagen leading to a paucity of anchoring fibrils. Anchoring fibrils are structures that anchor the epidermis and its underlying basement membrane zone (BMZ) onto the dermis (Briggaman and Wheeler, 1975; Uitto and Christiano, 1994). In EBA, there is also a paucity of anchoring fibrils, but this is because EBA patients have IgG autoantibodies targeted against the type VII collagen within anchoring fibrils. EBA represents an acquired autoimmune mechanism by which anchoring fibrils can be compromised rather than by a gene defect. Since EBA has become defined as autoimmunity to type VII collagen, it has become evident that EBA may also present with clinical manifestations reminiscent of bullous pemphigoid (BP), cicatricial pemphigoid (CP), and Brunsting-Perry pemphigoid.

In the early 1970s, Roenigk et al. (1971) reviewed the EBA world literature, reported three new cases and established the first diagnostic criteria for EBA: (1) spontaneous or trauma-induced blisters resembling hereditary DEB, (2) adult onset, (3) a negative family history for EB, and (4) the exclusion of all other bullous diseases. In the 1980's Yaoita et al. (1981) and Nieboer et al. (1980) found that EBA, like BP, exhibited IgG deposits at the dermal-epidermal junction (DEJ). In EBA, however, the IgG deposits are found within and below the lamina densa compartment of the BMZ, whereas in BP they are located higher, within hemidesmosomes and the lamina lucida. The sub-lamina densa location of the IgG deposits in EBA was understandable when it was recognized that the skin protein targeted by the IgG autoantibodies was type VII collagen within anchoring fibrils which emanate perpendicularly from the lamina densa into the high papillary dermis (Woodley et al., 1984, 1988). The primary unit of type VII collagen is a 290 kDa alpha chain which is the "EBA auto-antigen".

Etiology and Pathogenesis

Etiology and Epidemiology

The etiology of EBA is not completely clear. Because the disease features IgG autoantibodies directed against type VII collagen, it is thought that EBA has an autoimmune pathogenesis (Woodley et al., 1984, 1988). Similar to EBA, patients with bullous systemic lupus erythematosus (SLE) also develop auto-antibodies against type VII collagen (SLE) (Gammon et al., 1985). Both EBA and bullous SLE patients often have a common human leukocyte antigen (HLA) major histocompatibility (MHC) class II cell surface protein, HLA-DR2 (Gammon et al., 1988b). This HLA phenotype has been associated with hyperimmunity which again suggests an autoimmune etiology for EBA.

EBA is a rare disease with an incidence of 0.17–0.26 per million people in Western Europe (Bernard et al., 1995; Zillikens et al., 1995). EBA appears to be less common than BP, but it may be at least as common as CP, pemphigoid gestationis and linear IgA bullous dermatosis. Although there is no definite racial or gender predilection (Gammon and Briggaman, 1993), it has recently been suggested to have higher predilection in the Korean population (Lee, 1998). The age of onset varies widely from early childhood to late adult life, but most cases begin between the fourth and fifth decades (Gammon, 1988a; Arpey et al., 1991).

Type VII collagen is composed of three identical alpha chains wound into a triple helical structure. Each alpha chain is 290 kDa. However, half of the size of each alpha chain is consumed by a large, globular, non-collagenous domain at the amino end of the molecule. This globular domain is 145 kDa and is called the non-collagenous 1 domain (NC1). At the other end of the alpha chain, the carboxyl terminus, there is a much smaller non-collagenous globular domain called NC2 which is only 34 kDa. In between these two globular domains, there is a long rod-shaped, helical, collagenous domain characterized by repeating Gly-X-Y amino acid sequences (Fig. 1) (Sakai et al., 1986; Burgeson, 1993).

Within the extracellular space, type VII collagen molecules form antiparallel, tail-to-tail dimers stabilized by disulfide bonding through the small carboxyl-terminal NC2 overlap between two type VII collagen molecules. A portion of the NC2 domain is then proteolytically removed (Bruckner-Tuderman et al., 1995). The antiparallel dimers then aggregate laterally to form anchoring fibrils with large globular NC1 domains at both ends of the structure (Fig. 1).

Pathogenesis

Autoantibodies against type VII collagen have long been suspected a potential cause of EBA. The NC1 domain contains the major antigenic epitopes for EBA and bullous SLE

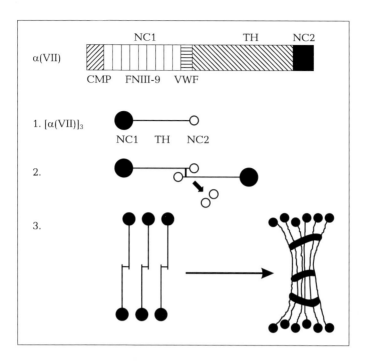

Fig. 1. A schematic representation of the type VII collagen alpha chain and assembly into anchoring fibril structures. The NC1 non-collagenous domain at the amino terminus has several segments with homologies to adhesive proteins including cartilage matrix protein (CMP), nine fibronectin type III like repeats (FNIII-9), and von Willibrand factor A (VWF). Then, there is a long triple helical collagenous segment (TH) and a smaller second non-collagenous globular domain called NC2. 1. Three type VII collagen alpha chains form a homotrimer $[\alpha(C\text{-}VII)]^3$. 2. In the extracellular space, two procollagen molecules align to form antiparallel dimers which are stabilized by the formation of disulfide bonds. The NC2 domain is then proteolytically cleaved. 3. Several of these dimer molecules laterally aggregate to assemble into anchoring fibrils

autoantibodies (Gammon et al., 1993; Jones et al., 1995; Lapiere et al., 1996). Recent passive transfer studies have offered more direct evidence that EBA autoantibodies are pathogenic. Antibodies raised in immunized rabbits against the NC-1 domain of both human and murine type VII collagen caused blister formation when injected in immune competent mice (Woodley et al., 2005; Sitaru et al., 2005). The mice developed skin changes reminiscent of EBA with sub-epidermal blisters and nail dystrophy. Similarly, injection of affinity purified human EBA autoantibodies against a NC-1 column into mice led to the development of a blistering disease with clinical, histologic, immunologic and ultrastructural features akin to human EBA (Woodley et al., 2006). These successful passive transfer experiments strongly suggest that EBA autoantibodies are pathogenic and capable of causing epidermal-dermal separation in skin.

The mechanism by which autoantibodies cause disease has not been completely elucidated. The NC1 domain contains a series of domains within it that have homology with adhesive proteins such as cartilage matrix protein, fibronectin and the A domain of von Willebrand factor (VWF-A) (Christiano et al., 1994). Therefore, the NC1 domain may facilitate binding of type VII collagen to other BMZ and matrix components. Because EBA often occurs with minimal clinical or histologic inflammation, it has been hypothesized that autoantibodies target and compromise functional epitopes on the NC1 domain. This then interferes with the normal interactions between NC1 and its extracellular matrix ligands such as laminin 5 and fibronectin and disrupt epidermal-dermal adherence (Chen et al., 1997a, 1999). In addition, there may be an interruption in the type VII collagen-fibronectin interaction in the collagenous domain which may be important for the adherence of basement membrane and the overlying epidermis onto the papillary dermis (Lapiere et al., 1994). The recent observation that some EBA autoantibodies from children with EBA target other domains within the alpha chain besides NC1 suggests that the helical collagenous domain and perhaps the NC2 domain may also play important roles in maintaining fully functional type VII collagen and anchoring fibrils (Tanaka et al., 1997). For example, some EBA patients' autoantibodies recognize antigenic epitopes within both the NC1 and NC2 domains, and the latter domain appears to be important in the formation of antiparallel dimers and anchoring fibril assembly (Chen et al., 2000). These mechanisms are attractive possibilities for explaining skin fragility and trauma-induced blisters in patients with classical EBA who lack significant inflammation but have markedly defective epidermal-dermal adherence.

We now understand that EBA does not always present as a non-inflammatory mechanobullous disease reminescent of DEB. Although less common, EBA may present as an inflammatory, widespread, vesiculobullous disease that clinically resembles BP. Therefore, it is possible that autoantibody recognition of one or several domains of type VII collagen may invoke an inflammatory cascade which could result in proteolytic degradation of matrix components within the DEJ that are essential for epidermal-dermal adherence. EBA autoantibodies may generate blisters by inducing localized inflammation with or without the amplification of complement fixation. The induced inflammatory response then causes tissue damage at DEJ, which results in blister formation (Gammon et al., 1984). This mechanism may explain those EBA and bullous SLE patients with acute inflammation at the BMZ, particularly when neutrophils are predominant in the inflammatory response because that type of inflammation is characteristic of experimental forms of immune complex and complement-mediated inflammation.

Clinical Manifestations

There is great diversity in the clinical presentation of EBA. The common denominator for patients with EBA is autoimmunity to type VII (anchoring fibrils) collagen and diminished anchoring fibrils (Woodley, 1988; Woodley et al., 1988). Although the clinical spectrum of EBA is still being defined, it appears that there are at least five clinical presentations of EBA (Fig. 2):

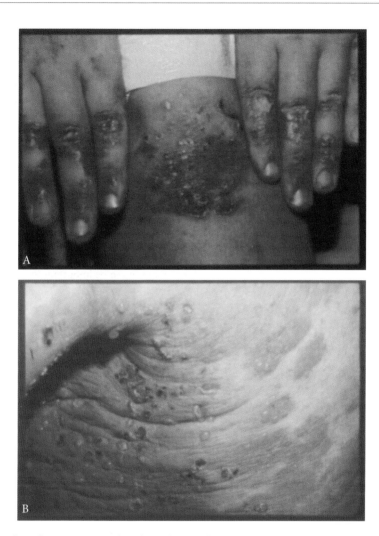

Fig. 2. Clinical presentations of Epidermolysis Bullosa Acquisita. **A.** Classical presentation in a white woman. **B.** Presentation of EBA that is highly inflammatory and appears like BP

1) "Classical" presentation that was initially described in EBA and closely resembles the features seen in patients with inherited forms of DEB
2) BP-like presentation
3) CP-like presentation
4) Brunsting-Perry Pemphigoid-like presentation
5) Linear IgA bullous dermatosis (LABD)-like disease. Its childhood presentation can be reminiscent of Chronic Bullous Disease of Childhood.

Classical EBA

This form of EBA presents as a mechanobullous noninflammatory disease with an acral distribution. The blisters and erosions heal with scarring and milia formation. This presentation in its mild form is reminiscent of porphyria cutanea tarda, and in its more severe forms is reminiscent of hereditary recessive DEB (Yaoita et al., 1981). Despite the similarities between EBA and porphyria cutanea tarda, patients with EBA do not present with hirsutism, photodistribution, scleroderma like changes and high levels of urinary porphyrins (Woodley, 1988; Woodley et al., 1998).

Classical EBA is a mechanobullous disease marked by skin fragility over trauma prone surfaces. Blisters, erosions and scars occur over the back of the hands, knuckles, elbows, knees, sacral area, and feet (Fig. 2A). There is often significant involvement of the oral mucosa with erosions and frank blisters. On the glabrous skin, the vesicles and bullae appear tense on non-inflamed or scarred skin. They can be hemorrhagic and can result in erosions, crusts, scales, scars, scarring alopecia, milia cysts and nail dystrophy. The lesions heal with scarring and frequently with the formation of pearl-like milia cysts within the scarred areas. In severe cases, there may be fibrosis of the hands and fingers and esophageal stenosis (Stewart et al., 1991; Harman et al., 1998). The histology shows dermal-epidermal separation at the BMZ and minimal inflammation.

BP-like Presentation

These patients present with features characteristic of the autoimmune bullous disease, BP, or a mixture of features characteristic of both BP and classic EBA presentation (Gammon et al., 1982, 1984b). This form of EBA manifests as a widespread inflammatory vesiculobullous eruption involving the trunk, extremities and skin folds usually accompanied by pruritus (Fig. 2B). Tense bullae are situated on inflamed and/or urticarial skin. In contrast to classical EBA, skin fragility is not prominent and scarring and milia formation may be minimal or absent. The distribution of the lesions is not confined to trauma-prone sites. The histology shows a moderate to dense polymorphic infiltrate of mononuclear cells and granulocytes. Neutrophils are often the predominant granulocyte, but occasionally eosinophils are seen.

CP-like Presentation

The clinical features in these patients closely resemble those considered characteristic of CP. This form of EBA presents as a bullous disease with a predominance of mucosal involvement. The patient may present with erosions and scars of the mouth, upper esophagus, conjunctiva, anus, and vagina (Dahl, 1979; Stewart et al., 1991; Harman et al., 1998) with or without similar lesions on the glabrous skin. Recently, tracheal involvement has been reported in the CP-like presentation of EBA (Wieme et al., 1999). There is also one report of predominantly mucosal involvement with no scarring (Tokuda et al., 1998). Unlike classical EBA, patients with the CP-like presentation often do not show significant skin fragility, evidence of trauma-induced lesions, or a predilection for blistering on extensor skin surfaces. The histology shows subepidermal blisters and usually a mixed inflammatory infiltrate in the upper dermis and at the BMZ and microscopic scarring.

Brunsting-Perry Pemphigoid

Brunsting-Perry Pemphigoid is a chronic recurrent subepidermal scarring vesiculobullous eruption localized to the head and neck. In contrast to CP, it has minimal or no mucosal involvement (Kurzhals et al., 1991; Yancey, 1998). IgG autoantibodies are deposited at the BMZ, but the autoantigenic target for these autoantibodies has not been defined. Recently, several patients have been reported to have the clinical, histological and immunological features of Brunsting-Perry Pemphigoid but their IgG autoantibodies are targeted against type VII (anchoring fibril) collagen (Kurzhals et al., 1991; Joly et al., 1993; Choi et al., 1998; Woodley et al., 1998). Therefore, we believe that Brunsting Perry Pemphigoid may actually be a clinical presentation of EBA.

LABD-like Presentation

This form of EBA is manifested by a subepidermal bullous eruption, a neutrophilic infiltrate and linear IgA deposits at the BMZ when viewed by direct immunofluorescence microscopy. It may resemble Chronic Bullous Disease of Childhood and feature tense vesicles arranged in an annular fashion and involvement of mucous membranes (Callot-Mellot et al., 1997, Park et al., 1997). The autoantibodies are usually IgA, IgG or both.

The diagnostic category of these patients with IgA antibodies against type VII collagen deposited in a linear fashion along the BMZ is not clear. Some clinicians regard these patients as purely LABD (Hashimoto et al., 1996), while others regard these patients as a subset of EBA (Rusenko et al., 1989; Bauer et al., 1999). It is interesting to note that in a recent study (Lee, 2000), 20 EBA patients' sera were evaluated for serum IgA anti-type VII collagen antibodies by immunoblotting. The investigators detected low titers of IgA anti-type VII collagen antibodies in 80% of the patients in addition to IgG.

Childhood EBA is a rare disease with variable presentations. In a recent study of 14 children with EBA, five of the patients presented as a LABD – like disease and five patients presented with the BP-like form of EBA. The remaining four children presented with the classical mechanobullous form of EBA (Callot-Mellot et al., 1997). Eleven out of 14 had mucosal involvement and all had IgG deposits at the BMZ by direct immunofluorescence, in addition to other immunoreactants. Indirect immunofluorescence was positive in 10 out of 14 patient sera, and the predominant serum antibody was of the IgG class. Although mucosal involvement is frequent and severe in childhood EBA, the overall prognosis and treatment is more favorable than in adult EBA (Callot-Mellot et al., 1997; Edwards et al., 1998).

The clinical presentation of the EBA patient may change during the course of the disease or can show two different presentations simultaneously. About 25% of patients with EBA may appear with the BP-like clinical appearance (unpublished observation). With time, the disease of some patients will eventually smolder into a more noninflammatory classic form of EBA. Both the classical and the BP-like forms (Stewart et al., 1991), and the CP-like and BP-like forms of the disease may coexist in the same patient (Wieme et al., 1999). The clinical phenotype of EBA that is reminiscent of pure CP is probably more rare and occurs in fewer than 10% of all EBA cases.

The Relationship between EBA and Bullous SLE

There have been reports of patients having both EBA and bullous SLE (Gammon and Briggaman, 1993). In contrast to the classical presentation of EBA, bullous SLE patients by definition must fulfill the American Rheumatism Association criteria for SLE. The patients tend to be young women with a widespread nonscarring vesiculobullous eruption with a predilection for sun-exposed areas. EBA often presents in the fourth to fifth decades whereas bullous SLE usually presents earlier, in the second and third decades. EBA often lasts many years whereas bullous SLE is remitting and may resolve in less than a year. EBA does not respond as much as bullous SLE to treatment with dapsone or prednisone. Histologically there can also be differences. Bullous SLE may exhibit neutrophilic papillary microabscesses and vasculitis, which are seldom seen in EBA (Gammon and Briggaman, 1993). Mucin is not increased in the reticular dermis in EBA unlike bullous SLE (Ackerman et al., 1997).

The Relationship between EBA and other Systemic Diseases

In Roenigk's review of the EBA world literature (Roenick et al., 1971), it was noted that there were many anecdotal reports of EBA associated with sytemic diseases such as SLE, diabetes, inflammatory bowel disease, amyloidosis, autoimmune thyroiditis, multiple endocrinopathy syndrome, rheumatoid arthritis, pulmonary fibrosis, chronic lymphocytic leukemia, thymoma, diabetes, and others (Woodley et al., 1998). However, EBA is a relatively rare disease, and most of these are anecdotal reports. It appears that the most frequently associated disease with EBA is inflammatory bowel disease, with an estimate of 25% of 50 EBA patients reviewed by Chan and Woodley (1996). It has also been shown that patients with inflammatory bowel disease, especially Crohn's disease, have a high prevalence of circulating antibodies against type VII collagen (Chen et al., 1997). In addition, type VII collagen was recently shown to be present in the intestinal epithelium (Lohi et al., 1996). Because type VII collagen is the antigenic target for autoantibodies in patients with EBA, we speculate that autoimmunity to type VII collagen which exists in both gut and skin, may explain why these patients frequently have inflammatory bowel disease. The presence of type VII collagen antibodies in Crohn's disease patients may be an epitope spreading phenomenon whereby inflammation originally invoked by Crohn's disease could perturb the intestinal epithelial BMZ such that BMZ components could be altered, resulting in an ongoing autoimmunity to type VII collagen (Chan et al., 1998).

Pathology

Lesional skin histology initially shows papillary edema and vacuolar alteration along the DEJ and at a later stage, a subepidermal blister. Various degrees of dermal inflammatory infiltrate are seen in concordance with the clinical presentation. The classical presentation shows little inflammatory infiltrate within the dermis as opposed to the BP-like presentation (Lever and Schaumburg-Lever, 1990). The infiltrate can be found around vessels, around follicles and in the interstitium. In the inflammatory subtypes, the dermal infiltrate may be rich in neutrophils. The infiltrate may be mixed with variable numbers of eosinophils and mononuclear cells. Fibrosis may be seen in older lesions (Ackerman et al., 1997). Because of the variable clinical and histological presentations, it is difficult to diagnose EBA by clinical and histological parameters alone.

Ultrastructural studies of EBA skin have demonstrated a paucity of anchoring fibrils and an amorphous, electron-dense band just beneath the lamina densa (Richer and McNutt, 1979; Ray et al., 1982). Although the autoantibodies are directed against the anchoring fibrils in the sublamina densa region of the BMZ, it should be noted that the cleavage plane of the blister may be either in the lamina lucida or the sublamina densa region where anchoring fibrils are located (Fine et al., 1989). Immunomapping studies have shown that EBA blisters frequently separate above the immune deposits within the lamina lucida (Fine et al., 1989). This is because the lamina lucida is the Achilles' heel of the cutaneous BMZ and is more susceptible to disadherence than the sublamina densa zone (Briggaman and Wheeler, 1975; Briggaman et al., 1980). Briggaman et al. (1980) have shown that a variety of soluble inflammatory mediators and cytokines can readily induce epidermal disadhesion through the lamina lucida space. It is likely that when there is some level of inflammation in EBA, the lamina lucida is much more vulnerable than the sublamina densa area to proteolytic degradation. Therefore, the cleavage plane of the blister is not a good way to discriminate EBA from other subepidermal bullous diseases.

Diagnosis

Direct Immunofluorescence (DIF)

By definition, patients with EBA have IgG deposits within the DEJ of their skin (Yaoita et al., 1981). This is best detected by DIF of a biopsy specimen obtained from a perilesional site. The deposits are predominantly IgG, but, complement, IgA, IgM, Factor B and properidin may be detected as well (Kushniruk, 1973; Yaoita et al., 1981). The DIF staining demonstates an intense, linear fluorescent band at the DEJ. Yaoita et al. (1981) have suggested that a positive DIF and IgG deposits within the sublamina densa zone are necessary criteria for the diagnosis of EBA. However, in some LABD – like patients, the deposited antibody is IgA without IgG (Hashimoto et al. 1996; Bauer et al., 1999).

Patients with porphyria cutanea tarda (a syndrome that clinically may mimic EBA) frequently have IgG and complement deposits at the DEJ similar to EBA patients (Epstein et al., 1973). However, DIF of porphyria patients as opposed to EBA patients, also demonstrates immune deposits around dermal blood vessels in addition to the DEJ.

Indirect Immunofluorescence (IIF)

Patients with EBA may have autoantibodies in their blood directed against the DEJ (Woodley et al., 1984). These antibodies can be detected by IIF of the patient's serum on a substrate of monkey or rabbit esophagus or human skin. A positive test gives a linear fluorescent band along the DEJ that may be indistinguishable from BP sera. The autoantibodies in EBA patients will label basement membranes beneath stratified squamous epithelium (skin, upper esophagus, and mucosa of the mouth and vagina) and will not bind to basement membranes within most mesenchymal organs such as blood vessels, liver, or kidney. Therefore, there is no difference in labeling pattern and distribution between EBA and BP autoantibodies in this test (Paller et al., 1986).

Distinguishing between EBA and other autoimmune subepidermal bullous diseases may be a problem if patients are evaluated only on the basis of clinical presentation, routine lesional histology and routine DIF and IIF. EBA may share clinical, pathologic, and immunohistologic features with BP, CP or LABD. In addition to the usual laboratory tests for primary blistering disorders (such as routine DIF and IIF), other special tests are necessary to confirm the diagnosis of EBA. These may include direct and indirect salt-split skin immunofluorescence (SSSI), transmission electron microscopy, immunoelectron microscopy, Western blot analysis, and enzyme-linked immunosorbent assay (ELISA).

Transmission Electron Microscopy

Standard transmittion electron microscopy (EM) of the DEJ of human skin can suggest the diagnosis of EBA. As mentioned above, EM would reveal a decrease in the number of anchoring fibrils emanating downward into the papillary dermis from the lamina densa compartment of the DEJ. Further, electron microscopists have noted in EBA skin that there is amorphous, electron – dense, ill-defined material lying just beneath the lamina densa. Although never definitively proven, it is likely that this material corresponds to the IgG deposits in the area attached to anchoring fibrils. This would be suggestive of the diagnosis of EBA.

Immunoelectron Microscopy (IEM)

The "gold standard" for the diagnosis of EBA is IEM. The purpose of IEM is to localize precisely the immune deposits in the patient's skin (direct IEM) or to localize precisely the structure within normal skin to which autoantibodies in the patient's serum bind (indirect IEM). If the deposits are in the sublamina densa region where anchoring fibrils normally exist, this is strong evidence for EBA. If the deposits are higher up over the basal keratinocyte's hemidesmosomes or high within the lamina lucida zone, this is strong evidence for

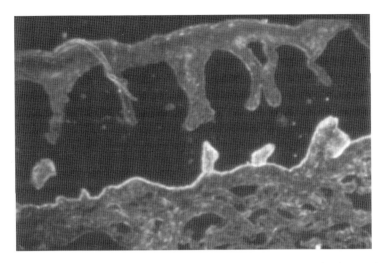

Fig. 3. Direct salt-split immunofluorescence microscopy of a perilesional skin biopsy showing IgG immune deposits remaining with the dermal floor and leaving the epidermis unstained

BP. The skin IgG deposited within the DEJ is demonstrated by a second antibody against human IgG. The second antibody is conjugated with an enzyme such as peroxidase. By incubating the preparation with a substrate such as diaminobenzadine, an electron dense reaction product is formed, thereby indicating the location of the immunoglobulin deposits by electron microscopy (Fig. 4). The second antibody may also be conjugated with electron dense gold particles instead of an enzyme. In EBA patients' tissue, immune deposits are demonstrated within the sublamina densa zone of the BMZ (Nieboer et al., 1980; Yaoita et al., 1981). This localization is distinct from deposits in BP, which are higher up in the hemidesmosome area (Schaumburg et al., 1975) or lamina lucida and from CP where the antigen is confined to the lamina lucida (Domloge-Hultsch et al., 1994).

Direct Salt Split Skin Immunofluorescence (SSSI)

This test is routine DIF performed on perilesional skin from patients that is fractured at the DEJ, through the lamina lucida zone by incubating the skin biopsy specimen with 1 M NaCl at 4 °C for approximately 3 days (Woodley et al., 1983). The direct SSSI test uses fluorescein-conjugated anti-human IgG to label the IgG deposits in the salt-split skin. If the labeling antibody detects the IgG deposits on the dermal floor of the salt-split skin, the diagnosis of EBA is suggested (Fig. 3). In contrast, if the dermal floor is unlabeled and the fluorescent label is observed along the epidermal roof of the salt split skin, EBA is effectively ruled out and the diagnosis of BP is suggested (Gammon et al., 1990).

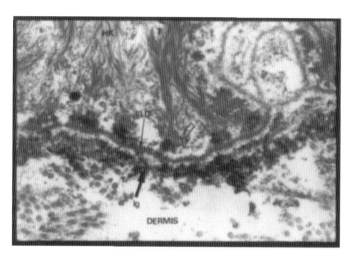

Fig. 4. Immunoelectron microscopy of a perilesional skin biopsy of a patient with EBA. The solid black arrow points to the IgG immune deposits which appear as a heavy, electron-dense band. Ig = immunoglobulin. LD = lamina densa. HK = human keratinocyte. TF = tonofilaments. Note that the IgG deposits are below the lamina densa leaving the lamina lucida unstained (hollow arrow)

Indirect SSSI

This test is designed to detect anti-BMZ autoantibodies in the serum of a patient. It is routine IIF performed on human skin substrate previously fractured through the lamina lucida by incubation of the skin slices with 1 M NaCl. This fracture places the BP antigen on the epidermal side of the split and all other BMZ components on the dermal side. When normal human skin is fractured through the DEJ by this method and used as a substrate for IIF to test the sera of patients with primary autoimmune bullous diseases (such as BP and EBA), the EBA autoantibodies bind to the dermal floor of the salt-split skin substrate, while BP autoantibodies bind to the epidermal roof (Gammon et al., 1984a). This test may be helpful in distinguishing rapidly EBA patients from BP patients. This is particularly important because EBA and BP may have clinical, histological and immunological parameters that are identical.

While the SSSI can be helpful in distinguishing autoantibodies in patients' sera and making the diagnosis of either BP or EBA, it should be noted that the dermal pattern of staining is no longer considered specific for EBA. In one study, a combined dermal-epidermal staining seen in 5% of 98 BP sera and 45% of 23 CP sera (Ghohestani et al., 1997). All of the EBA sera (10 patients), however, only showed dermal staining. Nevertheless, an exclusive dermal staining pattern using SSSI assay may be seen in several other subepidermal bullous diseases besides EBA. It may be seen in (1) bullous SLE (Gammon and Briggaman, 1993), (2) a BP-like disease in which the patients have autoantibodies to a 105 kDa laminia lucida glycoprotein that is unrelated to laminin-5 (Chan et al., 1993), (3) a subset of CP patients who have autoantibodies against laminin-5, a noncollagenous component of anchoring filaments within lamina lucida compartment (Domloge-Hultsch et al., 1994) and (4) in a newly described subepidermal bullous disease associated with a 200 kDa lower lamina lucida antigen designed "anti-p200 pemphigoid" (Mascaro et al., 2000). In contrast to EBA, the bullous diseases with autoantibodies to the novel p105 protein or the p 200 kDa protein respond promptly to topical or systemic corticosteroid treatment, and the lesions heal without scarring or milia formation.

About 50% to 80% of the EBA patients have both tissue-bound and circulating anti-BMZ antibodies (Gammon and Briggaman, 1993). Indirect SSSI test seems to be more sensitive than IIF performed on intact human skin showing higher antibody titers (Gammon et al., 1982; Woodley et al., 1984). At times, no circulating autoantibodies can be demonstrated by either routine IIF or indirect SSSI. In these cases, direct immunoelectron microscopy is needed to make a diagnosis of EBA (Hoang-Xuan et al., 1997).

Western Immunoblotting

Western blot analysis can be useful in making the diagnosis of EBA. In a Western blot, extracts of crude protein from skin basement membrane, amnion or cell culture may be used and subjected to SDS-PAGE and electrophoretically transferred to a membrane. Alternatively, recombinant type VII collagen or type VII collagen purified by biochemical methods can be used as substrate on Western blots. The membrane with immobilized proteins are incubated with EBA and control sera. EBA autoantibodies bind to either a 290 kDa band and/or a 145 kDa in Western blots of human skin basement membrane proteins, whereas sera from all other primary blistering diseases will not (Woodley et al., 1984). These proteins represent the full-length alpha chain of type VII collagen or its amino-terminal globular NC1 domain, the most frequent site of its antigenic epitopes of EBA and bullous SLE autoantibodies, respectively (Woodley et al., 1984; Gammon et al., 1993; Lapiere et al., 1993; Jones et al., 1995). Western immunoblot analysis using type VII collagen extracted from skin cells or from conditioned medium of skin cells may be difficult because of the background non-specific labeling of unrelated proteins when dealing with low titer sera. Alternatively, our recent success in producing unlimited supply of both purified recombinant full-length type VII collagen and the NC1 domain in the stably transfected human cells allows us to use purified recombinant proteins as substrate for Western analysis with virtually no non-specific background labeling (Chen et al., 1997a, 2000a).

Enzyme-Linked Immunosorbent Assay (ELISA)

Recently, Chen et al. (1997b) have produced milligram quantities of recombinant purified posttranslationally modified NC1 in stably transfected human 293 cells and have used this NC1 to develop an ELISA for autoantibody detection in sera from EBA and bullous SLE patients (Fig. 5). In contrast to other techniques such as IEM, IIF and immunoblot analysis, the NC1-based ELISA has several advantages as a screening assay: 1) It is faster and more efficient than IEM, IIF and Western immunoblot analysis, and the ELISA requires only 10–20 µl of serum. By storing batches of NC1-coated plates at −70 °C and using them as needed, the ELISA has an assay time of under 4 hrs. 2) It is easy to perform with a standardized technique. The complete reaction can be carried out in microtiter wells and a spectrophotometer reader allows quantitative measurement. 3) It is more sensitive than

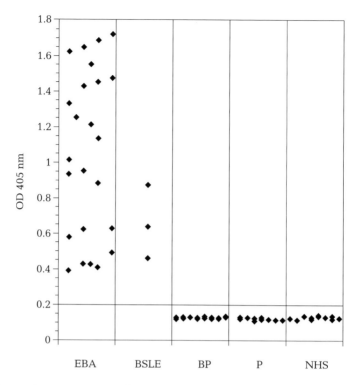

Fig. 5. Scatter plot representation of ELISA results using recombinant NC1. Patient and control sera (as indicated along the horizonal axis) (1:200 dilution) were incubated with immobilized purified recombinant NC1 domain of type VII collagen and the bound antibodies were detected with an alkaline-phosphatase-conjugated antibody against human IgG whole molecule. Each sample was run in triplicate and the points plotted on this graph is the average of the OD 405 obtained from study sera. Similar results were obtained in three other independent studies

conventional IEM or IIF methods, which make it very useful for detecting low titer EBA sera. 4) By using a standard amount of NC1 to coat the wells, one can easily quantitate the anti-NC1 autoantibodies. 5) While other methods (IIF, IEM, immunoblot) are qualitative, the ELISA provides an OD number for direct comparisons of sera, and 6) the ELISA detects autoantibodies which recognize the tertiary and quaternary structure of antigen (conformational epitope), because the assay is performed under native conditions. In contrast, Western immunoblot analysis would not detect autoantibodies requiring a tertiary or quaternary structure of the antigen, because the procedure requires denaturation of proteins with SDS. Thus, the ELISA using recombinant NC1 is a sensitive, specific assay and a useful tool for rapidly screening EBA and BSLE sera.

IIF Microscopy Using Substrate Deficient in Basement Membrane Molecules

IIF using a panel of skin samples which lack specific BMZ molecules, taken from subjects with inherited EB, is a relatively simple and useful tool to identify target antigens in immunobullous disorders. This IIF test is performed on a skin substrate from the most severe Hallopeau-Siemens type of recessive DEB patients, which is deficient in type VII collagen. In this test there was a lack of antibody labeling of the type VII collagen-deficient skin as compared to positive labeling on normal skin or BP180- and laminin-5 deficient skin when EBA sera were used (Vodegel et al., 1998; Jonkman et al., 2000). However, the major limitation of this technique is the availability of suitable skin samples from subjects with EB.

Suction Split Immunofluorescence

This test is similar to the SSSI staining assays, but instead of making the separation between the BMZ layers in vitro using 1 molar salt, it is made in vivo by suction. This method would be faster than salt-split skin substrate methods because the DEJ fracture can be accomplished in a matter of hours instead of days (Feliciani et al., 1998).

Fluorescent Overlay Antigen Mapping (FOAM)

This technique is not widely available. However, it may be less expensive and more rapid than ultrastructural studies using IEM. FOAM distinguishes between IgG deposits above the lamina densa as in BP, from those below, as in EBA (De Jong et al., 1996; Kazama et al., 1998). This technique demonstrates different antigens of the BMZ component by staining the perilesional skin of autoimmune skin disease patients with monoclonal antibodies to known BMZ components such as type VII collagen and staining the immune deposits with different markers. Using computer analysis, the stained BMZ antigens and the stained immune deposits are overlaid one on the other, with or without using confocal laser scanning microscopy, thereby giving the relation of the immune deposits to the BMZ structures.

As we reviewed the various complex diagnostic options, we were motivated to suggest slight modifications in the diagnostic criteria of Yaoita et al. (1981) to the following:

1. A bullous disorder within the clinical spectrum described.
2. Histology showing a subepidermal blister.
3. Deposition of IgG deposits at the DEJ in perilesional skin, i. e., a positive DIF of patient's skin
4. The IgG deposits are localized to the lower lamina densa and/or sublamina densa zone of the DEJ as demonstrated by direct IEM on perilesional skin.
5. Alternatives for item 4 are: indirect or direct salt-split or vacuum split skin immunofluorescence[1], IIF using substrate deficient in basement membrane molecules, Western blotting, FOAM, and ELISA.

When the EBA presentation is CP-like, the SSSI assay may not be sufficient to differentiate from true CP as it may show dermal deposition of antibodies in both diseases. In this instance, IEM is needed to distinguish the two diseases.

---

[1]   When the EBA presentation is CP-like, the SSSI assay may not be sufficient to differentiate from true CP as it may show dermal deposition of antibodies in both diseases. In this instance, IEM is needed to distinguish the two diseases.

Therapy

EBA is a chronic disease which is often refractory to treatment. EBA persists for at least several years in most patients and remission is unpredictable (Gammon and Briggaman, 1993). Because it is an incurable disease without a consistent therapeutic modality, supportive therapy is most important, including detailed and early wound care and antibiotic treatment for local skin infections. Exacerbating factors such as trauma, the use of harsh soaps, and sun exposure should be avoided (Jappe et al., 2000). The patient should be educated to recognize localized skin infections and to seek medical care and antibiotic therapy promptly when this occurs.

Colchicine

Because the responses to therapy are not consistent, the clinician often needs to take an empirical approach to therapy. It is reasonable for the clinician to try therapies in the order of using those therapies with the best side effect profile first. For example, there are several reports of patients with the classic and inflammatory phenotypes of EBA who responded to high doses of colchicine (Cunningham et al., 1996; Megahed and Scharfetter-Kochanek, 1994). Colchicine is a good first-line drug because its side effects are relatively benign compared with other therapeutic choices. One problem with colchicine is that many patients with EBA have inflammatory bowel disease, and the predictable, dose-dependent, gastrointestinal side effects of colchicine makes it unusable in these patients. Even patients without clinically defined inflammatory bowel disease may not be able to tolerate even the lowest doses of colchicine without suffering abdominal cramping and diarrhea. It is unclear how colchicine works in EBA, but there is evidence the colchicine can decrease the production of antibodies by plasma cells and may also inhibit antigen presenting cells from presenting antigen to T cells. Therefore, the drug may work at two levels – the inhibition of the initiation of autoimmunity and the inhibition of autoantibody production. Our experience has been that the patients who do the best on colchicine are those who are able to get up to 1.5–2.5 mg per day. We go up slowly starting at 0.4–0.6 mg per day and then double the dose every two weeks until the patient experiences gastrointestinal side-effects. We then back-off by one tablet with the hope of achieving the highest tolerable dose for the patient.

Immunosuppressive Agents

EBA patients, especially with the classical mechanobullous form, are often refractory to high doses of systemic glucocorticoids, azathioprine, methotrexate, and cyclophosphamide (Woodley et al., 1998). These agents may be somewhat helpful in controlling EBA when it appears as an inflammatory BP-like disease. Childhood EBA, a rare subset which is usually the inflammatory BP-like form of the disease, appears to respond more favorably to dapsone and prednisone than adult patients with EBA (Callot-Mellot et al., 1997).

Cyclosporin A

Cyclosporin, an immunosuppressive agent that is mainly used in organ transplantation, has been shown to be helpful in a number of EBA patients (Connolly and Sander, 1987; Crow et al., 1988). High doses of cyclosporin ($>6\,mg/kg$) are needed. Cyclosporin has a number of significant side-effects with its predictable nephrotoxicity being the most significant. The nephrotoxicity is time and dose dependent. Because EBA patients tend to be elderly with preexisting renal compromise due to age and because high doses of cyclosporine are needed to control the disease, the usage of cyclosporin in EBA is often problematic and limited. In most situations, the long-term toxicity of the drug makes its use warranted only as a last-resort measure.

High Dose Immunoglobulins

EBA has also been reported to respond to high and low dose intravenous immunoglobulins (Kofler et al., 1997), plasmapheresis in conjunction with immunoglobulins (Furue et al., 1986) and extracorporeal photochemotherapy (Gordon et al., 1997; Camara et al., 1999). Gammon and Briggaman (1993) reported having little or no success with phenytoin, gold, plasmapheresis, vitamin E or dapsone. Unfortunately, recent treatment trials with mycophenolate mofetil combined with autologous keratinocyte grafting were reported to be unsuccessful (Schattenkirchner et al., 1999).

Photopheresis

Photopheresis has been used in Sezary syndrome, mycosis fungoides, and a variety of autoimmune bullous diseases (Rook et al., 1990). One EBA patient in a life-threatening situation responded dramatically to photopheresis (Miller et al., 1995). In three other EBA patients, photopheresis improved some clinical parameters and significantly lengthened the suction blistering times of the patients, suggesting an improvement in their dermal-epidermal adherence (Gordon et al., 1997). All three patients also had reductions of anti-type VII collagen antibodies in their blood.

Rituximab

Rituximab is a monoclonal, chimeric antibody that specifically targets the mmune cell surface marker CD20, which is primarily expressed by B lymphocytes. Rituximab was originally used in the treatment of B-cell lymphomas but has also been used successfully in several autoimmune diseases. A small number of case reports have reported the successful treatment of treatment refractory EBA with rituximab as an adjuvant agent (Saha et al., 2009; Schmidt et al., 2006; Crichlow et al., 2007; Niedermeier et al., 2007). The clinical improvement was generally accompanied by reduction in immunosuppression necessary to control the disease as well as decreased anti-type VII collagen antibody titers.

3

Immune Adsorption

An unexplored and potentially productive approach to treatment that is now feasible is the utilization of fragments of recombinant type VII collagen to absorb autoantibodies from patients' sera or plasma. Previous studies have identified autoreactive epitopes within NC-1 domain. Peptides synthesized from these epitopes have been coupled to affinity matrices and shown to absorb autoantibodies to type VII collagen from patients' sera (Gammon et al., 1993). The recent method of Chen et al. (1997a) for producing milligram quantities of recombinant NC1 domain in human 293 cells makes affinity plasmapheresis of patients a feasible treatment approach. The rationale for this approach, particularly in patients with the inflammatory phenotype, is supported by the relationship between autoantibody levels and the development of inflammation at the DEJ in EBA and bullous SLE.

Summary

EBA is a clinically heterogeneous acquired, subepidermal bullous disease. In its classical form, it is a mechanobullous disease with skin fragility and trauma-induced blisters that have minimal inflammation and heal with scarring and milia – features that are highly reminiscent of hereditary dystrophic forms of epidermolysis bullosa. A hallmark of EBA are IgG autoantibodies targeted against the type VII collagen within anchoring fibrils. Anchoring fibrils are structures that anchor the epidermis and its underlying BMZ onto the dermis. However, it has also become evident that EBA may present with clinical manifestations reminiscent of bullous pemphigoid (BP), cicatricial pemphigoid (CP), and Brunsting-Perry pemphigoid. The diagnostic criteria for EBA are: (1) spontaneous or trauma-induced blisters resembling hereditary DEB, (2) adult onset, (3) a negative family history for EB, and (4) the exclusion of all other bullous diseases. Due to the pronounced skin fragility caused by the autoantibody-induced paucity of anchoring fibrils, EBA is difficult to treat. The BP-like inflammatory variants of EBA respond well to systemic corticosteroids and immunosuppressive adjuvants while the mechanobullous variant and the MMP-like variants do to a much lesser extent. Novel therapeutic strategies such as immunoadsorption and the anti-CD20 monoclonal antibody, rituximab, had beneficial effects in small case series.

References

Ackerman AB, Chongchitnant N, Sanchez J, Guo Y, Benin B, Reichel M, Randall MB (1997) Histologic diagnosis of inflammatory skin diseases: an algorithmic method based on pattern analysis. 2nd ed. Williams & Wilkins, Baltimore

Arpey CJ, Elewski BE, Moritz DK, Gammon WR (1991) Childhood epidermolysis bullosa acquisita: report of three cases and review of literature. J Am Acad Dermatol 24:706–714

Bauer JW, Schaeppi H, Metze D, Muss W, Pohla-Gubo G, Hametner R, Ruckhofer J, Grabner G, Hintner H (1999) Ocular involvement in IgA-epidermolysis bullosa acquisita. Br J Dermatol 141:887–892

Bernard P, Vaillant L, Labeille B, Bedane C, Arbeille B, Denoeux JP, Lorette G, Bonnetblanc JM, Prost C (1995) Incidence and distribution of subepidermal autoimmune bullous skin diseases in three French regions. Arch Dermatol 131:48–52

Borradori L, Caldwell JB, Briggaman RA, Burr CE, Gammon WR, James WD, Yancey KB (1995) Passive transfer of autoantibodies from a patient with mutilating epidermolysis bullosa acquisita induces specific alterations in the skin of neonatal mice. Arch Dermatol 131:590–595

Briggaman RA, Wheeler CE Jr (1975) The epidermal-dermal junction. J Invest Dermatol 65:71–84

Briggaman RA, Schechter NM, Fraki J, Lazarus GS (1980) Degradation of the epidermal-dermal junction by proteolytic enzymes from human skin and human polymorphonuclear leukocytes. J Exp Med 160:1027–1042

Bruckner-Tuderman L, Nilssen O, Zimmermann DR, Dours-Zimmermann MT, Kalinke DU, Gedde-Dahl TJr, Winberg JO (1995) Immunohistochemical and mutation analyzes demonstrate that procollagen VII is processed to collagen VII through removal of the NC-2 domain. J Cell Biol 131:551–559

Burgeson RE (1993) Type VII collagen, anchoring fibrils, and epidermolysis bullosa. J Invest Dermatol 101:252–255

Callot-Mellot C, Bodemer C, Caux F, Bourgault-Villada I, Fraitag S, Goudie G, Heller M, de Prost Y, Prost C (1997) Epidermolysis bullosa aquisita in childhood. Arch of Dermatol 133:1122–1126

Camara A, Becherel PA, Bussel A, Lagrange S, Chosidow O, Joly P, Piette JC, Frances C (1999) Resistant acquired bullous epidermolysis with severe ocular involvement: the success of extracorporeal photochemotherapy. Annal Dermatol Venereol 126:612–615

Chan LS, Fine JD, Briggaman RA, Woodley DT, Hammerberg C, Drugge RJ, Cooper KD (1993) Identification and partial characterization of a novel 105-kDalton lower lamina lucida autantigen associated with a novel immune-mediated subepidermal blistering disease. J Invest Dermatol 101:262–267

Chan LS, Woodley DT (1996) Pemphigoid: Bullous and cicatricial. In Current Therapy in Allergy, Immunology and Rhematology, 5th ed, edited by LM Lichtenstein, AS Fauci Mosby, St Louis, p 93

Chan LS, Vanderlugt CJ, Hashimoto T, Nishikawa T, Zones JJ, Black MM, Wojnarowask F, Stevens SR, Chen M, Failey JA, Miller SD, Gordon KB (1998) Epitope spreading: Lessons from autoimmune skin diseases. J Invest Dermatol 110:103–109

Chen M, Marinkovich MP, Veis A, O'Toole EA, Rao CN, Cai XY, Woodley DT (1997a) Interactions of the amino-terminal noncollagenous (NC1) domain of type VII collagen with extracellular matrix components: a potential role in epidermal-dermal adherence in human skin. J Biol Chem 272:14516–14522

Chen M, Chan LS, Cai X, O'Toole EA, Sample JC, Woodley DT (1997b) Development of an ELISA for rapid detection of anti-type VII collagen autoantibodies in epidermolysis bullosa acquisita. J Invest Dermatol 108:68–72

Chen M, O'Toole EA, Sanghavi J, Mahmud N, Kelleher D, Woodley DT (1997c) Type VII collagen exists in human intestine and serves as an antigenic target in patients with inflammatory bowel disease. J Invest Dermatol 108:542

Chen M, Marinkovich MP, Jones JC, O'Toole E, Li YY, Woodley DT (1999) NC1 domain of type VII collagen binds to the beta3 chain of laminin 5 via a unique subdomain within the fibronectin-like repeats. J Invest Dermatol 112:177–183

Chen M, Tahk SH, Costa FK, Kasahara N, Woodley DT (2000a) Recombinant expression of full-length type VII collagen alpha chain: structural and functional characterization and implication for gene therapy. J Invest Dermatol 114:756

Chen M, Wang J, Tahk SH and Woodley DT (2000b) Noncollagenous (NC2) domain of type VII collagen mediates the antiparallel-dimer formation of type VII collagen and constitutes a new antigenic epitope for EBA and BSLE autoantibodies. J Invest Dermatol 114:766

Cho HJ, Lee IJ, Kim SC (1998) Complement fixing abilities and IgG subclasses of autoantibodies in epidermolysis bullosa acquisita. Yonsei Medical Journal 39:339–344

Choi GS, Lee ES, Kim SC, Lee S (1998) Epidermolysis bullosa aquisita localized to the face. J Dermatol 25:19–22

Christiano AM, Greenspan DS, Lee S, and Uitto, J (1994) Cloning of human type VII collagen: complete primary sequence of the alpha 1(VII) chain and identification of intragenic polymorphisms. J Biol Chem 269:20256–20262

Connolly SM, Sander HM (1987) Treatment of epidermolysis bullosa acquisita with cyclosporin. J Am Acad Dermatol 16:890

Crichlow SM, Mortimer NJ, Harman KE (2007) A successful therapeutic trial of rituximab in the treatment of a patient with recalcitrant, high-titre epidermolysis bullosa acquisita. Br J Dermatol 156:194–196

Crow LL, Finkle JP, Gammon WR, Woodley DT (1988) Cleaning of epidermolysis bullosa acquisita on cyclosporin A. J Am Acad Dermatol 19:937–942

Cunningham BB, Kirchmann TT, Woodley DT (1996) Colchicine for epidermolysis bullosa (EBA). J Am Acad Dermatol 34:781–784

Dahl MG (1979) Epidermolysis bullosa acquisita – a sign of cicatricial pemphigoid? Br J Dermatol 101:475–483

De Jong MCJM, Bruins S, Heeres K, Jonkman MF, Nieboer C, Boorsma DM, Pas HH, van der Meer JB (1996) Bullous pemphigoid and epidermolysis bullosa acquisita: Differentiation by fluorescence overlay antigen mapping. Arch Dermatol 132:151–157

Domloge-Hultsch N, Anhalt GJ, Gammon WR, Lazarova Z, Briggaman R, Welch M, Jabs DA, Huff C, Yancey KB (1994) Antiepiligrin cicatricial pemphigoid: A subepithelial bullous disorder. Arch Dermatol 130:1521–1529

Edwards S, Wakelin SH, Wojnarowska F, Marsden RA, Kirtschig G, Bhogal B, Black MM (1998) Bullous pemphigoid and epidermolysis bullosa acquisita: presentation, prognosis, and immunopathology in 11 children. Pediatr Dermatol 15:184–190

Elliott GT (1895) Two cases of epidermolysis bullosa. J Cutan Genitourin Dis 13:10

Epstein JH, Tuffanelli DL, Epstein WL (1973) Cutaneous changes in the porphyrias. A microscopic study. Arch Dermatol 107:689–698

Feliciani C, Di Muzio M, Mohammad Pour S, Allegretti T, Amerio P, Toto P, Coscione G, Proietto G, Amerio P (1998) 'Suction split' as a routine method to differentiate epidermolysis bullosa acquisita from bullous pemphigoid. J Eur Acad Dermatol Venereol 10:243–247

Fine JD, Tyring S, Gammon WR (1989) The presence of intra-lamina lucida blister formation in epidermolysis bullosa acquisita: Possible role of leukocytes. J Invest Dermatol 92:27

Furue M, Iwata M, Yoon H-I, Kubota Y, Ohto H, Kawashima M, Tsuchida T, Oohara K, Tamaki K, Kukita A (1986) Epidermolysis bullosa acquisita: clinical response to plasma exchange therapy and circulating anti-BMZ antibody titer. J Am Acad Dermatol 14:873–878

Gammon WR, Briggaman RA, Wheeler CE Jr (1982) Epidermolysis bullosa acquisita presenting as an inflammatory bullous disease. J Am Acad Dermatol 7:382–387

Gammon WR, Briggaman RA, Inman AO, Queen LL, Wheeler CE (1984a) Differentiating anti-lamina lucida and antisublamina densa anti-BMZ antibodies by indirect immunofluorescence on 1.0 M sodium chloride-separated skin. J Invest Dermatol 82:139–144

Gammon WR, Briggaman RA, Woodley DT, Heald PW. Wheeler CE Jr (1984b) Epidermolysis bullosa acquisita – a pemphigoid like disease. J Am Acad Dermatol 11:820–832

Gammon WR, Woodley DT, Dole KC, Briggaman RA (1985) Evidence that basement membrane zone antibodies in bullous eruption of systemic lupus erythematosus recognize epidermolysis bullosa acquisita autoantigens. J Invest Dermatol 84:472–476

Gammon WR (1988a) Epidermolysis bullosa acquisita. Semin Dermatol 7:218–224

Gammon WR, Heise ER, Burke WA, Fine JD, Woodley DT, Briggaman RA (1988b) Increased frequency of HLA-DR2 in patients with autoantibodies to epidermolysis bullosa acquisita antigen: Evidence that the expression of autoimmunity to type VII collagen is HLA class II allele associated. J Invest Dermatol 91:228–232

Gammon WR, Kowalewski C, Chorzelski TP, Kumar V, Briggaman RA, Beutner EH (1990) Direct immunofluorescence studies of sodium chloride-separated skin in the differential diagnosis of bullous pemphigoid and epidermolysis bullosa acquisita. J Am Acad Dermatol 22:664–670

Gammon WR, Briggaman RA (1993) Epidermolysis bullosa acquisita and bullous systemic lupus erythematosus: disease of autoimmunity to type VII collagen. Dermatol Clin 11:535–547

Gammon WR, Murrell DF, Jenison MW, Padilla KM, Prisayanh PS, Jones DA, Briggaman RA, Hunt SW III (1993) Autoantibodies to type VII collagen recognize epitopes in a fibronectin-like region of the noncollagenous (NC1) domain. J Invest Dermatol 100:618–622

Ghohestani RF, Nicolas JF, Roussele P, Claudy AL (1997) Diagnostic value of indirect immunofluorescence on sodium chloride-split skin in differential diagnosis of subepidermal autoimmune bullous dermatoses. Arch Dermatol 133:1102–1107

Gordon KB, Chan LS, Woodley DT (1997) Treatment of refractory epidermolysis bullosa acquisita with extracorporeal photochemotherapy. Br J Dermatol 136:415–420

Harman KE, Whittam LR, Wakelin SH, Black MM (1998) Severe, refractory epidermolysis bullosa acquisita complicated by an oesophageal stricture responding to intravenous immune globulin. Br J Dermatol 139:1126–1127

Hashimoto T, Ishiko A, Shimizu H, Tanaka T, Dodd HJ, Bhogal BS, Black MM, Nishikawa T (1996) A case of linear IgA bullous dermatosis with IgA anti-type VII collagen autoantibodies. Br J Dermatol 134:336–339

Hoang-Xuan T, Robin H, Heller M, Caux F, Prost C (1997) Epidermolysis bullosa acquisita diagnosed by direct immunoelectron microscopy of the conjunctiva. Ophthalmology 104:1414–1420

Jappe U, Zillikens D, Bonnekoh B, Gollnick H (2000) Epidermolysis bullosa acquisita with ultraviolet radiation sensitivity. Br J Dermatol 142:517–520

Joly P, Ruto F, Thomine E, Delpech A, Balguerie X, Tron F, Lauret P (1993) Brunsting-Perry Cicatricial Bullous Pemphigoid: a clinical variant of localized acquired epidermolysis bullosa? J Am Acad Dermatol 28:89–92

Jones DA, Hunt SW III, Prisayanh PS, Briggaman RA, Gammon WR (1995) Immunodominant autoepitopes of type VII collagen are short, paired peptide sequences within the fibronectin type III homology region of the noncollagenous (NC1) domain. J Invest Dermatol 104:231–235

Jonkman MF, Schuur J, Dijk F, Heeres K, de Jong MC, van der Meer JB, Yancey KB, Pas HH (2000) Inflammatory variant of epidermolysis bullosa acquisita with IgG autoantibodies against type VII collagen and laminin α3. Arch Dermatol 136:227–231

Kazama T, Yamamoto Y, Hashimoto T, Komai A, Ito M (1998) Application of confocal laser scanning microscopy to differential diagnosis of bullous pemphigoid and epidermolysis bullosa acquisita. Br J Dermatol 138:593–601

Kofler H, Wambacher-Gasser B, Topar G, Weinlich G, Schuler G, Hintner H, Romani N, Fritsch P (1997) Intravenous immunoglobulin treatment in therapy – resistant epidermolysis bullosa acquisita. J Am Acad Dermatol 36:331–335

Kurzhals G, Stolz W, Meurer M, Kunze J, Braun-Falco O, Krieg T (1991) Acquired epidermolysis bullosa with the clinical feature of Brunsting-Perry cicatricial bullous pemphigoid. Arch Dermatol 127:391–395

Kushniruk W (1973) The immunopathology of epidermolysis bullosa acquisita. Can Med Assoc J 108:1143–1146

Lapiere JC, Woodley DT, Parente MG, Iwasaki T, Wynn KC, Christiano AM, Uitto J (1993) Epitope mapping of type VII collagen: identification of discrete peptide sequences recognized by sera from patients with acquired epidermolysis bullosa. J Clin Invest 92:1831–1839

Lapiere JC, Chen JD, Iwasaki T, Hu L, Uitto J, Woodley DT (1994) Type VII collagen specifically binds fibronectin via a unique subdomain within the collagenous triple helix. J Invest Dermatol 103:637–641

Lee CW (1998) Prevalences of subacute cutaneous lupus erythematosus and epidermolysis bullosa acquisita among Korean/oriental papulations. Dermatology 197:187

Lee CW (2000) Serum IgA autoantibodies in patients with epidermolysis bullosa acquisita: A high frequency of detection. Dermatology 200:83–84

Lever WF, Schaumburg-Lever G (1990) Congenital disease (genodermatoses). In Histopathology of the skin, edited by WF Lever, G Schaumburg-Lever. Philadephia, Lippincott, p 78

Lohi J, Leivo I, Tani T, Kiviluoto T, Kivilaakso E, Burgeson RE, Virtanen I (1996) Laminins, tenascin and type VII collagen in colorrectal mucosa. Histochem J 28:431–440

Mascaro JM Jr, Zillikens D, Giudice GJ, Caux F, Fleming MG, Katz HM, Diaz LA (2000) A subepidermal bullous eruption associated with IgG autoantibodies to a 200 kd dermal antigen: The first case report from the United States. J Am Acad Dermatol 242:309–315

Megahed M, Scharfetter-Kochanek K (1994) Epidermolysis bullosa acquisita-successful treatment with colchicine. Arch Dermatol Res 286:35–46

Miller JK, Stricklin GP, Fine JD, King LE, Arzubiaga MC, Ellis DL (1995) Remission of svere epidermolysis bullosa acquisita induced by extracoporeal photochemotherapy. Br J Dermatol 133:467–471

Niedermeier A, Eming R, Pfütze M, Neumann CR, Happel C, Reich K, Hertl M (2007) Clinical response of severe mechanobullous epidermolysis bullosa acquisita to combined treatment with immunoadsorption and rituximab (anti-CD20 monoclonal antibodies). Arch Dermatol 143:192–8

Nieboer C, Boorsma DM, Woerdeman MJ, Kalsbeek GL (1980) Epidermolysis bullosa acquisita: immunofluorescence, electron microscopic and immunoelectron microscopic studies in four patients. Br J Dermatol 102:383–392

Paller AS, Queen LL, Woodley DT, Lane AT, Gammon WR, Briggaman RA (1986) Organ specific, phylogenic and ontogenetic distribution of the epidermolysis bullosa acquisita antigen. J Invest Dermatol 86:376–379

Park SB, Cho KH, Youn JL, Hwang DH, Kim SC, Chung JH (1997) Epidermolysis bullosa aquisita in childhood – a case mimicking chronic bullous dermatosis of childhood. Clin Exp Dermatol 22:220–222

Ray TL, Levine JB, Weiss W, Ward PA (1982) Epidermolysis bullosa acquisita and inflammatory bowel disease. J Am Acad Dermatol 6:242–252

Richter BJ, McNutt NS (1979) The spectrum of epidermolysis bullosa acquisita. Arch Dermatol 115:1325–1328

Roenigk HH, Ryan JG, Bergfeld WF (1971) Epidermolysis bullosa acquisita: Report of three cases and review of all published cases. Arch Dermatol 103:1–10

Rook AH, Jegasothy BV, Heald P, Nahass GT, Ditre C, Witmer WK, Lazarus GS, Edelson RL (1990) Extracoporeal photochemotherapy for drug-resistant pemphigus vulgaris. Ann Intern Med 112:303–305

Rusenko KW, Gammon WR, and Briggaman RA (1989) Type VII collagen is the antigen recognized by IgA anti-sub lamina densa autoantibodies. J Invest Dermatol 92:510 Abstract

Saha M, Cutler T, Bhogal B, Black MM, Groves RW (2009) Refractory epidermolysis bullosa acquisita: successful treatment with rituximab. Clin Exp Dermatol 34: e979–980

Sakai LY, Keene DR, Morris NP, Burgeson RE (1986) Type VII collagen is a major structural component of anchoring fibrils. J Cell Biol 103:1577–1586

Schattenkirchner S, Eming S, Hunzelmann N, Krieg T, Smola H (1999) Treatment of epidermolysis bullosa acquisita with mycophenolate mofetil and autologous keratinocyte grafting. Br J Dermatol 141:932–933

Schaumburg-Lever G, Rule A, Schmidt-Ullrich B, Lever WF (1975) Ultrastructural localization of in vivo bound immunoglobulins in bullous pemphigoid – A prelimnary report. J Invest Dermatol 64:47–49

Schmidt E, Benoit S, Brocker EB, Zillikens D, Goebeler M. (2006) Successful adjuvant treatment of recalcitrant epidermolysis bullosa acquisita with anti-CD20 antibody rituximab. Arch Dermatol 142:147–150

Sitaru C, Mihai S, Otto C, Chiriac MT, Hausser I, Dotterweich B, Saito H, Rose C, Ishiko A, Zillikens D (2005) Induction of dermal-epidermal separation in mice by passive transfer of antibodies specific to type VII collagen. J Clin Invest 2005, 115:870–878

Stewart MI, Woodley DT, Briggaman RA (1991) Acquired epidermolysis bullosa and associated symptomatic esophageal webs. Arch Dermatol 127:373–377

Tanaka H, Ishida-Yamamoto A, Hashimoto T (1997) A novel variant of acquired epidermolysis bullosa with autoantibodies against the central triple-helical domain of type VII collagen. Lab Invest 77:623–632

Taniuchi K, Inaoki M, Nishimura Y, Mori T, Takehara K (1997) Nonscarring inflammatory epidermolysis bullosa acquisita with esophageal involvement and linear IgG deposits. J Am Acad Dermatol 36:320–322

Tokuda Y, Amagai M, Yaoita H, Kawachi S, Ito T, Matsuyama I, Tsuchiya S, Saida T (1998) A case of inflammatory variant of epidermolysis bullosa acquisita: Chronic bullous dermatosis associated with non scarring mucosal blisters and circulating IgG anti-type-VII-collagen antibody. Dermatology 197:58–61

Uitto J, Christiano AM (1994) Molecular basis for the dystrophic forms of epidermolysis bullosa: mutations in the type VII collagen gene. Arch Dermatol Res 287:16–22

Vodegel RM, Kiss M, De Jong MCJM, Pas HH, Altmayer A, Molnar K, Husz S, Van Der Meer JB, Jonkman MF (1998) The use of skin substrate deficient in basement membrane molecules for the diagnosis of subepidermal autoimmune bullous disease. Eur J Dermatol 8:83–85

Wieme N, Lambert J, Moerman M, Geerts ML, Temmerman L, Naeyaert JM (1999) Epidermolysis bullosa acquisita with combined features of bullous pemphigoid and cicatricial pemphigoid. Dermatology 198:310–313

Woodley DT, Sauder D, Talley MJ, Silver M, Grotendorst G, Qwarnstrom E (1983) Localization of basement membrane components after DEJ separation. J Invest Dermatol 81:149–153

Woodley DT, Briggaman RA, O'Keefe EJ, Inman AO, Queen LL, Gammon WR (1984) Identification of the skin basement-membrane autoantigen in epidermolysis bullosa acquisita. N Engl J Med 310:1007–1015

Woodley DT, O'Keefe EJ, Reese MJ, Mechanic GL, Briggaman RA, Gammon WR (1986) Epidermolysis bullosa acquisita antigen, a new major component of cutaneous basement membrane, is a glycoprotein with collagenous domains. J Invest Dermatol 86:668–672

Woodley DT (1988) Epidermolysis bullosa acquisita. Prog Dermatol 22:1

Woodley DT, Burgeson RE, Lunstrum G, Bruckner-Tuderman L, Reese MJ, Briggaman RA (1988) The epidermolysis bullosa acquisita antigen is the globular carboxyl terminus of type VII procollagen. J Clin Invest 81:683–687

Woodley DT, Gammon WR, Briggaman RA (1998) Epidermolysis bullosa acquisita. In: Fitzpatrick TB, Eisen AZ, Wolff K, Freedberg IM, Austen KF, editors. Dermatology in general medicine. 4th ed. Vols. I–II. McGraw-Hill, New York, 702–709

Woodley DT, Chang C, Saadat P, Ram R, Liu Z, Chen M (2005) Evidence that anti-type VII collagen antibodies are pathogenic and responsible for the clinical, histological, and immunological features of epidermolysis bullosa acquisita. J Invest Dermatol 124:958–964

Woodley DT, Ram R, Doostan A, Bandyopadhyay P, Huang Y, Remington J, Hou YP, Keene DR, Liu Z, Chen M (2006) Induction of epidermolysis bullosa acquisita in mice by passive transfer of autoantibodies from patients. J Invest Dermatol 126:1324–1330

Yancey KB. Cicatricial pemphigoid. In: Fitzpatrick TB, Eisen AZ, Wolff K, Freedberg IM, Austen KF (1998) Dermatology in general medicine. 4th ed. Vols. I – II. McGraw-Hill, New York, Inc., pp 674–679

Yaoita H, Briggaman A, Lawley TJ, Provost TT, Katz SI (1981) Epidermolysis bullosa acquisita: Ultrastructural and immunological studies. J Invest Dermatol 76:288–292

Zillikens D, Wever S, Roth A, Hashimoto T, Brocker EB (1995) Incidence of autoimmune subepidermal blistering dermatoses in a region of central Germany. Arch Dermatol 131:957–958

3

Scleroderma

4.1 Localized Scleroderma

4

Cristián Vera Kellet, Catherine H. Orteu, and Jan P. Dutz

Introduction

Definition

Localized scleroderma (LS) or morphea encompasses a group of disorders characterized by delimited and localized inflammatory sclerosis (thickening) and fibrosis of the skin, subcutaneous tissue, fascia and/or adjacent muscle. In contrast to systemic sclerosis, Raynaud's phenomenon, acrosclerosis and internal organ involvement do not usually occur. Morphea may be divided into 5 subtypes: plaque, generalized, bullous, linear and deep, based on the extent, form and depth of cutaneous sclerosis (Peterson et al., 1995). These subtypes frequently occur together in the same patient. Although morphea is rarely life threatening, significant morbidity and disability occur, particularly in the linear and deep forms.

Epidemiology

Most studies suggest that morphea is commoner in women, with female to male ratios of between 6 and 2.6:1 (Christianson et al., 1956; Jablonska, 1975b; Peterson et al., 1997; Silman et al., 1988). This female preponderance may be less marked in the linear group, in which ratios of 1:1 (Peterson et al., 1997) to 4:1 (Falanga et al., 1986) have been documented. The prevalence of morphea is not absolutely clear. A UK population based study in 1986, suggested prevalence rates of 13 and 48 per million in adult males and females respectively, with annual incidence rates of 1 and 6 per million (Silman et al., 1988). A second study, conducted over a 30 year period (1960–1993) by Peterson et al. (1997) in Olmsted County, USA, revealed 82 cases, an overall incidence of 2.7/100 000/year. Prevalence was estimated at 0.05% at age 18 years and at 0.22% at age 80 years. Interestingly, a progressive increase in the incidence of plaque morphea was noted over the 30 year period. In this study, plaque morphea was the commonest subtype (56% of cases), followed in order of frequency by linear (20%), generalized (13%), and deep (11%). Of the 11 patients with generalized morphea, 5 initially presented with morphea en plaque and progressed over 5 months to 3 years. Coexisting morphea subtypes occurred in 11% of patients.

4

In a large European referral-based series, Jablonska (1975b) found that plaque morphea was commoner in adults (28.5% of adult cases versus 15% for the linear group), and
that linear forms were commoner in children (31.5% and 21.3% of childhood cases respectively). These data are corroborated by those of Peterson et al. (1997): the mean age at onset of disease was 12.2 years in the linear group, 31.5 years in the plaque group, 39.9 years
in the generalized group, and 45.1years in the deep group. A retrospective analysis of 239
cases seen at an Italian referral center further confirmed these results: Children more commonly had linear or "mixed" linear and plaque-type forms of morphea (54/126 cases) than
adults (16/113 cases) (Marzano et al., 2003). Pediatric morphea (defined as onset under
age 16) was recently found to occur with an incidence of 3.4 per million/year in a study of
the UK and Ireland, again with linear forms predominating (71% of cases) (Herrick et al.,
2010) and with a mean age of onset (first assessment) of 10.4 years.

The duration of disease activity can vary from a few months up to 20–30 years, but is
usually 3–5 years (Christianson et al., 1956). Plaque lesions generally resolve earlier than
other subtypes. In the Olmsted county series, 50% of the patients had 50% softening (or
more), or resolution by 3.8 years after diagnosis. There was 50% resolution at 2.7 years in
the plaque group, at 5 years in generalized and linear groups and at 5.5 years in the deep
group (Peterson et al., 1997). Relapse can occur and may be more frequent with generalized, deep and "mixed" forms (Marzano et al., 2003).

The exact relationship between LS and systemic sclerosis (SSc) remains unclear, however, it has been compared to that between discoid and systemic lupus erythematosus
(Jablonska and Rodnan, 1979). LS in the absence of Raynaud's phenomenon and acral sclerosis rarely if ever evolves into SSc. In larger series, transition from morphea to SSc, was reported in 2/235 (Christianson et al., 1956) and 4/253 (Jablonska, 1975b) patients. Plaques
of morphea can be seen in association with true SSc, and occurred in 9/135 patients in a
Japanese study (Soma et al., 1993).

Histopathology

Scleroderma derives from the Greek terms *skleros,* hard, and *derma*, skin and means hard
skin. The different types of morphea do not differ in the elements of the histopathologic
findings but rather with regards to severity and depth of involvement. Both early inflammatory and late sclerotic changes have been described. Most biopsies will show an intermediate picture (Fig. 1).

In the early inflammatory phase, a moderately dense infiltrate of lymphocytes, plasma
cells and histiocytes, and occasionally, mast cells has been described (Fleischmajer and
Nedwich, 1972; O'Leary et al., 1957). This infiltrate may be found in the lower dermis, the
subcutaneous fat and around eccrine glands. The reticular dermis shows thickened collagen bundles. Large areas of subcutaneous fat may be replaced by wavy fibers of newly
formed collagen. Elastic fibers are preserved (Walters et al., 2009). The epidermis may be
normal or slightly acanthotic (Morley et al., 1985). Electron microscopy shows the deposition of collagen fibrils with decreased diameter when compared to mature collagen
(Fleischmajer and Prunieras, 1972). This is due, in part, to an increase in type III collagen

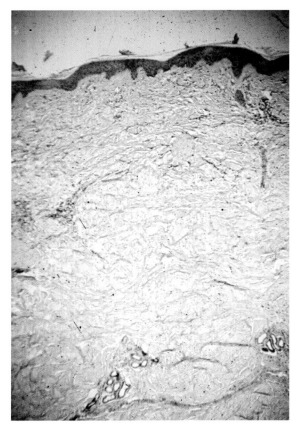

Fig. 1. Biopsy specimen showing normal epidermis, sclerosis of the papillary dermis, thickened sclerotic collagen bundles and periadnexal inflammation. (Original magnification × 40)

(Perlish et al., 1988). Vascular changes are mild in the dermis and subdermis and consist of endothelial swelling and edema of vessel walls (O'Leary et al., 1957).

In the sclerotic stage, there is little inflammation. Collagen bundles in the reticular dermis are thickened, eosinophilic and oriented horizontally. Eccrine glands are entrapped by collagen, and thus appear higher in the dermis. Fewer blood vessels are seen within the thickened collagen. The fascia and striated muscles underlying the lesions may likewise show fibrosis and sclerosis (Jaworsky, 1997).

Although the histology of involved skin is almost identical in LS and SSc (Young and Barr, 1985) inflammatory changes are more prominent in morphea (Torres and Sanchez, 1998). Sclerosis of the papillary dermis was noted in 10 / 32 morphea cases, but not in any of the 19 patients with SSc. Thus, simultaneous involvement of the superficial dermis with deep dermal changes may help differentiate localized from systemic scleroderma. Cases of morphea in which the sclerosis is limited to the superficial reticular dermis have also been described (McNiff et al., 1999). These changes were noted without any of the epidermal features of lichen sclerosus: epidermal thinning with vacuolar degeneration, lichenoid infiltrate or follicular plugging.

Etiopathogenesis

The cause of morphea is unknown. Proposed triggers for the development of morphea have included infectious and other environmental factors. Localised scleroderma has been reported after trauma (Falanga et al., 1986; Yamanaka and Gibbs, 1999), vaccination (Drago et al., 1998; Mork, 1981), ischemic injury (McColl and Buchanan, 1994) and radiation (Bleasel et al., 1999; Schaffer et al., 2000). Such triggers may have in common the generation of inflammatory and molecular "danger" signals that can activate the immune system and initiate fibrosis. There are rare cases of familial clustering suggesting a genetic component (Wuthrich et al., 1975). A possible association with Lyme borreliosis was proposed in 1985 (Aberer et al., 1985) but was not borne out by polymerase chain reaction analysis of affected tissues in North American patients (Dillon et al., 1995). Two possible explanations for the contradictory findings obtained in patients from Europe and Asia, and the USA have been offered (Weide et al., 2000): Either that *Borrelia burgdorferi* is not a causative agent for morphea, or that a subspecies present only in Europe and Asia, could cause morphea in a subset of patients.

Most studies on the pathophysiology of scleroderma focus on changes in patients with SSc. Here, we will focus on abnormalities detected in patients with LS. In both diseases three main themes have been pursued: vascular alterations, immune system activation and dysregulation, and changes in collagen metabolism and fibroblast biology. Abnormalities in these three areas are likely interrelated and contribute to the generation of the clinical phenotype.

Vascular activation in morphea

Endothelial swelling in early morphea lesions was first described by (O'Leary et al., 1957). Comparing biopsies from sclerotic centers, inflamed borders (lilac rings) and adjacent, clinically normal skin, (Kobayasi and Serup, 1985) described three patterns of vascular changes. Uninvolved skin as well as thickened skin showed vascular wall thickening and basal lamina duplication with associated mast cell and histiocyte infiltration. In clinically inflamed lesions, the outer surfaces of pericytes were thickened, and lymphocytes and plasma cells were present. Pericyte hypertrophy was noted in clinically inflamed as well as in sclerotic lesions. There is evidence for generalized vascular activation: Jones et al. (1996) noted low but increased levels of expression of the vascular adhesion molecules vascular cell adhesion molecule-1 (VCAM-1) and E-selectin on endothelium of uninvolved skin of morphea patients. More recently, increased serum levels of soluble VCAM-1 and E-selectin were found in a third of patients with generalized morphea and in approximately 10% of patients with linear and plaque type morphea (Yamane et al., 2000).

In addition to activation, the endothelium may be a primary site of damage in morphea: Endothelial cell apoptosis was noted in deep dermal vessels of 9/9 patients examined (Sgonc et al., 1996). Anti-endothelial cell antibody mediated antibody-dependent cytotoxicity has been suggested as a mechanism for the induction of endothelial cell death (Sgonc et al., 1996). Vascular damage by autologous complement activation has also been proposed as a mechanism of injury (Venneker et al., 1994). Lesional skin but not uninvolved skin showed decreased levels of endothelial membrane cofactor protein (MCP) and decay-accelerating factor (DAF) expression by immunohistochemistry. Both MCP and DAF inhibit the formation of the C3 / C5 convertases of the classical and alternative pathways and it was argued that this local deficiency could increase the susceptibility of the endothelium to damage by autologous complement. Potential consequences of enhanced endothelial cell apoptosis include pro-coagulant activity, and localized release of pro-inflammatory cytokines such as IL-1 with subsequent enhanced adhesion molecule display (Stefanec, 2000).

Immune system activation in morphea

Although only few cases of morphea have been examined by gene array technology, one study demonstrated that involved skin was associated with an inflammatory gene profile (Milano et al., 2008). Dermal inflammatory cell infiltrates are common and both B and T cells have been identified (Whittaker et al., 1989). A deficiency of regulatory T cells within lesional morphea skin has recently been reported (Antiga et al., 2010). Elevated levels of various cytokines, including IL-2, IL-4 and IL-6 have been detected, suggesting ongoing T cell activation (Ihn et al., 1995). The levels of these cytokines, as well as soluble IL-2 receptor, released following T cell activation, correlated with the extent of skin involvement (Ihn et al., 1996). Levels of soluble CD4 receptor but not soluble CD8 receptor are elevated in LS, in contradistinction to SSc, where elevated levels of sCD8 are noted (Sato et al., 1996b). TNF-α and IL-13 are cytokines than can be fibrogenic and that are elevated in roughly 25% of patients (Hasegawa et al., 2003). IL-8 is a chemotactic protein that is also detectable in increased amounts in sera from patients with morphea (Ihn et al., 1994). Lastly, soluble CD30 levels are increased and this may indicate possible involvement of T helper 2 (Th2) lymphocytes in the immunopathogenesis of disease (Ihn et al., 2000). Th2 cells promote humoral immunity and can secrete both IL-4 and IL-6. Consistent with this, elevated levels of IL-4 have been demonstrated in affected skin by immunohistochemistry (Salmon-Ehr et al., 1996). IL-4 and IL-6 have been shown to promote collagen synthesis by fibroblasts. B cell abnormalities have also been noted. Increased soluble CD23 indicates B cell activation (Sato et al., 1996a). The frequent detection of autoantibodies provides evidence of B cell dysregulation. Anti-histone and anti-single stranded DNA (ssDNA) antibodies are found most frequently (Falanga et al., 1985, 1987; Sato et al., 1994; Takehara et al., 1983) and suggest abnormal immune system handling of these antigens.

CD34+ dermal dendritic cells are markedly decreased in lesional skin (Aiba et al., 1994; McNiff et al., 1999; Skobieranda and Helm, 1995). This feature may be of diagnostic help in difficult cases, but its significance remains unknown. These CD34+ cells may be the target of autoimmune attack (Aiba et al., 1994) or they may function to regulate collagen synthesis (Skobieranda and Helm, 1995). CD34 expression correlates with progenitor cell characteristics and thus these cells have been characterized either as uncommitted mesenchymal cells (Narvaez et al., 1996) or as antigen presenting cells (Monteiro et al., 2000). Clarification of their function and the reason for their disappearance in sclerotic skin may shed light on the relationship between the immune alterations detailed here and fibrosis.

Altered collagen metabolism

Increased collagen deposition is an essential feature of scleroderma. Enhanced type I and type III collagen mRNA levels have been detected in lesional skin *in vivo* (Scharffetter et al., 1988). Fibroblasts cultured from lesional and inflamed morphea skin contain higher levels of type I collagen mRNA and synthesize more collagen relative to total protein than fibroblasts from uninvolved skin (Hatamochi et al., 1992). Synthesis of glycosaminoglycans (Moller et al., 1985) and fibronectin (Fleischmajer et al., 1981) is also increased. Alterations in the proportions of glycosaminoglycan-derived disaccharides have been described (Akimoto et al., 1992; Fleischmajer and Perlish, 1972; Passos et al., 2003). Enhanced expression of class II antigens on lesional fibroblasts has been interpreted as a sign of activation, likely secondary to cytokine stimulation (Branchet et al., 1992). Indeed, a subpopulation of fibroblasts shows increased type I and type III collagen mRNA expression (Kahari et al., 1988b) and these fibroblasts are often in proximity to mononuclear cells expressing transforming growth factor-β (Higley et al., 1994). Elevated circulating levels of TGF-β have also been documented (Higley et al., 1994) and TGF-β receptors are upregulated in dermal fibroblasts in the affected skin of patients with localized scleroderma (Kubo et al., 2001). TGF-β is known to induce collagen production by fibroblasts. Other cytokines that may directly mediate fibroblast activation include IL-1, PDGF (Zheng et al., 1998) and connective tissue growth factor (CTGF) (Igarashi et al., 1996). In addition to increased synthesis of collagen, there is evidence of decreased turnover of fibrotic dermal extracellular matrix. Inhibitors of matrix turnover such as tissue inhibitor of matrix metalloproteinases-3 (TIMP-3) are upregulated at the mRNA level in lesional skin (Mattila et al., 1998). Thus the fibrosis may be a net result of increased collagen deposition as well as decreased matrix turnover.

Clinical Appearance / Classification

Plaque Morphea

Morphea en plaque

This commonest form of LS is defined by the presence of lesions > 1 cm in diameter, occurring in 1 or 2 anatomical sites (Peterson et al., 1995; Peterson et al., 1997). The trunk is the most commonly involved site (41–74% patients), but plaques can occur anywhere, including the face and neck (12–13% of patients) (Christianson et al., 1956; Peterson et al., 1997). Onset is usually slow and insidious. Circumscribed oval patches may be erythematous and oedematous in the earliest stages, becoming indurated, yellowish-white or ivory coloured (Fig. 2a). A surrounding violaceous halo, the "lilac ring", suggests active inflammation, but was documented in only 43% of patients in one study (Peterson et al., 1997). The patches subsequently become waxy, shiny and sclerotic. Over months to years they

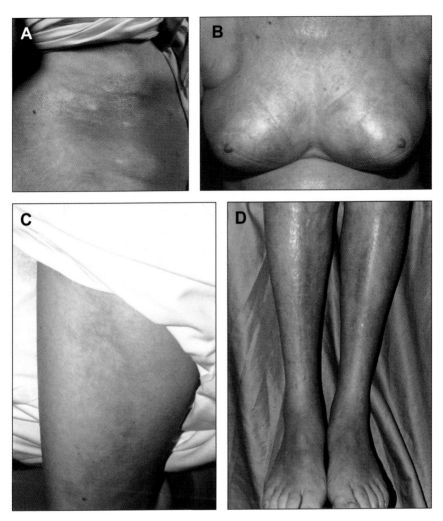

Fig. 2. a) Morphea en plaque with induration and pigmentary changes. b) Generalized morphea of the chest, with erythema, edema and induration. Note sparing of the areolae. c) Linear lesion on the thigh. d) Eosinophilic fasciitis showing erythema, swelling and induration (Peau d'orange).

soften, become atrophic and hypo- or hyperpigmented. Atrophy may involve the epidermis, dermis and/or subcutaneous tissue, producing wrinkling or depression of the skin surface. Lesions may be pruritic and/or paraesthetic. Loss of appendigeal structures results in reduced hair growth and decreased sweating.

Guttate morphea

These lesions resemble morphea en plaque, but are smaller (< 1 cm in diameter), and occur on the upper trunk as multiple, faintly erythematous oval lesions, which become yellowish, mildly indurated and which resolve leaving pigmentary changes. Winkelmann (1985) and Tuffanelli (1998) consider this to be a type of lichen sclerosis associated with morphea. The histologic features of lichen sclerosus and its frequent occurrence with other morphea sub-types (both in the same patients and the same biopsy specimen) suggest that these conditions share a common pathogenesis (Uitto et al., 1980). Interestingly, patients with lichen sclerosus specifically demonstrate antibodies to extracellular matrix protein 1 (Oyama et al., 2003; Oyama et al., 2004). Lesions of lichen sclerosis, but not of morphea, demonstrate discontinuities of the basement membrane zone (Kowalewski et al., 2004) possibly in relation to the presence of these auto-antibodies. Whether patients with morphea or clinical overlap with lichen sclerosus develop auto-antibodies with this specificity is still unknown.

Atrophoderma of Pasini and Pierini

Atrophoderma is uncommon and thought to represent a superficial abortive form of morphea with a benign course (Jablonska, 1975b; Kencka et al., 1995). It usually occurs in childhood, with lesions distributed symmetrically on the trunk (Canizares et al., 1958), but it may occur in a zosteriform distribution (Wakelin and James, 1995). Superficial morphea is a term coined by McNiff and colleagues in 1999 to describe patients with pigmentary changes, minimal cutaneous induration and superficial reticular dermal change (Mc-Niff et al., 1999) and that likely describes a condition that overlaps with atrophoderma (Jablonska and Blaszczyk, 2004). Atrophoderma of Moulin is a term used to describe clinically and histologically identical, but linear lesions, which follow the lines of Blaschko (Wollenberg et al., 1995). They consist of depressed areas of skin, typically with a sharply demarcated "cliff-drop" border, and grey or blue-brown pigmentation. The histology resembles the late atrophic stages of morphea. In a study of 139 patients followed for a mean of 10 years, areas of induration appeared within the lesions in 17% and plaques of morphea elsewhere on the body were found in 22% of cases (Kencka et al., 1995).

Keloid Nodular Morphea

This rare subtype is characterized by the presence of keloid-like nodules in patients with previous or co-existent morphea elsewhere. Lesions are commonest on the upper trunk and may coalesce or occur in a linear pattern (Hsu et al., 1999; Krell et al., 1995). Histology shows homogenization and thickening of collagen bundles with an increase in mucin (Micalizzi et al., 1994). Such keloidal and nodular reactions have also been described in the setting of progressive systemic sclerosis (Cannick et al., 2003; Labandeira et al., 2003; Rencic et al., 2003) and likely arise in patients with scleroderma (either localized or progressive) predisposed to keloid formation.

Generalized morphea

Morphea is referred to as "generalized" when plaque type lesions occur in 3 or more anatomical sites (Peterson et al., 1995). Commonest sites are the trunk, upper thighs and lumbosacral region. Plaques are often distributed symmetrically and may become confluent (Fig. 2b). Plaques at varying stages of evolution usually coexist.

Bullous morphea

This rare subtype is characterized by the presence of tense subepidermal bullae, which appear to develop as a result of subepidermal oedema, and which may occur in the presence of any of the subtypes of morphea (Daoud et al., 1994; Kobayasi et al., 1990; Su and Greene, 1986). In a study of 13 cases, bullae were most frequent on the legs, and lymphatic dilatation, attributed to obstruction from sclerosis, was observed in 77% of the patients (Daoud et al., 1994).

Linear morphea

Linear forms include linear morphea, en coup de sabre lesions and progressive hemifacial atrophy. Sclerotic lesions are distributed in a linear, band-like pattern (Fig. 2c). Clinical evidence of inflammation, the "lilac ring" is seen less often in this type (19%)(Peterson et al., 1997). Their distribution may be dermatomal, however, it has been argued that they follow Blashcko's lines and may thus occur partly as a result of postzygotic mosaicism (Hauser et al., 1996; Itin and Schiller, 1999). Frontoparietal lesions in particular, appear "Blaschkoid" rather than dermatomal (Itin and Schiller, 1999; Soma and Fujimoto, 1998). Trauma is more often sited as a possible precipitating factor in this type of morphea (Falanga et al., 1986; Yamanaka and Gibbs, 1999). Facial and limb asymmetry caused by impaired growth of the bones and soft tissues in the affected area, as well as multiple joint contractures, can cause severe cosmetic, orthopedic, and psychologic problems.

Acral Linear morphea

Unilateral lesions predominate, although bilateral lesions are described in 5.5% (Christianson et al., 1956)–46% (Falanga et al., 1986) of patients. They most often occur on the lower limbs. Multiple sites are involved in up to 60% of cases, and plaque forms often coexist on the trunk (Falanga et al., 1986). Generalised arthralgias and edema of the involved extremity can precede the onset of disease (Christianson et al., 1956). Induration can involve the dermis, subcutis, underlying muscle and bone. Multiple joint contractures, are common, occurring in 56% of cases in one study (Falanga et al., 1986). Myopathic changes, atrophy and weakness of involved and adjacent muscles may occur (Uziel et al., 1994b). Discrepancies of limb length are a frequent complication in children with limb involvement (Liu et al., 1994).

En coup de sabre

This type affects the face and scalp. Lesions generally follow one of two lines. The first descends vertically from the frontal scalp to the side of the nose, adjacent to the midline. The second starts close to the vertex and progresses forwards to the lateral forehead, and then medially towards the inner canthus (Blaszczyk and Jablonska, 1999; Soma and Fujimoto, 1998). Bilateral lesions occur rarely (Rai et al., 2000). Concomitant linear and plaque lesions at other sites are commoner (Falanga et al., 1986; Peterson et al., 1997). The sclerosis is thought to involve the skin and subcutis first, and later extend to underlying fascia and bone (Jablonska, 1975a). Epilepsy is the most frequent neurological complication occurring in up to 10% (Jablonska, 1975a). Ocular and auditory complications may also be present (David et al., 1991; Luer et al., 1990). Intracranial calcification and white matter abnormalities have been noted on CT and MR scans (Liu et al., 1994). One case study suggests sclerodermatous involvement of underlying brain tissue (Chung et al., 1995): dense sclerosis with increased collagen deposition, gliosis, scattered calcifications, and thickened sclerotic blood vessel walls were present in the involved dura and brain. The presence of oligoclonal banding on CSF examination, of lymphocytic inflammation on brain biopsy and of improvement in MRI white matter abnormalities following corticosteroid treatment all attest to the primary inflammatory nature of the underlying CNS lesions (Stone et al., 2001; Unterberger et al., 2003).

Progressive hemifacial atrophy (Parry-Romberg syndrome)

This is thought to be a primary atrophic disorder of the subcutaneous tissue, muscle and bone. The absence of skin induration distinguishes it from "en coup de sabre" lesions (Sakuraoka et al., 1992). Progressive hemifacial atrophy (PHA) often begins at the sites described above, and then extends to involve the cheek, tongue and mandible. Hypoplasia of the maxilla and mandible may cause marked facial asymmetry, particularly if lesions first develop in early childhood. There is overlap between the two conditions (Blaszczyk and Jablonska, 1999; Menni et al., 1997). In one series 20/58 cases of linear scleroderma of the face (en coup de sabre) showed transition to PHA (Jablonska, 1975a). Similar radiographic and clinical neurologic abnormalities and ocular complications are encountered, but may be commoner in PHA (Fry et al., 1992; Liu et al., 1994). Morphea lesions elsewhere have been noted in patients with PHA and both groups with PHA (without skin induration) and those with "en coup de sabre" lesions have abnormalities in cerebral blood flow as detected by SPECT analysis (Blaszczyk et al., 2003).

Deep Morphea

In deep morphea the sclerotic process occurs in the subcutaneous tissue, in other words, in the fat, fascia or superficial muscle. The various subtypes are classified according to the level of maximal involvement on a deep tissue biopsy. Lesions are frequently bilateral and symmetrical and involve the upper and lower limbs (Peterson et al., 1997).

Subcutaneous morphea

The primary site of involvement is the subcutaneous fat, although the fascia may also be involved, making it difficult to distinguish this form from "morphea profunda". In Person and Su's description of 16 cases, plaques were usually extensive, ill-defined and bound-down, and showed rapid centrifugal progression (Person and Su, 1979). Disease activity ranged from 6 months to 7 years. Five patients had coexistent plaques of morphea or lichen sclerosus, and five had a peripheral eosinophilia.

Morphea profunda

Su and Person (1981) originally suggested a number of diagnostic criteria: the presence of diffuse, taut, bound-down deep cutaneous sclerosis; of significant hyalinization and thickening of collagen bundles in both the subcutaneous fat and fascia; and a response to treatment with antimalarials or corticosteroid. Some authors do not distinguish between this subtype and subcutaneous morphea (Weedon, 1997). Solitary lesions have been described both in children (Kobayashi et al., 1991) and adults (Whittaker et al., 1989). Recently 3 unusual cases of deep linear, primarily atrophic lesions, without preceding inflammation or sclerosis, involving the subcutis and deeper tissues were described. They may have a more benign outcome. Their relationship to morphea is underscored by the coexistence of hemifacial atrophy in one case (Blaszczyk et al., 2000).

Eosinophilic fasciitis (Shulman syndrome)

This condition is characterized by a diffuse sclerosis, predominantly involving the fibrous septa of the subcutis and deep fascia, a high ESR, hypergammaglobulinaemia and peripheral eosinophilia (Mitchet et al., 1981; Shulman, 1974). Inflammatory changes may extend into the underlying muscle (Weedon, 1997). It usually occurs on the extremities, but spares the hands and feet (Fig. 2d). It can result in severe joint contractures and associated morbidity. Associated haematologic abnormalities including aplastic anemia, thrombocytopenia and leukaemia have been noted (Doyle and Ginsburg, 1989). Other subtypes of morphea may be present (Miller, 1992a).

Disabling pansclerotic morphea of childhood

This extremely rare variant is at the most severe end of the clinical spectrum. Rapid progression of deep cutaneous fibrosis occurs, extending to involve muscle, fascia and bone (Diaz-Perez et al., 1980). It usually results in severe joint contractures and cutaneous ulceration. Unlike other forms of LS, this disease does not undergo spontaneous remission. Increased serum IgG, a positive ANA and peripheral eosinophilia are documented (Scharffetter-Kochanek et al., 1995; Todd et al., 1998).

Associated symptoms

Arthralgias are relatively common (40% of patients) (Christianson et al., 1956; Uziel et al., 1994b). Synovitis has been documented mainly in deep forms (Peterson et al., 1997). Associated pulmonary and esophageal involvement can occur. Routine testing revealed that 7/41 (17%) patients had esophageal dysmotility and 9/53 (17%) had abnormal gas transfer on lung function testing. These abnormalities were asymptomatic over 4yrs follow up in all but 2 of the patients (Dehen et al., 1994). In a series of 16 cases of subcutaneous morphea, 4/10 and 3/10 patients investigated had asymptomatic abnormal lung function and esophageal dysmotility respectively (Person and Su, 1979). This suggests that the frequency of internal involvement may be underestimated. Other associated findings include carpal tunnel syndrome (Winkelmann et al., 1982) and vertebral anomalies (in particular spina bifida) present in 47% of 68 patients examined radiographically (Christianson et al., 1956). Associated cutaneous diseases include lichen sclerosus (see above), vitiligo, alopecia areata, and lichen planus (Uitto et al., 1980; Winkelmann, 1985). Morphea may also occur with other connective tissue diseases, including lupus erythematosus (Dubois et al., 1971; Ko et al., 2009; Umbert and Winkelmann, 1978), dermatomyositis and rheumatoid arthritis (Jablonska, 1975b). Morphea has also been associated with Hashimoto's thyroiditis (Lee et al., 2002), another auto-immune condition. A recent study pointed out the high prevalence of autoimmune syndromes associated with various types of morphea (Leitenberger et al., 2009). Morphea has also been noted to occur after TNF-α inhibitor treatment (Mattozzi et al., 2010). All these clinical situations have in common a high type 1 interferon signature (de Gannes et al., 2007), possibly predisposing to autoimmunity.

Laboratory abnormalities

Eosinophilia occurs in all types of morphea, but is more pronounced in patients with generalized and deep forms. Levels of eosinophilia may parallel disease activity (Falanga et al., 1986). A mean of 5.4% (percentage of total leukocytes) at diagnosis and 2.8% at last follow up was observed in Peterson's series (Peterson' et al., 1997). Polyclonal hypergammaglobulinemia and a positive rheumatoid factor were present in 50% and 26% respectively of 53 patients with linear or generalized morphea. Both were correlated with more extensive, active disease (Falanga et al., 1986). In studies using Hep2 cells, anti-nuclear antibody (ANA)-positivity occurred in 46–76% of cases, in decreasing order of frequency in generalized, linear and plaque forms (Falanga et al., 1986; Rosenberg et al., 1995; Uziel et al., 1994b). Antibodies to ssDNA are usually of the IgM subtype (Ruffatti et al., 1991), and are seen mainly in patients with longstanding, extensive linear or generalized disease (Falanga et al., 1986; Rosenberg et al., 1995). Antihistone antibodies may also be present but anti-Scl 70 (polymerase III) and anticentromere antibodies are rare. Levels of anti-histone antibodies and antibodies to ssDNA correlate with disease severity in linear disease (Arkachaisri et al., 2008). Anti-phospholipid antibodies of both the IgM and IgG subtypes are detected with increased frequency in patients with generalized and linear morphea, in the absence of increased thrombotic events (Sato et al., 2003). The similarity in auto-antibody specificities between drug-induced lupus and morphea has prompted the suggestion that morphea, like drug-induced lupus, is an environmentally driven disease. Recent studies have identified serum autoantibodies to fibrillin 1 (Arnett et al., 1999), the major component of microfibrils in the extracellular matrix, and to Hsp73 (Fujimoto et al., 1995). It is likely that these autoantibodies are by-products of the underlying pathologic process, rather than being primarily pathogenic. Unique disease-associated auto-antibody profiles may nevertheless give a clue to pathogenesis. In this regard, 76% of patients with localized disease and 85% of patients with generalized disease are found to have antibodies to anti DNA topoisomerase IIα in contrast to only 14% of patients with progressive systemic sclerosis (Hayakawa et al., 2004). This is a ubiquitous enzyme that modulates the topologic state of DNA and it was hypothesized that, as this protein is selectively cleaved during Fas-mediated apoptotic cell death, it may be presented to the immune system during the endothelial cell apoptosis detected in early morphea lesions. Most patients (41 / 46) with morphea and 13 / 13 patients with generalized morphea were recently shown to have antibodies to a cytosolic form of superoxide dismutase (Cu / Zn SOD or SOD1) (Nagai et al., 2004). In patients with generalized disease, the presence of IgM antibodies to Cu / Zn SOD correlated with severity of disease. These observations suggest that reactive oxygen species may participate in disease pathogenesis.

Diagnosis and Measurement of Disease Activity

The diagnosis is based on characteristic clinical findings and histology. Characteristic cutaneous ultrasound images may aid in diagnosis (Cosnes et al., 2003). No reliable laboratory markers of disease activity are available. Clinical features suggestive of active disease include extension of lesions, appearance of new lesions and the presence of a violaceous or erythematous halo. More objective assessments can be made using modified Rodnan skin scores (Rodnan et al., 1979). Ideally this should be combined with the use of a durometer (Seyger et al., 1997) or 20 MHz ultrasound (Levy et al., 1993) to assess skin thickness and elasticity. Recently, thermography has been used to aid in the assessment of disease activity (Birdi et al., 1992; Martini et al., 2002). These apparatus are unfortunately not widely available. A global skin damage and activity index has recently been proposed that may aid in following disease activity and response to treatment (Arkachaisri et al., 2010). Significant psychological stress has been identified in patients with active disease and measurement of psychological parameters is thus encouraged (Kroft et al., 2009b). It has been suggested that serum IL-2 receptor levels may distinguish between active and inactive disease (Uziel et al., 1994a) but the utility of this test in clinically following disease activity has not been independently confirmed. Serial determinations of eosinophilia, hypergammaglobulinaemia and ANA titers may be of value in patients with extensive disease as these values may fluctuate with disease activity.

Therapy

There is no uniformly accepted or effective therapy for LS. Assessing the efficacy of treatments can be sometimes challenging because LS is a rare condition with heterogeneity of disease severity; trials are small, most of them uncontrolled and they lack of uniform outcomes; the difficulty to differentiate active versus inactive disease and finally the disease in most patients will remit spontaneously making it difficult to appreciate the role of treatment.

Immune cell activation is believed to underlie the development of skin sclerosis, and both topical and systemic immunosuppressants have been used. Unfortunately, few controlled studies are available with which to objectively assess the benefits obtained. In a majority of older studies the improvements described are based on poorly documented clinical observations. Recently more objective outcome measures have been employed. Patients with LS need to be treated because the disease may cause cosmetic and functional sequelae and patients that are treated at an early stage respond better. Given the propensity for skin thickening to improve in morphea, larger controlled studies are needed to confirm the efficacy of both traditional and newer treatments.

Topical corticosteroids

Although high potency topical corticosteroids have been the "first-line" treatment for patient with plaque morphea for many years, no prospective or controlled studies of their effectiveness alone in LS have been published. They have, however, retrospectively been shown to be useful in children with active plaque morphea (Bodemer et al., 1999a; Bodemer et al., 1999b), and to be highly effective in the treatment of lichen sclerosis (Garzon and Paller, 1999) a clinically associated and possibly related condition.

Ultraviolet A

Ultraviolet light A_1(340–400 nm) (UVA$_1$) is increasingly being used to treat morphea. Different dosage regimens have been proposed for UVA$_1$ phototherapy: low dose (10–20 J/cm^2 per single dose), medium dose (50–70 J/cm^2 per single dose) or high dose (90–130 J/cm^2 per single dose) (Sator et al., 2009). Different studies on the optimal therapeutic UVA$_1$ dose for the treatment of LS have obtained equivocal results. Some authors such as Kerscher et al. (Kerscher et al., 1998) reported excellent results with low-dose UVA$_1$, while others such as Stege et al. (Stege et al., 1997) and Kreuter et al. (Kreuter et al., 2001) found no response with low-dose UVA$_1$, but good response to either high or medium dose of UVA$_1$. Published reports detailed in Table 1 suggest that medium-dose UVA$_1$ treatment is as effective as high-dose UVA$_1$ and is the most efficacious form of ultraviolet light, followed in order, by low-dose UVA$_1$ (20 J/cm^2/treatment), UVA in conjunction with other treatments such as topical and systemic psoralens (PUVA) and calcipotriol. These effects were also seen in darker skin tones, despite the fact that most reports evaluating the benefits of UVA_1 phototherapy focuses on a predominantly Caucasian population (Jacobe et al., 2008).

Effective therapy with UVA_1 has been reported in 162/169 treated patients, with disease durations of up to 25 years (Andres et al., 2009; Gruss et al., 1997a; Gruss et al., 1997c; Kerscher et al., 1995; Kerscher et al., 1998; Kreuter et al., 2001; Kreuter et al., 2006b; Sator et al., 2009; Stege et al., 1997). Deep forms appear least responsive. Outcome measures have included assessment of lesion size and induration, and ultrasonographic and biopsy assessments of dermal thickness and elasticity. In one study, a direct comparison of high-dose UVA_1 versus low-dose therapy showed that high-dose was superior for all the parameters assessed (Stege et al., 1997). The effects may be seen as early as after 4–10 treatments. Maximal responses may require 25 or more treatments. The use of medium dose UVA_1 ($48 J/cm^2/$ treatment) in 8 patients was associated with improved skin scores and increased skin elasticity as measured by a cutometer in all patients after 20 treatments. In an effort to limit UVA_1 dosing, low-dose UVA_1 therapy has been combined with topical calcipotriol ointment therapy for childhood morphea. A 19-patient uncontrolled trial of this therapy showed a 67% improvement in skin scores (Kreuter et al., 2001).

Sator et al. (Sator et al., 2009) published the first study to use intra-patient comparisons to investigate the relative efficacy of medium-dose (MD) UVA_1 and low-dose (LD) UVA_1 phototherapy for LS, avoiding inter-individual differences in treatment response as a confounding factor. In this study, all time points of the study, a greater decrease in skin thickness measured by 20-MHz ultrasound assessment was found in the irradiated plaques with medium and low-dose as compared with the un-irradiated control side. This study was also the first to provide data on a long-term outcome (patients were followed up for a 1-year period after cessation of therapy). A randomized control trial that compared the safety and efficacy of LD UVA_1, MD UVA_1, and narrowband (NB) UVB phototherapy in the treatment of 64 patients with LS, showed that MD UVA_1 was significantly more effective than NB UVB ($P < 0.05$). There were no significant differences between LD UVA_1 and NB UVB and the former and MD UVA_1 (Kreuter et al., 2006b).

Limited access to UVA_1 light sources remains a major obstacle. This has prompted trials of broadband UVA therapy. In 13 patients with disease durations of 1 month to 3 years (El-Mofty et al., 2000; Steger and Matthews, 1999) clinical improvement (without objective skin scoring) was observed in all cases. Those with early disease were said to respond best. A significant reduction in upper dermal collagen concentration was seen on biopsy in 9/12 cases. At follow up 1 year later two patients had relapsed. Improved skin thickness as assessed by ultrasound was detected in 3 out of 4 patients with morphea after 30–60 treatments of broadband UVA (Oikarinen and Knuutinen, 2001). When treatments with $20 J/cm^2/$ session, $10 J/cm^2/$ session and $5 J/cm^2/$ session of broadband UVA were compared, a significant clinical dose-response association was not demonstrated despite UV dose-related decreases in collagen and TGF-β mRNA levels (El-Mofty et al., 2004). 6/16 (38%) patients receiving 20 sessions of $5 J/cm^2$ were perceived to have a good to very-good response compared to 15/26 (58%) receiving 20 sessions of $20 J/cm^2$ prompting the authors to conclude that lower doses of broadband UVA may also be beneficial.

Psoralens increase the overall cytotoxicity of UVA, but reduce the total number of joules required for effective therapy in other cutaneous inflammatory diseases. The effects of bath PUVA have been documented in 20 patients. 80% or more of the sclerotic plaques

Table 1. UVA treatment for localized morphea

Treatment	Morphea type	Number published	Dose and duration	Improved	Comment	Reference
High dose UVA1	P G L	12 3 2	130 J/cm² /Rx x4/wk for 5 wks and x2/wk for 5 wks	12 3 2	Effective and superior to low dose, 38% vs 15% decrease in skin thickness, but high total irradiation (3900 J/cm²).	{{789 Stege, H. 1997}}
Medium dose UVA1	P	30	50 J/cm² / Rx x5/wk for 3–6 weeks	25	Retrospective and prospective study. 82% of improvement of skin elasticity and 84% of reduction of skin thickness measured by ultrasound.	{{720 Andres, C. 2009}}
Medium dose UVA1 v/s Low Dose UVA1	P	14	70 J/cm² /Rx x4/wk for 5 weeks all body 20 J/cm² /Rx x4/wk for 5 weeks on 1 plaque	14	Ultrasound showed that the median decrease in skin thickness was greater for 70 J/cm² (0.270 mm) than for 20 J/cm² (0.195 mm) or no irradiation (0.090 mm). Intra-patient control	{{722 Sator, P.G. 2009}}
Medium dose UVA1 v/s Low dose UVA1 v/s narrowband UVB	P G L D	50 9 3 2	27 patients with UVA1 (20 J/cm²), 18 patients UVA1 (50 J/cm²), and 19 patients with NB UVB 5 times weekly for 8 weeks	50 9 3 2	Randomized control study. Medium-dose UVA1 was significantly more effective than NB UVB (P < 0.05).	{{726 Kreuter, A. 2006}}
Low dose UVA1	P/G L D	24 16 4	20 J/cm²/Rx x4/wk for 5–6 wks +/– x1-2/wk for 5–6 wks	24 16 2	Effective, 50–80% clearance, 15–37% decrease in skin thickness, lower total exposure (600 J/cm²)	{{790 Gruss, C. 1997; 791 Gruss, C. 1997}} {{792 Kerscher, M. 1995; 788 Kerscher, M. 1998}} {{787 Stege, H. 1997}}

4

Table 1. (continued) UVA treatment for localized morphea

Treatment	Morphea type	Number published	Dose and duration	Improved	Comment	Reference
Low dose UVA1 + calcipotriol	P	8	20J/cm² /Rx x4/wk for 10 wks and calcipotriol 0.005% ung BID	8	67% improvement in clinical score, improvement in skin thickness in 4/4 tested, no comparison to either treatment alone	{{728 Kreuter, A. 2001}}
	L	9		9		
	D	2		2		
Low dose broadband UVA	P	3	20J/cm² x3/wk, 20 Rx or x4/wk for 6 wks and x1/wk for 6 wks	3	Possibly as effective as low dose UVA1, but no objective clinical scores, lower total exposures effective (400J/cm²)	{{794 El-Mofty, M. 2000}} {{795 Steger, J.W. 1999}}
	G	7		7		
	L (ECS)	3 (1)		3		
Bath PUVA	G	10	1.2–3.5 J/cm² 25–35 Rx	8	Slightly less effective, but up to 40% decrease in skin thickness and up to 80% clearance in some patients (10–60J/cm²)	{{797 Kerscher, M. 1994; 796 Kerscher, M. 1996}} {{798 Schiener, R. 2000}}
	P	3		3		
	L	5		4		
	D	2		1		
PUVA Cream	P	4	0.001%–0.0025% 8MOP + 30% H$_2$O in oil emulsion x4/week, 30 Rx	4	84% reduction in skin thickness, useful if small number of plaques/area involved. Lower total irradiance (121 J/cm²)	{{799 Grundmann-Kollmann, M. 2000}}
Systemic PUVA	P/G	5	0.4–0.6mg/kg 8MOP, 3–4 x/wk 1–9 months	4	Less effective and prolonged Rx often required (total doses up to 840J/cm²), few objective outcome measures reported	{{800 Garcia-Bustinduy, M. 1998}} {{801 Kanekura, T. 1996}} {{802 Todd, D.J. 1998}} {{803 Yamaguchi, K. 1998}}
	L	2		2		
	D	2		1		

P = plaque, G = generalized, L = linear, D = deep morphea, Rx = treatment, ECS = bullous morphea regressed in 15 / 19 patients within 3 months, based on clinical skin scores, ultrasound and histologic evaluations (Kerscher et al., 1995; Kerscher et al., 1996). The effect lasted 1year in 15 / 17 patients. Cream psoralen plus UVA has been used in 4 patients alone with excellent response judged by 20 MHz ultrasound and lesional biopsy (Grundmann-Kollmann et al., 2000), or in two children with linear scleroderma 'en coup de saber in association with calcipotriol (Gambichler et al., 2003) judged by 20 MHz ultrasound.

Systemic PUVA therapy may be somewhat less effective. Of 9 patients reported (Garcia-Bustinduy et al., 1998; Kanekura et al., 1996; Morison, 1997; Scharffetter-Kochanek et al., 1995; Todd et al., 1998; Yamaguchi et al., 1998), all but one showed some clinical improvement. However, prolonged or maintenance treatment was often required, increasing the risks of long-term toxicity.

All forms of UVA therapy appear to act via a direct effect on the irradiated skin area, since plaques covered during treatment fail to show any improvement. The mechanism of action of UVA is suggested by studies which show that it induces apoptosis in skin-infiltrating T cells (Morita et al., 1997) depletion of skin-infiltrating T cells and pro-inflammatory cytokines such as IL-1, IL-6, IL-8, human β-defensins (Kreuter et al., 2006a) and upregulates collagenase I (MMP1) mRNA expression both in vitro and in vivo (Gruss et al., 1997b; Stege et al., 1997; Wlaschek et al., 1995). Treatment has also resulted in partial normalization in the number of CD34+ dermal dendritic cells (Camacho et al., 2001). While the long-term oncogenic potential of PUVA is well documented, the potential long-term toxicity of long wave UVA is still unknown. Controlled studies are required to establish the safest and most efficacious form of UVA therapy, both in terms of dosage and duration of therapy.

Vitamin D derivatives

Both oral calcitriol (Caca-Biljanovska et al., 1999; Elst et al., 1999; Hulshof et al., 1994; Humbert et al., 1995; Humbert et al., 1990) and topical calcipotriol either alone (Cunningham et al., 1998; Koeger et al., 1999; Tay, 2003) or associated with psoralen cream + UVA (Gambichler et al., 2003) or with betamethasone dipropionate (Dytoc et al., 2007) have been used effectively in small, uncontrolled series of patients with all forms of LS (see Table 2). Systemic treatment with 0.25 µg / day is increased by 0.25 µg weekly up to a maximum of 2.5 µg / day (Humbert et al., 1995). Documented effects include improved well-being and joint mobility, a reduction in the appearance of new lesions, and of induration in existing lesions. Improvement occurred within 2–6 months, suggesting a therapeutic effect. A randomized, double-blind, placebo-controlled study of 9 months' duration with a 6-month follow-up was performed on a total of 27 patients (7 patients with SSc and 20 with LS) comparing oral calcitriol (0.75 µg / day for 6 months plus 1.25 µg / day for 3 months) or placebo for 9 months. The skin score in patients with morphea showed no significant difference between the placebo and calcitriol groups, implying that calcitriol at that dose was not superior than placebo in patients with morphea (Hulshof et al., 1994).

The mechanism of action of vitamin D derivatives in morphea remains uncertain. Receptors for 1,25 dihydroxyvitamin D3 have been detected on human dermal fibroblasts, keratinocytes and lymphocytes (Clemens et al., 1983; Holick et al., 1987) as well as dendritic cells (Maruotti and Cantatore, 2010). It may inhibit antigen induced T cell activation and proliferation, both by inhibiting T cell-monocyte interactions, and reducing IL-2 and

IFN γ synthesis (Rigby et al., 1987; Rigby and Waugh, 1992) and by activating regulatory T cells (Jeffery et al., 2009). In addition, it causes a dose dependant inhibition of fibroblast growth and collagen synthesis (Boelsma et al., 1995; Bottomley et al., 1995). Vitamin D analogues may thus have immunomodulatory, antisynthetic and antiproliferative effects.

Methotrexate

Anecdotal evidence of benefit was initially reported in a child with linear disease and in an adult with eosinophilic fascitis (Foeldvari, 1998; Janzen et al., 1995). A few observational studies have since been published, but none of them are randomized trials. In one of them, 9 adults were treated (Seyger et al., 1998). Improvement in skin thickness scores was noted in 6/9 patients. Durometer readings, skin itch scores, and levels of type III procollagen propeptide showed no significant improvement. In a second study, 9 children were treated with methotrexate and pulsed intravenous methylprednisolone (Uziel et al., 2000). A good response, defined as skin softening, and lack of progression or appearance of new lesions, occurred in all 9 patients. The median time to response was 3 months, was fastest in those with early disease, and persisted over the treatment period. The authors suggested treating patients for at least 1 year of inactive disease before tapering the dose of methotrexate. It is of note that a total of 4/18 patients were withdrawn from the two studies because of significant side effects (raised liver enzymes, stomatitis, weight loss and leukopenia). In a retrospective study in 34 children with LS, pulsed intravenous methylprednisolone was given, followed by oral prednisolone on a reducing regimen and maintenance treatment with methotrexate (Weibel et al., 2006). The disease stopped progressing in 94% of the patients. All patients demonstrated significant clinical improvement within a mean time of 5.7 ± 3.9 months. Mean duration of follow-up over the treatment period and beyond was 2.9 ± 2.0 years. In 16 (47%) patients therapy was discontinued when the disease was considered to be inactive clinically; however, seven (44%) of the 16 developed a relapse, needing to repeat treatment. At last follow-up, 24 (71%) of the 34 patients had completely inactive disease.

The largest retrospective case series of patients with sclerotic skin diseases treated with MTX was published by Kroft in, 2009 (Kroft et al., 2009a). MTX was given alone or either in combination with corticosterois in 58 patients with sclerotic skin diseases, whereas 49 of them had LS. Both treatment strategies (MTX and MTX + CS) were effective. No difference in median weekly MTX dose was found between the two treatment strategies. Patients who showed a relapse had received a lower cumulative dose of MTX in the first course (MTX, 443 mg; MTX + CS, 658 mg) compared with the patients who reached remission status (MTX, 708 mg; MTX + CS, 1070 mg). This difference was not statistically significant, but it may suggest a role for the total cumulative MTX dose in achieving definitive remission (Kroft et al., 2009a). This study was without a control group and was retrospective, requiring caution in interpretation as pointed out in an editorial (Jessop and Whitelaw, 2009).

Methotrexate, possibly by enhancing monocyte differentiation (Seitz et al., 1998), has been shown to reduce serum levels of soluble IL-2 receptors (Rose et al., 1994), and of IL-1β, IL-6, IL-8 and TNF-α (Barrera et al., 1995; Seitz et al., 1995). It may thus modulate cytokine production and T cell-monocyte interactions, in addition to its well-docu-

Table 2. Systemic and topical therapies for localized scleroderma

Treatment	Morphea type	Number published	Dose and duration	Improved	Comment	Reference
Oral Calcitriol	G D L Unspecified	5 2 7 7	0.25–1.25 µg OD 3–10.5 months 0.25–2.5 mg/day 2–36 months	5 2 6 7	Significant objective improvement in skin extensibility documented in 12 patients, relatively non toxic	{{837 Caca-Biljanovska, N.G. 1999}} {{841 Elst, E.F. 1999}} {{842 Hulshof, M.M. 1994}} {{838 Humbert, P.G. 1990; 844 Humbert, P. 1995}}
	SSc Unspecified	7 20	0.75 µg/day for 6 months plus 1.25 µg/day for 3 months or placebo for 9 months	20/20	Calcitriol at this dose was not more effective than placebo in patients with morphea. Small sample size.	{{737 Hulshof, M.M. 2000}}
Topical calcipotriol	P/G and L	13	0.005% ointment or cream BID +/– occlusion nocte 3–6 months	13	44% improvement in skin scores, safe and non toxic	{{840 Cunningham, B.B. 1998}} {{843 Koeger, A.C. 1999}}
Corticosteroids	G L D	5 28 9	Prednisone 0.5–1 mg/kg/day for up to 70 months	5 9 8	Benefits appear greatest in deep group, few objective outcome measures	{{831 Balat, A. 1999}} {{832 Bodemer, C. 1999}} {{834 Castanet, J. 1994}} {{836 Gordon, G.V. 1981}} {{830 Joly, P. 1994}} {{835 Miller, J.J.,3rd 1992}}
Methotrexate	G P	7 2	15 mg/wk–25 mg/wk 24 weeks	5/6	Moderate effect, 20% reduced skin scores in responders	{{851 van den Hoogen, F.H. 1996}}

SSc = systemic sclerosis

Table 2. (continued) Systemic and topical therapies for localized scleroderma

Treatment	Morphea type	Number published	Dose and duration	Improved	Comment	Reference
Methotrexate + IV Methylprednisolone (IVMP)	G L	5 4	0.3–0.6 mg/kg/wk 22.3 months + 30 mg/kg/day x3 days, monthly for the 1st 3 months	9/9	Combination promising but, needs larger studies and more objective outcome measures	{{748 Kreuter, A. 2005; 824 Uziel,Y. 2000}}
	G L	10 5	15 mg/week of MTX 1000 mg for 3 days/week of IVMP for at least 6 months	14/15		{{748 Kreuter, A. 2005}}
	G L P	2 31 1	Two courses of high-dose IVMP (30 mg·kg day, max 500 mg), each containing three pulses, given on two consecutive weeks. Oral prednisolone was started after the first course of IVMP(initial dose 0.5 mg·kg), and then continued on a reducing regimen. MTX 10 mg/week	34/34	Risk of relapse after discontinuing therapy	{{745 Weibel, L. 2006}}
Aminoquinoline antimalarials	P/G D	4 7	Hydroxychloroquine 200–400 mg Chloroquine 250 mg OD Duration not specified	2/4 4/7	No objective outcome measures but may be of benefit in deep group	{{819 Person, J.R. 1979}} {{817 Winkelmann, R.K. 1982}} {{818 Wuthrich, R.C. 1975}}
D-penicillamine	G L	3 14	2–7.5 mg/kg/day 13–53 months	14	Effects unproven, few objective outcome measures, mean 24% decrease in skin scores where documented	{{811 Curley, R.K. 1987}} {{815 Falanga.V. 1990}} {{813 Moynahan, E.J. 1973}} {{814 van Bergen, B.H. 1997}}
Sulphasalazine	P/G Bullous	6 1	1–5 g/day 7–13 months	4/6 1	Effects unproven, based on subjective assessments	{{759 Czarnecki, D.B. 1982}} {{758 Micalizzi, C. 1996}} {{760 Stava, Z. 1977}} {{757 Taveira, M. 1999}}

mented anti-metabolite action. Elevated levels of tenascin in the center and margins of lesional skin and numbers of mast cells at the margins of lesions were found to be decreased by methotrexate treatment (Seyger et al., 2001).

Systemic corticosteroids

Systemic therapy has rarely been described in patients with rapidly progressive generalized disease and linear forms. It has variably been reported to be of benefit (Joly et al., 1994) or not (Balat et al., 1999; Bodemer et al., 1999b). The need for prolonged treatment, associated with well documented side effects, and the significant risk of relapse on withdrawal (Joly et al., 1994), are all factors which should be taken into account when considering using this treatment modality, particularly as monotherapy. It may be of greater benefit when used in combiation with other therapies such as methotrexate or plasmapheresis (Uziel et al., 2000; Wach et al., 1995). Kreuter et al. in a prospective, nonrandomized, open pilot study in fifteen patients with severe LS, confirmed sustained response to oral methotrexate (15 mg/wk) combined with pulsed intravenous methylprednisolone (1000 mg for 3 days monthly) for at least 6 months. Response was sustained in all cases, except for one, and resulted in a significant decrease of visual analog score, 20-MHz ultrasonographic measurement and modified skin score, whereas the body is divided into 7 regions and skin thickness is assessed on a 0- to 3-point scale (0, normal skin; 1, thickened skin; 2, decreased ability to pinch or move skin; and 3, unable to pinch or move skin) (Kreuter et al., 2005). A possible exception may be eosinophilic fasciitis for which anecdotal evidence suggests greater steroid responsiveness (Castanet et al., 1994; Gordon, 1981; Miller, 1992b).

D Penicillamine

Isolated case reports and small series have suggested benefit, predominantly in patients with severe, progressive, linear disease (Curley et al., 1987; Moynahan, 1973; van Bergen et al., 1997). In the largest published study of 11 patients, improvement was noted in 7 and began within 3–6 months (Falanga and Medsger, 1990). There were no new or active lesions, skin softening occurred in 5/7 and normalization of growth of the affected limb in 2/3 children. Significant, but reversible side effects (nephrotic syndrome, milder proteinuria, leukopenia, thrombocytopenia) occurred in 4 patients. In a further study of six children with eosinophilic fascitis and morphea en plaque elsewhere on the body, addition of long term penicillamine, following initial treatment with prednisone, produced little additional benefit (Miller, 1992a).

Antimalarials

Aminoquinolone antimalarials are relatively safe and well tolerated. They were of benefit in 12/20 reported patients (Brownell et al., 2007; Person and Su, 1979; Tollefson and Witman, 2007; Winkelmann et al., 1982; Wuthrich et al., 1975). Although not studied in morphea, the use of combination antimalarial therapy, i. e., either hydroxychloroquine or chloroquine with quinacrine, can be of benefit in patients with cutaneous lupus refractory to single agent therapy alone (Chung and Hann, 1997). This may be a safe and worthwhile strategy in generalized morphea, but requires clinical studies.

Interferon-γ

Interferon-γ (IFN-γ) has a strong inhibitory effect on collagen synthesis by normal and scleroderma fibroblasts in vitro (Kahari et al., 1988a), which provides a rationale for it's use in morphea. Unfortunately, in one of the rare double-blind controlled studies conducted in 24 patients, no significant differences were found between intralesional IFN-γ and placebo when considering fibrosis, lesion size or collagen mRNA expression (Hunzelmann et al., 1997).

Other therapies

The description of a large number of anecdotal therapies for morphea attests, in part, to their lack of efficacy. Phenytoin (200 mg/day) resulted in skin softening within 2–3 months in 5/5 patients with linear disease (Neldner, 1978). Interestingly these patients all received concomitant vitamin D supplements, which may have contributed to the observed effects. 5/7 patients with progressive plaque or generalized disease responded to sulphasalazine (Czarnecki and Taft, 1982; Micalizzi et al., 1996; Stava and Kobikova, 1977; Taveira et al., 1999). Benefit was seen within 4 weeks of starting cyclosporine therapy (5 mg/kg/day tapered to 1.5 mg/kg/day after 8 months) in 2 patients (Peter et al., 1991). It has also been used as an inductor treatment followed by methotrexate as maintenance treatment in a girl with linear morphea (Crespo et al., 2009) and in a girl with rapidly progressing linear morphea despite the use of high potency steroids (Strauss et al., 2004). Some improvement has also been seen after 3 months of intravenous immunoglobulin therapy (5 g alpha-globulin/day ×5 days, then monthly for 1 year) in a child with pansclerotic morphea (Wollina et al., 1998). Prior reports in the use of extracorporeal photochemotherapy (ECP) in 2 patients have shown poor or incomplete responses (Cribier et al., 1995), but recently, a case of a patient with severe disabling generalized deep morphea showed a marked clinical response to treatment with ECP (Neustadter et al., 2009). Acitretin has been used with success in 9 patients (Neuhofer and Fritsch, 1984) one of them a patient with psoriasis and morphea (Bilen et al., 1999), and topical tocoretinate in 4 patients (Mizutani et al., 1999). Topical photodynamic therapy (PDT) using 5-aminolaevulinic acid (ALA), has shown before to be effective in 5/5 patients with progressive disease (Karrer et al., 2000), but recently studies performed on 7 patients has not confirmed the efficacy of PDT (Batchelor et al., 2008). A single report suggests the efficacy of repeated treatment with a 585 nm pulsed dye laser (Eisen and Alster, 2002) but a case reported in 2009 of a patient with en coup de saber who was given an initial diagnosis of acquired port-wine stain and treated with pulsed dye laser presented with unanticipated blistering because of the use of the laser (Kakimoto et al., 2009). Penicillin, used because of the possible association with *borrelia* infection, and a suggested effect on collagen fibrillogenesis was also recently shown to reduce skin thickness in a child with linear disease (Mohrenschlager et al., 1999). Tacrolimus ointment 0.1% applied topically twice daily with plastic wrap occlusion was of benefit in 2 patients over 12 weeks (Mancuso and Berdondini, 2003). It has also been used in thirteen patients with morphea without occlusion for 4 months, showing that thick, well-established lesions responded more poorly in comparison to other less thick and more erythematous ones (Stefanaki et al., 2008). There is one randomized, double-blind, emollient-controlled pilot study performed in 10 patients with plaque morphea showing reduction in durometer and clinical feature scores (Kroft et al., 2009a). Imiquimod cream 5% may have been of benefit in 15/15 reported cases (Campione et al., 2009; Dytoc et al., 2005; Man and Dytoc, 2004). Mycofenolate mofetil has been used in association with extracorporeal photopheresis with success in a patient with recalcitrant generalized bullous morphea (Schlaak et al., 2008) and in two patients with disabling pansclerotic morphoea, three patients with generalized morphoea, five patients with linear scleroderma and in three patients with coup de sabre, all of them in association with methotrexate or oral corticosteroids (Martini et al., 2009).

Summary

Morphea is an uncommon but potentially disabling condition. Abnormalities in immune system parameters, endothelial activation and fibroblast metabolism have been described, but a unifying pathophysiologic model remains to be tested. The clinician is faced with considerable uncertainty when choosing a treatment modality for LS. Given the benign natural progression of plaque type morphea, treatment with topical modalities such as superpotent corticosteroids or calcipotriol is prudent. For more generalized forms of morphea, as well as the linear forms, UVA is currently the best-documented therapeutic modality. In the absence of access to UVA treatment, oral calciferol or systemic immunosuppression may be contemplated. Recent studies support the use of methotrexate with systemic corticosteroids for the management of aggressive disease. The authors have had variable success with PUVA, broadband UVA, and methotrexate in severe disease. Resolution of therapeutic uncertainty must await the organization and completion of controlled trials.

References

Aberer E, Neumann R, Stanek G (1985) Is localised scleroderma a borrelia infection? [letter]. Lancet 2 (8449):278

Aiba S, Tabata N, Ohtani H, Tagami H (1994) Cd34+ spindle-shaped cells selectively disappear from the skin lesion of scleroderma. Arch Dermatol 130 (5):593–597

Akimoto S, Hayashi H, Ishikawa H (1992) Disaccharide analysis of the skin glycosaminoglycans in systemic sclerosis. Br J Dermatol 126 (1):29–34

Andres C, Kollmar A, Mempel M, Hein R, Ring J, Eberlein B (2010) Successful ultraviolet a1 phototherapy in the treatment of localized scleroderma: A retrospective and prospective study. Br J Dermatol 162 (2):445–447

Antiga E, Quaglino P, Bellandi S, Volpi W, Del Bianco E, Comessatti A, Osella-Abate S, De Simone C, Marzano A, Bernengo MG, Fabbri P, Caproni M (2010) Regulatory T cells in the skin lesions and blood of patients with systemic sclerosis and morphoea. Br J Dermatol 162 (5):1056–1063

Arkachaisri T, Fertig N, Pino S, Medsger TA, Jr. (2008) Serum autoantibodies and their clinical associations in patients with childhood- and adult-onset linear scleroderma. A single-center study. J Rheumatol 35 (12):2439–2444

Arkachaisri T, Vilaiyuk S, Torok KS, Medsger TA, Jr. (2010) Development and initial validation of the localized scleroderma skin damage index and physician global assessment of disease damage: A proof-of-concept study. Rheumatology (Oxford) 49 (2):373–381

Arnett FC, Tan FK, Uziel Y, Laxer RM, Krafchik BR, Antohi S, Bona C (1999) Autoantibodies to the extracellular matrix microfibrillar protein, fibrillin 1, in patients with localized scleroderma. Arthritis Rheum 42 (12):2656–2659

Balat A, Akinci A, Turgut M, Mizrak B, Aydin A (1999) Eosinophilic fasciitis – progression to linear scleroderma: A case report. Turk J Pediatr 41 (3):381–385

Barrera P, Haagsma CJ, Boerbooms AM, Van Riel PL, Borm GF, Van de Putte LB, Van der Meer JW (1995) Effect of methotrexate alone or in combination with sulphasalazine on the production and circulating concentrations of cytokines and their antagonists. Longitudinal evaluation in patients with rheumatoid arthritis. Br J Rheumatol 34 (8):747–755

Batchelor R, Lamb S, Goulden V, Stables G, Goodfield M, Merchant W (2008) Photodynamic therapy for the treatment of morphoea. Clin Exp Dermatol 33 (5):661–663

Bilen N, Apaydin R, Ercin C, Harova G, Basdas F, Bayramgurler D (1999) Coexistence of morphea and psoriasis responding to acitretin treatment. J Eur Acad Dermatol Venereol 13 (2):113–117

Birdi N, Shore A, Rush P, Laxer RM, Silverman ED, Krafchik B (1992) Childhood linear scleroderma: A possible role of thermography for evaluation. J Rheumatol 19 (6):968–973

Blaszczyk M, Jablonska S (1999) Linear scleroderma en coup de sabre. Relationship with progressive facial hemiatrophy (pfh). In: Uitto Ma (ed) Rheumaderm. Kluwer Academic / Plenum Publishers, New York, pp 101–104

Blaszczyk M, Krolicki L, Krasu M, Glinska O, Jablonska S (2003) Progressive facial hemiatrophy: Central nervous system involvement and relationship with scleroderma en coup de sabre. J Rheumatol 30 (9):1997–2004

Blaszczyk M, Krysicka-Janiger K, Jablonska S (2000) Primary atrophic profound linear scleroderma. Report of three cases. Dermatology 200 (1):63–66

Bleasel NR, Stapleton KM, Commens C, Ahern VA (1999) Radiation-induced localized scleroderma in breast cancer patients. Australas J Dermatol 40 (2):99–102

Bodemer C, Amoric JC, Hamel-Teillac D, De Prost Y (1999a) Localized scleroderma in children and a therapeutic trial using calcitriol: A therapeutic possibility to define. Ann Dermatol Venereol 126 (10):725–726

Bodemer C, Belon M, Hamel-Teillac D, Amoric JC, Fraitag S, Prieur AM, De Prost Y (1999b) [scleroderma in children: A retrospective study of 70 cases]. Ann Dermatol Venereol 126 (10):691–694

Boelsma E, Pavel S, Ponec M (1995) Effects of calcitriol on fibroblasts derived from skin of scleroderma patients. Dermatology 191 (3):226–233

Bottomley WW, Jutley J, Wood EJ, Goodfield MD (1995) The effect of calcipotriol on lesional fibroblasts from patients with active morphoea. Acta Derm Venereol 75 (5):364–366

Branchet MC, Boisnic S, Bletry O, Robert L, Charron D, Frances C (1992) Expression of hla class ii antigens on skin fibroblasts in scleroderma. Br J Dermatol 126 (5):431–435

Brownell I, Soter NA, Franks AG, Jr. (2007) Familial linear scleroderma (en coup de sabre) responsive to antimalarials and narrowband ultraviolet b therapy. Dermatology online journal 13 (1):11

Caca-Biljanovska NG, Vlckova-Laskoska MT, Dervendi DV, Pesic NP, Laskoski DS (1999) Treatment of generalized morphea with oral 1,25-dihydroxyvitamin d3. Adv Exp Med Biol 455:299–304

Camacho NR, Sanchez JE, Martin RF, Gonzalez JR, Sanchez JL (2001) Medium-dose uva1 phototherapy in localized scleroderma and its effect in cd34-positive dendritic cells. J Am Acad Dermatol 45 (5):697–699

Campione E, Paterno EJ, Diluvio L, Orlandi A, Bianchi L, Chimenti S (2009) Localized morphea treated with imiquimod 5% and dermoscopic assessment of effectiveness. The Journal of dermatological treatment 20 (1):10–13

Canizares O, Sachs P, Jaimovich L, Torres V (1958) Idiopathic atrophoderma of pasini and pierini. Arch Dermatol 77:42–59

Cannick L, 3rd, Douglas G, Crater S, Silver R (2003) Nodular scleroderma: Case report and literature review. J Rheumatol 30 (11):2500–2502

Castanet J, Lacour JP, Perrin C, Taillan B, Dubois D, Ortonne JP (1994) Association of eosinophilic fasciitis, multiple morphea and antiphospholipid antibody. Dermatology 189 (3):304–307

Christianson H, Dorsey C, O'Leary P, Kierland R (1956) Localized scleroderma: A clinical study of twohundred thirty-five cases. Arch Dermatol 74:629–639

Chung H, Hann S (1997) Lupus panniculitis treated by a combination therapy of hydroxycvhloroquine and quinacrine. J Dermatol 24 (9):569–572

Chung MH, Sum J, Morrell MJ, Horoupian DS (1995) Intracerebral involvement in scleroderma en coup de sabre: Report of a case with neuropathologic findings. Ann Neurol 37 (5):679–681

Clemens TL, Adams JS, Horiuchi N, Gilchrest BA, Cho H, Tsuchiya Y, Matsuo N, Suda T, Holick MF (1983) Interaction of 1,25-dihydroxyvitamin-d3 with keratinocytes and fibroblasts from skin of normal subjects and a subject with vitamin-d-dependent rickets, type ii: A model for study of the mode of action of 1,25-dihydroxyvitamin d3. J Clin Endocrinol Metab 56 (4):824–830

Cosnes A, Anglade MC, Revuz J, Radier C (2003) Thirteen-megahertz ultrasound probe: Its role in diagnosing localized scleroderma. Br J Dermatol 148 (4):724–729

Crespo MP, Mas IB, Diaz JM, Costa AL, Nortes IB (2009) Rapid response to cyclosporine and maintenance with methotrexate in linear scleroderma in a young girl. Pediatr Dermatol 26 (1):118–120

Cribier B, Faradji T, Le Coz C, Oberling F, Grosshans E (1995) Extracorporeal photochemotherapy in systemic sclerosis and severe morphea. Dermatology 191 (1):25–31

Cunningham BB, Landells ID, Langman C, Sailer DE, Paller AS (1998) Topical calcipotriene for morphea/linear scleroderma. J Am Acad Dermatol 39 (2 Pt 1):211–215

Curley RK, Macfarlane AW, Evans S, Woodrow JC (1987) The treatment of linear morphoea with d-penicillamine. Clin Exp Dermatol 12 (1):56–57

Czarnecki DB, Taft EH (1982) Generalized morphoea successfully treated with salazopyrine. Acta Derm Venereol 62 (1):81–82

Daoud MS, Su WP, Leiferman KM, Perniciaro C (1994) Bullous morphea: Clinical, pathologic, and immunopathologic evaluation of thirteen cases. J Am Acad Dermatol 30 (6):937–943

David J, Wilson J, Woo P (1991) Scleroderma "En coup de sabre". Ann Rheum Dis 50:260–262

de Gannes GC, Ghoreishi M, Pope J, Russell A, Bell D, Adams S, Shojania K, Martinka M, Dutz JP (2007) Psoriasis and pustular dermatitis triggered by tnf-{alpha} inhibitors in patients with rheumatologic conditions. Arch Dermatol 143 (2):223–231

Dehen L, Roujeau JC, Cosnes A, Revuz J (1994) Internal involvement in localized scleroderma. Medicine (Baltimore) 73 (5):241–245

Diaz-Perez J, Connolly S, Winkelmann R (1980) Disabling pansclerotic morphea of children. Arch Dermatol 116:169–173

Dillon WI, Saed GM, Fivenson DP (1995) Borrelia burgdorferi DNA is undetectable by polymerase chain reaction in skin lesions of morphea, scleroderma, or lichen sclerosus et atrophicus of patients from north america. J Am Acad Dermatol 33 (4):617–620

Doyle JA, Ginsburg WW (1989) Eosinophilic fasciitis. Med Clin North Am 73 (5):1157–1166

Drago F, Rampini P, Lugani C, Rebora A (1998) Generalized morphoea after antitetanus vaccination [letter]. Clin Exp Dermatol 23 (3):142

Dubois EL, Chandor S, Friou GJ, Bischel M (1971) Progressive systemic sclerosis (pss) and localized scleroderma (morphea) with positive le cell test and unusual systemic manifestations compatible with systemic lupus erythematous (sle): Presentation of 14 cases including one set of identical twins, one with scleroderma dn the other with sle. Review of the literature. Medicine (Baltimore) 50 (3):199–222

Dytoc M, Ting PT, Man J, Sawyer D, Fiorillo L (2005) First case series on the use of imiquimod for morphoea. Br J Dermatol 153 (4):815–820

Dytoc MT, Kossintseva I, Ting PT (2007) First case series on the use of calcipotriol-betamethasone dipropionate for morphoea. Br J Dermatol 157 (3):615–618

Eisen D, Alster TS (2002) Use of a 585 nm pulsed dye laser for the treatment of morphea. Dermatol Surg 28 (7):615–616

El-Mofty M, Mostafa W, El-Darouty M, Bosseila M, Nada H, Yousef R, Esmat S, El-Lawindy M, Assaf M, El-Enani G (2004) Different low doses of broad-band uva in the treatment of morphea and systemic sclerosis. Photodermatol Photoimmunol Photomed 20 (3):148–156

El-Mofty M, Zaher H, Bosseila M, Yousef R, Saad B (2000) Low-dose broad-band uva in morphea using a new method for evaluation. Photodermatol Photoimmunol Photomed 16 (2):43–49

Elst EF, Van Suijlekom-Smit LW, Oranje AP (1999) Treatment of linear scleroderma with oral 1,25-dihydroxyvitamin d3 (calcitriol) in seven children. Pediatr Dermatol 16 (1):53–58

Falanga V, Medsger TA, Jr. (1990) D-penicillamine in the treatment of localized scleroderma. Archives of Dermatology 126 (5):609–612

Falanga V, Medsger TA, Jr., Reichlin M (1987) Antinuclear and anti-single-stranded DNA antibodies in morphea and generalized morphea. Arch Dermatol 123 (3):350–353

Falanga V, Medsger TA, Jr., Reichlin M, Rodnan GP (1986) Linear scleroderma. Clinical spectrum, prognosis, and laboratory abnormalities. Ann Intern Med 104 (6):849–857

Falanga V, Medsger TA, Reichlin M (1985) High titers of antibodies to single-stranded DNA in linear scleroderma. Arch Dermatol 121 (3):345–347

Fleischmajer R, Nedwich A (1972) Generalized morphea. I. Histology of the dermis and subcutaneous tissue. Arch Dermatol 106 (4):509–514

Fleischmajer R, Perlish JS (1972) Glycosaminoglycans in scleroderma and scleredema. J Invest Dermatol 58 (3):129–132

Fleischmajer R, Prunieras M (1972) Generalized morphea. Ii. Electron microscopy of collagen, cells, and the subcutaneous tissue. Arch Dermatol 106 (4):515–524

Fleischmajer R, Perlish JS, Krieg T, Timpl R (1981) Variability in collagen and fibronectin synthesis by scleroderma fibroblasts in primary culture. J Invest Dermatol 76 (5):400–403

Foeldvari I (1998) Progressive linear scleroderma and morphea in a child. J Pediatr 133 (2):308

Fry A, Alvarellos A, Fink C, Blaw M, Roach E (1992) Intracranial findings in progressive facial hemiatrophy. J Rheumatol 19:956–958

Fujimoto M, Sato S, Ihn H, Takehara K (1995) Autoantibodies to the heat-shock protein hsp73 in localized scleroderma. Arch Dermatol Res 287 (6):581–585

Gambichler T, Kreuter A, Rotterdam S, Altmeyer P, Hoffmann K (2003) Linear scleroderma 'en coup de sabre' treated with topical calcipotriol and cream psoralen plus ultraviolet a. J Eur Acad Dermatol Venereol 17 (5):601–602

Garcia-Bustinduy M, Noda A, Sanchez R, Gonzalez de Mesa MJ, Guimera F, Garcia-Montelongo R (1998) Puva therapy in localized scleroderma [letter]. J Eur Acad Dermatol Venereol 10 (3):283–284

Garzon M, Paller A (1999) Ultrapotent topical corticosteroids treatment of childhood genital lichen sclerosus. Arch Dermatol 135 (5):525–528

Gordon GV (1981) Eosinophilic fasciitis. A case report and review of the literature. Cutis 28 (3):268, 271–263

Grundmann-Kollmann M, Ochsendorf F, Zollner TM, Spieth K, Sachsenberg-Studer E, Kaufmann R, Podda M (2000) Puva-cream photochemotherapy for the treatment of localized scleroderma. J Am Acad Dermatol 43 (4):675–678

Gruss C, Reed JA, Altmeyer P, McNutt NS, Kerscher M (1997a) Induction of interstitial collagenase (mmp-1) by uva-1 phototherapy in morphea fibroblasts. Lancet 350 (9087):1295–1296

Gruss C, Reed JA, Altmeyer P, McNutt NS, Kerscher M (1997b) Induction of interstitial collagenase (mmp-1) by uva-1 phototherapy in morphea fibroblasts [letter]. Lancet 350 (9087):1295–1296

Gruss C, Stucker M, Kobyletzki G, Schreiber D, Altmeyer P, Kerscher M (1997c) Low dose uva1 phototherapy in disabling pansclerotic morphoea of childhood [letter]. Br J Dermatol 136 (2):293–294

Hasegawa M, Sato S, Nagaoka T, Fujimoto M, Takehara K (2003) Serum levels of tumor necrosis factor and interleukin-13 are elevated in patients with localized scleroderma. Dermatology 207 (2):141–147

Hatamochi A, Ono M, Arakawa M, Takeda K, Ueki H (1992) Analysis of collagen gene expression by cultured fibroblasts in morphoea. Br J Dermatol 126 (3):216–221

Hauser C, Skaria A, Harms M, Saurat JH (1996) Morphoea following blaschko's lines [letter]. Br J Dermatol 134 (3):594–595

Hayakawa I, Hasegawa M, Takehara K, Sato S (2004) Anti-DNA topoisomerase iialpha autoantibodies in localized scleroderma. Arthritis Rheum 50 (1):227–232

Herrick AL, Ennis H, Bhushan M, Silman AJ, Baildam EM (2010) Incidence of childhood linear scleroderma and systemic sclerosis in the uk and ireland. Arthritis Care Res (Hoboken) 62 (2):213–218

Higley H, Persichitte K, Chu S, Waegell W, Vancheeswaran R, Black C (1994) Immunocytochemical localization and serologic detection of transforming growth factor beta 1. Association with type i procollagen and inflammatory cell markers in diffuse and limited systemic sclerosis, morphea, and raynaud's phenomenon. Arthritis Rheum 37 (2):278–288

Holick MF, Smith E, Pincus S (1987) Skin as the site of vitamin d synthesis and target tissue for 1,25-dihydroxyvitamin d3. Use of calcitriol (1,25-dihydroxyvitamin d3) for treatment of psoriasis. Arch Dermatol 123 (12):1677–1683a

Hsu S, Lee MW, Carlton S, Kramer EM (1999) Nodular morphea in a linear pattern. Int J Dermatol 38 (7):529–530

Hulshof MM, Pavel S, Breedveld FC, Dijkmans BA, Vermeer BJ (1994) Oral calcitriol as a new therapeutic modality for generalized morphea. Arch Dermatol 130 (10):1290–1293

Hulshof MM, Bouwes Bavinck JN, Bergman W, Masclee AA, Heickendorff L, Breedveld FC, Dijkmans BA (2000) Double-blind, placebo-controlled study of oral calcitriol for the treatment of localized and systemic scleroderma. J Am Acacd Dermatol 43 (6):1017–1023

Humbert P, Aubin F, Dupond JL, Delaporte E (1995) Oral calcitriol as a new therapeutic agent in localized and systemic scleroderma. Archives of Dermatology 131 (7):850–851

Humbert PG, Dupond JL, Rochefort A, Vasselet R, Lucas A, Laurent R, Agache P (1990) Localized scleroderma – response to 1,25-dihydroxyvitamin d3. Clin Exp Dermatol 15 (5):396–398

Hunzelmann N, Anders S, Fierlbeck G, Hein R, Herrmann K, Albrecht M, Bell S, Muche R, Wehner-Caroli J, Gaus W, Krieg T (1997) Double-blind, placebo-controlled study of intralesional interferon gamma for the treatment of localized scleroderma. J Am Acad Dermatol 36 (3):433–435

Igarashi A, Nashiro K, Kikuchi K, Sato S, Ihn H, Fujimoto M, Grotendorst GR, Takehara K (1996) Connective tissue growth factor gene expression in tissue sections from localized scleroderma, keloid, and other fibrotic skin disorders. J Invest Dermatol 106 (4):729–733

Ihn H, Sato S, Fujimoto M, Kikuchi K, Takehara K (1994) Demonstration of interleukin 8 in serum samples of patients with localized scleroderma [letter]. Arch Dermatol 130 (10):1327–1328

Ihn H, Sato S, Fujimoto M, Kikuchi K, Takehara K (1995) Demonstration of interleukin-2, inter-leukin-4 and interleukin-6 in sera from patients with localized scleroderma. Arch Dermatol Res 287 (2):193–197

Ihn H, Sato S, Fujimoto M, Kikuchi K, Takehara K (1996) Clinical significance of serum levels of soluble interleukin-2 receptor in patients with localized scleroderma. Br J Dermatol 134 (5):843–847

Ihn H, Yazawa N, Kubo M, Yamane K, Sato S, Fujimoto M, Kikuchi K, Soma Y, Tamaki K (2000) Circulating levels of soluble cd30 are increased in patients with localized scleroderma and cor-related with serological and clinical features of the disease. J Rheumatol 27 (3):698–702

Itin PH, Schiller P (1999) Double-lined frontoparietal scleroderma en coup de sabre. Dermatology 199 (2):185–186

Jablonska S (1975a) Facial hemiatrophy and it's relation to localized scleroderma. In: Jablonska S (ed) Scleroderma and pseudoscleroderma. PZWL, Warsaw, pp 537–548

Jablonska S (1975b) Localised scleroderma. In: Jablonska S (ed) Scleroderma and pseudosclero-derma. 2nd edn. Polish Medical Publishers, Warsaw, pp 277–303

Jablonska S, Rodnan G (1979) Localized forms of scleroderma. Clin Rheumatol Dis 5:215–241

Jablonska S, Blaszczyk M (2004) Is superficial morphea synonymous with atrophoderma pasini-pierini? J Am Acad Dermatol 50 (6):979–980

Jacobe HT, Cayce R, Nguyen J (2008) Uva1 phototherapy is effective in darker skin: A review of 101 patients of fitzpatrick skin types i-v. Br J Dermatol 159 (3):691–696

Janzen L, Jeffery JR, Gough J, Chalmers IM (1995) Response to methotrexate in a patient with idio-pathic eosinophilic fasciitis, morphea, igm hypergammaglobulinemia, and renal involvement. J Rheumatol 22 (10):1967–1970

Jaworsky C (1997) Connective tissue diseases. In: Elder D (ed) Lever's histopathology of the skin. Lippincott-Raven, Philadelphia, pp 253–285

Jeffery LE, Burke F, Mura M, Zheng Y, Qureshi OS, Hewison M, Walker LS, Lammas DA, Raza K, Sansom DM (2009) 1,25-dihydroxyvitamin d3 and il-2 combine to inhibit t cell production of inflammatory cytokines and promote development of regulatory t cells expressing ctla-4 and foxp3. J Immunol 183 (9):5458–5467

Jessop S, Whitelaw D (2009) Methotrexate for sclerotic skin disorders: No evidence for effective-ness. Br J Dermatol 161 (5):1205

Joly P, Bamberger N, Crickx B, Belaich S (1994) Treatment of severe forms of localized sclero-derma with oral corticosteroids: Follow-up study on 17 patients. Archives of Dermatology 130 (5):663–664

Jones SM, Mathew CM, Dixey J, Lovell CR, McHugh NJ (1996) Vcam-1 expression on endothe-lium in lesions from cutaneous lupus erythematosus is increased compared with systemic and localized scleroderma. Br J Dermatol 135 (5):678–686

Kahari VM, Heino J, Vuorio T, Vuorio E (1988a) Interferon-alpha and interferon-gamma reduce excessive collagen synthesis and procollagen mrna levels of scleroderma fibroblasts in culture. Biochim Biophys Acta 968 (1):45–50

Kahari VM, Sandberg M, Kalimo H, Vuorio T, Vuorio E (1988b) Identification of fibroblasts re-sponsible for increased collagen production in localized scleroderma by in situ hybridization. J Invest Dermatol 90 (5):664–670

Kakimoto CV, Victor Ross E, Uebelhoer NS (2009) En coup de sabre presenting as a port-wine stain previously treated with pulsed dye laser. Dermatol Surg 35 (1):165–167

Kanekura T, Fukumaru S, Matsushita S, Terasaki K, Mizoguchi S, Kanzaki T (1996) Successful treatment of scleroderma with puva therapy. J Dermatol 23 (7):455–459

Karrer S, Abels C, Landthaler M, Szeimies RM (2000) Topical photodynamic therapy for localized scleroderma. Acta Derm Venereol 80 (1):26–27

Kencka D, Blaszczyk M, Jablonska S (1995) Atrophoderma pasini-pierini is a primary atrophic abortive morphea. Dermatology 190 (3):203–206

Kerscher M, Dirschka T, Volkenandt M (1995a) Treatment of localised scleroderma by uva1 phototherapy. Lancet 346 (8983):1166

Kerscher M, Meurer M, Sander C, Volkenandt M, Lehmann P, Plewig G, Rocken M (1996) Puva
bath photochemotherapy for localized scleroderma. Evaluation of 17 consecutive patients. Arch
Dermatol 132 (11):1280–1282

Kerscher M, Volkenandt M, Gruss C, Reuther T, von Kobyletzki G, Freitag M, Dirschka T, Altmeyer P (1998b) Low-dose uva phototherapy for treatment of localized scleroderma. J Am
Acad Dermatol 38 (1):21–26

Ko JY, Kim YS, Lee CW (2009) Multifocal lesions of morphoea in a patient with systemic lupus
erythematosus. Clin Exp Dermatol 34 (8):e676–679

Kobayashi KA, Lui H, Prendiville JS (1991) Solitary morphea profunda in a 5-year-old girl: Case
report and review of the literature. Pediatr Dermatol 8 (4):292–295

Kobayasi T, Serup J (1985) Vascular changes in morphea. Acta Derm Venereol 65 (2):116–120

Kobayasi T, Willeberg A, Serup J, Ullman S (1990) Generalized morphea with blisters. A case report. Acta Derm Venereol 70 (5):454–456

Koeger AC, Rozenberg S, Fautrel B (1999) Effectiveness of topical calcitriol for localized scleroderma [letter]. J Rheumatol 26 (1):239–240

Kowalewski C, Kozlowska A, Zawadzka M, Wozniak K, Blaszczyk M, Jablonska S (2004) Alterations of basement membrane zone in bullous and non-bullous variants of extragenital lichen
sclerosus. Am J Dermatopathol 26 (2):96–101

Krell JM, Solomon AR, Glavey CM, Lawley TJ (1995) Nodular scleroderma. J Am Acad Dermatol
32 (2 Pt 2):343–345

Kreuter A, Gambichler T, Avermaete A, Jansen T, Hoffmann M, Hoffmann K, Altmeyer P, von
Kobyletzki G, Bacharach-Buhles M (2001) Combined treatment with calcipotriol ointment and
low-dose ultraviolet a1 phototherapy in childhood morphea. Pediatr Dermatol 18 (3):241–245

Kreuter A, Gambichler T, Breuckmann F, Rotterdam S, Freitag M, Stuecker M, Hoffmann K, Altmeyer P (2005) Pulsed high-dose corticosteroids combined with low-dose methotrexate in severe localized scleroderma. Arch Dermatol 141 (7):847–852

Kreuter A, Hyun J, Skrygan M, Sommer A, Bastian A, Altmeyer P, Gambichler T (2006a) Ultraviolet a1-induced downregulation of human beta-defensins and interleukin-6 and interleukin-8
correlates with clinical improvement in localized scleroderma. Br J Dermatol 155 (3):600–607

Kreuter A, Hyun J, Stucker M, Sommer A, Altmeyer P, Gambichler T (2006b) A randomized controlled study of low-dose uva1, medium-dose uva1, and narrowband uvb phototherapy in the
treatment of localized scleroderma. J Am Acad Dermatol 54 (3):440–447

Kroft EB, Creemers MC, van den Hoogen FH, Boezeman JB, de Jong EM (2009a) Effectiveness, side-
effects and period of remission after treatment with methotrexate in localized scleroderma and
related sclerotic skin diseases: An inception cohort study. Br J Dermatol 160 (5):1075–1082

Kroft EB, de Jong EM, Evers AW (2009b) Psychological distress in patients with morphea and eosinophilic fasciitis. Arch Dermatol 145 (9):1017–1022

Kubo M, Ihn H, Yamane K, Tamaki K (2001) Up-regulated expression of transforming growth
factor beta receptors in dermal fibroblasts in skin sections from patients with localized scleroderma. Arthritis Rheum 44 (3):731–734

Labandeira J, Leon-Mateos A, Suarez-Penaranda JM, Garea MT, Toribio J (2003) What is nodular-
keloidal scleroderma? Dermatology 207 (2):130–132

Lee HJ, Kim MY, Ha SJ, Kim JW (2002) Two cases of morphea associated with hashimoto's thyroiditis. Acta Derm Venereol 82 (1):58–59

Leitenberger JJ, Cayce RL, Haley RW, Adams-Huet B, Bergstresser PR, Jacobe HT (2009) Distinct
autoimmune syndromes in morphea: A review of 245 adult and pediatric cases. Arch Dermatol
145 (5):545–550

Levy JJ, Gassmuller J, Audring H, Brenke A, Albrecht-Nebe H (1993) [imaging subcutaneous atrophy in circumscribed scleroderma with 20 mhz b-scan ultrasound]. Hautarzt 44 (7):446–451

Liu P, Uziel Y, Chuang S, Silverman E, Krafchik B, Laxer R (1994) Localized scleroderma: Imaging features. Pediatr Radiol 24:207–209

Luer W, Jockel D, Henze T, Schipper HI (1990) Progressive inflammatory lesions of the brain parenchyma in localized scleroderma of the head. J Neurol 237 (6):379–381

Man J, Dytoc MT (2004) Use of imiquimod cream 5% in the treatment of localized morphea. J Cutan Med Surg 8 (3):166–169

Mancuso G, Berdondini RM (2003) Topical tacrolimus in the treatment of localized scleroderma. Eur J Dermatol 13 (6):590–592

Martini G, Murray KJ, Howell KJ, Harper J, Atherton D, Woo P, Zulian F, Black CM (2002) Juvenile-onset localized scleroderma activity detection by infrared thermography. Rheumatology (Oxford) 41 (10):1178–1182

Martini G, Ramanan AV, Falcini F, Girschick H, Goldsmith DP, Zulian F (2009) Successful treatment of severe or methotrexate-resistant juvenile localized scleroderma with mycophenolate mofetil. Rheumatology (Oxford, England) 48 (11):1410–1413

Maruotti N, Cantatore FP (2010) Vitamin d and the immune system. J Rheumatol 37 (3):491–495

Marzano AV, Menni S, Parodi A, Borghi A, Fuligni A, Fabbri P, Caputo R (2003) Localized scleroderma in adults and children. Clinical and laboratory investigations on 239 cases. Eur J Dermatol 13 (2):171–176

Mattila L, Airola K, Ahonen M, Hietarinta M, Black C, Saarialho-Kere U, Kahari VM (1998) Activation of tissue inhibitor of metalloproteinases-3 (timp-3) mrna expression in scleroderma skin fibroblasts. J Invest Dermatol 110 (4):416–421

Mattozzi C, Richetta AG, Cantisani C, Giancristoforo S, D'Epiro S, Gonzalez Serva A, Viola F, Cucchiara S, Calvieri S (2010) Morphea, an unusual side effect of anti-tnf-alpha treatment. Eur J Dermatol 20 (3):400–401

McColl G, Buchanan RR (1994) Unilateral scleroderma following ischemic hand injury [letter]. J Rheumatol 21 (2):380–381

McNiff JM, Glusac EJ, Lazova RZ, Carroll CB (1999) Morphea limited to the superficial reticular dermis: An underrecognized histologic phenomenon. Am J Dermatopathol 21 (4):315–319

Menni S, Marzano AV, Passoni E (1997) Neurologic abnormalities in two patients with facial hemiatrophy and sclerosis coexisting with morphea. Pediatr Dermatol 14 (2):113–116

Micalizzi C, Parodi A, Rebora A (1994) Morphea with nodular lesions. Br J Dermatol 131:298–300

Micalizzi C, Parodi A, Rebora A (1996) Generalized bullous morphoea. Efficacy of salazopyrin. Clin Exp Dermatol 21 (3):246–247

Milano A, Pendergrass SA, Sargent JL, George LK, McCalmont TH, Connolly MK, Whitfield ML (2008) Molecular subsets in the gene expression signatures of scleroderma skin. PLoS One 3 (7):e2696

Miller J (1992a) The fasciitis-morphea complex in children. Am J Dis Child 146 (6):733–736

Miller JJ, 3rd (1992b) The fasciitis-morphea complex in children. American Journal of Diseases of Children (1960) 146 (6):733–736

Mitchet C, Doyle J, Ginsburg W (1981) Eosinophilic fascitis: Report of 15 cases. Mayo Clin Proc 56:27–34

Mizutani H, Yoshida T, Nouchi N, Hamanaka H, Shimizu M (1999) Topical tocoretinate improved hypertrophic scar, skin sclerosis in systemic sclerosis and morphea. J Dermatol 26 (1):11–17

Mohrenschlager M, Jung C, Ring J, Abeck D (1999) Effect of penicillin g on corium thickness in linear morphea of childhood: An analysis using ultrasound technique. Pediatr Dermatol 16 (4):314–316

Moller R, Serup J, Ammitzboll T (1985) Glycosaminoglycans in localized scleroderma (morphoea). Connect Tissue Res 13 (3):227–236

Monteiro MR, Murphy EE, Galaria NA, Whitaker-Menezes D, Murphy GF (2000) Cytological alterations in dermal dendrocytes in vitro: Evidence for transformation to a non-dendritic phenotype. Br J Dermatol 143 (1):84–90

Morison WL (1997) Psoralen uva therapy for linear and generalized morphea. J Am Acad Dermatol 37 (4):657–659

Morita A, Werfel T, Stege H, Ahrens C, Karmann K, Grewe M, Grether-Beck S, Ruzicka T, Kapp A, Klotz LO, Sies H, Krutmann J (1997) Evidence that singlet oxygen-induced human t helper cell apoptosis is the basic mechanism of ultraviolet-a radiation phototherapy. J Exp Med 186 (10):1763–1768

Mork NJ (1981) Clinical and histopathologic morphea with immunological evidence of lupus erythematosus: A case report. Acta Derm Venereol 61 (4):367–368

Morley SM, Gaylarde PM, Sarkany I (1985) Epidermal thickness in systemic sclerosis and morphoea. Clin Exp Dermatol 10 (1):51–57

Moynahan EJ (1973) Morphoea (localized cutaneous scleroderma) treated with low-dosage penicillamine (4 cases, including coup de sabre). Proc R Soc Med 66 (11):1083–1085

Nagai M, Hasegawa M, Takehara K, Sato S (2004) Novel autoantibody to cu/zn superoxide dismutase in patients with localized scleroderma. J Invest Dermatol 122 (3):594–601

Narvaez D, Kanitakis J, Faure M, Claudy A (1996) Immunohistochemical study of cd34-positive dendritic cells of human dermis. Am J Dermatopathol 18 (3):283–288

Neldner KH (1978) Treatment of localized linear scleroderma with phenytoin. Cutis 22 (5):569–572

Neuhofer J, Fritsch P (1984) Treatment of localized scleroderma and lichen sclerosus with etretinate. Acta Derm Venereol 64 (2):171–174

Neustadter JH, Samarin F, Carlson KR, Girardi M (2009) Extracorporeal photochemotherapy for generalized deep morphea. Arch Dermatol 145 (2):127–130

O'Leary P, Montgomery H, Ragsdale W (1957) Dermatohistopathology of various types of scleroderma. Arch Dermatol 75:78–87

Oikarinen A, Knuutinen A (2001) Ultraviolet a sunbed used for the treatment of scleroderma. Acta Derm Venereol 81 (6):432–433

Oyama N, Chan I, Neill SM, Hamada T, South AP, Wessagowit V, Wojnarowska F, D'Cruz D, Hughes GJ, Black MM, McGrath JA (2003) Autoantibodies to extracellular matrix protein 1 in lichen sclerosus. Lancet 362 (9378):118–123

Oyama N, Chan I, Neill SM, South AP, Wojnarowska F, Kawakami Y, D'Cruz D, Mepani K, Hughes GJ, Bhogal BS, Kaneko F, Black MM, McGrath JA (2004) Development of antigen-specific elisa for circulating autoantibodies to extracellular matrix protein 1 in lichen sclerosus. J Clin Invest 113 (11):1550–1559

Passos CO, Werneck CC, Onofre GR, Pagani EA, Filgueira AL, Silva LC (2003) Comparative biochemistry of human skin: Glycosaminoglycans from different body sites in normal subjects and in patients with localized scleroderma. J Eur Acad Dermatol Venereol 17 (1):14–19

Perlish JS, Lemlich G, Fleischmajer R (1988) Identification of collagen fibrils in scleroderma skin. J Invest Dermatol 90 (1):48–54

Person JR, Su WP (1979) Subcutaneous morphoea: A clinical study of sixteen cases. Br J Dermatol 100 (4):371–380

Peter RU, Ruzicka T, Eckert F (1991) Low-dose cyclosporine a in the treatment of disabling morphea. Arch Dermatol 127 (9):1420–1421

Peterson LS, Nelson AM, Su WP (1995) Classification of morphea (localized scleroderma). Mayo Clin Proc 70 (11):1068–1076

Peterson LS, Nelson AM, Su WP, Mason T, O'Fallon WM, Gabriel SE (1997) The epidemiology of morphea (localized scleroderma) in olmsted county 1960–1993. J Rheumatol 24 (1):73–80

Rai R, Handa S, Gupta S, Kumar B (2000) Bilateral en coup de sabre-a rare entity. Pediatr Dermatol 17 (3):222–224

Rencic A, Brinster N, Nousari CH (2003) Keloid morphea and nodular scleroderma: Two distinct clinical variants of scleroderma? J Cutan Med Surg 7 (1):20–24

Rigby WF, Denome S, Fanger MW (1987) Regulation of lymphokine production and human t lymphocyte activation by 1,25-dihydroxyvitamin d3. Specific inhibition at the level of messenger rna. J Clin Invest 79 (6):1659–1664

Rigby WF, Waugh MG (1992) Decreased accessory cell function and costimulatory activity by 1,25-dihydroxyvitamin d3-treated monocytes. Arthritis Rheum 35 (1):110–119

Rodnan GP, Lipinski E, Luksick J (1979) Skin thickness and collagen content in progressive systemic sclerosis and localized scleroderma. Arthritis Rheum 22 (2):130–140

Rose CD, Fawcett PT, Gibney K, Doughty RA, Singsen BH (1994) Serial measurements of soluble interleukin 2 receptor levels (sil2-r) in children with juvenile rheumatoid arthritis treated with oral methotrexate. Ann Rheum Dis 53 (7):471–474

Rosenberg AM, Uziel Y, Krafchik BR, Hauta SA, Prokopchuk PA, Silverman ED, Laxer RM (1995) Antinuclear antibodies in children with localized scleroderma. J Rheumatol 22 (12):2337–2343

Ruffatti A, Peserico A, Rondinone R, Calligaro A, Del Ross T, Ghirardello A, Germino M, Todesco S (1991) Prevalence and characteristics of anti-single-stranded DNA antibodies in localized scleroderma. Comparison with systemic lupus erythematosus. Arch Dermatol 127 (8):1180–1183

Sakuraoka K, Tajima S, Nishikawa T (1992) Progressive facial hemiatrophy: Report of five cases and biochemical analysis of connective tissue. Dermatology 185 (3):196–201

Salmon-Ehr V, Serpier H, Nawrocki B, Gillery P, Clavel C, Kalis B, Birembaut P, Maquart FX (1996) Expression of interleukin-4 in scleroderma skin specimens and scleroderma fibroblast cultures. Potential role in fibrosis. Arch Dermatol 132 (7):802–806

Sato S, Fujimoto M, Hasegawa M, Takehara K (2003) Antiphospholipid antibody in localised scleroderma. Ann Rheum Dis 62 (8):771–774

Sato S, Fujimoto M, Ihn H, Kikuchi K, Takehara K (1994) Clinical characteristics associated with antihistone antibodies in patients with localized scleroderma. J Am Acad Dermatol 31 (4):567–571

Sato S, Fujimoto M, Kikuchi K, Ihn H, Tamaki K, Takehara K (1996a) Elevated soluble cd23 levels in the sera from patients with localized scleroderma. Arch Dermatol Res 288 (2):74–78

Sato S, Fujimoto M, Kikuchi K, Ihn H, Tamaki K, Takehara K (1996b) Soluble cd4 and cd8 in serum from patients with localized scleroderma. Arch Dermatol Res 288 (7):358–362

Sator PG, Radakovic S, Schulmeister K, Honigsmann H, Tanew A (2009) Medium-dose is more effective than low-dose ultraviolet a1 phototherapy for localized scleroderma as shown by 20-mhz ultrasound assessment. J Am Acad Dermatol 60 (5):786–791

Schaffer JV, Carroll C, Dvoretsky I, Huether MJ, Girardi M (2000) Postirradiation morphea of the breast presentation of two cases and review of the literature. Dermatology 200 (1):67–71

Scharffetter K, Lankat-Buttgereit B, Krieg T (1988) Localization of collagen mrna in normal and scleroderma skin by in-situ hybridization. Eur J Clin Invest 18 (1):9–17

Scharffetter-Kochanek K, Goldermann R, Lehmann P, Holzle E, Goerz G (1995) Puva therapy in disabling pansclerotic morphoea of children [letter]. Br J Dermatol 132 (5):830–831

Schiener R, Behrens-Williams SC, Gottlober P, Pillekamp H, Peter RU, Kerscher M (2000) Eosinophilic fasciitis treated with psoralen-ultraviolet a bath photochemotherapy. Br J Dermatol 142 (4):804–807

Schlaak M, Friedlein H, Kauer F, Renner R, Rogalski C, Simon JC (2008) Successful therapy of a patient with therapy recalcitrant generalized bullous scleroderma by extracorporeal photopheresis and mycophenolate mofetil. J Eur Acad Dermatol Venerol 22 (5):631–633

Seitz M, Loetscher P, Dewald B, Towbin H, Rordorf C, Gallati H, Baggiolini M, Gerber NJ (1995) Methotrexate action in rheumatoid arthritis: Stimulation of cytokine inhibitor and inhibition of chemokine production by peripheral blood mononuclear cells. Br J Rheumatol 34 (7):602–609

Seitz M, Zwicker M, Loetscher P (1998) Effects of methotrexate on differentiation of monocytes and production of cytokine inhibitors by monocytes. Arthritis Rheum 41 (11):2032–2038

Seyger MM, van den Hoogen FH, de Boo T, de Jong EM (1997) Reliability of two methods to assess morphea: Skin scoring and the use of a durometer. J Am Acad Dermatol 37 (5 Pt 1):793–796

Seyger MM, van den Hoogen FH, de Boo T, de Jong EM (1998) Low-dose methotrexate in the treatment of widespread morphea. J Am Acad Dermatol 39 (2 Pt 1):220–225

Seyger MM, van den Hoogen FH, van Vlijmen-Willems IM, van de Kerkhof PC, de Jong EM (2001) Localized and systemic scleroderma show different histological responses to methotrexate therapy. J Pathol 193 (4):511–516

Sgonc R, Gruschwitz MS, Dietrich H, Recheis H, Gershwin ME, Wick G (1996) Endothelial cell apoptosis is a primary pathogenetic event underlying skin lesions in avian and human scleroderma. J Clin Invest 98 (3):785–792

Shulman L (1974) Diffuse fasciitis with hypergammaglobulinemia and eosinophilia: A new syndrome? Clinical Reaserch 23:443A

Silman A, Jannini S, Symmons D, Bacon P (1988) An epidemiological study of scleroderma in the west midlands. Br J Rheumatol 27 (4):286–290

Skobieranda K, Helm KF (1995) Decreased expression of the human progenitor cell antigen (cd34) in morphea. Am J Dermatopathol 17 (5):471–475

Soma Y, Fujimoto M (1998) Frontoparietal scleroderma (en coup de sabre) following blaschko's lines. J Am Acad Dermatol 38 (2 Pt 2):366–368

Soma Y, Tamaki T, Kikuchi K, Abe M, Igarashi A, Takehara K, Ishibashi Y (1993) Coexistence of morphea and systemic sclerosis. Dermatology 186:103–105

Stava Z, Kobikova M (1977) Salazopyrin in the treatment of scleroderma. Br J Dermatol 96 (5):541–544

Stefanaki C, Stefanaki K, Kontochristopoulos G, Antoniou C, Stratigos A, Nicolaidou E, Gregoriou S, Katsambas A (2008) Topical tacrolimus 0.1% ointment in the treatment of localized scleroderma. An open label clinical and histological study. J Dermatol 35 (11):712–718

Stefanec T (2000) Endothelial apoptosis: Could it have a role in the pathogenesis and treatment of disease? Chest 117 (3):841–854

Stege H, Berneburg M, Humke S, Klammer M, Grewe M, Grether-Beck S, Boedeker R, Diepgen T, Dierks K, Goerz G, Ruzicka T, Krutmann J (1997) High-dose uva1 radiation therapy for localized scleroderma [see comments]. J Am Acad Dermatol 36 (6 Pt 1):938–944

Steger JW, Matthews JH (1999) Uva therapy for scleroderma. Journal of the American Academy of Dermatology 40 (5 Pt 1):787–788

Stone J, Franks AJ, Guthrie JA, Johnson MH (2001) Scleroderma «En coup de sabre»: Pathological evidence of intracerebral inflammation. J Neurol Neurosurg Psychiatry 70 (3):382–385

Strauss RM, Bhushan M, Goodfield MJ (2004) Good response of linear scleroderma in a child to ciclosporin. The British journal of dermatology 150 (4):790–792

Su WP, Greene SL (1986) Bullous morphea profunda. Am J Dermatopathol 8 (2):144–147

Su WP, Person JR (1981) Morphea profunda. A new concept and a histopathologic study of 23 cases. Am J Dermatopathol 3 (3):251–260

Takehara K, Moroi Y, Nakabayashi Y, Ishibashi Y (1983) Antinuclear antibodies in localized scleroderma. Arthritis Rheum 26 (5):612–616

Taveira M, Selores M, Costa V, Massa A (1999) Generalized morphea and lichen sclerosus et atrophicus successfully treated with sulphasalazine [letter]. J Eur Acad Dermatol Venereol 12 (3):283–284

Tay YK (2003) Topical calcipotriol ointment in the treatment of morphea. J Dermatolog Treat 14 (4):219–221

Todd DJ, Askari A, Ektaish E (1998) Puva therapy for disabling pansclerotic morphoea of children [letter]. Br J Dermatol 138 (1):201–202

Tollefson MM, Witman PM (2007) En coup de sabre morphea and parry-romberg syndrome: A retrospective review of 54 patients. Journal of the American Academy of Dermatology 56 (2):257–263

Torres JE, Sanchez JL (1998) Histopathologic differentiation between localized and systemic scleroderma. Am J Dermatopathol 20 (3):242–245

Tuffanelli DL (1998) Localized scleroderma. Semin Cutan Med Surg 17 (1):27–33

Uitto J, Santa Cruz DJ, Bauer EA, Eisen AZ (1980) Morphea and lichen sclerosus et atrophicus. Clinical and histopathologic studies in patients with combined features. J Am Acad Dermatol 3 (3):271–279

Umbert P, Winkelmann RK (1978) Concurrent localized scleroderma and discoid lupus erythematosus. Cutaneous 'mixed' or 'overlap' syndrome. Arch Dermatol 114 (10):1473–1478

Unterberger I, Trinka E, Engelhardt K, Muigg A, Eller P, Wagner M, Sepp N, Bauer G (2003) Linear scleroderma "En coup de sabre" Coexisting with plaque-morphea: Neuroradiological manifestation and response to corticosteroids. J Neurol Neurosurg Psychiatry 74 (5):661–664

Uziel Y, Feldman BM, Krafchik BR, Yeung RS, Laxer RM (2000) Methotrexate and corticosteroid therapy for pediatric localized scleroderma. J Pediatr 136 (1):91–95

Uziel Y, Krafchik BR, Feldman B, Silverman ED, Rubin LA, Laxer RM (1994a) Serum levels of soluble interleukin-2 receptor. A marker of disease activity in localized scleroderma. Arthritis Rheum 37 (6):898–901

Uziel Y, Krafchik BR, Silverman ED, Thorner PS, Laxer RM (1994b) Localized scleroderma in childhood: A report of 30 cases. Semin Arthritis Rheum 23 (5):328–340

van Bergen BH, van Dooren-Greebe RJ, Fiselier TJ, Koopman RJ (1997) [d-penicillamine in treatment of scleroderma "En coup de sabre"]. Hautarzt 48 (1):42–44

van den Hoogen FH, Boerbooms AM, Swaak AJ, Rasker JJ, van Lier HJ, van de Putte LB (1996) Comparison of methotrexate with placebo in the treatment of systemic sclerosis: A 24 week randomized double-blind trial, followed by a 24 week observational trial. Br J Rheumatol 35 (4):364–372

Venneker GT, Das PK, Naafs B, Tigges AJ, Bos JD, Asghar SS (1994) Morphoea lesions are associated with aberrant expression of membrane cofactor protein and decay accelerating factor in vascular endothelium. Br J Dermatol 131 (2):237–242

Wach F, Ullrich H, Schmitz G, Landthaler M, Hein R (1995) Treatment of severe localized scleroderma by plasmapheresis – report of three cases. Br J Dermatol 133 (4):605–609

Wakelin SH, James MP (1995) Zosteriform atrophoderma of pasini and pierini. Clin Exp Dermatol 20 (3):244–246

Walters R, Pulitzer M, Kamino H (2009) Elastic fiber pattern in scleroderma / morphea. J Cutan Pathol 36 (9):952–957

Weedon D (1997) Disorders of collagen. In: Skin pathology. 1st edn. Churchill Livingstone, Hong-Kong, pp 288–293

Weibel L, Sampaio MC, Visentin MT, Howell KJ, Woo P, Harper JI (2006) Evaluation of methotrexate and corticosteroids for the treatment of localized scleroderma (morphoea) in children. The British journal of dermatology 155 (5):1013–1020

Weide B, Walz T, Garbe C (2000) Is morphoea caused by borrelia burgdorferi? A review. Br J Dermatol 142 (4):636–644

Whittaker SJ, Smith NP, Jones RR (1989) Solitary morphoea profunda. Br J Dermatol 120 (3):431–440

Winkelmann R (1985) Localized cutaneous scleroderma. Seminars in Dermatology 4 (2):90–103

Winkelmann RK, Connolly SM, Doyle JA (1982) Carpal tunnel syndrome in cutaneous connective tissue disease: Generalized morphea, lichen sclerosus, fasciitis, discoid lupus erythematosus, and lupus panniculitis. J Am Acad Dermatol 7 (1):94–99

Wlaschek M, Briviba K, Stricklin GP, Sies H, Scharffetter-Kochanek K (1995) Singlet oxygen may mediate the ultraviolet a-induced synthesis of interstitial collagenase. J Invest Dermatol 104 (2):194–198

Wollenberg A, Baumann L, Plewig G (1995) Linear atrophoderma of moulin: A disease which follows blaschko's lines. Br J Dermatol 135:277–279

Wollina U, Looks A, Schneider R, Maak B (1998) Disabling morphoea of childhood-beneficial effect of intravenous immunoglobulin therapy [letter]. Clin Exp Dermatol 23 (6):292–293

Wuthrich RC, Roenigk HH, Steck WD (1975) Localized scleroderma. Arch Dermatol 111 (1):98–100

Yamaguchi K, Takeuchi I, Yoshii N, Gushi A, Kanekura T, Kanzaki T (1998) The discrepancy in hardness between clinical and histopathological findings in localized scleroderma treated with puva. J Dermatol 25 (8):544–546

Yamanaka CT, Gibbs NF (1999) Trauma-induced linear scleroderma. Cutis 63 (1):29–32

Yamane K, Ihn H, Kubo M, Yazawa N, Kikuchi K, Soma Y, Tamaki K (2000) Increased serum levels of soluble vascular cell adhesion molecule 1 and e-selectin in patients with localized scleroderma. J Am Acad Dermatol 42 (1 Pt 1):64–69

Young EM, Jr., Barr RJ (1985) Sclerosing dermatoses. J Cutan Pathol 12 (5):426–441

Zheng XY, Zhang JZ, Tu P, Ma SQ (1998) Expression of platelet-derived growth factor b-chain and platelet-derived growth factor beta-receptor in fibroblasts of scleroderma. J Dermatol Sci 18 (2):90–97

4

Scleroderma

4.2 Progressive Systemic Scleroderm

4

Nicolas Hunzelmann and Thomas Krieg

Introduction

Systemic sclerosis (SSc) belongs to the group of "diffuse inflammatory connective tissue diseases" or "collagen vascular diseases" comprising a variety of severe, sometimes life-threatening systemic diseases which often have a chronic, debilitating course. SSc is characterized by the involvement of the skin and various internal organs (e. g. kidney, lung, heart). The inflammatory and fibrotic process destroys the normal architecture of the affected organs leading to dysfunction and failure. The disease activity is highly variable and often unpredictable. The severity of the disease process in SSc leads to a reduced lifespan, impaired mobility and loss of autonomy.

SSc mainly evolves along pathological changes of the vascular system, the immune system and of the extracellular matrix including its major cell type, the fibroblast. The resulting fibrosis leading to atrophy and failure of the affected organs largely determines the outcome of the disease process. However, despite intense research efforts the relationship and interaction between the pathophysiological processes affecting the vascular system, the immune system and the extracellular matrix are only incompletely understood.

Immune Dysregulation

One of the hallmarks of SSc is a perturbed immunoregulation (resulting in the presence of autoantibodies), which appears to be influenced by additional factors such as genetic and exogenous factors. Autoimmunity in SSc is characterized by HLA gene restricted autoantibody responses against nuclear and nucleolar antigens. The mechanisms inducing the antibody production are unknown but clinical associations with autoantibody specificities suggest that these antigen-restricted responses are involved in disease specific pathology. In 2006 a pathogenetic role of cell surface specific antibodies recognizing the PDGF receptor has been described in SSc. These antibodies bind to the receptors, stimulate respective signalling pathways and lead to increased type I collagen gene expression in fibroblasts (Baroni et al., 2006). Antibodies directed to cell surface molecules inducing thereby signal transduction pathways are an intriguing concept, which is currently discussed in the pathophysiology of several unrelated diseases e. g. rejection of renal allografts, preeclampsia, hypertrophic cardiomyopathy. These autoimmune phenomena are in a not well understood way related to the inflammatory process with lymphocytic perivascular infiltrates in the skin and lung evident early on in the disease process and preceding the development of fibrosis (Gabrielli et al., 2009). The similarity of the condition with some aspects of graft versus host disease has frequently been noted. Recently it was suggested that microchimerism, i. e. the persistence of foetal cells in the maternal bone marrow and other organs like the skin might be a risk factor, also explaining the female excess (Artlett et al., 1998; Evans et al., 1999). However, subsequent studies found similar frequencies of microchimerisms compared to normal controls but nevertheless an increased number of microchimeric fetal cells in patients (Burastero et al., 2003).

Vascular Pathology

The relationship between autoimmune responses and the vascular pathology is unclear, as Raynaud's syndrome and vascular abnormalities may be evident many years prior to the onset of disease (Blockmans et al., 1996). The morphological changes that can be observed on a ultrastructural level, i. e. basement membrane thickening, intimal hyperplasia and inflammatory cell infiltration have been interpreted as a sign indicating microvascular injury as a primary event in this disease (Prescott et al., 1992).

Depending on the study population and statistical methodology, between 5 and 20% of all individuals presenting with Raynaud's phenomenon are reported to subsequently develop SSc. A constellation of additional signs and symptoms indicative of microvascular damage separates SSc patients from others presenting with Raynaud's phenomenon. These include nailfold capillaroscopic changes (Maricq et al., 1980), hand / foot edema, digital ulcers, calcifications and teleangiectasia. The combination of a fibrotic microvascular and hyperreactive vasoconstrictor status is thought to represent the primary lesion responsible for the vasospastic episodes. Tissue hypoxia normally induces new blood vessel growth by induction of a variety of angiogenic factors. Recently, hypoxia has been linked to the induction of epithelial-mesenchymal transition, an evolving concept for the pathogenesis of fibrosis of the lung. In SSc, loss of capillaries is a typical and early disease manifestation which has been related to an increase in angiostatic factors and programmed endothelial cell death (apoptosis) where a number of possible mechanisms have been proposed (Kahaleh and Fan, 1997; Hebbar et al., 2000; Beyer et al., 2009). Interestingly, a very recent study on patients followed up after stem cell therapy for SSc indicates for the first time, that the observed loss of capillaries, a well known (usually interpreted as end stage) hallmark of the disease, may be reversible (Fleming et al., 2008).

Dysregulation of Extracellular Matrix Synthesis

The dysregulation of extracellular matrix synthesis is the third major pathophysiologic change, with the extent and progression of the fibrotic process being important prognostic factors in the disease process. It has been well established by in situ hybridization and by fibroblast cultures obtained from involved tissue (e. g. skin or lung) that scleroderma fibroblasts display an activated phenotype producing increased amounts of various collagens and expressing adhesion molecules such as ICAM-1 (LeRoy et al., 1974; Uitto et al., 1979; Scharffetter et al., 1988; Majewski et al., 1995). The newly synthesized extracellular matrix is deposited particularly around skin appendages and at the border of the dermis to the subcutaneous tissue, partially replacing the latter (Perlish et al., 1985). The collagen bundles running parallel with the skin surface show swelling and variation in thickness. Although the biosynthesis of collagens has been investigated in detail, its metabolism and turnover in vivo is not yet fully understood. In physiological situations involving increased collagen synthesis, as e. g. in wound healing, the amount of collagen in the tissue is obviously tightly controlled by its similarly increased degradation. Similarly, in a fibrotic disease, the net gain of collagens must thus involve a disturbed balance between the synthetic and degradative processes. The most commonly used approach to study collagen degradation is the study of collagen degrading enzymes (Herrmann et al., 1991; Mauch et al., 1998). However, the results are difficult to interpret in terms of the in vivo situation, as a combination of several enzymes including the corresponding inhibitors are likely to be involved in the degradation of a single collagen fiber. A different approach to this question is to study the degradation products as they appear in vivo. Interestingly, we and others could demonstrate that increased levels of ICTP, a degradation product of cross-linked type I collagen, are common in patients with SSc (Heickendorff et al., 1995; Hunzelmann et al., 1998b). They correlate well with the skin score, a commonly used indicator of the severity of the disease (Subcommittee of the ARA 1980; Kahaleh et al., 1986). This indicates that the concentrations of circulating ICTP reflect the type I collagen load in this disease. We found the highest values in patients with very active and extensive disease. Furthermore these crosslinks can usually only be detected in bone, suggesting that occurence of these crosslinks in the skin is related to the sclerotic process. Of interest, in microarray analyses of SSc skin a marked upregulation of a number of bone and cartilage associated proteins as e. g. collagens X, XI and Cartilage oligomeric protein (COMP) was reported. The deposition of molecules which are not organotypic may contribute to the resistance to remodelling which is a characteristic feature of fibrosis.

The factors which finally lead to the activated phenotype of scleroderma fibroblasts are not entirely clear. Several studies suggest the contribution of transforming growth factor-ß (TGF-ß) (Kulozik et al., 1990). TGF-ß is the most potent inducer of collagen synthesis, suppresses the production of matrix degrading metalloproteinases and is regarded as a master regulator of the fibrotic process in the pathogenesis of systemic sclerosis. Nearly all cells involved in the pathophysiology of SSc, i. e. endothelial cells, fibroblasts, platelets and a variety of immune cells synthesize TGF-ß. Furthermore, fibroblasts of SSc patients express increased numbers of TGF-ß receptors, thereby enhancing the potential cellular response to TGF-ß. This notion is further supported by the detection of connective tissue growth factor (CTGF) gene expression in skin biopsies of SSc patients (Igarashi et al., 1995) and SSc fibroblasts (Shi-Wen et al., 2000) as TGF-ß is also known to induce CTGF. Recent studies indicate that a deficiency in SMAD-7 an inhibitory protein in the TGF-ß signalling pathway is characteristic of scleroderma fibroblasts (Dong et al., 2002). In the fibrotic process, however, besides TGF-ß several other profibrotic mediators are known to play an important role including PDGF, CTGF, IL-4, Il-13, Il-17, MCP-1, Endothelin-1. Recently, it could be demonstrated that the activation of PDGF- and TGF-ß receptors can be impaired by tyrosine kinase inhibitors resulting in a reduced synthesis of extracellular matrix proteins by dermal fibroblasts (Distler et al., 2007). This result could also be extended to mouse models and initial clinical observations on the use of TRK-inhibitors in different fibrotic diseases as Scleroderma and GvHD begin to be reported.

4

Clinical Appearence / Classification

The incidence of SSc is reported to be 2–20 / million population and the prevalence 4–290 / million population. The disease is much commoner in females than males for reasons that are not entirely clear with a female-to-male ratio of 3–9:1. There are some populations at high risk as e. g. the Choctaw Indians from Oklahoma suggesting that genetic factors are critical. However, twin studies are inconclusive and familial aggregation is rare.

Based on distinct clinical aspects and courses of the disease an internationally accepted classification was established with two forms: limited cutaneous SSc (lSSc) and diffuse cutaneous SSc (dSSc). Both forms, however, lead to life threatening involvement of internal organs and are associated with marked excess mortality. The quality of life is severely reduced and the patients require continous medical support. The two major clinical variants are distinguished primarily on the degree and extent of skin involvement. However, during recent years it became apparent that in clinical practice this classification fails to address a number of patients presenting with SSc symptoms (Hunzelmann et al., 2008). For instance, a significant number of patients belongs to a subgroup with symptoms of systemic sclerosis occuring simultaneously with those of other connective tissue diseases like myositis, Sjögren's syndrome or lupus erythematodes. These patients are often classified as scleroderma overlap-syndrome and are characterized by typical auto-antibodies e. g. most frequently anti-U1-RNP- or anti-PmScl-antibodies. Furthermore, due to improved health care, patients present earlier in the course of the disease with symptoms suggestive of, but not conclusive for a diagnosis of definite systemic sclerosis, e. g. RP and scleroderma-specific antinuclear antibodies; these symptomes have been described as undifferentiated connective tissue disease (UCTD) [19, 20].

The hallmark of SSc is fibrosis of the skin resulting early on in oedema, often the first indication of SSc skin involvement, which is followed by fibrotic induration and finally atrophy. Several skin scoring methodologies have been developed with the modified Rodnan skin score having the broadest distribution (Kahaleh et al., 1986; Furst et al., 1998). It is assessed by palpation of skin using a 0–3 scale (normal, mild, moderate or severe thickening) at seventeen areas. Following the skin score and the distribution of cutaneous induration is of major clinical importance, as patients with diffuse cutaneous scleroderma are much more likely to have significant heart and / or renal disease than those with the limited form of SSc. Furthermore early disability and premature mortality are observed in this group (Clements et al., 1990). The period when skin thickening is most rapidly is also a time in which decline in visceral function is most likely to occur (Seibold, 1994) (Fig. 1).

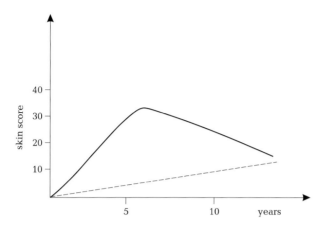

Fig. 1. Longitudinal development of skin score in patients with diffuse systemic sclerosis (——) and limited systemic sclerosis (- - - -)

Diffuse cutaneous SSc (dSSc)

dSSc is characterized by distal and proximal extremity and truncal skin thickening. Usually the elbows and knees are considered the dividing line. Leading symptoms of dSSC are: 1) onset of Raynaud's syndrome within 1 year of onset of skin changes (puffy or hidebound); 2) presence of tendon friction rubs; 3) early and significant incidence of interstitial lung disease, oliguric renal failure, diffuse gastrointestinal disease, and myocardial involvement; 4) absence of anti CENP-B antibodies; 5) nailfold capillary dilatation and capillary destruction; 6) anti-DNA-topoisomerase I antibodies (30%). In two large epidemiological studies this subset accounted for about 30% of all SSc patients (Walker et al., 2007; Hunzelmann et al., 2008).

Limited Cutaneous SSc (lSSc)

Leading symptoms of lSSc are the following: 1) Raynaud's syndrome for years (occasionally decades); 2) skin involvement limited to hands, face, and forearms (acral) or absent; 3) a significant late incidence of pulmonary hypertension, with or without interstitial lung disease; 4) a high incidence of anti centromer (CENP-B) antibodies (70–80%); 5) dilated nailfold capillary loops, usually without capillary dropout; 6) skin calcifications and teleangiectasia particularly affecting the face and hands; 7) occasional late development of small bowel malabsorption.

Recent studies suggest that systemic sclerosis sine scleroderma is a rare subset of SSc (around 1% of SSc patients) which should be included into the spectrum of SSc with limited cutaneous involvement and should not be considered as a distinct disorder (Poormoghim et al., 2000; Hunzelmann et al., 2008). Except for the absence of skin thickening, the group of patients with systemic sclerosis sine scleroderma had no significant differences in individual internal organ involvements, laboratory features, serum autoantibody type (e.g. anti-centromer) or survival rate compared with lSSc patients. There was a tendency but no significant difference toward more pronounced pulmonary arterial hypertension and reduced carbon monoxide diffusing capacity (<70% of predicted).

Scleroderma Overlap Syndromes

The most common overlap syndromes are Mixed Connective Tissues Disease (MCTD), Scleromyositis (PM-Scl-associated) and the Synthetase Syndrome (Jo 1-associated). Overlap syndromes account for about 10% of patients presenting with symptoms compatible with SSc (Hunzelmann et al., 2008). MCTD and the Synthetase Syndrome are more extensively dealt with in Chap. 7.

Scleromyositis is a scleroderma/polymyositis or scleroderma/dermatomyositis overlap disorder associated with antibodies directed to the nucleolar PM-Scl complex and associated with HLA-DR3 (Genth et al., 1990). In a recent study of 108 cases, 83% of patients had characteristic manifestations (Jablonska and Blasczyk, 1999). These findings include Raynaud's syndrome, scleroderma-like and dermatomyositis-like cutaneous changes of the face and hands including hyperkeratotic changes on the fingers, myalgia and arthritis. Pulmonary involvement occurs in about 30 to 60% of the patients (Marguerie et al., 1992). This syndrome is also a rather common subtype in children as about one third of the reported cases in the study of Jablonska (1999) are children with a mean age of onset at nine years. The course of this overlap syndrome is considered to be benign and usually responds to small or moderate doses of corticosteroids.

Environmentally Related Scleroderma-Like Syndromes

A broad variety of environmental factors have been reported to induce scleroderma (reviewed in Straniero et al., 1989). However, with few exceptions (contaminated tryptophan, contaminated rape seed oil, vinyl chloride, trichloroethylene and most recently gadolinium as the elicitor of a new disease entity i.e. nephrogenic systemic fibrosis) these cases are likely to represent random occurences. These scleroderma-like disorders often lack several features of SSc, in particular the autoimmune phenomena (autoantibody synthesis). In this respect, there has been much concern and publicity on the role of silicone (e.g. in the form of surgical implants) as a possible environmental factor for connective tissue diseases such as SSc, but despite several epidemiological studies, no link has been established (Janowsky et al., 2000).

In contrast, several studies indicate that silica dust-associated scleroderma can not be distinguished from SSc in terms of antibody profile and phenotype (Haustein and Anderegg, 1998). This is supported by experimental data suggesting that silica dust induces pathophysiological events similar to SSc (Haustein and Anderegg, 1998).

Diagnosis

As in many other chronic diseases, diagnosis is in general readily performed once the illness has fully developed. Due to the often smoldering disease onset and the uncharacteris-
tic changes ocurring early on in SSc, including Raynaud's phenomenon, joint pain or swelling, the clinical diagnosis of SSc and the differentiation from other diffuse inflammatory
connective tissue diseases (rheumatoid arthritis, systemic lupus erythemtosus, polymyositis) or disorders characterised by abnormal extracellular deposition (e. g. amyloidosis) may
be difficult. Although each of the diffuse inflammatory connective tissue diseases are clinically distinct entities, they share some general analogies and often display a high level of
clinical variability resulting not uncommonly in overlap syndromes which pose a particular diagnostic and therapeutic challenge.

Investigations related to the autoimmune phenomena and the vascular changes (e. g. capillaroscopy) are therefore necessary to perform. In some cases, follow up of the patient over
time will indicate whether the patient finally develops inflammatory connective tissue disease, overlap syndrome etc. or may experience remission of an early flare up of autoimmune
phenomena reflecting undifferentiated connective tissue disease (Williams et al., 1999).

Autoantibody Profile

The identification of autoantibodies is mandatory in establishing the correct diagnosis, indicating the prognosis and providing a guide to treatment and follow up (Fritzler, 1993). In
several studies, more than 95% of patients show antinuclear antibodies (ANA) (Bunn et al.,
1998, Hunzelmann et al., 2008), thus making the diagnosis of SSc in a patient without ANA
quite unlikely. Although there is no antibody which can be related to disease activity like
the presence of anti-ds DNA antibodies in systemic lupus erythematosus, patient classification according to serologic subsets can be meaningful. Nearly 85% of patients can be associated to one of seven SSc related antibodies (Table 1) and each of these antibodies describes
a subset which to a different degree has characteristic clinical manifestations (Fig. 2).

Clinical Presentation

At clinical presentation, sclerodactily is present in about 95% of patients and Raynaud's
syndrome is present in about 90%. If none of these features (including ANA) is present, the
patient is likely to have a disorder other than SSc.

Differential diagnosis includes in particular the generalized form of localized scleroderma, eosinophilic fasciitis, scleromyxoedema, scleroderma adultorum Buschke, amyloidosis, porphyria cutanea tarda, nephrogenic systemic fibrosis and acrodermatitis chronica
atrophicans in the inflammatory phase (Table 2) and rarely sclerodermiform genodermatoses. Furthermore, one has to be aware of the vast differential diagnoses of Raynaud's phenomenon in the patients presenting in the initial phase of the disease.

Table 1. Clinical Characteristics of Autoantibodies Associated with Progressive Systemic Sclerosis

Antibody	Antigen	Comments	Frequency
Scl-70	DNA-topoisomerase I	increased risk for tumors	up to 70% of dSSc; 10 to 20% of SSc
U1 RNP	U1 small nuclear ribonucleo-protein	overlap syndrome to SLE	
Fibrillarin	U3 RNP	poor prognosis	10–20% of dSSc
RNA Polymerase I, III	sub units of RNA polymerase		20% of dSSc
centromere	kinetochores, CENP-A, B, C, E	limited disease	60–80% of lSSc; 15% of SSc
Th/To	Rnase P	limited disease	2%
PM-Scl	nuclear protein-complex	characteristic skin changes	15% of overlap syndromes
Ku	Nucleolar heterodimer	overlap syndrome	< 10% of overlap syndromes
Jo1	histidyl-tRNA synthetase	SSc/polymyositis overlap	10% of overlap syndromes

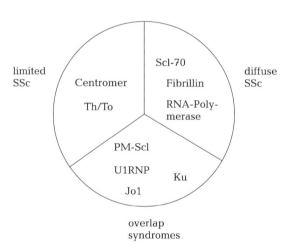

Fig. 2. Antibody profile and clinical classification of progressive systemic sclerosis and overlap syndromes

Table 2. Scleroderma-Like Disorders

I. Sclerotic disorders	Scleredema adultorum Buschke
	Scleredema diabeticorum
	Scleredema amyloidosum
	Scleromyxedema
	Environmentally related scleroderma-like syndromes (i. e. nephrogenic systemic fibrosis)
	Graft versus host disease
	Porphyria cutanea tarda
	Acrodermatitis chronica atrophicans
II. Sclerodermiform genodermatoses	Werner Syndrome
	Progeria
	Acrogeria / Metageria

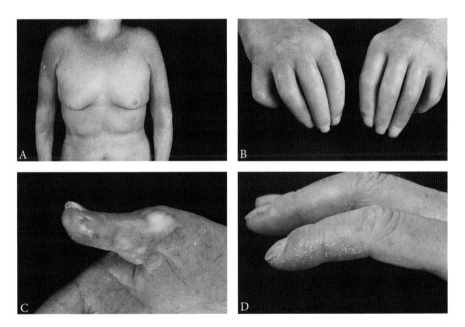

Fig. 3. Clinical phenotype of progressive systemic sclerosis and overlap syndromes. **A.** Diffuse systemic scleroderma: diffuse sclerosis with hyperpigmentation of the trunk. **B.** Sclerodactyly with contractures and atrophy of the fingers. **C.** Cutaneous calcinosis. **D.** PM-Scl overlap syndrome: mechanic hands with hyperkeratosis of the fingers

Associated Diseases

Association of SSc with other autoimmune diseases is relatively common including primary biliary cirrhosis, Sjogren-syndrome (including the detection of anti-Ro / La antibodies) and in the subset of overlap syndromes, dermatomyositis and polymyositis.

Therapy

The treatment of SSc is challenging due to the complex disease process and the difficulty to specifically treat distinct subgroups. SSc poses a particular problem to the medical system due to the relative rarity of the disease requiring specialised care by the general practicioner. Therefore, diagnosis and care should be at least in part in the hands of specialists who have daily exposure to this disease and have access to a laboratory trained in autoimmune serology, to dermatohistopathology, and modern diagnostic radiologic procedures (e. g. CT, MRT, angiography). Cooperation with different subspecialties is often necessary to provide optimal care due to the nature of the disease affecting other organ systems than the skin (e. g. rheumatology, pulmonary medicine, nephrology, neurology). Specialized care should be provided in a setting where the outpatient facilities have also access to hospital beds to ensure timely and appropriate treatment for patients presenting with exacerbation of their disease. Physical therapy which has access to treatment facilities to prevent loss of function is another prerequisite for these specialised facilities. Patient support groups which to date in part make up for these shortcomings play an increasing role in communicating the special needs of these patients to society. In recent years the internet has become a routine resource for the information of patients and recruitement for ongoing studies (e. g. http://www.sclero.org). Furthermore, the development of competence and communication based networks on a national (e. g. DNSS in Germany) and international level (e. g. Eustar) has helped to significantly improve the level of care and the dissipation of information. In 2009, for the first time evidence based recommendations for treatment of SSc have been published by the Eular Scleroderma trials and research group (Eustar) (Kowal-Bielecka et al., 2009) where most of the recommendations given below are described in more detail.

Immunosuppressive Agents

For most of the drugs with immunosuppressive properties, which have been used in the treatment of SSc, large well-controlled prospective clinical trials are lacking. To date in systemic sclerosis (SSc) little evidence for the effectiveness of corticosteroid and immunosuppressive therapy exists with the exception of cyclophosphamide demonstrating a modest effect on lung and skin involvement. Nevertheless, these potentially harmful drugs are frequently prescribed to patients with all forms of SSc (Hunzelmann et al., 2009). For instance, d-penicillamine seems to affect both collagen and the immune system thus making it an ideal candidate to treat SSc. Interestingly, it took until the mid 90s to start a double blind randomized trial to investigate the effect of D-penicillamine in SSc. Unfortunately, no difference was found between a dose of 62.5 mg and 750 mg D-penicillamine daily indicating lack of efficacy (Clements et al., 1999). Also photopheresis (extracorporeal photochemotherapy) that has shown promise in several uncontrolled studies (Rook et al., 1992), failed in a recent crossover study to demonstrate a favourable effect (Enomoto et al., 1999). Several smaller trials investigated the use of cyclosporin A, which unfortunately was associated with considerable toxicity, especially nephropathy (Denton et al., 1994). Methotrexate, although its toxicity profile in patients with SSc was better than exspected, produced inconsistent results in two controlled studies (van den Hoogen et al., 1996; Pope et al., 1998). The best available data exist for cyclophosphamide, which showed a modest, statistically significant benefit in a randomized controlled double blind trial (Tashkin et al., 2006) on both, lung and skin fibrosis.

Antifibrotic Agents

Interferon-γ is the most potent cytokine known to inhibit collagen synthesis. Several uncontrolled studies applying the cytokine over up to one year have been performed to investigate the potential role of interferon-γ in the treatment of SSc showing no major effect on the disease course (Hunzelmann et al., 1997). Interferon-α has also been shown to inhibit collagen synthesis (Duncan et al., 1995). However, a placebo controlled study of early diffuse SSc found no benefit for skin sclerosis and pulmonary function, but a greater mortality in the active treatment arm (Black et al., 1998). Relaxin is a pregnancy-related hormone that has tissue remodeling and antifibrotic effects. Relaxin has been tested in a phase 2 trial where in the low dose group a significant improvement of the modified Rodnan skin score was found ($p = 0.049$) wheras in the high dose group no such effect was seen (Seibold et al., 2000).

Organ-Specific Therapies

Skin Involvement

General measures include skin protection from cold and trauma, skin care with moistening creams, lymph drainage and active physiotherapy. Calcium channel blockers or angiotensin II receptor type 1 antagonists can be given to decrease symptoms of Raynaud's syndrome (Dziaio et al., 1999). In severe cases of finger tip ulcerations and impending digit amputation, intravenous prostacycline analogues may be of value (Zachariae et al., 1996; Pope et al., 2000). Bosentan, a dual endothelin receptor antagonist was shown in two randomized studies to significantly reduce the number of new digital ulcers. The efficacy of phosphodiesterase-inhibitors concerning raynauds syndrome and digital ulcer healing is still under investigation. Ectopic calcifications or calcinosis when compromising blood circulation or causing symptoms may be removed surgically or by the use of CO^2-laser (Bottomly et al., 1996). Laser (i. e. argon or flashlamp pumped dye laser) therapy is the treatment of choice to remove teleangiectasias, which may also involve the mucosa.

UV radiation (UVA1 or bath-PUVA) with small patients numbers in uncontrolled studies has been reported to be beneficial. In localized scleroderma, evidence for the efficacy of UVA1 or bath-PUVA is increasing although no double blind prospective study is available (Kerscher et al., 1996). Recent studies have shown that UVA irradiation alone, and more so in conjunction with photosensitizing agents, increases the expression, synthesis and activation of metalloproteinases. In addition, a variety of cytokines and soluble factors in vitro and in vivo are modulated by UVA and can affect connective tissue remodeling (Scharffetter et al., 1991; Herrmann et al., 1993). Clinical and ultrasound evaluation revealed that the sclerotic lesions disappeared or markedly improved during PUVA bath photochemotherapy in 13 of the 17 enrolled patients within less than three months. We have additional experience in 14 patients suffering from localized scleroderma who improved substantially from bath PUVA therapy as monitored by skin score, cutaneous elastometry and evaluation of skin thickness by ultrasound analysis (Hunzelmann et al., 1998b). In a recent publication, the therapeutic potential of UVA1 therapy has been evaluated in localized scleroderma (Stege et al., 1998). This study corroborates and extends previous observations that in vivo UVA1 irradiation exposure of healthy human skin is associated with the induction of interstitial collagenase RNA expression in situ which may play a role in the remodelling of the fibrotic connective tissue.

Musculosceletal Involvement

Musculosceletal involvement, arthralgia and musculosceletal pain being the most frequent complaints, is common in scleroderma and may lead to secondary fibromyalgia. Muscle weakness and some increase in serum creatine kinase levels are quite common. Inflammatory arthritis can occur but raises the suspicion of the presence of an overlap syndrome and only rarely results in mutilating arthritis. Corticosteroids should be avoided due to their long term side effects and association with nephropathy in higher doses exceeding 15 mg prednisone equivalents (Steen et al., 1998). Non steroidal anti-inflammatory agents should also be prudently chosen due to their potential side effects on renal function, blood pressure and gastrointestinal function. The superiority of the use of cyclo-oxygenase 2 inhibitors remains to be proven.

Renal Involvement

Acute renal crisis is a serious and potentially fatal SSc complication associated with an acute reduction on cortical blood flow, hyperreninemia, hypertension which occurs most likely in diffuse cutaneous scleroderma of less than four years duration. Many of these patients will progress to renal failure and dialysis or renal transplantation. Thus regular control of blood pressure (at least twice a week) is recommended to detect acute renal involvement early on. Chronic renal involvement is associated with a slowly progressive obliterative vasculopathy. Before the advent of ACE inhibitor therapy and other improvements in the management of advanced renal disease, survival for longer than 3–6 months was almost unknown. Particularly in acute renal crisis, ACE inhibitors are the mainstay of treatment significantly prolonging patient survival (Steen et al., 1990). Additional administration of intravenous prostacyclin may be considered. Nevertheless, prognosis of established renal crisis is still relatively poor with about one third of patients progressing to renal replacement therapy. Here, a five year kidney graft survival rate of 47% was reported comparable to that of patients with SLE (Chang and Spiera, 1999).

Pulmonary Involvement

Pulmonary fibrosis in SSc affects to different degrees the parenchymal and the vascular system. In early disease, inflammatory alveolitis may precede and / or accompany interstitial fibrosis leading to loss of pulmonary function as evidenced by decreased diffusing capacity and vital capacity. Bronchoalveolar lavage (in experienced hands) and high resolution chest computertomography will help to determine the degree of inflammation. Several studies indicate that alveolitis can be treated successfully with cyclophosphamide (White et al., 2000, Tashkin et al., 2006).

Pulmonary hypertension may most prominently develop in patients with limited cutaneous scleroderma of long duration with relatively little interstitial disease determining markedly the prognosis of these patients. Yearly screening investigations by echo are therefore strongly recommended in all SSc patients (Kowal-Bielecka et al., 2009; Hunzelmann et al., 2009). In case of a positive echocardiography or strong clinical suspicion right heart catheterization is mandatory.

Besides the infusion or inhalation of prostacycline analogues, new drugs targeting different aspects of vascular pathology have become available, e. g. endothelin receptor antagonists and phosphodiesterase-5 (PDE-5) inhibitors (Pigula et al., 1997; Badesch et al., 2000; Hoeper et al., 2000; Rubin et al., 2002). Here, very recently treatment has been approved also for the WHO functional class II, extending previous approval for the use of bosentan and sildenafil in functional class for class III and IV (McLaughlin et al., 2009).

Gastrointestinal Involvement

The gastrointestinal tract is frequently involved with a frequency for the oesophagus in about 80%, the stomach, small intestine and large intestine in about 40–70% (Walker et al., 2007; Hunzelmann et al., 2008). The pathology is characterized both by atrophy of the smooth muscles that line the gastrointestinal tract and involvement of the myenteric nerve plexus. Main symptoms associated are heartburn, esophageal dysfunction in the upper gastrointestinal tract, diarrhoea due to bacterial overgrowth, and fetal incontinence in the distal tract. Prokinetics (e. g. octreotide) are of limited use in severe constipation and recently, the prokinetic cisapride has been withdrawn from the market due to associated cardiac arrythmias leading to death. Proton pump inhibitors and to a lesser extent H2-blockers are effective in controlling reflux esophagitis apart from typical conservative measures (no late meals etc.). Barretts esophagus is a late sequel of reflux disease. Bacterial overgrowth and fungal infections (e. g. candida esophagitis) can be dealt with by intermittent antimicrobial therapy and antimycotics. Rarely, teleangiectasias may also be present on the mucosa representing a potential source of occult intestinal bleeding.

Cardiac Involvement

The nature and severity of cardiac disease depends on the extent of myocardial fibrosis, a primary component of this disorder, and on the extent to which concurrent fibrosis of the lung and thickening and fibrosis of the small pulmonary arteries place an additional burden on the circulation. Large perfusion abnormalities on thallium scans are predictive of shortened survival and an increased number of cardiac events (Steen et al., 1996). Also, intermittent vascular ischemia is observed which probably reflects similar pathophysiological changes as observed in the peripheral vasculature (Raynaud's syndrome). Arrhythmias are quite common in SSc but seldom meet the definition of severe arrhythmia.

Novel Therapeutic Perspectives

The understanding of the pathophysiology of scleroderma still relies on the vascular, immune system and the connective tissue as the most relevant components of the disease process. In recent years, research on SSc has particularly evolved along a better understanding of the interdependence of these components. This is reflected by the concept of trans-differentiation of fibroblasts to myofibroblasts, the recognition of hypoxia as a major pathogenic factor, the potential role of surface receptor specific autoantibodies in SSc and the use of a variety of intracellular and extracellular strategies to inhibit the activity of TGF-ß in vivo including tyrosine kinase inhibitors and high dose immunosuppression (for review see Hunzelmann et al., 2010). Although until recently fibrosis was considered an end stage process which is not amenable to treatment, results of stem cell transplantation in patients with severe, rapidly progressing disease as well as clinical observation and animal studies clearly indicate, that fibrosis is at least in part reversible.

Summary

Despite intense research efforts and major advances in the understanding of particular aspects of the disease process, the etiology of SSc is still unknown and the pathogenesis only partly understood. Survival has markedly improved over the past two decades, with the 10-year survival rate approaching 80%, although to date with the exception of cyclophosphamide there is no effective disease-modifying treatment of SSc. The introduction of drugs that treat organ complications has changed markedly, the mortality and life quality of subgroups of SSc. The associated side effects and lack of efficacy in certain subgroups of organ involvement indicate however, that the available treatment options are still unsatisfactory (e. g. in pulmonary fibrosis or kidney failure). Therefore, future treatments should be designed to specifically target **distinct** pathogenetic pathways in SSc.

References

Alarcon GS (2000) Unclassified or undifferentiated connective tissue disease. Baillieres Best Pract Res Clin Rheumatol 14:125–37

Artlett CM, Smith CB, Jimenez SA (1998) Identification of fetal DNA and cells in skin lesions from women with systemic sclerosis. N Engl J Med 338:1186–1191

Badesch D, Tapson VF, McGoon MD (2000) Continuous intravenous epoprostenol for pulmonary hypertension due to the scleroderma spectrum of disease. Ann Int Med 132:425–434

Baroni SS, Santillo M, Bevilacqua F, Luchetti M, Spadoni T, Mancini M et al. (2006) Stimulatory autoantibodies to the PDGF receptor in systemic sclerosis. N Engl J Med 22;354(25):2667–76

Beyer C, Schett G, Gay S, Distler O, Distler JH (2009) Hypoxia. Hypoxia in the pathogenesis of systemic sclerosis. Arthritis Res Ther 11(2):220

Black CM, Silman SJ, Herrick AI (1998) Interferon-alpha does not improve outcome at one year in patients with diffuse cutaneous scleroderma: results of a randomized, double blind, placebo-controlled trial. Arthritis Rheum 42:299–305

Blockmans D, Beyens G, Verhaege R (1996) Predictive value of nailfold capillaroscopy in the diagnosis of connective tissue diseases. Clin Rheumatol 15:148–153

Bottomley WW, Goodfield MJ, Sheehan-Dare RA (1996) Digital calcification in systemic sclerosis: effective treatment with good tissue preservation using the carbon dioxide laser. Br J Dermatol 135:302–304

Bunn CC, Denton CP, Shi-Wen X, Knight C, Black CM (1998) Anti-RNA Polymerases and other autoantibody specificities in systemic sclerosis. Br J Rheumatol 37:15–20

Burastero SE, Galbiati S, Vassallo A, Sabbadini MG, Bellone M, Marchionni L et al. (2003) Cellular microchimerism as a lifelong physiologic status in parous women: an immunologic basis for its amplification in patients with systemic sclerosis. Arthiritis Rheum 48:1109–1116

Chang YJ, Spiera H (1999) Renal transplantation in scleroderma. Medicine 78:382–385

Clements PJ, Lachenbruch PA, Ng SC (1990) Skin score. A semiquantitative measure of cutaneous involvement that improves prediction of prognosis in systemic sclerosis. Arthritis Rheum 33:1256–1263

Clements PJ, Furst DE, Wong WK (1999) High dose versus low dose D-penicillamine in early diffuse systemic sclerosis: analysis of a two year, double blind, randomized, controlled clinical trial. Arthritis Rheum 42:1194–203

Denton CP, Sweny P Abdulla A, Black CM (1994) Acute renal failure occurring in scleroderma treated with cyclosporin A: a report of three cases. Br J Rheumatol 33:90–92

Dong C, Zhu S, Wang T, Yoon W, Li Z, Alvarez RJ et al. (2002) Deficient Smad 7 expression: aputative molecular defect in scleroderma. PNAS 99:3908–13

Distler JH, Jüngel A, Huber LC et al. 2007 Imatinib mesylate reduces production of extracellular matrix and prevents development of experimental dermal fibrosis. Arthritis Rheum; 56(1):311–22

Duncan MR, Hasan A, Berman B (1995) Pentoxifylline, pentifylline and interferons decrease type I and III procollagen mRNA levels in dermal fibroblasts: evidence for mediation by nuclear factor 1 downregulation. J Invest Dermatol 104:282–286

Dziadzio M, Denton CP Smith R (1999) Losartan therapy for raynauds phenomenon and scleroderma: clinical and biochemical findings in a fifteen-week, randomized, parallel group, controlled trial. Arthritis Rheum 42:2646–2455

Enomoto, Mekkes JR, Bossuyt PM (1999) Treatment of patients with systemic sclerosis with extracorporeal photochemotherapy (photopheresis). J Am Acad Dermatol 41:915–922

Evans PC, Lambert N, Maloney S (1999) Long term fetal microchimerism in peripheral blood mononuclear scell subsets in healthy women and women with scleroderma. Blood 93:2033–2037

Fleming JN, Nash RA, McLeod DO, Fiorentino DF, Shulman HM, Connolly MK et al. (2008)
Capillary regeneration in scleroderma: stem cell therapy reverses phenotype? PLoS One
16;3(1):e1452

Fritzler MJ (1993) Autoantibodies in scleroderma. J Dermatol 20:257–268

Furst DE, Clements PJ, Steen VD (1998) The modified rodnan skin score is an accurate reflection
of skin biopsy thickness in systemic sclerosis. J Rheumatol 25:84–88

Gabrielli A, Avvedimento EV, Krieg T (2009) Scleroderma. N Engl J Med 7;360(19):1989–2003

Genth E, Mierau R, Genetzky P (1990) Immunogenetic associations of scleroderma-related antinuclear antibodies. Arthritis Rheum 33:657–665

Jablonska S, Blaszyk M (1999) Scleroderma Overlap Syndromes. Adv Exp Med Biol 455:85–92

Janowsky EC, Kupper LL, Hulka BS (2000) Meta-analyses of the relation between silicone breast
implants and the risk of connective tissue. N Engl J Med 342:781–790

Haustein UF, Anderegg U (1998) Silica induced scleroderma – clinical and experimental aspects.
J Rheumatol 25:1917–1926

Hebbar M, Peyrat JP, Hornez L, Hatron PY, Hachulla E, Devulder B. (2000) Increased concentrations of the circulating angiogenesis inhibitor endostatin in patients with systemic sclerosis.
Arthritis Rheum 43:889–93

Heickendorff L, Zachariae H, Bjerring P, Halkier-Sorensen L, Sondergaard K (1995) The use of
serologic markers for collagen synthesis and degradation in systemic sclerosis. J Am Acad Dermatol 32:584–588

Herrmann K, Heckmann M, Kulozik M, Haustein UF, Krieg T (1991) Steady state mRNA levels
of collagens I,III, fibronectin and collagenase in skin biopsies of systemic sclerosis patients.
J Invest Dermatol 97:219–225

Herrmann G, Wlaschek M, Lange TS, Prenzel K, Goerz G, Scharffetter-Kochanek K (1993) UVA
irradiation stimulates the synthesis of various matrix-metalloproteinases (MMPs) in cultured
human fibroblasts. Exp Dermatol 2:92–97

Hoeper MM et al. (2000) Long term treatment of primary pulmonary hypertension with aerolized
iloprost, a prostacyclin analogue. N Engl J Med 342:1866–70

Hunzelmann N, Anders S, Fierlbeck G, Hein R, Herrmann K, Albrecht M et al. (1997) Systemic
scleroderma: multicenter trial of one year treatment with recombinant interferon-gamma. Arch
Dermatol 133:609–613

Hunzelmann N, Risteli J, Risteli L, Sacher C, Black CM, Krieg T (1998a) Increased circulating
concentrations of the type I collagen specific degradation product ICTP in systemic sclerosis
reflect the extent of skin involvement: A new serum marker for clinical severity in SSc patients.
Br J Dermatol 139:1020–1025

Hunzelmann N, Scharfetter-Kochanek K, Hager C, Krieg T (1998b) Management of localized scleroderma. Sem Cutan Med Surg 17:34–41

Hunzelmann N, Genth E, Krieg T, Lehmacher W, Melchers I, Meurer M et al.; Registry of the
German Network for Systemic Scleroderma (2008) The registry of the German Network for
Systemic Scleroderma: frequency of disease subsets and patterns of organ involvement. Rheu-
matology (Oxford) Aug;47(8):1185–92

Hunzelmann N, Genth E, Krieg T, Meurer M, Melchers I, Moinzadeh P et al.; German Network for
Systemic Sclerosis (2008) Organ-specific diagnosis in patients with systemic sclerosis: Recommendations of the German Network for Systemic Sclerosis (DNSS). Z Rheumatol 67(4):334–6,
337–40

Hunzelmann N, Moinzadeh P, Genth E, Krieg T, Lehmacher W, Melchers I et al.; German Network for Systemic Scleroderma Centers (2009) High frequency of corticosteroid and immunosuppressive therapy in patients with systemic sclerosis despite limited evidence for efficacy. Arthritis Res Ther 11(2):R30

Hunzelmann N, Brinckmann J (2010) What are the new milestones in the pathogenesis of systemic sclerosis? Ann Rheum Dis 69 Suppl 1:i52–56

Igarashi A, Nashiro K, Kikuchi K (1995) Significant correlation between connective tissue growth factor gene expression and skin sclerosis in tissue sections from patients with systemic sclerosis. J Invest Dermatol 105:280–284

Kahaleh MB, Sultany GL, Smith EA, Huffstetter JE, Loadholt CB, LeRoy EC (1986) A modified scleroderma skin scoring method. Clin Exp Rheumatol 4:367–369

Kahaleh M, Fan PS (1997) Mechanism of serum mediated endothelial injury in scleroderma: identification of a granular enzyme in scleroderma skin and sera. Clin Immunol Immunopathol 83:32–40

Kerscher M, Meurer M, Sander C, Volkenandt M, Lehmann P, Plewig G, Röcken M (1996) PUVA bath photochemotherapy for localized scleroderma. Arch Dermatol 132:1280–1282

Kowal-Bielecka O, Landewé R, Avouac J, Chwiesko S, Miniati I, Czirjak L et al.; EUSTAR Co-Authors (2009) EULAR recommendations for the treatment of systemic sclerosis: a report from the EULAR Scleroderma Trials and Research group (EUSTAR). Ann Rheum Dis 68(5):620–8

Kulozik M, Hogg A, Lankat-Buttgereit B, Krieg T (1990) Co-localization of transforming growth factor ß2 with a1(1) procollagen mRNA in tissue sections of patients with systemic sclerosis. J Clin Invest 86:917–921

LeRoy EC (1974) Increased collagen synthesis by scleroderma fibroblasts in vitro. J Clin Invest 54:880–889

LeRoy EC, Maricq HR, Kahaleh MB (1980) Undifferentiated connective tissue syndromes. Arthritis Rheum 23:341–3

Majewski S, Hunzelmann N, Johnson JP, Jung C, Mauch C, Ziegler-Heitbrock H et al. (1991) Expression of intercellular adhesion molecule-1 (ICAM-1) on fibroblasts in the skin of patients with systemic sclerosis. J Invest Dermatol 97:667–671

Marguerie C (1992) The clinical and immunogenetic features of patients with autoantibodies to the nucleolar anitgen PM-Scl. Medicine 71:327–336

Maricq H, LeRoy E, Dangelo W (1980) Diagnostic potential of in vivo capillary microscopy in scleroderma and related disorders. Arthritis Rheum 23:183–189

Mauch C (1998) Regulation of connective tissue turnover by cell-matrix interactions. Arch Dermatol Res 290: S30–36

McCormick LL, Zhang Y, Tootell E, Gilliam AC (1999) Anti-TGF-beta treatment prevents skin and lung fibrosis in murine sclerodermatous graft-versus-host disease: a model for human scleroderma. J Immunol 163:5693–5699

McLaughlin V, Humbert M, Coghlan G, Nash P, Steen V (2009) Pulmonary arterial hypertension: the most devastating vascular complication of systemic sclerosis. Rheumatology (Oxford) 48 Suppl 3:iii25–31

Perlish JS, Lemlich G, Fleischmajer R (1988) Identification of collagen fibrils in scleroderma skin. J Invest Dermatol 90:48–54

Pigula FA, Griffith BP, Zenati MA (1997) Lung transplantation for respiratory failure resulting from systemic disease. Ann Thorac Surg 64:1630–1634

Poormoghim H, Lucas M, Fertig N, Medsger TA (2000) Systemic sclerosis sine scleroderma: demographic, clinical, and serologic features and survival in forty eight patients. Arthritis Rheum 43:444–451

Pope J, Bellamy N, Seibold J (1998) A controlled trial of methotrexate versus placebo in early diffuse scleroderma – preliminary analysis. Arthritis Rheum 41: S420

Pope J, Fenlon D, Thompson A (2000) Iloprost and cisaprost for Raynaud's phenomenon in progressive systemic sclerosis. Cochrane Database Syst Rev 2: CD000953

Prescott RJ, Freemont A, Jones C (1992) Sequential dermal microvascular and perivascular changes in the development of scleroderma. J Pathol 166:255–263

Rook AH, Freundlich B, Jegasothy BV (1992) Treatment of systemic sclerosis with extracorporeal photochemotherapy. Results of a multicenter trial. Arch Dermatol 128:337–346

Rubin LJ, Badesch DB, Barst RJ, Galie N, Black CM et al. (2002) Bosentan therapy for pulmonary hypertension. NEJM 346:896–903

Scharffetter K, Lankat-Buttgereit B, Krieg T (1988) Localization of collagen mRNA in normal and scleroderma skin by in situ hybridization. Eur J Clin Invest 18:9–17

Scharffetter K, Wlaschek M, Hogg A, Bolsen K, Schothorst A, Goerz G, Krieg T, Plewig G (1991) UVA irradiation induces collagenase in human dermal fibroblasts in vitro and in vivo. Arch Dermatol Res 283:506–511

Seibold J (1994) Systemic sclerosis. In: Klipped J, Dieppe P, Mosby St. Louis (Eds) Rheumatology, 8.1–8.14

Seibold J, Korn J, Simms R (2000) Recombinant human relaxin in the treatment of scleroderma. A randomized, double blind, placebo-controlled study. Ann Int Med 132:871–879

Sgonc R, Gruschwitz M, Dietrich H (1996) Endothelial cell apoptosis is a primary pathogenetic event underlying skin lesions in avian and human scleroderma. J Clin Invest 98:785–792

Shi-Wen X, Pennington D, Holmes A (2000) Autocrine overexpression of CTGF maintains fibrosis: RDA analysis of fibrosis genes in systemic sclerosis. Exp Cell Res 25:213–224

Steen VD, Constantino JP, Shapiro AP, Medsger TA (1990) Outcome of renal crisis in systemic sclerosis: relation to availability of angiotensin converting enzyme (ACE) inhibitors. Ann Int Med 113:352–357

Steen VD, Follansbee WP, Conte CG, Medsger TA (1996) Thallium perfusion defects predict subsequent cardiac dysfunction in patients with systemic sclerosis. Arthritis Rheum 39:677–681

Steen VD, Medsger TA (1998) Case-control study of corticosteroids and other drugs that either precipitate or protect from the development of scleroderma renal crisis. Arthritis Rheum 41:1613–1619

Stege H, Berneburg M, Humke S (1997) High-dose UVA1 radiation therapy for localized scleroderma. J Am Acad Dermatol 36:938–944

Straniero NR, Furst DE (1989) Environmentally induced systemic sclerosis like illness. Baillieres Clin Rheumatol 3:63–79

Subcommittee for Scleroderma Criteria of the American Rheumatism Association Diagnosis and Therapeutic Criteria Committee (1980) Preliminary criteria for the classification of systemic sclerosis (scleroderma). Arthritis Rheum 23:581–590

Tashkin DP, Elashoff R, Clements PJ, Goldin J, Roth MD, Furst DE et al.; Scleroderma Lung Study Research Group (2006) Cyclophosphamide versus placebo in scleroderma lung disease. N Engl J Med 22;354(25):2655–66

Tyndall A, Black C, Finke J, Peter H, Gratwohl A (1997) Treatment of systemic sclerosis with autologous hemopoetic stem cell transplantation. The Lancet 349:254–356

Uitto J, Bauer EA, Eisen AZ (1979) Scleroderma. Increased biosynthesis of triple helical type I and type III procollagen associated with unaltered expression of collagenase by skin fibroblasts in culture. J Clin Invest 64:921–930

van den Hoogen FH, Boerbooms AM, Swaak AJ (1996) Comparison of methotrexate with placebo in the treatment of systemic sclerosis: a 24 week randomized double blind trial, followed by a 24 week observation trial. Br J Rheumatol 35:364–372

Walker UA, Tyndall A, Czirják L, Denton C, Farge-Bancel D, Kowal-Bielecka O et al. (2007) Clinical risk assessment of organ manifestations in systemic sclerosis: a report from the EULAR Scleroderma Trials And Research group database. Ann Rheum Dis 66(6):754–63

White B, Moore WC, Wigley FM (2000) Cyclophosphamide is associated with pulmonary function and survival benefit in patients with scleroderma and alveolitis. Ann Int Med 132:947–954

Williams HJ, Alarcon GS, Joks R (1999) Early undifferentiated connective tissue disease. VI an inception cohort after 10 years: disease remissions and changes in diagnoses in well established and undifferentiated CTD. J Rheumatol 26:816–825

Zachariae H, Halkier-Sorensen L, Bjerring P, Heickendorff L (1996) Treatment of ischemic digital ulcers and prevention of gangrene with intravenous iloprost in systemic sclerosis. Acta Derm Venereol 76:236–238

Introduction

The skin represents one of the major organs afflicted by lupus erythematosus (LE). LE was in fact first described as a skin disease in the mid and late 19th century (Talbot, 1993) and denominated for the characteristic mutilations seen in some subtypes of the disorder. Ever since in 1936 systemic manifestation without skin symptoms was appreciated as a disease entity, the subject has differentially been dealt with in the dermatological and rheumatological literature. Malar rash and discoid lesions are listed among the criteria defined by the American College of Rheumatology (ACR) for the diagnosis of systemic lupus erythematosus (SLE) (Tan et al., 1982). Characteristic and defined entities encompassing various forms of acute, subacute and chronic cutaneous LE can be opposed to less characteristic skin manifestations like rashes and symptoms of cutaneous vasculitis (Provost, 2004). Both groups of symptoms may however be present at any stage of the disease development. 20% of all SLE cases present with initial skin manifestations and 50–70% of all SLE patients will eventually show skin symptoms during the course of their disease (Costner et al., 2003).

Classification

Chronic cutaneous lupus erythematosus (CCLE) comprises different clinical entities with discoid lupus erythematosus (DLE) as the most common form (Kuhn et al., 2007, Rothfield et al., 2006). In contrast to acute cutaneous LE (ACLE) and subacute cutaneous LE (SCLE), lesions are long-lasting for up to decades with occasional spontaneous remissions. Disfiguring atrophy and scarring with emotional discomfort for patients as well as an increased risk to develop into squamous cell carcinoma in long-standing DLE pose distinct medical problems (Costner et al., 2003, Patel and Werth, 2002). In many cases, symptoms are restricted to the skin without major systemic inflammatory or autoimmune manifestations. This used to be undiscriminately called DLE until thirty years ago when it was clearly dissected from other forms, especially from what is now referred to as SCLE (Gilliam, 1977, Gilliam, Sontheimer, 1981). The term DLE should nowadays be restricted to thoses subsets of CCLE with morphologically distinct plaques irrespective of systemic involvement.

In other, rather rare cases, DLE as well as further subsets of CCLE may present as the first or intercurrent manifestations of SCLE and SLE and will eventually result in systemic disease. Exact epidemiological data of the different CCLE subtypes as well as their relation to SLE and SCLE are not available partly due to the different perception over the last couple of decades and within dermatology and rheumatology. CCLE may be underestimated within rheumatological literature and in case of absent systemic manifestations not be amply diagnosed at all. CCLE lesions, especially DLE lesions are found in up to 20% of SCLE patients and may predate manifestation of systemic disease. Further support of the relation as well as distinction of DLE and SLE is provided by the finding that DLE is present in 15–30% of SLE patients at any time during their disease course and is the prominent feature in 5–10% of such patients (Parodi and Rebora, 1997; Tebbe et al., 1997, Rothfield et al., 2006). Classical DLE as termed at the time of first diagnosis will progress into SLE in 5–10% of cases (Parodi and Rebora, 1997; Tebbe et al., 1997). Such courses may account for different criteria of diagnosing SLE and varying medical check-up among different medical specialists. Generalized DLE and DLE associated with high autoantibody titers have a higher chance to develop into systemic disease. However, the overall incidence of DLE is estimated ten-fold higher than that of SLE. At the same time, the female to male ratio of 3:2 to 3:1 for DLE is quite distinct from 9:1 in SLE indicating separate entities. Similarly, the age of disease manifestation (20–40 years) is slightly higher in DLE than in SLE. The other CCLE subtypes show varying correlations to SLE and will be discussed below (Costner et al., 2003).

The issue of CCLE as a distinct and separate entity at the benign end of a spectrum of LE or a limited stage or concurrent manifestation within the chronological evolution of SLE has to be further evaluated. Especially, characteristic etiopathogenic factors as well as prognostic markers for CCLE remain to be elucidated. The final diagnosis of a distinct subset of LE can only be made following careful case history, clinical manifestations at the skin and other organs and laboratory findings encompassing the criteria defined by the American College of Rheumatology (ACR). Alternative classification criteria for cutaneous lesions have been suggested by the European Academy of Dermatology and Venereology (EADV) and are currently debated. Being more specific, however less sensitive than the ACR criteria, they have so far not found their way into the rheumatologic literature (Parodi and Rebora, 1997).

Pathogenesis

Various causes and resulting *inflammatory and immunological processes* have been identified as relevant for the induction of cutaneous LE (reviewed by Lee and Sinha, 2006, Pelle, 2006, Kuhn and Bijl, 2008). However, their particular role in individual clinical subsets of CCLE with respect to quantitative or qualitative differences has been barely addressed nor

Table 1. Pathogenetically Relevant Factors for CCLE

Genetics	HLA-antigens
	Cytokine-polymorphisms
	Cytokine-receptor-polymorphisms
	Complement deficiency
	Deficiency of 21-hydroxylase-A
Inflammatory dysregulation	Overinduction of cytokines
	ICAM-1 expression
	Matrix metalloproteinase expression
	Heat shock protein expression
	Apoptosis-related markers (e. g. bcl-2, Fas)
Environmental	Viral infections (alpha-virus, CMV as co-factor, paramyxovirus, Hep. C)
	UV-radiation
	Isomorphic phenomenon (Köbner phenomenon)
	Cigarette smoking
	Estrogen
	Certain drugs (questionable)

clarified. Factors suspected to precipitate or aggravate cutaneous LE lesions are listed in Table 1. Regarding a *genetic background*, various markers have been detected or suspected in LE (Lee and Sinha, 2006). These include HLA antigens, complement factor polymorphisms or deficiencies, namely C4 and C5 in DLE (Asghar et al., 1991; Nousari et al., 1999), cytokine and receptor-polymorphisms (Jacob, 1992), a deficiency of 21-hydroxylase-A with subsequent alterations of steroid homeostasis, isoforms of glutathione-S-transferase as well as genetically fixed varying responses to inflammatory stimuli regarding cytokine expression (Wenzel et al., 2009, Sontheimer, 2009), ICAM-1 or stress protein expression as well as matrix metalloproteinases (Jarvinen et al., 2007). Recently, the impact of apoptosis-related molecules and receptors like bcl-2 or Fas in LE has been addressed (see below) (Bachmann et al., 2002; Baima and Sticherling; 2001, Kuhn et al., 2006). Their dysregulation in either keratinocytes (exaggerated apoptosis) or lymphocytes (decreased apoptosis with persistance of autoreactive lymphocytes) may be related to genetic factors as well. Regarding DLE, rather conclusive data have been found for a correlation to extended HLA phenotypes such as HLA-B7, Cw7, DR3 or HLA-Cw7, DR3, DQw1 as well as DQA1*0102 with relative risks of 7.4 and 4.7, respectively. The role that genetic factors may play in the pathogenesis of DLE is stressed by the observed association of DLE with X-linked granulomatous disease, a disorder that is characterized by deficient or reduced NADPH oxidase (Rupec et al., 2000).

Evidence for virus infections as etiologic factors for LE is provided by the detection of viral material like alphavirus or paramyxovirus in skin lesions, the aggravation of LE fol-

Table 2. Specific LE Skin Symptoms

Acute cutaneous lupus erythematosus (ACLE)	Localized (classical butterfly rash)
	Generalized
Subacute cutaneous lupus erythematosus (SCLE)	Annular
	Papulosquamous
Chronic cutaneous lupus erythematosus (CCLE)	Discoid (DLE)
	Localized (above neck)
	Generalized (above and below neck)
	follicular
	Hypertrophic DLE
	Mucosal LE
	Lupus panniculitis
	Lupus profundus (Panniculitis and DLE)
	Chilblain lupus
	Papulous mucinosis
Intermittent cutaneous lupus erythematosus (ICLE)	Lupus erythematosus tumidus

lowing cytomegalovirus infections as well as a clinical, but probably accidental correlation of disseminated DLE lesions and SCLE with chronic hepatitis C. Altogether, evidence for viral induction is circumstantial and may in some cases be related to the induction of pro-inflammatory cytokines like interferon-γ and a subsequent triggering of the disease rather than direct involvement of virus.

In contrast to SLE and SCLE, distinct drugs do not seem to be relevant for the induction of CCLE lesions. However, the environmental factor smoking is associated to the persistence of DLE lesions as well as to a lack of therapeutic response to chloroquine (Gallego et al., 1999; Jewell and McCauliffe, 2000, Kreuter et al., 2009). A relation of CCLE to hormones like estrogen has been reported but seems to be less important than in SLE and SCLE. Nonspecific injury to the skin (*isomorphic response or Köbner phenomenon*) was found to induce DLE lesions similar to psoriasis and lichen planus and may explain manifestations at unusual locations (Ueki, 2005).

A huge body of literature is in support of the influence of ultraviolet radiation in LE, the subsequent induction of inflammatory processes and its relation to autoantibody formation (Kind et al., 1993; Costner et al., 2003; Kuhn and Beissert, 2005, Bijl and Kallenberg, 2006). As photosensitivity is a feature in up to 70% of SLE patients, it has been included as a criterion for diagnosis of SLE by the ACR. Regarding UV radiation and skin manifestations, 70% of SCLE patients are photosensitive and develop typical lesions after prolonged exposure to a combination of UVA and UVB (53%), UVB (33%) or UVA (14%) (Kind et al., 1993). An increased expression of Ro/SSA antigen and nuclear antigens as well as anti-Ro/SS-A antibodies have been related to UV-sensitivity in both cutaneous inflammation as well as in SLE (Mond et al., 1989, Oke et al., 2009, Reich et al., 2009).

UV-light is able to induce pro-inflammatory cytokines like TNF-α and IL-1 in both keratinocytes and lymphocytes. This leads to the induction of local inflammatory mediators like chemokines and lipid mediators which focus and amplify the subsequent inflammatory response to the local level. Both resident skin cells (endothelial cells, fibroblasts, mast cells) are activated as well as migratory cells like monocytes and lymphocytes attracted to the dermal and epidermal compartment through an induction of different adhesion molecules in a characteristic sequence of events (Bijl and Kallenberg, 2006).

The central involvement of autoantibodies in the pathogenesis of LE like anti-Ro / SS-A has been fostered by recent results on the expression and / or release of intracellular antigens like the nucleoprotein SS-A on the keratinocyte surface upon UV radiation (Casciola-Rosen et al., 1995; Bachmann et al., 2002, Reich et al., 2009). Alternatively, these antigens are expressed on keratinocytes undergoing apoptosis upon UV-irradiation. Recent results correlated keratinocyte apoptosis with local disease activity at a low rate in CDLE and a high rate in ACLE (Baima and Sticherling, 2001, Kuhn et al., 2006). Consequently, keratinocytes are killed by antibody-dependent cellular cytotoxicity and the humoral immune response is triggered and boosted by antigenic challenge (Tan, 1994; Bachmann et al., 2002). Immune complex formation at the onset of LE seems to be of minor importance as immune complexes are detected at the dermo-epidermal junction only as late as six weeks after UV-irradiation. At that stage, influx of inflammatory cells like monocytes and other changes characteristic for LE has already taken place. According to this concept, inflammatory and immunological pathways are overreacting or insufficiently counterbalanced due to a variety of environmental or genetic factors or a combination of both (Hussein et al., 2008, Wenzel et al., 2009).

However, the concept of a UV-induced pathogenesis elaborated for cutaneous LE like ACLE and SCLE seems less conclusive for CCLE and does not yet convincingly explain its clinical characteristics and distinction from other forms of cutaneous LE. In DLE, photosensitivity (predominently to UVB, but also UVA radiation) is found in only 40% of the patients and anti-SS-A antibodies are rarely detected. If positive, they may indicate incipient systemic disease. Other antibody specificities and pathogenic mechanisms have been suggested, but not yet been proven to be relevant. Only few studies address specific differences of CCLE to other forms of cutaneous LE. Immunohistochemical analysis of activated cutaneous lymphocytes has demonstrated a local T helper 2 response with the preferential activation of dermal T cells (Furukawa et al., 1996; Denfeld et al., 1997; Stein et al., 1997). Expression of various cellular and extracellular proteins like keratins (de Berker et al., 1995), adhesion molecules (Tebbe et al., 1997) and extracellular matrix proteins (de Jong et al., 1997) point to inflammatory processes common for chronic, hyperproliferative diseases with only partial distinction from other lichenoid skin reactions (McCauliffe, 1998, Hussein et al., 2008, Sontheimer, 2009, Wenzel et al., 2009). The immunohistochemical demonstration of the membrane attack complex (C5b-9) may further subdivide different subsets of CCLE and suggests a pathogenic involvement (Magro et al., 1996). With respect to different subsets of inflammatory cells, CD4- and CD8-positive lymphocytes as well as macrophages constitute a major portion of the skin infiltrate in both SCLE and SLE (Hasan et al., 1999, Hussein et al., 2008) whereas dermal Langerhans cells are absent in both entities (Sontheimer and Bergstresser, 1982). Recent results demonstrate the involvement of plasmacytoid dendritic cells (Obermoser et al., 2009). However, an increased frequency of

5

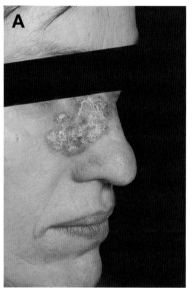

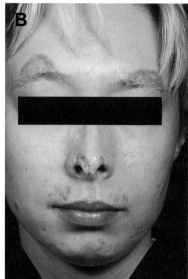

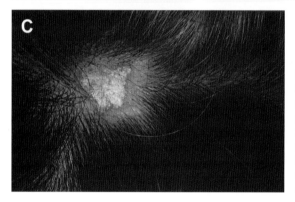

Fig. 1. A. Clinical presentation of chronic discoid lupus erythematosus. Typical sharply demarcated elevated erythematous plaque. **B.** Chronic atrophic lesions of the face lead to disfiguration. **C.** Involvement of the scalp leads to cicatricial alopecia

TCRγ/δ-positive T cells in DLE (Volc-Platzer et al., 1993) as well as the presence of granzyme B-expressing CD-8-positive T cells (Grassi et al., 2009) suggest specific T-cell mediated epidermal cytotoxicity in cutaneous LE.

Clinical Appearance / Classification

Several distinctly different clinical entities can be allocated to the group of CCLE (Table 2). They may be found as the one and only manifestation or associated with other forms of CCLE, localized or disseminated, both with and without systemic manifestations and a varying relation to SLE (Kuhn et al., 2007, Renner and Sticherling, 2009). The most common form is chronic discoid lupus erythematosus (CDLE or DLE). It is characterized by persistent, sharply demarcated, elevated erythematous plaques with adherent scales which may rarely ulcerate (Fig. 1A). Early stages are characterized by erythema and *hyperpigmentation*. The characteristic painful sensation upon touching is caused by follicular plugging resulting in the so-called carpet-tack sign. Apart from that, atrophy and scarring can be found in the center of untreated lesions and may result in considerable disfiguration particularly when present in the face (Fig. 1B). A characteristic pitted, acneiform scarring is also a common residual feature of the perioral area including the lips.

DLE lesions predominantly occur in the light-exposed areas of skin like face, ears, neck and arms, but may be found in sun-protected areas as well as inguinal folds, palmo-plantar locations and the scalp. At the latter location, DLE may even be the only cutaneous manifestation in 10% of cases and thus presents a classical differential diagnosis of scarring alopecia. Altogether an involvement of the scalp can be found in about 60% of DLE patients (Costner et al., 2003) (Fig. 1C). With a distribution above the neck, the so-called *localized form of DLE* can be separated from a *generalized DLE* if present below the neck as well. Small, follicularly orientated erythematous papules of less than 1 cm in diameter present as *follicular DLE* at the elbows, but may occur at any other part of the body as well. Precipitation of DLE lesions by physical trauma (Köbner phenomenon) has already been mentioned above and may explain occurance at unusual locations.

If DLE lesions are distinctly proliferative, they are referred to as *hypertrophic or verrucous DLE*. They have to be separated from spinous cell carcinoma, keratoacanthoma and lichen planus by histology and immunohistochemistry (Perniciaro et al., 1995; Uy et al., 1999, Sontheimer, 2009, Wenzel et al., 2009).

Another rare manifestation of CCLE is *lupus profundus or lupus panniculitis*, also referred to as *Kaposi-Irgang disease* (Caproni et al., 1995; Watanabe and Tsuchida, 1996; Kundig et al., 1997; Uy et al., 1999; Martens et al., 1999, Massone et al., 2005, Kuhn et al., 2007). It can be found in about 2% of SLE patients, but presents more commonly without further or only mild signs of systemic manifestation in about 50% of patients. Severe nephritis is an uncommon event. In contrast to DLE, mainly women are affected by painful, firm subcutaneous nodules of red-bluish colour and up to 1–3 cm diameter. Their main locations are the upper arms, buttocks and thighs, but chest, head and neck can be affected as well (Fig. 2A). The inflammatory process in the deeper dermis and subcutaneous tissue results in saucer-like depressions sometimes resembling lipathrophy. When DLE lesions are found on the overlying skin as is the case in 70% of patients, it is referred to as *lupus profundus*.

Chilblain or perniotic lupus is characterized by bluish-red patches and plaques at acral locations like nose, ears, fingers, toes, knees and elbows (Su et al., 1994; Fisher and Everett, 1996). These are painful upon pressure, especially when located at heels and knuckels where fissuring is quite common (Fig. 2B). It mainly occurs in cold climates and is possibly caused by the Köbner phenomenon. During further disease process, typical DLE lesions may appear and patches may ulcerate. As in lupus profundus, mild systemic symptoms like arthralgia can be found to fulfil three to four ACR criteria for diagnosis of SLE in up to 20% of patients. Due to its rare occurence, no definite association to SLE can be made. The term lupus pernio is often used synonymously for this entity, should however be restricted to cutaneous sarcoidosis as a totally unrelated disease and important differential diagnosis.

Another rare manifestation of CCLE, *lupus tumidus*, is characterized by excessive dermal mucin deposition resulting in urticarial plaques (Ruiz and Sanchez, 1999; Dekle et al.,

5

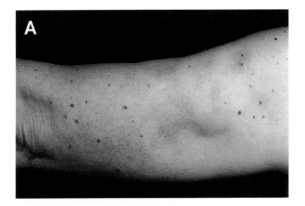

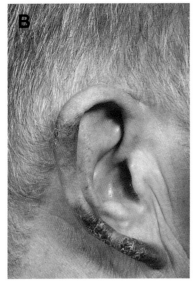

Fig. 2. A. Rare manifestations of chronic cutaneous lupus erythematosus. Lupus profundus or lupus panniculitis lead to saucer-like depressions resembling lipatrophy. **B.** Chilblain or perniotic lupus is characterized by bluish-red patches and plaques located at the acra, such as the ears

1999, Kuhn et al., 2003; Schmitt et al., 2010). Compared to other CCLE types, it is characterized by distinct photosensitivity which explains its main occurence at sun-exposed areas and the induction of lesions upon photoprovocation. Recently a clear distinction from the other CLE subsets was made and the name intermittent cutaneous lupus erythematosus suggested for this new entity (Kuhn et al., 2009). With a male preponderance its peak incidence is around the 30–40th year of age. Differential diagnosis to lymphocytic infiltration and polymorphous light eruption can be very difficult both clinically and histologically (Costner et al., 2003).

Mucous membrane involvement (*mucosal DLE*) can be found among CCLE patients in up to 25% (Burge et al., 1989; Botella et al., 1999). It does not necessarily reflect systemic manifestation, specific or high antibody titers or high disease activity. It is, however, included in the list of 11 diagnostic criteria for SLE defined by the ACR. Oral, mainly buccal manifestations are most common (Fig. 3), but nasal, conjunctival and anogenital mucous

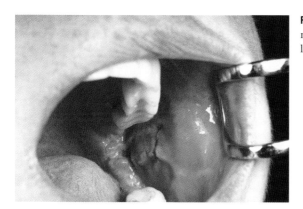

Fig. 3. Ulcers of the buccal mucosa in chronic cutaneous lupus erythematosus

membranes may be affected as well. They present as painful erythematous patches which may ulcerate and cause atrophy in the long run. Sometimes mucosal DLE resembles lichen planus with honeycomb appearance. Squamous cell carcinoma as a long-term complication should be suspected and excluded in any case of asymmetrical induration of either mucosal or cutaneous lesions. Affliction of the lips (vermillion border, diffuse cheilitis especially of lower lip) can cause considerable discomfort and disfiguration. Mucosal DLE of the nose may result in nasal septum perforation especially in association with SLE. Similarly, ocular affections which are mainly located to the palpebral conjunctiva and lower eyelids can cause permanent loss of eye lashes, ectropion and stromal keratitis (Uy et al., 1999).

Annular erythema has in the past been regarded as a rare manifestion of CCLE. It will not be dealt with in this chapter since it is generally associated with SCLE and Sjogren's syndrome (Watanabe et al., 1997).

Papular mucinosis may occur as early or only manifestation of CCLE and shows similarities to *lupus tumidus* in respect to dermal mucin deposition (Kanda et al., 1997; Williams and Ramos-Caro, 1999, Sonntag et al., 2003, Kuhn et al., 2003). In contrast to *lupus tumidus*, more papular than plaque appearance and lack of inflammatory erythema can be found. Asymptomatic isolated or multiple lesions are located to the trunk, upper limbs and the face with less apparent photosensitivity than in *lupus tumidus*. The definite diagnosis may be only made upon immunohistochemical detection of linear or granular depositions of IgG, IgM and complement C3 at the dermo-epidermal junction whereas other histological traits of LE are absent. Accordingly, differential diagnosis to other cutaneous mucinoses can be difficult.

Diagnosis

In contrast to skin manifestations associated with overt SCLE and SLE, patients with the different subtypes of CCLE will primarily present to dermatologists as long as systemic manifestations are missing. Once an internal organ involvement has occurred, these patients will be referred to general practitioners or rheumatologists for exclusion of systemic disease. Alternatively, general practitioners or rheumatologists may ask dermatologists to search for typical skin manifestations of LE in a suspected patient or to evaluate present skin symptoms as typical for or related to LE. In cases of CCLE, first line efforts will head at their definite diagnosis which as already outlined above may be sometimes difficult to establish.

The case history has to focus on LE-related symptoms like photosensitivity, arthralgia or arthritis, diffuse or areata-like alopecia, Raynaud's phenomenon, Sicca symptoms, morning stiffness of joints, thrombosis, spontaneous abortion, atypical pneumonia and carditis as well as neurological disorders. To support the clinical diagnosis, histological as well as immunohistochemical examinations of skin lesions will be performed. Depending on the stage and acuity of LE, the typical histological findings include epidermal hyperkeratosis, epidermal atrophy, basal cell degeneration, thickening of the epidermal basement membrane, liquefaction degeneration and mononuclear cell infiltrate at the dermo-epidermal junction as well as around blood vessels and adnexial structures. The dermato-histological features of different LE types (ACLE, SCLE, DLE) may be very similar (Costner et al., 2003; Ackerman, 2005). Often these parameters do not allow to clearly distinguish the different entities apart from quantitative differences in epidermal or especially follicular hyperkeratosis which are characteristic for DLE. Special histological features can be found in *LE tumidus* with its characteristic abundant, partly focal deposition of mucin among collagenous fibers of the reticular dermis. *Lupus panniculitis* presents with a lobular pattern of perivascular and periadnexial mononuclear infiltration and partially necrobiotic changes of fatty tissue with fibrinoid deposits as well as focal calcinosis in the deep dermis.

Direct Immunofluorescence

The characteristic findings in direct immunohistochemical examination of lesional skin are granular immune deposits of mostly IgG, IgM and complement factor C3 in a continuous line along the dermo-epidermal junction (so-called lesional *lupus band test*) (George et al., 1995; Cardinali et al., 1999). They will be only found in lesions of more than four to six weeks duration, an aspect which argues against their pathogenic relevance and the immediate involvement of immune complex mechanisms. Furthermore, the incidence of positive lupus band tests is higher in biopsies from upper body sites as more likely in biopsies from the face than from the trunk. However, neither does their absence exclude CCLE nor is their presence specific for LE. They may be found in sun-damaged skin, rosacea and polymorphic light eruption, often with deposits of IgM only. The significance of immune deposits in non-lesional skin (*non-lesional lupus band test*) is much debated (George et al., 1995; Cardinali et al., 1999, Sticherling et al., 2008) and seems specific for SLE when IgG and two additional immunoglobulin subtypes (IgM, IgA) are detected. Skin biopsies for non-lesional skin may be taken from the the inner aspect of the upper arm (sun-protected) and the extensor aspect of the forearm (sun-exposed). In CCLE with no extracutaneous manifestations the latter two biopsies should be negative. The findings of the lupus band test have to be carefully interpreted together with other serological examinations. The currently available anti-DNA detection assays with both high sensitivity and specificity may substitute the classical lupus band test at three site for all but lesional skin. Epidermal dust-like particles in a specific fine speckled pattern are generally associated with SCLE and anti-SS-A antibodies rarely detected in DLE. If present they may indicate more severe disease with progression to systemic manifestations (Costner et al., 2003). In patients with high titered anti-nuclear antibodies, especially anti-U1-RNP (which is typically associated with mixed connective tissue disease), positive epidermal nuclei can be found by direct immunofluorescence microscopy. This phenomenon most probably derives from an in vitro binding of high titer or high affinity antibodies. In vivo penetrating autoantibodies may be found as well. However, their significance for the disease manifestation as well as diagnostic procedures remains to be elucidated (Golan et al., 1997). Using specific monoclonal antibodies, the membrane attack complex (C5b-9) could be demonstrated in the epidermis of different subsets of CCLE and may allow further distinction (Magro et al., 1996). In lupus profundus as well as in SLE granular deposits of IgG and C3 may be occasionally found in dermal vessel walls indicating immune complex vasculitis.

Serological Tests

Serological tests are critical for the confirmation of CCLE. Antinuclear antibodies of high titers and characteristic specificity will rarely be found without systemic manifestation. They may, however, be present in cases of generalized DLE which in turn has a greater risk to progress to SLE. Anti-Ro/SS-A antibodies can sometimes be detected by ELISA techniques, may however lack precipitating activity, i. e. immunodiffusion techniques are negative (Provost et al., 1996). Anti-DNA-antibodies are negative in classical DLE and other subsets of CCLE and if present indicate systemic disease (Provost et al., 1996; Costner et al., 2003; Tebbe et al., 1997, Sticherling et al., 2008). Anti-cardiolipin antibodies are mostly not detectable. They may be found in cases of lupus panniculitis and chilblain lupus indicating secondary antiphospholipid syndrome and progession to systemic disease (Ruffati et al., 1995). Similarly, tests for complement consumption (e. g. CH50 test), detection of complement fragments and circulating immune complexes will mostly be negative or only slightly altered and should only be performed in cases of suspected systemic disease. Serum levels of other serological molecules like soluble adhesion markers, neopterin and soluble IL-2 receptor are related to disease activity (Costner et al., 2003), but have not yet been established as routine parameters.

Apart from the above examinations, basic clinical routine laboratory tests should be performed to exclude anemia, leukopenia, renal involvement (proteinuria, hematuria) and systemic inflammation. Accordingly, blood sedimentation rate (BSR), blood cell count, hepatic enzymes, urine sediment and serum immunoglobulins should be checked. Pathologic findings are substantiated by further tests if necessary. Additional clinical tests like chest X-ray and evaluation of organ involvement (e. g. in ophthalmology, neurology, cardiology) should only be performed based on clues in the individual case history or pathologic results of physical or laboratory examinations. The indication for routine testing of cutaneous sensitivity to ultraviolett light as well as photoprovocation is much debated in CCLE (Kuhn et al., 2001, Callen, 2006). However, the impact of these examinations with regard to stringency of sun protection and consequences for life-style supports their usefulness in the clinical routine (Kind et al., 1993; Costner et al., 2003, Kuhn et al., 2001, Kuhn and Beissert, 2005).

CCLE patients should be monitored at 6 to 12-months intervals for further signs of systemic disease, especially when anemia or leukopenia, persistent high ANA titers or elevated blood sedimentation rates are found. Evaluated activity scores based on these clinical and laboratory findings become increasingly available to monitor patients in a clinical or more likely study setting. These include the Systemic Lupus Activity Measure (SLAM) (Parodi et al., 2000) for SLE or the Cutaneous Lupus Erythematosus Disease Activity and Severity Index (Krathen et al., 2008, Bonilla-Martinez et al., 2008, Anonymous, 2007).

Therapy

Many of the following drugs have been extensively used in SCLE which is different in respect to a more pronounced inflammatory and less hyperproliferative activity (Table 3) (Wallace, 2002, Callen, 2006, Sticherling et al., 2008). They will accordingly be discussed in detail in the context of SCLE. Therapy regimens and their intensity will be dictated by the extent of cutaneous as well extracutaneous involvement and thus have to depend on ample diagnostic procedures as outlined above. The scarring potential of CCLE demands early and aggressive treatment to avoid cosmetically and emotionally disturbing and irreversible disfiguration (Costner et al., 2003; Drake et al., 1996). Individual cases may require combinations of different therapy regimens and frequently, disease relapses after lowering daily doses of drugs or stopping the treatment.

In cases of solitary or only few DLE lesions and absent systemic manifestations local therapy may suffice (Wallace, 2002, Callen, 2006, Ting and Sontheimer, 2001). This comprises local application of glucocorticosteroids (e. g. clobetasol propionate 0.05%, betamethasone dipropionate 0.05%, triamcinolone acetonide 0.1%, fluocinonide) twice daily for 10–14 days as ointment, fluid (propylenglykol), tape / occlusive dressing or focal infiltration. Tazarotene which has been successfully used topically in a case of DLE with distinct hyperproliferation (Edwards and Burke, 1999) is no longer available. The calcineurin inhibitors pimecrolimus and tacrolimus have shown conflicting results upon topical use in cases of discoid and subacute cutaneous lupus erythematosus. The only limited number of studies of mostly low evidence levels advocate their use in SCLE and less convincingly in DLE (Sardy et al., 2009, Sticherling, 2010).

In more severe or disseminated cases, antimalarials have been successfully used either alone or in combination (hydroxychloroqine, chloroquine, quinacrine) especially in DLE (Costner et al., 2003; Drake et al., 1996, Kalia and Dutz, 2007, Cooper and Magwere, 2007, Lesiak et al., 2009) with a delayed effect after a treatment period of three to four weeks. Hydroxychloroqine is usually used first-line starting with 400 mg/d or better dosed according to ideal weight and tapered after four to eight weeks to 200 mg/d upon clinical improvement. In cases of insufficient response, it may be combined with 100 mg/d quinacrine, especially in lupus profundus and hypertrophicus (Cavazzana et al., 2009). Alternatively, chloroquine may be used at 250 mg/d. Glucose-6-phosphate deficiency should be excluded prior to therapy to minimize the risk of idiosyncratic reactions. Otherwise, neurotoxicity as well as muscular and hepatic toxicity may occur. Retinal toxicity should be monitored

Table 3. Therapeutic Options for CCLE

Local therapy	glucocorticosteroids
	retinoids
	calcineurin inhibitors
	inferferons
	laser
	cryotherapy
	cosmetic surgery
	camouflage
Systemic therapy	antimalarials
	glucocorticosteroids
	dapsone
	methotrexate
	azathioprine
	mycophenolate mofetil / mycophenolic acid
	thalidomide
	retinoids
	ciclosporin
	interferons
	clofazimine
	gold
	cyclophosphamide
	sulfasalazine
	intravenous immunoglobulins
	photopheresis
	biologics?

by initial examination of the ocular fundus and thereafter every 6–12 months during therapy. Retinal toxicity is low at daily doses below 6 mg/kg/d hydroxychloroquine (4 mg/kg/d chloroquine) with no apparent maximal total life time dosis (Ochsendorf, 2004). Recently, the inhibitory effect of cigarette smoking on the therapeutic efficacy of antimalarials has been demonstrated (Gallego et al., 1999; Jewell and McCauliffe, 2000, Kreuter et al., 2009). This may be explained by the induction of hepatic microsomal enzymes leading to an accelerated metabolism of antimalarials. Initially, especially in cases of high inflammatory activity or generalized disease, antimalarials may be combined with oral glucocorticosteroids well below 1 mg/kg/d prednisolone-equivalent which should be tapered within two to three weeks. Classical CCLE will however seldomly require such a regimen.

Dapsone (diaminodiphenylsulfone) may be alternatively used at 50–200 mg/d (Drake et al., 1996; Wozel, 1996, Costner et al., 2003, Abe et al., 2008). As with antimalarials, glucose-6-phosphate deficiency should be excluded. Regular monitoring for hemolytic anemia as well as hepatic disturbances and eventually methemoglobulinemia should be performed at two week intervals during the first three months of therapy and monthly thereafter. The incidence and severity of anemia can be reduced by adding cimetidin or vitamin C/E.

Thalidomide in a dose of 100 to 200 mg/d or even less, has been shown to be effective in DLE and especially lupus panniculitis (Drake et al., 1996; Warren et al., 1998; Georgala et al., 1998; Ordi-Ros et al., 2000; Kyriakis et al., 2000, Costner et al., 2003, Sticherling et al., 2008). Peripheral irreversible neuropathy and fatigue present limiting side-effects in up to 50% of the patients. Furthermore, amenorrhoea or thromboembolic events may occur (Ordi et al., 1998). Regarding the well-known teratogenic effects of thalidomide, strict contraception is mandatory. To avoid relapses, slow reduction of therapeutic doses or long-term treatment with low doses are recommended.

Retinoids present another therapeutic option in cases of insufficient response to above mentioned approaches. All three ever clinically available compounds (isotretinoin, etretinate, acitretin) have been used in LE, at a dosage of 0.5–1 mg/kg/d (Marks, 1995, Sticherling et al., 2008). The teratogenic effects limit their use in women of childbearing age and require strict contraceptive measures. Apart from that, dryness of mucous membranes as well as skin, peeling of palms and soles and transient hair loss, hepatic disturbances including drug-induced hepatitis, hypertriglyceridemia and hypercholesterinemia as well as phototoxic effects present common and therapy-limiting side effects.

Controversial results have been reported on the use of interferons in LE. Both local and systemic interferon-α 2A have successfully been used in SCLE and DLE (Thivolet et al., 1990; Costner et al., 2003). However, interferon-α treatment of chronic inflammatory and malignant diseases resulted in precipitation or exacerbation of SLE (Garcia-Porrua et al., 1998). This potential adverse side effect stresses the importance to distinguish SLE from CCLE before starting the therapy.

Case reports demonstrated the beneficial effects of *clofazimine* (100 mg/d), oral or parenteral *gold* (cave: mucocutaneous toxicity, hematological, renal and pulmonary toxicity), *methotrexate* (Bottomley and Goodfield, 1995, Kuhn et al., 2002), *cyclophosphamide* and *azathioprine*. Recently positive experience has been published on the use of mycophenolate mofetil (Mok, 2007). Sulfasalazine at a dose of up to 2 g/d has also been used successfully (Sabbagh et al., 1997) as well as immunomodulatory substances like ciclosporin (Saeki et al., 2000), leflunomide (Furst, 1999), systemic tacrolimus or fumaric acid esters (Jayne, 1999). Intravenous immunoglobulins have been effective in recalcitrant CCLE as adjuvant therapy (Wallace, 2002, Callen, 2006). The impact of "biologics" namely antibodies, fusion proteins and soluble receptors still need to be evaluated in the context of CCLE (Lateef and Petri, 2010). Monoclonal antibodies against e.g. CD4 (Prinz et al., 1996), CD 20 or TNFα have only anecdotically been used in CCLE or in SLE only. As their efficacy still needs to be evaluated especially for CCLE they should be used only in cases of disseminated and refractory disease as last resort. Recently, positive effects of extracorporeal photopheresis have been reported in widespread and recalcitrant DLE (Richter et al., 1998; Wollina and

Looks, 1999). The therapeutic use of UV exposure in lupus is still controversial regarding photosensitivity and should be restricted to individual cases (Millard and Hawk, 2001).

UV protection should be performed in all cases of CCLE as supportive measure. Its stringency does not need to be enforced as strictly as in SCLE in all but cases of proven UV sensitivity. This includes avoidance of the sun especially during midday and summer months, wearing of sun-protective clothing and application of broad-spectrum sun-screen with high UV protection factor. Titanium dioxide containing sun-screens have become available as convenient and very efficient physical sun-protection.

In case of disfiguration camouflage is recommended (Boehncke et al., 2002; Penso-Assathiany et al., 2010). Alopecia may be hidden by ample hair dressing or hair pieces. Surgical approaches including hair transplantation or cosmetic surgery should only be initiated when the inflammatory disease activity has totally subsided or was stopped by therapeutic measures. Different approaches with laser therapy (Nunez et al., 1996; Nurnberg et al., 1996; Walker and Harland, 2000) and cryotherapy (Molin, 1999) have been used with varying success. However, when therapeutically applying physical procedures, one has to take into account the possibility of isomorphic provocation and aggravation of cutaneous disease.

Summary

Skin, to a similar extent as the joints, represents the most common organ involved in LE either as primary manifestation or during the course of disease. Nonspecific symptoms can be separated from the distinct and specific manifestations of acute, subacute, chronic and intermitted cutaneous LE. The latter may present as a disease confined to the skin or as a manifestation of systemic disease. In several subtypes of CCLE, mild involvement of the internal organs may be present which does not suffice for diagnosing SLE. The risk of further development into systemic disease is, however, present in 5–10% of CCLE. The pathogenesis of the different CCLE entities is not as conclusively known as for ACLE and SCLE. The impact of photosensitivity is comparatively low as are evident systemic autoimmune phenomena like high titered antinuclear antibodies. Similar to systemic disease, lesional skin of CCLE is characterized by positive immune deposits at the dermo-epidermal junction. The major subtypes of CCLE can present as solitary disease or combined with other subtypes. These are discoid lupus erythematosus (DLE), hypertrophic DLE, mucous membrane DLE, chilblain lupus, lupus tumidus and lupus panniculitis/profundus. In contrast to SCLE, lesions tend to show atrophy and scarring. Typical DLE lesions are represented by sharply demarcated erythematous plaques with hyperkeratosis and follicular plugging. In lupus panniculitis, deep inflammatory processes in the dermis and subcutis result in saucer-like defects often associated with typical overlying epidermal changes. Entities most intimately associated with systemic disease are chilblain lupus and lupus panniculitis. Diagnostic procedures have to substantiate cutaneous and to exclude underlying systemic disease. Histological and immunohistochemical examinations have to be combined with autoimmune serological tests as well as additional clinical laboratory tests depending on the findings of clinical examinations. Accordingly, therapeutic measures depend on the extent of cutaneous involvement and the accompanying systemic manifestations. Early and aggressive treatment has to prevent irreversible scarring and disfiguration. Local therapy with glucocorticosteroids, retinoids, laser and cryotherapy may not suffice and has to be accompanied or substituted by systemic therapy. Antimalarial drugs, possibly in combination with short term oral glucocorticosteroids, oral retinoids, dapsone, thalidomide and supportive UV protection are the most common regimens. Alternatively, clofazimine, gold, interferons, methotrexate and azathioprine may be used. The impact of biologics is still a matter of debate.

References

Abe M, Shimizu A, Yokoyama Y, Takeuchi Y, Ishikawa O (2008). A possible inhibitory action of diaminodiphenyl sulfone on tumour necrosis factor-alpha production from activated mononuclear cells on cutaneous lupus erythematosus. Clin Exp Dermatol 33:759–63

Ackerman AB (2005) Lupus erythematosus. In: Ackerman AB (ed) Histologic diagnosis of inflammatory skin diseases. 3rd ed. Williams & Wilkins, Baltmore pp 525–546

Anonymous. Response criteria for cutaneous SLE in clinical trials (2007). Clin Exp Rheumatol 25:666–671,

Asghar SS, Venneker GT, van Meegen M, Meinardi MM, Hulsmans RF, de Waal LP (1991) Hereditary deficiency of C5 in association with discoid lupus erythematosus. J Am Acad Dermatol 24:376–378

Bachmann MP, Gross JA, Pan Z, Farris AD (2002). Apoptosis, a mechanism to break tolerance? In: Conrad K, Fritzler M, Meurer M, Sack U, Shoenfeld Y (eds) From proteomics to molecular epidemiology: relevance of autoantibodies. Pabst Science Publishers, Lengerich, pp 203–219–186

Baima B, Sticherling M (2001) Apoptosis in different manifestations of cutaneous lupus erythematosus. Br J Dermatol 144:958–966

Bijl M, Kallenberg CGM (2006). Ultraviolet light and cutaneous lupus. Lupus; 15:724–727

Boehncke WH, Ochsendorf F, Paeslack I, Kaufmann R, Zollner TM (2002) Decorative cosmetics improve the quality of life in patients with disfiguring skin diseases. Eur J Dermatol; 12:577–80

Bonilla-Martinez ZL, Albrecht J, Troxel AB, Taylor L, Okawa J, Dulay S, Werth VP (2008). The cutaneous lupus erythematosus disease area and severity index: a responsive instrument to measure activity and damage in patients with cutaneous lupus erythematosus. Arch Dermatol 144:173–180

Botella R, Alfonso R, Silvestre JF, Ramon R (1999) Discoid lupus erythematosus-like lesions and stomatitis. Arch Dermatol 135:847, 850

Bottomley WW, Goodfield MJ (1995) Methotrexate for the treatment of discoid lupus erythematosus. Br J Dermatol 133:655–656

Burge SM, Frith PA, Juniper RP, Wojnarowska F (1989) Mucosal involvement in systemic and chronic cutaneous lupus erythematosus. Br J Dermatol 121:727–741

Callen JP (2006) Cutaneous lupus erythematosus: a personal approach to management. Australas J Dermatol; 47:13–27

Caproni M, Palleschi GM, Papi C, Fabbri P (1995) Discoid lupus erythematosus lesions developed on lupus erythematosus profundus nodules. Int J Dermatol 34:357–359

Cardinali C, Caproni M, Fabbri P (1999) The utility of the lupus band test on sun-protected non-lesional skin for the diagnosis of systemic lupus erythematosus. Clin Exp Rheumatol 17:427–432

Casciola-Rosen LA, Anhalt G, Rosen A (1994) Autoantigens targeted in systemic lupus erythematosus are clustered in two populations of surface structures on apoptotic keratinocytes. J Exp Med 179:1317–1330

Cavazzana I, Sala R, Bazzani C, Ceribelli A, Zane C, Cattaneo R, Tincani A, Calzavara-Pinton P, Franceschini F (2009). Treatment of lupus skin involvement with quinacrine and hydroxychloroquine. Lupus 18:735–9

Cooper RG, Magwere T (2007) Chloroquine has not disappeared. Afr Health Sci 7:185–186

Costner MI, Sontheimer RD, Provost TT (2003). Lupus erythematosus. In: Sontheimer RD, Provost TT: Cutaneous manifestations of rheumatic diseases. Philadelphia: Williams & Wilkins, 15–64

de Berker D, Dean D, Leigh IM, Burge S (1995) Keratin expression in discoid lupus erythematosus. Exp Dermatol 4:350–356

de Jong EM, van der Vleuten CJ, van Vlijmen-Willems IM (1997) Differences in extracellular matrix proteins, epidermal growth and differentiation in discoid lupus erythematosus, lichen planus and the overlap syndrome. Acta Derm Venereol 77:356–360

Dekle CL, Mannes KD, Davis LS, Sangueza OP (1999) Lupus tumidus. J Am Acad Dermatol 41:250–253

Denfeld RW, Kind P, Sontheimer RD, Schöpf E, Simon JC (1997) In situ expression of B7 and CD28 receptor families in skin lesions of patients with lupus erythematosus. Arthritis Rheum 40:814–821

Drake LA, Dinehart SM, Farmer ER, Goltz RW, Graham GF, Hordinsky MK, Lewis CW, Pariser DM, Skouge JW, Webster SB, Whitaker DC, Butler B, Lowery BJ, Sontheimer RD, Callen JP, Camisa C, Provost TT, Tuffanelli DL (1996) Guidelines of care for cutaneous lupus erythematosus. American Academy of Dermatology. J Am Acad Dermatol 34:830–836

Edwards KR, Burke WA (1999) Treatment of localized discoid lupus erythematosus with tazarotene. J Am Acad Dermatol 41:1049–1050

Fisher DA, Everett MA (1996) Violaceous rash of dorsal fingers in a woman. Diagnosis: chilblain lupus erythematosus (perniosis). Arch Dermatol 132:459–462

Furst DE (1999) Leflunomide, mycophenolic acid and matrix metalloproteinase inhibitors. Rheumatology (Oxford) 38:14–18

Furukawa F, Tokura Y, Matsushita K, Iwasaki-Inuzuka K, Onagi-Suzuki K, Yagi H, Wakita H, Takigawa M (1996) Selective expansions of T cells expressing V beta 8 and V beta 13 in skin lesions of patients with chronic cutaneous lupus erythematosus. J Dermatol 23:670–676

Gallego H, Crutchfield CE 3rd, Lewis EJ, Gallego HJ (1999) Report of an association between discoid lupus erythematosus and smoking. Cutis 63:231–234

Garcia-Porrua C, Gonzales-Gay MA, Fernandez-Lamelo F, Paz-Carreira JM, Lavilla E, Gonzales-Lopez MA (1998) Simultaneous development of SLE-like syndrome and autoimmune thyroiditis following alpha-interferon treatment. Clin Exp Rheumatol 16:107–108

Georgala S, Katoulis AC, Hasapi V, Koumantaki-Mathioudaki E (1998) Thalidomide treatment for hypertrophic lupus erythematosus. Clin Exp Dermatol 23:141

George R, Kurian S, Jacob M, Thomas K (1995) Diagnostic evaluation of the lupus band test in discoid and systemic lupus erythematosus. Int J Dermatol 34:170–173

Gilliam JN (1977). The cutaneous signs of lupus erythematosus. Cont Educ Fam Phys. 6:37–40

Gilliam JN, Sontheimer RD (1981). Distinctive cutaneous subsets in the spectrum of lupus erythematosus. J Am Acad Dermatol 4:471–5

Golan TD, Sigal D, Sabo E, Shemuel Z, Guedj D, Weinberger A (1997) The penetrating potential of autoantibodies into live cells in vitro coincides with the in vivo staining of epidermal nuclei. Lupus 6:18–26

Grassi M, Capello F, Bertolino L, Seia Z, Pippione M (2009) Identification of granzyme B-express-ing CD-8-positive T cells in lymphocytic inflammatory infiltrate in cutaneous lupus erythema-tosus and in dermatomyositis. Clin Exp Dermatol 34:910–4

Hasan T, Stephansson E, Ranki A (1999) Distribution of naive and memory T-cells in photopro-voked and spontaneous skin lesions of discoid lupus erythematosus and polymorphous light eruption. Acta Derm Venereol 79:437–442

Hussein MR, Aboulhagag NM, Atta HS, Atta SM (2008). Evaluation of the profile of the immune cell infiltrate in lichen planus, discoid lupus erythematosus, and chronic dermatitis. Pathology 40:682–93

Jarvinen TM, Kanninen P, Jeskanen L, Koskenmies S, Panelius J, Hasan T, Ranki A,. Saarialho-Kere U (2007) Matrix metalloproteinases as mediators of tissue injury in different forms of cutane-ous lupus erythematosus. Br J Dermatol 157:970–980

Jayne D (1999) Non-transplant uses of mycophenolate mofetil. Curr Opin Nephrol Hypertens 8:563–567

Jewell ML, McCauliffe DP (2000) Patients with cutaneous lupus erythematosus who smoke are less responsive to antimalarial treatment. J Am Acad Dermatol 42:983–987

Kalia S, Dutz JP (2007) New concepts in antimalarial use and mode of action in dermatology. Dermatol Ther. 20:160–174

Kanda N, Tsuchida T, Watanabe T, Tamaki K (1997) Cutaneous lupus mucinosis: a review of our cases and the possible pathogenesis. J Cutan Pathol 24:553–558

Kind P, Lehmann P, Plewig G (1993) Phototesting in lupus erythematosus. J Invest Dermatol 100:53S–57S

Krathen MS, Dunham J, Gaines E, Junkins-Hopkins J, Kim E, Kolasinski SL, Kovarik C, Kwan-Morley J, Okawa J, Propert K, Rogers N, Rose M, Thomas P, Troxel AB, Van Voorhees A, Feldt JV, Weber AL, Werth VP (2008). The Cutaneous Lupus Erythematosus Disease Activity and Severity Index: expansion for rheumatology and dermatology. Arthritis Rheum 59:338–344

Kreuter A, Gaifullina R, Tigges C, Kirschke J, Altmeyer A, Gambichler T (2009). Lupus erythema-tosus tumidus: response to antimalarial treatment in 36 patients with emphasis on smoking. Arch Dermatol 145:244–8,

Kuhn A, Sonntag M, Richter-Hintz D, Oslislo C, Megahed M, Ruzicka T, Lehmann P (2001) Pho-totesting in lupus erythematosus: a 15-year experience. J Am Acad Dermatol 45:86–95

Kuhn A, Specker C, Ruzicka T, Lehmann P (2002) Methotrexate treatment for refractory subacute cutaneous lupus erythematosus. J Am Acad Dermatol 46:600–603

Kuhn A, Sonntag M, Ruzicka T, Lehmann P, Megahed M (2003) Histopathologic findings in lupus erythematosus tumidus: review of 80 patients. J Am Acad Dermatol 48:901–908

Kuhn A, Beissert S (2005). Photosensitivity in lupus erythematosus. Autoimmunity. 38:519–29

Kuhn A, Herrmann M, Kleber S, Beckmann-Welle M, Fehsel K, Martin-Villalba A, Lehmann P, Ruzicka T, Krammer PH, Kolb-Bachofen V (2006) Accumulation of apoptotic cells in the epi-dermis of patients with cutaneous lupus erythematosus after ultraviolet irradiation. Arthritis Rheum 54:939–50

Kuhn A, Sticherling M, Bonsmann G (2007) Clinical manifestations of cutaneous lupus erythema-tosus. J Deutsch Dermatol Ges 5:1124–40

Kuhn A, Bijl M (2008) Pathogenesis of cutaneous lupus erythematosus. Lupus. 17:389–93

Kuhn A, Bein D, Bonsmann G (2009) The 100th anniversary of lupus erythematosus tumidus. Autoimmun Rev 8:441–8

Kundig TM, Trueb RM, Krasovec M (1997) Lupus profundus/panniculitis. Dermatology 195:99–101

Kyriakis KP, Kontochristopoulos GJ, Panteleos DN (2000) Experience with low-dose thalidomide therapy in chronic discoid lupus erythematosus. Int J Dermatol 39:218–222

Lateef A, Petri M (2010) Biologics in the treatment of systemic lupus erythematosus. Curr Opin Rheumatol 22:504–9

Lee HJ, Sinha AA (2006) Cutaneous lupus erythematosus: understanding of clinical features, genetic basis, and pathobiology of disease guides therapeutic strategies. Autoimmunity 39:433–444

Lesiak A, Narbutt J, Kobos J, Kordek R, Sysa-Jedrzejowska A, Norval M, Wozniacka A (2009) Systematic administration of chloroquine in discoid lupus erythematosus reduces skin lesions via inhibition of angiogenesis. Clin Exp Dermatol 34:570–5

Magro CM, Crowson AN, Harrist TJ (1996) The use of antibody to C5b-9 in the subclassification of lupus erythematosus. Br J Dermatol 134:855–862

Marks R (1995) Lichen planus and cutaneous lupus erythematosus. in: Lowe N, Marks R (eds) Retinoids. A clinician's guide. Martin Dunitz, London, pp 113–117

Martens PB, Moder KG, Ahmed I (1999) Lupus panniculitis: clinical perspectives from a case series. J Rheumatol 26:68–72

Massone C, Kodama K, Salmhofer W, Abe R, Shimizu H, Parodi A, Kerl H, Cerroni L (2005) Lupus erythemtaosus panniculitis (lupus profundus): clinical, histopathological and molecular analysis of nine cases. J Cutan Pathol 32:396–404

McCauliffe DP (1998) Distinguishing subacute cutaneous from other types of lupus erythematosus. Lancet 351:1527–1528

Millard TP, Hawk JLM (2001) Ultraviolet therapy in lupus. Lupus 10:185–187

Mok CC (2007) Mycophenolate mofetil for non-renal manifestations of systemic lupus erythematosus: a systematic review. Scand J Rheumatol 36:329–337

Molin L (1999) Discoid lupus erythematosus lesions treated with cryosurgery. Adv Exp Med Biol 455:375–376

Mond CB, Peterson MG, Rothfield NF (1989) Correlation of anti-Ro antibody with photosensitivity rash in systemic lupus erythematosus patients. Arthritis Rheum 32:202–204

Nousari HC, Kimyai-Asadi A, Provost TT (1999) Generalized lupus erythematosus profundus in a patient with genetic partial deficiency of C4. J Am Acad Dermatol 41:362–364

Nunez M, Boixeda P, Miralles ES, de Misa RF, Ledo A (1996) Pulsed dye laser treatment of teleangiectatic chronic erythema of cutaneous lupus erythematosus. Arch Dermatol 132:354–355

Nurnberg W, Algermissen B, Hermes B, Henz BM, Kolde G (1996) Erfolgreiche Behandlung des chronisch-diskoiden Lupus erythematodes mit dem Argon Laser. Hautarzt 47:767–770

Obermoser G, Schwingshackl P, Weber F, Stanarevic G, Zelger B, Romani N, Sepp N (2009). Recruitment of plasmacytoid dendritic cells in ultraviolet irradiation-induced lupus erythematosus tumidus. Br J Dermatol 160(1):197–200, 2009

Ochsendorf FR (2004) Antimalarials. In: Kuhn A, Lehmann P, Ruzicka T, editors. *Cutaneous lupus erythematosus*. Heidelberg: Springer; p. 347–72.

Oke V, Vassilaki I, Espinosa A, Strandberg L, Kuchroo VK, Nyberg F, Wahren-Herlenius M (2009) High Ro52 expression in spontaneous and UV-induced cutaneous inflammation. J Invest Dermatol 129:2000–10.

Ordi J, Cortes F, Martinez N, Mauri M, De Torres I, Vilardell M (1998) Thalidomide induces amenorrhea in patients with lupus disease. Arthritis Rheum 41:2273–2275

Ordi-Ros J, Cortes F, Cucurull E, Mauri M, Bujan S, Vilardell M (2000) Thalidomide in the treatment of cutaneous lupus refractory to conventional therapy. J Rheumatol 27:1429–1433

Parodi A, Rebora A (1997) ARA and EADV criteria for classification of systemic lupus erythematosus in patients with cutaneous lupus erythematosus. Dermatology 194:217–220

Parodi A, Massone C, Cacciapuoti M, Aragone MG, Bondavalli P, Cattarini G, Rebora A (2000) Measuring the activity of the disease in patients with cutaneous lupus erythematosus. Br J Dermatol 142:457–460

Patel PP, Werth V (2002) Cutaneous lupus erythematosus: a review. Dermatol Clin 20:373–385

Pelle MT (2006) Issues and advances in the management and pathogenesis of cutaneous lupus erythematosus. Adv Dermatol 22:55–65

Penso-Assathiany D, Cribier B, Petit A, Wolkenstein P, Consoli S; pour le groupe d'éthique de la Sociètè francaise de dermatologie (2010) [How far can we go in diseases that make life difficult: the example of disfiguring dermatoses] Ann Dermatol Venerol 137:72–7

Perniciaro C, Randle HW, Perry HO (1995) Hypertrophic discoid lupus erythematosus resembling squamous cell carcinoma. Dermatol Surg 21:255–257

Prinz JC, Meurer M, Reiter C, Rieber EP, Plewig G, Riethmuller G (1996) Treatment of severe cutaneous lupus erythematosus with a chimeric CD4 monoclonal antibody, cM-T412. J Am Acad Dermatol 34:244–252

Provost TT, Watson R, Simmons-O'Brien E (1996) Significance of the anti-Ro (SS-A) antibody in evaluation of patients with cutaneous manifestations of a connective tissue disease. J Am Acad Dermatol 35:147–169

Provost TT (2004) Nonspecific cutaneous manifestations of systemic lupus erythematosus. In: Kuhn A, Lehmann P, Ruzicka T, editors. *Cutaneous lupus erythematosus.* Heidelberg: Springer. p. 93–106

Reich A, Meurer M, Viehweg A, Muller DJ (2009) Narrow-band UVB-induced externalization of selected nuclear antigens in keratinocytes: implications for lupus erythematosus pathogenesis. Photochem Photobiol 85:1–7

Renner R, Sticherling M (2009). The different faces of cutaneous lupus erythematosus. G Ital Dermatol Venereol 144:135–47

Richter HI, Krutmann J, Goerz G (1998) Extrakorporale Photopherese bei therapie-refraktärem disseminiertem diskoiden Lupus erythematodes. Hautarzt 49:487–491

Rothfield N, Sontheimer RD, Bernstein M (2006) Lupus erythematosus: systemic and cutaneous manifestations. Clin Dermatol 24:348–62

Ruffatti A, Veller-Fornasa C, Patrassi GM, Sartori E, Tonello M, Tonetto S, Peserico A, Todesco S (1995) Anticardiolipin antibodies and antiphospholipid syndrome in chronic discoid lupus erythematosus. Clin Rheumatol 14:402–404

Ruiz H, Sanchez JL (1999) Tumid lupus erythematosus. Am J Dermatopathol 21:356–360

Rupec RA, Petropoulou T, Belohradsky BH, Walchner M, Liese JG, Plewing G, Messer G (2000) Lupus erythematosus tumidus and chronic discoid lupus erythematosus in carriers of X-linked chronic granulomatous disease. Eur J Dermatol 10:184–189

Sabbagh N, Delaporte E, Marez D, Lo-Guidice JM, Piette F, Broly F (1997) NAT2 genotyping and efficacy of sulfasalazine in patients with chronic discoid lupus erythematosus. Pharmacogenetics 7:131–135

Sárdy M, Ruzicka T, Kuhn A (2009). Topical calcineurin inhibitors in cutaneous lupus erythematosus. Arch Dermatol Res 301:93–8

Saeki Y, Ohshima S, Kurimoto I, Miura H, Suemura M (2000) Maintaining remission of lupus erythematosus profundus (LEP) with cyclosporin A. Lupus 9:390–392

Schmitt V, Meuth AM, Amler S, Kuehn E, Haust M, Messer G, Bekou V, Sauerland C, Metze D, Köpcke W, Bonsmann G, Kuhn A (2010) Lupus erythematosus tumidus is a separate subtype of cutaneous lupus erythematosus. Br J Dermatol 162:64–73

Sonntag M, Lehmann P, Megahed M, Ruzicka T, Kuhn A (2003) Papulonodular mucinosis associated with subacute cutaneous lupus erythematosus. Dermatology 206:326–329

Sontheimer RD, Bergstresser PR (1982) Epidermal Langerhans cell involvement in cutaneous lupus erythematosus. J Invest Dermatol 79:237–243

Sontheimer RD (2009). Lichenoid tissue reaction / interface dermatitis: clinical and histological perspectives. J Invest Dermatol 129:1088–99

Stein LF, Saed GM, Fivenson DP (1997) T-cell cytokine network in cutaneous lupus erythematosus. J Am Acad Dermatol 36:191–196

Sticherling M., Bonsmann G., Kuhn A (2008).: Cutaneous lupus erythematosus – diagnostics and therapy. JDDG 6:48–61 (2008)

Sticherling M (2010) Update on the use of topical calcineurin inhibitors in cutaneous lupus erythematosus. Biologics: Targets & Therapy (in press)

Su WP, Perniciaro C, Rogers RS 3rd, White JW Jr (1994) Chilblain lupus erythematosus (lupus pernio): clinical review of the Mayo Clinic experience and proposal of diagnostic criteria. Cutis 54:395–399

Talbot JH (1993) Historical background of discoid and systemic lupus erythematosus. In: Wallace DJ, Hahn BH (eds) Dubois' Lupus Erythematosus. 4th ed. Lea and Fiebiger, Philadelphia, pp 3–12

Tan EM, Cohen AS, Fries JF, Masi AT, McShane DJ, Rothfield NF, Schaller JG, Talal N, Winchester RJ (1982) The 1982 revised criteria for the classification of systemic lupus erythematosus. Arthritis Rheum 25:1271–1277

Tan EM (1994) Autoimmunity and apoptosis. J Exp Med 179:1083–1086

Tebbe B, Mansmann U, Wollina U, Auer-Grumbach P, Licht-Mbalyohere A, Arensmeier M, Orfanos CE (1997) Markers in cutaneous lupus erythematosus indicating systemic involvement. A multicenter study on 296 patients. Acta Derm Venereol 77:305–308

Thivolet J, Nicolas JF, Kanitakis J, Lyonnet S, Chouvet B (1990) Recombinant interferon alpha 2a is effective in the treatment of discoid and subacute cutaneous lupus erythematosus. Br J Dermatol 122:405–409

Ting WW, Sontheimer RD (2001) Local therapy for cutaneous and systemic lupus erythematosus: practical and theoretical considerations. Lupus 10:171–184

Ueki H (2005) Koebner phenomenon in lupus erythematosus with special consideration of clinical findings. Autoimmunity Reviews 4:219–223

Uy HS, Pineda R 2nd, Shore JW, Polcharoen W, Jakobiec FA, Foster CS (1999) Hypertrophic discoid lupus erythematosus of the conjunctiva. Am J Ophthalmol 127:604–605

Volc-Platzer B, Anegg B, Milota S, Pickl W, Fischer G (1993) Accumulation of gamma delta T cells in chronic cutaneous lupus erythematosus. J Invest Dermatol 100:84S–91S

Walker SL, Harland CC (2000) Carbon dioxide laser resurfacing of facial scarring secondary to chronic discoid lupus erythematosus. Br J Dermatol 143:1101–1102

Wallace DJ (2002) Management of lupus erythematosus: recent insights. Curr Opin Rheumatol 14:212–219

Warren KJ, Nopper AJ, Crosby DL (1998) Thalidomide for recalcitrant discoid lesions in a patient with systemic lupus erythematosus. J Am Acad Dermatol 39:293–295

Watanabe T, Tsuchida T (1996) Lupus erythematosus profundus: a cutaneous marker for a distinct clinical subset? Br J Dermatol 134:123–125

Watanabe T, Tsuchida T, Ito Y, Kanda N, Ueda Y, Tamaki K (1997) Annular erythema associated with lupus erythematosus/Sjogren's syndrome. J Am Acad Dermatol 36:214–218

Wenzel J, Zahn S, Bieber T, Tüting T (2009) Type I interferon-associated cytotoxic inflammation in cutaneous lupus erythematosus. Arch Dermatol Res. 301:83–6

Williams WL, Ramos-Caro FA (1999) Acute periorbital mucinosis in discoid lupus erythematosus. J Am Acad Dermatol 41:871–873

Wollina U, Looks A (1999) Extracorporeal photochemotherapy in cutaneous lupus erythematosus. J Eur Acad Dermatol Venereol 13:127–130

Wozel G (1996) Dapson – Pharmakologie, Wirkmechanismus und klinischer Einsatz. Thieme Stuttgart, New York 1996

Lupus Erythematosus

5.2 Subacute Cutaneous and Systemic Lupus Erythematosus

5

Donna M. Pellowski, Jane E. Kihslinger, and Richard D. Sontheimer

Definition and Classification

Lupus erythematosus (LE) is a polyclonal T and B lymphocyte autoimmune disease thought to result from a complex interplay of genetic and environmental factors. Clinical expression of LE ranges in continuum from minor cutaneous lesions to life-threatening vital organ dysfunction. Throughout this continuum skin manifestations are variable and common. In 1981 Gilliam and Sontheimer developed a classification system that divides lesions into LE specific and LE non-specific cutaneous disease. LE specific cutaneous disease includes three clinically, immunologically and genetically distinct disorders: acute cutaneous LE (ACLE), subacute cutaneous LE (SCLE) and chronic cutaneous LE (CCLE). Histopathological differentiation between especially the first two disorders can be difficult.

This chapter focuses on the clinical features of SCLE and its management. SCLE is clinically characterized by nonscarring, nonindurated, erythematous, papulosquamous and / or annular skin lesions occurring in a symmetric, photodistributed pattern. Patients with SCLE tend to exhibit milder systemic symptoms than those with unselected systemic LE (SLE). Although not mandatory for diagnosis, the majority of SCLE patients produce anti-Ro / SSA autoantibodies.

Epidemiology

SCLE patients comprise approximately 3–32% of worldwide LE populations with the lowest reported rates in Korean and Chinese populations (Sontheimer, 1989; Tebbe and Orfanos, 1997; Lee, 1998). SCLE is most frequent in young to middle-aged Caucasian females, but it can occur at any age and onset over age 60 years is possible (Chlebus et al., 1998). Seventy percent of the original SCLE cohort reported by Sontheimer et al. (1979) was female with a mean age of onset of 43.3 years and a range of 16–67 years. Eighty-five percent of the initial SCLE cohorts was Caucasian and 15% was African American or Hispanic, whereas the latter two groups comprised approximately 50% of the regional populations (Sontheimer et al., 1979). Other authors have reported similar demographic data (Callan and Klein, 1988, Black et al., 2002). There have been five case reports of SCLE occurring in children 18 months to 9 years old (Buckley and Barnes, 1995, Siamopoulou-Mavridou et al., 1989, Parodi et al., 2000, Ciconte et al., 2002, Amato et al., 2003).

Etiology and Pathomechanisms

Programmed epidermal keratinocyte death in association with a lymphohistiocytic infiltrate is a hallmark histopathological feature of -LE specific skin disease. Abnormally high rates of epidermal keratinocyte apoptosis occurs in patient with cutaneous LE when exposed to a precipitating environmental stressors such as ultraviolet light (Orteu et al., 2001). Abnormal exposure of autoantigens associated with apoptosis occurring within in a pro-inflammatory environment is thought to result in loss of immunological tolerance to such autoantigens. Cytokines, cytotoxic drugs, cytotoxic T cells and UV light can induce keratinocyte apoptosis (Millard and McGregor, 2001). Apoptotic keratinocytes undergo programmed intracellular proteolysis and present Ro autoantigen, DNA, ribonucleoproteins, and calreticulin on surface membrane blebs as they disintegrate. (Millard and McGregor, 2001; Racila et al., 2003). It has been proposed that anti-Ro / SSA and anti-La / SSB may bind to exposed autoantigen resulting in complement-mediated lysis or antibody-dependent cell-mediated cytotoxicity (ADCC) and cytotoxic T lymphocytes can induce keratinocyte lysis causing further release of epidermal cytokines. Partial / relative C1q deficiency may inhibit clearance of apoptotic debris and may lead to increased autoantibody production (Racila et al., 2003). The TNF-α G-308A polymorphism can lead to increased apoptosis and leukocyte migration into the skin and may promote the inflammatory pathway of apoptotic debris clearance. Inducible nitric oxide synthases in endothelial cells and keratinocytes may also be associated with dysregulated keratinocyte apoptosis and inflammation, but its role in the pathogenesis of photosensitive LE remains unclear (Orteu et al., 2001). Expression of the adhesion molecules ICAM-1, VCAM-1, E-selectin, and P-selectin is increased in cutaneous endothelial cells of CLE patients (Kuhn et al., 2002a). Local T-cell and endothelial activation are possibly involved in the persistence and extension of lesions (Norris, 1993). (Fig. 1 and Fig. 2).

Immunogenetics

The earliest immunogenetic studies on SCLE patients suggested an association with several HLA class II phenotypes. HLA-DR3, a phenotype found in 25% of Caucasians in the US (Ahearn et al., 1982), was reported in some studies in at least half of SCLE patients (Sontheimer, 1989; Vasquez-Doval et al., 1992), while others reported a lower frequency (Callen and Klein, 1988; Drosos et al., 1990; Cohen and Crosby, 1994). HLA-DR3 expression has been associated with annular more than papulosquamous SCLE lesions

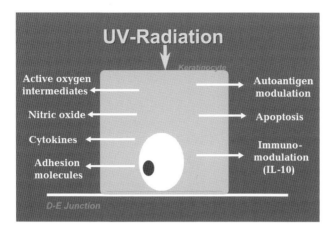

Fig. 1. Potential factors involved in the pathogenesis of UV-induced cutaneous LE

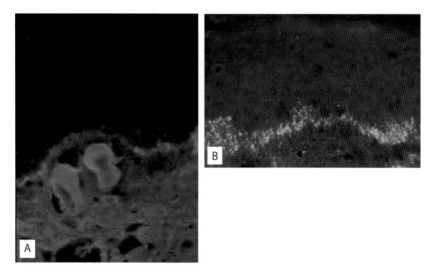

Fig. 2. Cutaneous immune phenomena in lupus erythematosus.
Apoptotic epidermal keratinocytes (Cytoid bodies) underneath the dermo-epidermal base-ment membrane (A) and deposits of polyclonal immunoglobulins along the dermo-epider-mal basement membrane (B)

(Sontheimer et al., 1982; Herrero et al., 1988) and HLA class II phenotype expression has been even more closely associated with autoantibody production than with skin changes (Watson et al., 1991). HLA-DR3 and HLA-DR2 were first associated with the presence of anti-Ro/SSA antibody (Bell and Madisson, 1980; Sontheimer et al., 1982; Watson et al., 1991), and subsequent work revealed that DQ alleles are the most frequent class II al-leles associated with anti-Ro/SSA (Maddison, 1999). Very high levels of anti-Ro/SSA pro-duction have been associated with the extended haplotype HLA-B8, DR3, DRw6, DQ2, DRw52 (Harley et al., 1986). (Fig 3).

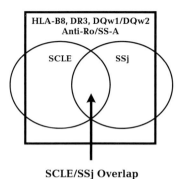

Fig. 3. Suggested algorithm for prescribing systemic medications in SCLE

SCLE/SSj Overlap

5

A distinct extended haplotype called the "high human immune responder" 8.1 ancestral haplotype (A*01, B*08, DRB1*0301, DQB1*0201, TNFAB*a2b3, C2*C) has also been
linked with anti-Ro / SSA production (Price et al., 1999, Lio et al., 2001). Located on human
chromosome 6, the 8.1 ancestral haplotype is in linkage disequilibrium with the gene for
tumor necrosis factor-alpha (TNF-α), an important proinflammatory mediator of the cutaneous innate immune response. A single nucleotide polymorphism in the promoter region of TNF-α, G-308A, has been found to be associated with the SCLE phenotype (Werth
et al., 2000, Millard et al., 2001a). Following exposure to UVB radiation in the presence of
IL-1α, this promoter polymorphism produced exaggerated levels of TNF-α in human keratinocytes, which may have a priming effect on the adaptive component of the LE autoimmune response (Werth et al., 2000).

Inherited deficiencies of C1q, C2, C3, and C4 complement have also been associated
with SCLE (Callen et al., 1987; Johansson-Stephansson et al., 1989; M van Hees et al., 1992).
It has been shown that homozygous complete congenital deficiency of C1q is the strongest single genetic risk factor yet identified for the development of SLE (Korb and Ahearn,
1997, Fishelson et al., 2001, Topaloglu et al., 2000, Walport et al., 1998, Barilla-LaBarca
and Atkinson, 2000). Approximately 93% of individuals with a congenital C1q deficiency
have developed early onset severe SLE with photosensitive cutaneous forms of LE among
the most common disease presentation. Racila et al. (2003) recently reported a highly significant association between a C1q coding region single nucleotide polymorphism (SNP),
C1QA-Gly70GGA, and the SCLE phenotype. This SNP does not encode a different amino
acid, but may alter C1q expression through an alternative splicing mechanism. Its presence
correlates inversely with serum levels of C1q antigenic protein in SCLE patients. Since C1q
binds calreticulin and is involved in clearance of cellular debris, C1q deficiency may result
in decreased clearance of immunogenic material (Racila et al., 2003).

Environmental Factors

Photosensitivity. Photosensitivity is seen in the majority of SCLE patients. UV light can induce the release of inflammatory mediators such as IL-1, TNF-α, IL-10 and oxygen free

Table 1. Medications that may induce SCLE lesions

Diuretics	Thiazides	Antimicrobials	Griseofulvin
	Spironolactone		Terbinafine
Calcium Channel Blockers	Diltiazem	Antihistamines	Cinnarizine/
	Verapamil		Thiethylperazine
	Nifedipine		
	Nitrendipine		
ACE inhibitors	Captopril	Sulfonylureas	Glyburide
	Cilazapril		
Acid Blockers	Ranitidine	Chemotherapy	Taxotere
	Omeprazole		
NSAIDS	Naproxen	Others	Interferon beta-1a
	Piroxicam		Interferon alfa
			Etanercept
			Phenytoin
Beta Blocker	Oxprenolol		Procainamide
			d-penicillamine
Lipid-lowering	Pravastatin		Psoralen-UVA
	Simvastatin		Insecticides

radicals at the level of the epidermis and dermis. In addition to natural light, cutaneous LE lesions have been provoked by exposure to psoralen with UVA (Dowdy et al., 1989; McGrath et al., 1990), UVB via unshielded fluorescent light (Rihner and McGrath, 1992; Kuhn et al., 2001), radiation therapy (Balabanova et al., 1997), and even photocopier light (Klein et al., 1995). In addition, many drugs which have been reported to induce SCLE lesions often have photosensitization as a side effect of their use. Several researchers have used standardized phototesting protocols which involve exposing specific patches of skin to precise amounts of UVR or natural light in order to demonstrate photosensitivity in these patients (Sanders et al., 2003; as reviewed in Kuhn et al., 2001). One such study was able to diagnose photosensitivity in 100% of SCLE patients despite the use of steroids, antimalarials, or methotrexate in several patients tested (Sanders et al., 2003). Their testing also demonstrated that the majority of skin reactions appeared after more than a 1-week delay, which the authors postulated, could explain why many patients who reported a negative history of photosensitivity were found to have a positive phototest. This evidence reaffirmed the need to encourage all SCLE patients to use photoprotective measures despite history.

Drugs. Several drugs are associated with the induction of SCLE lesions (Table 1). Thiazide diuretics (Reed et al., 1985; Fine, 1989; Parodi et al., 1989; Brown and Deng, 1995), calcium channel blockers (Crowson and Magro, 1997; Gubinelli et al., 2003; Marzano et al., 2003a) and angiotensin-converting enzyme (ACE) inhibitors (Patri et al., 1985; Fernan-

dez-Diaz et al., 1995) have most commonly been reported. Others include spironolactone (Leroy et al., 1987), interferon beta-1a (Nousari et al., 1998), procainamide (Sheretz,
1988), d-penicillamine (Sontheimer, 1989), sulfonylureas (Sontheimer, 1989), terbinafine
(Brooke et al., 1998; Callen et al., 2001; Bonsmann et al., 2001), oxprenolol (Gange and
Levene, 1979), griseofulvin (Miyogawa et al., 1994), naproxen (Parodi et al., 1992), piroxicam (Roura et al., 1991), phenytoin (Ross et al., 2002), etanercept (Bleumink et al., 2001)
and PUVA (McGrath et al., 1990). The combination of the antihistamines cinnarizine and
thiethylperazine was cited as the cause of annular SCLE lesions in one patient (Toll et al.,
1998). Personal anecdotal experience has suggested acid inhibitors such as omeprazole and
ranitidine may also be a trigger for SCLE (RDS). Some hypothesize that hormones play a
significant enough role in SCLE and that it may be reasonable to recommend that cutaneous LE patients avoid estrogen-containing contraceptives (Tebbe and Orfanos, 1997).
However, no cases of SCLE have been reported as a result of oral estrogen use. A recent retrospective study showed an association between certain medications and the onset of disease in 15 of 70 patients with Ro positive cutaneous lupus (Srivastava et al., 2003). Antihy-
pertensives were most commonly identified as possible triggers, in addition to statins, interferon alfa, and interferon beta. In that review, clinical disease began between 4 and 20
weeks, and improved 6–12 weeks after discontinuation of the offending drug.

Drug-induced SCLE should be differentiated from classical drug-induced SLE. The former is associated with Ro / SSA autoantibodies and a characteristic photodistributed rash,
whereas the latter is dominated by histone autoantibodies and systemic symptoms such as
fever, arthritis, myalgias, and serositis (Brogan and Olsen, 2003). A lupus-specific skin rash
is rarely present in the drug-induced form of SLE, and is much more commonly seen in
idiopathic SLE (Rubin, 2002). The medications which typically trigger SCLE (Table 1) are
distinct from those that trigger classical SLE (e. g., hydralazine, procainamide, isoniazid,
minocycline, sulfasalazine, etanercept), with exceptions, probably reflecting different underlying disease mechanisms.

Cutaneous Manifestations

Before Gilliam and Sontheimer classified it as a distinct entity, lesions of SCLE were referred to with varied nomenclature including symmetric erythema centrifugum, disseminated DLE, autoimmune annular erythema, subacute disseminated LE, superficial disseminated LE, psoriasiform LE, pityriasiform LE, and maculopapular photosensitive LE
(Sontheimer et al., 1979). (Fig 4).

Cutaneous lesions of SCLE typically begin with red macules or papules which evolve
into psoriasiform and / or annular plaques on sun-exposed skin, characteristically the
shoulders, upper back, extensor arms, V of the lower neck and upper chest, and back of
the neck. The face is less commonly affected. Annular lesions tend to expand with central
clearing and trailing scale. When active inflammation resolves, hypopigmentation is common, especially in the inactive centers of annular lesions. In Sontheimer's original cohort
half presented with predominantly papulosquamous and half were predominantly annular

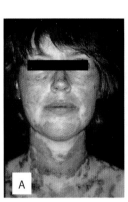
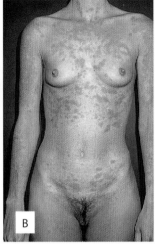
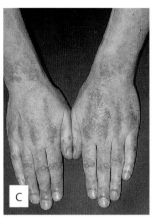

Fig. 4. Subacute lupus erythematosus: Volatile erythemato-papular exanthem of the entire integument. Predilection sites are the UV-exposed skin areas (A, C).

lesions. Parodi reported similar findings (Parodi et al., 2000), whereas some cohorts have had a majority of annular lesions (Herrero et al., 1988; Chlebus et al., 1998; Black et al., 2002) and some have had a majority of papulosquamous lesions (Molad et al., 1987; Callen and Klein, 1988; Cohen and Crosby, 1994).

Atypical presentations of SCLE occur, including vesiculo-bullous forms. Well before the classification of SCLE as a subset of LE, Rowell et al. (1963), described EM-like (erythema multiforme) lesions in four so-called DLE patients who had a speckled ANA, rheumatoid factor and precipitating antibodies to the saline extract of human tissues (anti-Sj-T). Whereas EM and DLE can coexist, it has been suggested that Rowell's syndrome should now be reclassified as SCLE (Roustan et al., 2000). Lyon et al. (1998) reported two cases of delayed diagnosis of SCLE because of the clinical and histologic similarities between SCLE and EM. Additional cases of EM-like SCLE lesions have been reported (Massone et al., 2000). In one patient the lesions developed changes similar to toxic epidermal necrolysis (Bielsa et al., 1987). Marginal vesicles were clinically evident in 38% of annular SCLE lesions that Herrero et al. observed (1988).

Rarer presentations of SCLE have also been reported including a morbilliform exanthem (Sontheimer, 1985), exfoliative erythroderma (DeSpain and Clark, 1988; Parodi et al., 2000), pityriasiform lesions (Sontheimer, 1989; Parodi et al., 2000; Caproni et al., 2001), peculiar acral annular plaques (Scheinman, 1994), progressive generalized poikiloderma (Pramatarov et al., 2000; Marzano et al., 2003b), sunlight induced papulonodular mucinosis (Sonntag et al., 2003), generalized erythroderma with acral bullae preceeding SCLE (Mutasim, 2003) and annular SCLE lesions that were eventually replaced by morphea (Rao et al., 1990).

SCLE patients may have other LE specific skin lesions. Localized ACLE not uncommonly occurs in the setting of SCLE and is characterized by an erythematous, edematous malar rash in a butterfly pattern that usually spares the nasolabial folds (Sontheimer, 1989).

Localized ACLE is usually more transient than SCLE and usually heals without scarring or pigmentary changes. Sontheimer has anecdotally suggested that the individuals who developed ACLE following SCLE might be predisposed to eventually developing findings of SLE such as nephritis (Sontheimer, 1989).

Classical DLE is the most common form of CCLE and may be seen in some SCLE patients. DLE lesions are more common on the scalp and face and have more hypopigmentation, hyperpigmentation, scarring, follicular plugging, and adherent scale than SCLE lesions. Induration was the most important clinical feature differentiating DLE from SCLE lesions (David-Bajar et al., 1992). Lupus panniculitis, often reported in association with DLE, has recently been reported in association with SCLE (Morgan & Callen, 2001).

SCLE patients may also have LE nonspecific skin findings. The most common are diffuse alopecia, mucositis, livedo reticularis, periungual telangiectasias, small vessel vasculitis, Raynaud's phenomenon, cutaneous sclerosis (Sontheimer, 1989), and red lunulae (Wollina et al., 1999). Dystrophic calcinosis cutis (Marzano et al., 1999), multiple HPV-11 cutaneous squamous cell carcinomas (Cohen et al., 1992), and erythema gyratum repens, a rare paraneoplastic eruption (Hochedez et al., 2001), have been case reported.

Systemic Disease

Thirty to 63% of SCLE patients have four or more American College of Rheumatology (ACR) diagnostic criteria for SLE (Sontheimer, 1989; Parodi et al., 2000; Chlebus et al., 1998, Black et al., 2002). Musculoskeletal symptoms such as arthritis and arthralgias are the most common systemic manifestations observed. Overall, most patients with SCLE tend to have mild systemic disease and it appears that isolated joint symptoms are a marker for milder disease. Some authors have reported musculoskeletal symptoms in 100 percent of their SCLE cohorts (Molad et al., 1987; Johansson-Stephansson et al., 1989). Renal and central nervous system (CNS) disease has been seen in 20% or less of SCLE cohorts (Cohen and Crosby, 1994; Sontheimer, 1989; Johansson-Stephansson et al., 1989; Chlebus et al., 1998; Parodi et al., 2000, Black et al., 2002). SCLE cohorts who have nephritis, papulosquamous lesions, high ANAs (> 1:640), or who require high dose immunosuppressive therapy may have a worse prognosis (Sontheimer, 1985, Cohen and Crosby, 1994, Tebbe et al., 1997, Chlebus et al., 1998). Fatalities have rarely been reported in patients with severe systemic manifestations (Sontheimer, 1989; Gunmundsen et al., 1992).

Sjogren's syndrome is the most common autoimmune disease associated with SCLE. The HLA-B8, DR3, DRw6, DQ2, and DRw52 extended haplotype is common to both Sjogren's syndrome and SCLE cohorts (Provost et al., 1988). The association with HLA-DR is probably more related to high circulating Ro / SS-A autoantibodies rather than to SCLE skin lesions. High Ro / SS-A antibody titers have also been associated in Sjogren's and LE patients with HLA-DQw1 / DQw2 (Harley et al., 1986; Hamilton et al., 1988). (Fig. 2). In early studies twelve percent of SCLE cohorts developed Sjogren's syndrome. (Sontheimer et al., 1981). Subsequent studies with longer observation periods have reported the coincidence of Sjogren's syndrome to be as high as 43% (Black et al., 2002). In SCLE patients, the presentation of Sjogren's syndrome may be atypical. Rapidly progressive hypokalemic flaccid tetraparesis caused by a distal renal tubular acidosis was attributed to unrecognized Sjogren's syndrome in an SCLE patient (De Silva et al., 2001). Furthermore, annular erythema of Sjogren's syndrome is considered to be the Asian counterpart of SCLE in white persons. These patients have annular lesions similar to SCLE; however, they lack histopathologic findings at the dermal-epidermal junction of LE. It has been suggested that this is a subset of SCLE and that the relative absence of HLA DR3 in Japanese patients may account for the differences in disease expression (Haimowitz et al., 2000).

Other autoimmune disorders associated with SCLE include rheumatoid arthritis (Cohen et al., 1986; Sontheimer, 1989, Pantoja et al., 2002), autoimmune thyroiditis (Sontheimer, 1989; Ilan and Ben Yahuda, 1991), hereditary angioedema (Gudat and Bork, 1989), and autoimmune polyglandular syndrome type II (Schmidt's syndrome) (Wollina and Schreiber, 2003).

SCLE has been associated with various malignancies and some authors have suggested that SCLE is a paraneoplastic dermatosis (Brenner et al., 1997). Reported malignancies include lung, gastric, breast, uterine and hepatocellular carcinoma (Brenner et al., 1997, Ho et al., 2001), Hodgkin's disease (Castenet et al., 1995), malignant melanoma (Modley et al., 1989), and meningioma (Richardson and Cohen, 2000). The significance of these anecdotal observations remains to be determined and the authors do not routinely screen new SCLE patients for occult malignancy.

SCLE has been associated with a myriad of other diseases. Polymorphic light eruption (PLE), an inherited photosensitivity disorder, has frequently been associated with SCLE and they may have a common genetic predisposition (Millard et al., 2001b). Two-thirds of SCLE cohorts develop PLE and PLE cohorts have an increased relative risk of SCLE (Millard et al., 2001). Case reports of prophyria cutanea tarda (Camp and Davis, 1997), Sweet's syndrome (Goette, 1985), Crohn's disease (Ashworth, 1992), gluten sensitive enteropathy (Messenger and Church, 1986), and X-linked Chronic Granulomatous Disease Carrier Status (Cordoba-Guijarro et al., 2000) have been associated with SCLE. Because of the infrequency of the latter reports, they may be incidental.

Differential Diagnosis

The clinical diagnosis of SCLE is not always obvious. Annular lesions can be confused with erythema annulare centrifugum, granuloma annulare, erythema gyratum repens, autoinvolutive photoexacerbated tinea corporis (Dauden et al., 2001), or EM. Papulosquamous lesions may be confused with photosensitive psoriasis, lichen planus, eczema, pitiryiasis rubra pilaris, disseminated superficial actinic porokeratosis, contact dermatitis, tinea faciei (Meymandi et al., 2003) and dermatomyositis. Lesional photodistribution, characteristic histopathology and Ro / SS-A autoantibodies are useful in distinguishing SCLE from its differential diagnosis.

Table 2. Serological Findings in Patients with SCLE

Serology	Frequency range (percent)
ANA	60–88
Anti-Ro / SS-A	40–82
Anti-La / SS-B	12–71
Anti-dsDNA	1–33
Anti-U1RNP	0–53
Anti-Sm	0–12
Anticardiolipin	10–16
Rheumatoid factor	36–48
VDRL (false positive)	7–33
Antithyroid	18–44
Antilymphoyte	33

Data obtained from Sontheimer et al. (1982); Sontheimer (1989); Johansson-Stephensson et al. (1989); Marschalko et al. (1989); Konstadoulakis et al. (1993); Cohen and Crosby (1994); Chlebus et al. (1998); Parodi et al. (2000); Ng et al. (2000); Wenzel et al. (2000) and Black et al. (2002)

Laboratory Findings

Serology. Whereas various autoantibodies have been found in SCLE cohorts, the Ro / SS-A autoantibody is the characteristic laboratory marker. Anti-Ro / SSA is present in approximately 70% of SCLE cohorts by the classical Ouchterlony double immunodiffusion technique (Sontheimer, 1989; Lee et al., 1994; Chlebus et al., 1998; Parodi et al., 2000) with its frequency ranging from 40–82% depending on the method of assay. ELISA (enzyme-linked immunosorbent assay) has been shown to be the most sensitive test for determining Ro / SS-A autoantibodies (Lee et al., 1994) and is the assay technique currently used in most clinical laboratories in the USA. Anti-Ro / La autoantibodies have to be monitored carefully in affected women of childbearing age since they are considered the primary cause of neonatal LE (Fig 5). Unfortunately, up to 10% of the normal population demonstrate Ro antibodies by such commercial ELISA techniques. Anti-La / SS-B usually occurs with less frequency and is seldom seen in the absence of anti-Ro / SS-A. Anti-nuclear antibody (ANA) tested with human substrate was found in 60–88% of SCLE cohorts and less frequent when animal substrate was used (Callen and Klein, 1988; Herrero et al., 1988; Ng et al., 2000; Reichlin, 2000). Other autoantibodies are present with varying frequencies in SCLE (Table 2).

Miscellaneous laboratory. Particularly if they have concomitant SLE, many SCLE patients have laboratory abnormalities including leukopenia, lymphocytopenia (Wenzel et al., 2002), thrombocytopenia, anemia, elevated erythrocyte sedimentation rate, elevated BUN and creatinine, hypergammaglobulinemia, proteinuria, hematuria, and urine casts.

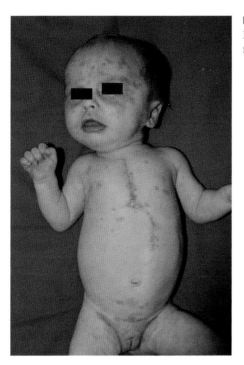

Fig. 5. Neonatal lupus erythematosus: Disseminated erythematous plaques at the face and trunk

Complement levels may be depressed as a result of either genetic deficiency or consumption secondary to immune complex formation.

Histopathology

The histopathologic features of LE specific skin disease include hyperkeratosis, epidermal atrophy, liquifactive vacuolar basal cell degeneration, and nodular perivascular and perifollicular mononuclear cell infiltrates. Some authors have reported degrees of LE specific features among LE subsets. SCLE has more epidermal atrophy, but less hyperkeratosis, basement membrane thickening, follicular plugging and inflammatory cell infiltrates when compared to DLE (David-Bajar and Bangert, 1997; Davis et al., 1984). Since the histologic findings typically mirror the clinical findings, this is expected, and corresponds to the fine less adherent scale, lack of induration and less frequent alopecia of SCLE . Herrero et al. biopsied the border of annular vesicular lesions in a SCLE cohort group with a high frequency of anti-Ro / SSA and the HLA DR3 phenotype (Herrero et al., 1988). Epidermal necrolysis was prominent and the authors suggested this immunophenotype may correlate with the histologic findings. However, other authors have reported variable success in differentiating LE subsets. Bangert et al. (1984) were unable to distinguish the histology between papulosquamous and annular SCLE lesions.

Immunopathology

Lesional skin. Direct immunofluorescence (DIF) is an adjunctive diagnostic test for all subsets of LE. DIF of lesional skin shows immunoglobulins (IgG, IgA, IgM) and complement components in a granular band-like pattern at the epidermal basement membrane (DEJ). In the original cohort (Sontheimer et al., 1979), 40 percent of SCLE patients had a negative DIF. Therefore a positive DIF can help to confirm the diagnosis of LE, but a negative test cannot rule it out.

Nieboer et al. (1988) observed a distinctive "dust-like particle" pattern of IgG deposition near the DEJ of lesional skin in 30% of SCLE patients. Valeski et al. (1992) correlated this pattern with the presence of Ro/SSA autoantibodies. However, Lipsker et al. (1998) retrospectively reviewed 4374 cutaneous DIF specimens and found a dust-like particle pattern in only 66 specimens from 60 individuals. Of those 60 persons 85% had some form of connective tissue disease, 53% had SCLE and 36% had Ro/SSA antibodies. Lipsker et al. concluded that whereas these particles are highly suggestive of connective tissue disease in general, the dust-like pattern is not specific for SCLE. Furthermore, since some investigators have not been able to appreciate this DIF pattern due probably to differences in immunofluorescence microscopy techniques, its meaning remain controversial (David-Bajar and Davis, 1997).

Nonlesional Lupus Band Test (LBT). A 'positive' LBT shows a 'band' of immunoglobulin and complement reactants at the DEJ of nonlesional skin. The diagnostic and prognostic significance of the LBT is the subject of ongoing debate (Sontheimer and Provost, 1996; David-Bajar and Davis, 1997). Twenty-six percent of a SCLE cohort had a positive LBT when sun-protected flexor forearm skin was biopsied (Sontheimer and Gilliam, 1979). When three or more immunoreactants are present in the LBT of sun-protected skin, the diagnostic specificity for SLE is very high (Velthuis et al., 1992) and a positive LBT correlates with a higher risk of lupus nephritis (Davis and Gilliam, 1984). It is unclear if the LBT provides added value to more available, less invasive testing such as serologic assays for double-stranded DNA autoantibodies. The greatest utility of the LBT may be in patients with atypical clinical and laboratory presentations of SLE.

Evaluation and management

Effective management of SCLE patients relies upon adequate baseline evaluation and ongoing surveillance during treatment. The initial history and physical should include a comprehensive review of systems in order to uncover evidence of systemic disease. Additionally, laboratory workup should include a complete blood count with differential, platelet count, erythrocyte sedimentation rate, urinalysis, and blood chemistry profile. In addition to histopathology and ANA, Ro / SS-A autoantibodies, determination of C3, C4 and CH50 may also be helpful depending on clinical symptoms. Follow-up intervals for re-examination and laboratory monitoring should be customized to the individual patient as well as selected treatment modality.

Adequate patient education is essential. Disease-provoking factors such as sunlight, artificial ultraviolet (UV) exposure, photosensitizing drugs and even tobacco use are all modifiable factors, and alteration of these may be of value in the course of the disease. If possible, potentially offending drugs should be eliminated. Initial medical therapy should focus on maximizing local measures before systemic agents are introduced.

Local Therapy

Protection from UV exposure. The importance of avoiding direct sunlight especially during midday hours and summer months should be stressed. A relatively lower danger from UV radiation while outdoors can be realized if one's shadow is longer than one is tall. SCLE patients should also be advised to avoid use of artificial tanning devices. Tightly woven clothing and broad-brimmed hats should be worn when outdoors. Specialty clothing lines which offer maximal UV protection are currently being marketed over the internet for those anticipating prolonged sun exposure. Examples of internet sites include www.sunprecautions.com, www.sunproof.com and www.sunprotectiveclothing.com.

In order to achieve maximal shielding from sunlight, broad spectrum sunscreens should be used in conjunction with photo-protective clothing. Water resistant or waterproof agents that block both UVA and UVB with a sun protection factor (SPF) of 30 or greater should be selected and generously applied. Since it has been shown that the amount of sunscreen that consumers put on is less than that applied under laboratory conditions when determining SPF ratings (Azurdia et al., 1999) it is important to use high SPF products to insure adequate protection under real-life conditions. Additionally, products with Parsol, 1789 (avobenzone), zinc oxide or titanium dioxide provide broad UVA protection, offering a possible added value for SCLE patients (Callen et al., 1991a). Standardized testing to determine the best sunscreen for maximal protection in SCLE patients is needed. Stege et al. (2000) tested 3 commercially available sunscreens via photoprovocative testing with UVA and UVB and showed that while all three sunscreens tested were at least somewhat beneficial, they differed significantly in their abilities to protect against development of skin lesions and against the corresponding upregulation of ICAM-1 in exposed skin. These differences were found in spite of the fact that all 3 contained both Parsol, 1789 and Titanium Dioxide. Sunscreens should be applied 30 min. before sun exposure and reapplied after bathing or significant perspiration. Stick-type sunscreens formulated for the lips may be better tolerated around the eyes than other sun blocking products. UV blocking films such as Llumar® UV Shield™ (www.uv-shield.com) should be placed over home and automobile windows. Plastic films or shields may be applied over fluorescent lighting, which can be a small source of UV irradiation. Corrective camouflage cosmetics such as Dermablend® (www.dermablend.com) and Covermark® (www.covermark.com) offer the dual benefit of being highly effective physical sunscreens as well as aesthetically pleasing cosmetic masking agents which can provide great psychological benefit for these patients.

Topical agents. Superpotent topical class I agents are appropriate initial agents in the management of SCLE. Twice daily application to lesional skin for two weeks followed by a two week rest period is recommended in order to minimize the risk of steroid atrophy and telangiectasia. Intralesional steroids are not as effective in the treatment of SCLE as they are in DLE. Additionally, most SCLE patients have lesions that are too numerous to be managed in this manner. Topical tacrolimus may be of some benefit especially on the face and on skin lesions with less hyperkeratosis (Bohm et al., 2003), without the skin atrophy side effect seen with topical steroids. A speculative review concerning the utility in SCLE of new technology for defecting the stratum corneum barrier has recently been presented (Ting and Sontheimer, 2001). Unfortunately, the majority of patients do not respond adequately to local therapy, and systemic therapy is usually required.

Systemic Therapy

Antimalarials. The aminoquinolone antimalarial agents have been the most efficacious of systemic agents used in the treatment of SCLE and represent first-line systemic therapy (see Fig. 3). Up to 75 percent of patients have responded to one or a combination of drugs within this class (Furner, 1990a). Initial treatment should begin with hydroxychloroquine sulfate not to exceed a dose of 6 mg / kg lean body mass/day. It requires 6–8 weeks to achieve equilibrium blood levels. If an adequate clinical response is achieved, the dose can be decreased to 3 mg / kg lean body mass/day for maintenance for at least one year in order to minimize recurrence. If there is no significant improvement by 2 months, quinacrine hydrochloride 100 mg/day can be added (Feldman et al., 1994). If there is an inadequate response to this combination regimen after 4–6 weeks, chloroquine diphosphate 3 mg / kg lean body mass/day can be substituted for hydroxychloroquine while continuing quinacrine.

A rare, but well-known side effect of the antimalarial agents is retinal toxicity. When using either hydroxychloroquine or chloroquine, ophthalmologic evaluation is required. The current surveillance guidelines recommend follow-up ophthalmologic examination 5 years after an initial baseline exam in uncomplicated individuals on hydroxychloroquine. Complicated individuals (i. e. those who have taken antimalarials for greater than 5 years, those taking larger than recommended daily doses, those with high body fat levels, those greater than 60 years of age, and those with liver or kidney disease) should have yearly screening examinations. (Marmor et al., 2002, Marmor, 2003) Examination should include fundoscopic assessment, visual field testing (including central fields with a red object) and visual acuity testing. The use of an Amsler grid at home may allow early self-detection of visual field defects. This is important since retinal changes may become irreversible if not found early. The risk of retinal toxicity may be minimized if certain daily doses of hydroxychloroquine (6 mg / kg / day) and chloroquine (3 mg / kg / day) are not exceeded (Lanham and Hughes, 1982). Hydroxychloroquine and chloroquine should not be used together because of an enhanced risk of retinal toxicity. Quinacrine has not been shown to cause retinal toxicity. However, it is associated with a higher incidence of side effects than the others, including headaches, gastrointestinal intolerances, hematologic and dermatologic manifestations. Quinacrine is more likely to induce hemolysis in patients who are glucose-6-phosphate dehydrogenase (G6PD) deficient (Trenholme and Carson, 1978).

All of the antimalarials have dermatologic side effects. Blue-black pigmentation of sun-exposed skin, the palatal mucosa and nails has been seen with these agents. They can rarely cause a bleaching of lightly pigmented hair. The antimalarials can also induce a lichenoid hypersensitivity drug reaction in the skin which can be confused with the appearance of true cutaneous LE lesions including SCLE. Thus, if new skin lesions appear in an SCLE patient on antimalarial therapy, one should consider the possibility of a superimposed lichenoid drug reaction. Quinacrine can cause diffuse reversible yellowing of the skin, especially in fair-skinned individuals. Other potential side effects of the antimalarials include hematologic (e. g. bone marrow suppression, aplastic anemia), neuropsychiatric (e. g. toxic psychosis, grand mal seizures), cardiac (e. g. arrhythmias, cardiomyopathy) and muscular. These are less common than in the past, when higher daily dosage regimens of antimalarials were used. Periodic laboratory monitoring of hematological and hepatic function is helpful in identifying any patient who might suffer an idiosyncratic reaction. Johansen and Gran (1998) reported two cases of ototoxicity associated with hydroxychloroquine. Hearing loss has been associated with chloroquine and quinine in the past, but this was the first report of such with hydroxychloroquine.

There is evidence that patients with cutaneous LE who smoke are less likely to respond to antimalarial therapy than nonsmokers (Rahman et al., 1998; Jewell and McCauliffe, 2000). In addition to the well-known dangers of smoking, this represents another reason to strongly encourage tobacco cessation in the SCLE patient. Appropriate referrals should be made if counseling or drug therapy is needed to accomplish this goal.

Thalidomide. Thalidomide is a potent anti-inflammatory agent which acts in part via downregulation of TNF-α, a proinflammatory cytokine which may be involved in the pathogenesis of SCLE as discussed above. Treatment with 50–300 mg / day can be very effective in otherwise-refractory cutaneous LE (Stevens et al., 1997; Georgala et al., 1998; Warren et al., 1998; Duong et al., 1999; Ordi-Ros et al., 2000). In general, about 75 percent of cutaneous LE patients will respond to antimalarial monotherapy or combination therapy. It appears that thalidomide can be effective in 75 percent of antimalarial-refractory cutaneous LE. Because of the high rate (approximately 75 percent) of relapse after withdrawal of the medication, it has been suggested that low maintenance doses for long periods of time may be necessary (Ordi-Ros et al., 2000). Alternatively, other forms of therapy such as antimalarials can be used to maintain thalidomide-induced remissions. Since thalidomide is a potent teratogen, special precautions must be taken when prescribing the drug. Other second-line drugs should be considered in females of child-bearing potential. Thalidomide is available in the United States under the name Thalomid. Physicians and pharmacies are required to register with the manufacturer, the Celgene Corporation. Once registered, Celgene will send the physician specially developed materials (System for Thalidomide Education and Prescribing Safety (STEPS) to educate patients in the prevention of birth defects.

Another important adverse effect of thalidomide is sensory neuropathy, which is sometimes irreversible. Routine clinical assessment for neuropathy is the single most effective means to detect the early development of neuropathy (Duong et al., 1999). Nerve conduction tests are recommended at baseline and periodically during treatment, but the role of these is not well defined. Evidence of neuropathy, by either high clinical suspicion or by electrophysiologic data is an indication to withdraw the drug (Stevens et al., 1997). Other side effects of thalidomide include amenorrhea, drowsiness, weight gain, vomiting, constipation, migraine headaches, and skin eruptions. Some of these side effects are improved on lower daily doses and when the drug is given at bedtime. A case of toxic pustuloderma secondary to thalidomide was reported in a patient with refractory cutaneous LE (Rua-Figueroa et al., 1999). While clear evidence of thrombosis in SCLE patients on thalidomide is lacking, Piette et al. (2002) also warned about the potential thrombotic risk associated with thalidomide therapy. There are known cases of thrombosis in cancer, Bechet's syndrome, and SLE patients including one SCLE patient with antiphospholipid antibodies (Flageul et al., 2000) on thalidomide therapy. The authors emphasized the need for increased surveillence in SCLE patients treated with thalidomide. These concerns are especially valid since SCLE patients often have additional prothrombotic risk factors such as smoking, estrogen-containing contraceptive use, antiphospholipid antibodies, or stopping antimalarial therapy like hydroxychloroquine which has anti-thrombotic properties.

Dapsone. Dapsone (Diaminodiphenylsulfone) has been used successfully in some antimalarial-refractory SCLE cases (McCormack et al., 1984; Holtman et al., 1990; Neri et al., 1999) but overall experience with this agent for cutaneous LE has been disappointing (Sontheimer and Provost, 1996; Callen, 1997). An initial dose of 25 mg twice daily can be increased to 200–300 mg/day as needed. Frequent monitoring is required to evaluate for potential renal, hepatic, and hematologic toxicity, including hemolysis and/or methemoglobinemia that occur especially in patients deficient in G6PD enzyme activity.

Retinoids. The synthetic retinoids, isotretinoin and acitretin, have been shown to significantly improve SCLE lesions in doses of 1/2–1 mg/kg/day (Furner, 1990b; Richardson and Cohen, 2000). Their long-term use may be limited by the potential for teratogenicity, mucocutaneous dryness, photosensitivity, hepatitis, hypertriglyceridemia, mood alteration, psuedotumor cerebri, and bony changes consistent with diffuse idiopathic skeletal hyperostosis (DISH) syndrome.

Clofazimine and Gold. Although these agents have been successfully used in the treatment of refractory cutaneous LE (Costner et al., 2004; Crovato, 1981), they are both limited by their potential for toxic side effects.

Systemic corticosteroids and other immunosuppressive agents. These agents are usually reserved for those patients who have not responded to less toxic therapies. However, they may be needed before an adequate trial of less toxic drugs is completed in those patients with severe disease. Pulsed intravenous methylprednisolone at a dose of 1 g for three consecutive days provided improvement of SCLE patients in the presence of systemic LE (Goldberg and Lidsky, 1984). The side effects of steroids, especially when used over long periods of time are worrisome. They are more appropriately used as adjunctive treatment and tapered off if possible. Steroid-sparing agents that may be of benefit in refractory SCLE include methotrexate (Boehm et al., 1998, Kuhn et al., 2002b), azathioprine (Callen et al., 1991b), cyclosporine, and mycophenolate. Mycophenolate is increasingly being reported as an effective option for refractory SCLE. Hanjani and Nousari (2002) reported one SCLE patient treated with 3 g/day of mycophenolate with complete resolution at 3 months and no flare by 10 months after failing multiple prednisone tapers and antimalarials. Schanz et al. (2002) presented two additional cases of antimalarial, azathioprine, and high dose steroid refractory SCLE which completely resolved within a few weeks on 2 g/day of mycophenolate. In one patient this response was successfully maintained for over 24 months on a lower dose of at least 1 g/day. Mycophenolate offers a lower toxicity profile than some of the other immunosuppressants. A thorough understanding of potentially harmful side effects is imperative with all of these medications, and close monitoring is essential.

Immune regulation. Five patients, including one SCLE patient with refractory cutaneous LE, who received infusions of chimeric CD4 monoclonal antibody showed improvement and became more responsive to conventional treatments (Prinz et al., 1996). Intravenous immunoglobulin may lead to improvement of cutaneous LE lesions (Genereau et al., 1999; Goodfield et al., 2004), but its study and use is limited mostly by cost-prohibitiveness. Recombinant IFN-α 2a, allowed a complete response in two of four SCLE patients (Thivolet et al., 1990). However, the use of IFN-α has also been associated with the induction and/or exacerbation of SCLE (Srivistava et al., 2003) and SLE. Caution should therefore be used in this setting.

Fautrel et al. (2002) reported the resolution of SCLE in a rheumatoid arthritis patient using etanercept, an anti-TNFα recombinant biologic agent. Etanercept and infliximab have both been associated with the development of anti-double-stranded DNA antibodies and a lupus-like syndrome in some RA and Crohn's patients. A small number of case reports suggests the possibility of etanercept-induced SCLE (Bleumink et al., 2001). Thus, there is some concern regarding the induction or unmasking of cutaneous or systemic LE with the use of either of these agents in cutaneous LE. Rituximab (Rituxan), a recombinant monoclonal antibody which inhibits CD20 expressing B cells, has shown efficacy in small numbers of systemic and cutaneous LE patients (Perotta et al., 2002; Kneitz et al., 2002). Finally, other biologic drugs which inhibit antigen presenting cell-T cell interaction are speculated to be of benefit in SCLE, although more study is needed. Some examples include alefacept (Amevive), an inhibitor of the LFA3:CD2 interaction, and efalizumab (Raptiva), an inhibitor of the LFA-1:ICAM-1 interaction.

Other. Two antineoplastic drugs, cyclophosphamide and cytarabine, were beneficial in refractory SCLE (Schulz and Menter, 1971; Yung and Richardson, 1995). Although sulfasalazine, phenytoin, danazol, dehydroepiandrosterone sulfate (DHEAS) and cefuroxime axetil have all been suggested in the treatment of cutaneous lupus, they have not been effectively used by the authors.

Ultraviolet A-1 phototherapy (UVA-1). Finally, it has been suggested that cutaneous lupus patients may benefit from low doses of longer wavelength (340–400 nm) UV irradiation (Sonnichsen et al., 1993; McGrath, 1997). According to McGrath (1997), this modality reduced the need for medication and attenuated autoimmune antibody levels. These results should be interpreted with caution. Conflicting data indicate that UVA, including long wave UVA, may play a role in cutaneous LE (Lehmann et al., 1990; Nived et al., 1993). Additionally, in an SLE murine model, UVA-1 irradiation was associated with increased renal disease and death (Cai et al., 2000).

Prognosis

Because SCLE has been recognized for little over two decades, long-term outcomes of patients are not yet known. Most patients tend to have intermittent recurrent skin lesions without significant disease progression, while some may experience permanent remissions. Approximately 15 percent of patients developed active SLE in the original cohort. More recent studies addressing prognosis have revealed similar findings (Chlebus, 1998). In addition, an informal long-term prospective follow-up study of SCLE patients who presented from 1971–1995 in the Department of Dermatology at UT Southwestern Medical Center in Dallas was initiated by one of the authors (RDS, unpublished observation). To date, 18 of 130 patients have been evaluated. Mean duration of follow-up was 12.6 years. Thirty-nine percent had inactive skin and systemic disease at follow-up. The most common complaints other than skin lesions and photosensitivity were fatigue, arthralgias and Raynaud's phenomenon. In addition, many patients had a subjective history of depression. Lesions were predominantly papulosquamous in this particular population. Facial involvement, hypopigmentation and telangiectasias were common, while true scarring rarely occurred. At least one, and possibly three, out of 130 died of causes related to SLE (pancreatic vasculitis). A larger number of SCLE patients needs to be examined in a prospective study to more firmly establish its course, ANA and Ro / SS-A prevalence, overlap with other connective tissue diseases, as well as prognosis.

Summary

Lupus erythematosus is a multi-organ autoimmune disease which presumably results from a complex interplay of genetic and environmental factors. The clinical phenotype of LE ranges in continuum from minor cutaneous lesions to life-threatening vital multi organ dysfunction. Throughout this continuum, skin manifestations are variable and common. There is a commonly accepted classification system that divides lesions into LE specific and LE non-specific cutaneous disease. LE specific cutaneous disease includes three clinically, immunologically and genetically distinct disorders: acute cutaneous LE (ACLE), subacute cutaneous LE (SCLE) and chronic cutaneous LE (CCLE). Histopathological differentiation between especially the first two disorders can be difficult. SCLE is clinically characterized by non-scarring, non-indurated, erythematous, papulo-squamous and / or annular skin lesions occurring in a symmetric, photodistributed pattern. Patients with SCLE tend to exhibit milder systemic symptoms than those with unselected systemic LE (SLE). Although not mandatory for diagnosis, the majority of SCLE patients produce anti-Ro / SSA autoantibodies. In SLE, musculoskeletal symptoms such as arthritis and arthralgias are the most common systemic manifestations observed. Overall, most patients with SCLE tend to have mild systemic disease and it appears that isolated joint symptoms are a marker for milder disease. The clinical diagnosis of SCLE is not always obvious. Annular lesions can be confused with erythema annulare centrifugum, granuloma annulare, erythema gyratum repens, tinea corporis or erythema multiforme. Lesional photodistribution, characteristic histopathology and Ro / SS-A autoantibodies are useful in distinguishing SCLE from its differential diagnosis. Most SCLE patients tend to have intermittent recurrent skin lesions without significant disease progression, while some may experience permanent remissions. Approximately 15 percent of patients develop active SLE. The most common complaints other than skin lesions and photosensitivity were fatigue, arthralgias and Raynaud's phenomenon. In addition, many patients had a subjective history of depression. The real prognosis of SCLE needs to be evaluated in a larger number of patients to more firmly establish its course, ANA and Ro / SS-A prevalence, overlap with other connective tissue diseases, as well as prognosis.

References

Ahearn JM, Provost TT, Dorsch CA, Stevens MB, Bias WB, Arnett FC (1982) Interrelationships of HLA-DR, MB and MT phenotypes, autoantibody expression, and clinical features in systemic lupus erythematosus. Arthritis Rheum 25:1031–1040

Amato L, Coronella G, Berti S, Moretti S, Fabbri P (2003) Subacute cutaneous lupus erythematosus in childhood. Pediatric Dermatol 20(1):31–4

Ashworth J (1992) Subacute cutaneous lupus erythematosus in a patient with Crohn's disease. Clin Exp Dermatol 17:135–136

Azurdia RM, Pagliaro JA, Diffey BL, Rhodes LE (1999) Sunscreen application by photosensitive patients is inadequate for protection. Br J Dermatol 140:255–258

Balbanova MB, Botev IN, Michailoba JI (1997) Subacute cutaneous lupus erthematosus induced by radiation therapy. Br J Dermatol 137:648–649

Bangert JL, Freeman RG, Sontheimer RD, Gilliam JN (1984) Comparative histopathology of subacute cutaneous lupus erythematosus and discoid lupus erythematosus. Arch Dermatol 120:332

Barilla-LaBarca ML, Atkinson JP (2000) Rheumatic syndromes associated with complement deficiency. Current Opinion in Rheumatol 15:55–60

Bell DA, Maddison PJ (1980) Serologic subsets in systemic lupus erythematosus. Arthritis Rheum 23:1268–1273

Bielsa I, Herrero C, Font J, Mascaro JM (1987) Lupus erythematosus and toxic epidermal necrolysis. J Am Acad Dermatol 16:1265–1267

Black DR, Hornung CA, Schneider PD, Callen JP (2002) Frequency and severity of systemic disease in patients with subacute cutaneous lupus erythematosus. Arch Dermatol 138(9):1175–8

Bleumink GS, ter Borg EJ, Ramselaar CG, Ch Stricker BH (2001) Etanercept-induced subacute cutaneous lupus erythematosus Rheumatology 40(11):1317–9

Boehm IB, Boehm GA, Bauer R (1998) Management of cutaneous lupus erythematosus with low-dose methotrexate: indication for modulation of inflammatory mechanisms. Rheumatol Int 18:59–62

Bohm M, Gaubitz M, Luger TA, Metze D, Bonsmann G (2003) Topical tacrolimus as a therapeutic adjunct in patients with cutaneous lupus erythematosus – A report of three cases. Dermatology 207:381–385

Bonsmann,G., Schiller M, Luger TA, and Stander S (2001) Terbinafine-induced subacute cutaneous lupus erythematosus. Journal of the American Academy of Dermatology 44:925–931

Brenner S, Golan H, Gat A, Bialy-Golan A (1997) Paraneoplastic subacute cutaneous lupus erythematosus: report of a case associated with cancer of the lung. Dermatology 194:172–174

Brogan BL, Olsen NJ (2003) Drug-induced rheumatic syndromes. Curr Opin Rheumatol. 15(1):76–80

Brooke R, Coulson IH, al-Dawoud A (1998) Terbinafine-induced subacute cutaneous lupus erythematosus. Br J Dermatol 139:1132–1133

Brown CW, Jr. and Deng JS (1995) Thiazide diuretics induce cutaneous lupus-like adverse reaction. J Toxicol Clin Toxicol 33:729–733

Buckley D and Barnes L (1995) Childhood subacute cutaneous lupus erythematosus associated with homozygous complement 2 deficiency. Pediatr. Dermatol. 4:327–30

Cai W, Maldonado M, Werth VP (2000) Differential effects of UVA1 and UVB on skin lesions of MRL/lpr lupus mice. (Abstract) J Invest Dermatol 114:884

Callen JP (1997) Management of antimalarial-refaractory cutaneous lupus erythematosus. Lupus 6:203–208

Callen JP, Hodge SJ, Kulick KB, Stelzeer G, Buchino JJ (1987) Subacute cutaneous lupus erythematosus in multiple members of a family with C2 deficiency. Arch Dermatol 123:66–70

Callen JP, Klein J (1988) Subacute cutaneous lupus erythematosus. Clinical, serologic, immunogenetic, and therapeutic considerations in 72 patients. Arthritis Rheum 31:1007–1013

Callen JP, Roth DE, McGrath C, Dromgoole SH (1991a) Safety and efficacy of a broad-spectrum sunscreen in patients with discoid or subacute cutaneous lupus erythematosus. Cutis 47:130–132, 135–136

Callen JP, Spencer LV, Burruss JB, Holtman J (1991b) Azathioprine. An effective, corticosteroid-sparing therapy for patients with recalcitrant cutaneous lupus erythematosus or with recalcitrant cutaneous leukocytoclastic vasculitis. Arch Dermatol 127:515–522

Callen JP, Hughes AP, and Kulp-Shorten C (2001) Subacute cutaneous lupus erythematosus induced or exacerbated by terbinafine – A report of 5 cases. Archives of Dermatology 137:1196–1198

Camp PB, Davis LS (1997) Coexistence of subacute cutaneous lupus erythematosus and porphyria cutanea tarda: a case report [letter; comment]. Cutis 59:216E

Caproni M, Cardinali C, Salvatore E, Fabbri P (2001) Subacute cutaneous lupus erythematosus with pityriasis-like cutaneous manifestations Int J Dermatol 40(1):59–62

Castenet J, Taillan B, Lacour JP, Garnier G, Perrin C, Ortonne JP (1995) Subacute cutaneous lupus erythematosus associated with Hodgkin's disease. Clin Rheumatol 14:692–694

Chlebus E, Wolska H, Blaszczyk M, Jablonska S (1998) Subacute cutaneous lupus erythematosus versus systemic lupus erythematosus – Diagnostic criteria and therapeutic options. J Am Acad Dermatol 38:405–412

Ciconte A, Mills AE, Shipley A, Marks R (2002) Subacute cutaneous lupus erythematosus presenting in a child Australasian J Dermatol 43(1):62–4

Cohen LM, Tyring SK, Rády P, Callen JP (1992) Human papillomavirus type II in multiple squamous cell carcinomas in a patient with subacute cutaneous lupus erythematosus. J Am Acad Dermatol 26 Suppl:840–845

Cohen MR, Crosby D (1994) Systemic disease in subacute cutaneous lupus erythematosus: A controlled comparison with systemic lupus erythematosus. J Rheumatol 21:1665–1669

Cohen S, Stastny P, Sontheimer RD (1986) Concurrence of subacute cutaneous lupus erythematosus and rheumatoid arthritis. Arthritis Rheum 29:421–425

Cordoba-Guijarro S, Feal C, Dauden E, Fraga J, Garcia-Diez A (2000) Lupus erythematosus-like lesions in a carrier of X-linked chronic granulomatous disease J Euro Acad Dermatol & Venereol 14(5):409–11

Costner MI, Provost TT, and Sontheimer RD (2004) Lupus erythematosus. Chapter 2. In, *Cutaneous Manifestations of Rheumatic Diseases*. 2nd edition. Lippincott Williams and Wilkins, Philadelphia

Crowson AN, Magro CM (1997) Subacute cutaneous lupus erythematosus arising in the setting of calcium channel blocker therapy. Human Pathol 28:67–73

Crovato F (1981) Clofazimine in the treatment of annular lupus erythematosus. Arch Dermatol 117:249–250

Dauden E, Bartolome B, Pascual M, Fraga J, Garcia-Diez A (2001) Autoinvolutive photoexacerbated tinea corporis mimicking a subacute cutaneous lupus erythematosus Acta Dermato-Venereologica 81(2):141–2

David-Bajar KM, Bennion SD, DeSpain JD, Golitz LE, Lee LA (1992) The clinical, histologic and immunofluorescent distinctions between subacute cutaneous lupus erythematosus and discoid lupus erythematosus. J Invest Dermatol 99:251–257

David-Bajar KM, Davis BM (1997) Pathology, immunopathology and immunohistochemistry in cutaneous lupus erythematosus. Lupus 6:145–157

Davis BM, Gilliam JN (1984) Prognostic significance of subepidermal immune deposits in uninvolved skin of patients with systemic lupus erythematosus: a 10-year longitudinal study. J Invest Dermatol 83:242–247

De Silva BD, Plant W, Kemmett D (2001) Subacute cutaneous lupus erythematosus and life-threatening hypokalaemic tetraparesis: a rare complication Br J Dermatol 144(3):622–4

DeSpain J, Clark DP (1988) Subacute cutaneous lupus erythematosus presenting as erythroderma. J Am Acad Dermatol 19:388–392

Dowdy MJ, Nigra TP, Barth WF (1989) Subacute cutaneous lupus erthematosus during PUVA therapy for psoriasis: Case report and review of the literature. Arthritis Rheum 32:343–346

Drosos AA, Dimou GS, Siamopoulou-Mavridou A, Hatzis J, Moutsopoulos HM (1990) Subacute cutaneous lupus erythematosus in Greece. A clinical, serological and genetic study. Ann Med Interne (Paris) 141:421–424

Duong DJ, Spigel GT, Moxley RT, Gaspari AA (1999) American experience with low-dose thalidomide therapy for severe cutaneous lupus erythematosus. Arch Dermatol 135:1079–1087

Fautrel B, Foltz V, Frances C, Bourgeois P, Rozenberg S (2002) Regression of subacute cutaneous lupus erythematosus in a patient with rheumatoid arthritis treated with a biologic tumor necrosis factor alpha-blocking agent: comment on the article by Pisetsky and the letter from Aringer et al. Arthritis & Rheumatism 46(5):1408–9

Feldmann R, Salomon D, Saurat J-H (1994) The association of the two antimalarials chloroquine and quinacrine for treatment-resistant chronic and subacute cutaneous lupus erythematosus. Dermatology 189:425–427

Fernandez-Diaz ML, Herranz P, Suarez-Marrero MC, Borbujo J, Manzano R, Casado M (1995) Subacute cutaneous lupus erythematosus associated with cilazapril [letter]. Lancet 345:398

Fine RM (1989) Subacute cutaneous lupus erythematosus associated with hydrochlorothiazide therapy. Int J Dermatol 28:375–376

Fishelson Z, Attali G, Mevorach D (2001) Complement and apoptosis. Molecular Immunol 38:207–219

Flageul B, Wallach D, Cavelier-Balloy B, Bachelez H, Carsuzaa F, Dubertret L (2000) Thalidomide and thrombosis Annales de Dermatologie et de Venereolgie 127(2):171–4

Furner BB (1990a) Treatment of subacute cutaneous lupus erythematosus. Int J Dermatol 29:542–547

Furner BB (1990b) Subacute cutaneous lupus erythematosus response to isotretinoin. Int J Dermatol 29:587–590

Gange KW, Levene GM (1979) A distinctive eruption in patients receiving oxprenolol. Clin Exp Dermatol 4:87–97

Genereau T, Chosidow O, Danel C, Cherin P, Herson S (1999) High-dose intravenous immunoglobulin in cutaneous lupus erythematosus. Arch Dermatol 135:1124–1125

Georgala S, Katoulis AC, Hasapi V, Koumantaki-Mathioudaki E (1998) Thalidomide treatment for hypertrophic lupus erythematosus [letter]. Clin Exp Dermatology. 23:141

Gilliam JN, Sontheimer RD (1981) Distinctive cutaneous subsets in the spectrum of lupus erythematosus. J Am Acad Dermatol 4:471–475

Goette DK (1985) Sweet's syndrome in subacute cutaneous lupus erythematosus. Arch Dermatol 121:789–791

Goldberg JW, Lidsky MD (1984) Pulse methylprednisolone therapy for persistent subacute cutaneous lupus. Arthritis Rheum. 27:837–838

Goodfield M, Davison K, Bowden K (2004) Intravenous immunoglobulin (IVIg) for therapy-resistant cutaneous lupus erythematosus (LE). J Dermatolog Treat. 15(1):46–50

Gubinelli E, Cocuroccia B, and Girolomoni G (2003) Subacute cutaneous lupus erythematosus induced by nifedipine. J Cutan Med Surg. February 10

Gudat W, Bork K (1989) Hereditary angioedema associated with subacute cutaneous lupus erythematosus. Dermatologica 179:211–213

Gundmundsen K, Otridge B, Murphy GM (1992) Fulminant fatal lupus erythematosus. Br J Dermatol 126:303–304

Gupta G, Roberts DT (1999) Pulsed dye laser treatment of subacute cutaneous lupus erythematosus. Clin Exp Dermatol 24:498–499

Haimowitz JE, McCauliffe DP, Seykora J, Werth V (2000) Annular erytherma of Sjogren's syndrome in a white woman. J Am Acad Dermatol 42:1069–1073

Hamilton RG, Harley JB, Bias WB, Roebber M, Reichlin M, Hochberg MC, Arnett FC (1988) Two Ro (SS-A) autoantibody responses in systemic lupus erythematosus. Correlation of HLA-DR/DQ specificities with quantitative expression of Ro (SS-A) autoantibody. Arthritis Rheum 31(4):496–505

Hanjani NM, Nousari CH (2002) Mycophenolate mofetil for the treatment of cutaneous lupus erythematosus with smoldering systemic involvement. Arch Dermatol 138(12):1616–8

Harley JP, Reichlin M, Arnett FC, Alexander EL, Bias WB, Provost TT (1986) Gene interaction at the HLA-DQ locus enhances autoantibody production in primary Sjogren's syndrome. Science 232:1145–1147

Herrero C, Bielsa I, Font J, Lozano F, Ericilla G, Lecha M, Ingelman M, Mascaro JM (1988) Subacute cutaneous lupus erythematosus: Clinical pathologic findings in 13 cases. J Am Acad Dermatol 19:1057–1062

Ho C, Shumack SP, Morris D (2001) Subacute cutaneous lupus erythematosus associated with hepatocellular carcinoma Australasian J Dermatol 42(2):110–3

Hochedez P, Vasseur E, Staroz F, Morelon S, Roudier Pujol C, Saiag P (2001) Subacute cutaneous lupus gyratus repens Annales de Dermatologie et de Venereologie 128(3 Pt1):244–6

Holtman JH, Neustadt DH, Klein J, Callen JP (1990) Dapsone is an effective therapy for the skin lesions of subacute cutaneous lupus erythematosus and urticarial vasculitis in a patient with C2 deficiency. J Rheumatol 17:1222–1225

Ilan Y, Ben Yehuda A (1991) Subacute cutaneous lupus associated with Hashimoto's thyroiditis. Neth J Med 39:105–107

Jewell M, McCauliffe DP (2000) Cutaneous lupus erythematosus patients that smoke are less responsive to antimalarial treatment. J Am Acad Dermatol 42:983–987

Johansen PB, Gran JT (1998) Ototoxicity due to hydroxychloroquine – report of two cases. Clin Exper Rheumatol 16:472–474

Johansson-Stephansson E, Koskimes S, Partanen J, Kariniemi AL (1989) Subacute cutaneous lupus erythematosus: Genetic markers and clinical and immunological findings in patients. Arch Dermatol 125:791–796

Klein LR, Elmets CA, Callen JP (1995) Photoexacerbation of cutaneous lupus erythematosus due to ultraviolet A emissions from a photocopier. Arthritis Rheum 38:1152–1156

Kneitz C, Wilhelm M, Tony HP (2002) Effective B cell depletion with rituximab in the treatment of autoimmune diseases. Immunobiology 206:519–27

Konstadoulakis MM, Kroubouzos G, Tosca A, Piperingos G, Marafelia P, Konstadoulakis M, et al. (1993) Thyroid autoantibodies in the subsets of lupus erythematosus: Correlation with other autoantibodies and thyroid function. Thyroidol Clin Exp 5:1–7

Korb LC, Ahearn JM (1997) C1q binds directly and specifically to surface blebs of apoptotic human keratinocytes – complement deficiency and systemic lupus erythematosus revisited. J Immunol 158:4525–4528

Kuhn A, Sonntag M, Richter-Hintz D, Oslislo C, Megahed M, Ruzicka T, Lehmann P (2001) Phototesting in lupus erythematosus: a 15-year experience. J Am Acad Dermatol 45(1):86–95

Kuhn A, Sonntag M, Lehmann P, Megahed M, Vestweber D, Ruzicka T (2002a) Characterization of the inflammatory infiltrate and expression of endothelial cell adhesion molecules in lupus erythematosus tumidus. Arch Dermatol Res 294:6–13

Kuhn A, Specker C, Ruzicka T, Lehmann P (2002b) Methotrexate treatment for refractory sub-acute cutaneous lupus erythematosus. J Am Acad Dermatol 46(4):600–3

Lanham JG, Hughes GRV (1982) Antimalarial therapy in SLE. Clin Rheumat Disease 8:279–299

Lee LA, Roberts CM, Frank MB, McCubbin VR, Reichlin M (1994) The autoantibody response to Ro / SSA in cutaneous lupus erythematosus. Arch Dermatol 130:1262–1268

Lee CW (1998) Prevalences of subacute cutaneous lupus erythematosus and epidermolysis bullosa acquisita among Korean / Oriental populations. Dermatology 197:187

Lehmann P, Holzle E, Kind P, Goerz G, Plewig G (1990) Experimental reproduction of skin lesions in lupus erythematosus by UVA and UVB radiation [see comments]. J Am Acad Dermatol 22:181–187

Leroy DA, Dompmartin A, Le Jean SGJLMJC, Deschamps P (1987) Toxidermie A L'aldactone a type d'erytheme annulaire centrifuge lupique. Ann Dermatol Venereol 114:1237–1240

Lio D, Candore G, Colombo A, et al. (2001) A genetically determined high setting of TNF-alpha influences immunologic parameters of HLA-B8, DR3 positive subjects: implications for auto-immunity. Hum Immunol 62:705–713

Lipsker D, Dicesare MP, Cribier D, Grosshans E, Heid E (1998) The significance of the 'dust-like particles' pattern of immunofluorescence. Br J Dermatol 138:1039–1042

Lyon CC, Blewitt R, Harrison PV (1998) Subacute cutaneous lupus erythematosus: Two cases of delayed diagnosis. Acta Derm Venereol 78:57–59

M VanHees CL, Boom BW, Vermeer BJ, Daha MR (1992) Subacute cutaneous lupus erythematosus in a patient with inherited deficiency of the third component of complement. Arch Dermatol 128:700–701

Maddison PJ (1999) Nature and nurture in systemic lupus erythematosus. Adv Exp Med Biol 455:7–13

Marmor MF, Carr RE, Easterbrook M, et al. (2002) Recommendations on screening for chloro-quine and hydroxychloroquine retinopathy: a report by the American Academy of Ophthal-mology. Opthalmology 190:1377–82

Marmor, MF (2003) New American Academy of Ophthalmology recommendations on screening for hydroxychloroquine retinopathy. Arthritis and Rheumatism 48:1764

Marschalko M, Dobozy E, Daroczy J, Gyimesi E, Horvath A (1989) Subacute cutanous lupus ery-thematosus: A study of 15 cases. Orvosi Hetilap 130:2623–2628

Marzano AV, Kolesnikova LV, Gasparini G, Alessi E (1999) Dystrophic calcinosis cutis in subacute lupus. Dermatology 198:90–92

Marzano AV, Borghi A, Mercogliano M, Facchetti M, Caputo R (2003a) Nitrendipine-induced sub-acute cutaneous lupus erythematosus. Eur. J. Dermatol. 13:213–216

Marzano AV, Facchetti M, Alessi E (2003b) Poikilodermatous subacute cutaneous lupus erythema-tosus. Dermatology 207(3):285–90

Massone C, Parodi A, Rebora A (2000) Erythema multiforme-like subacute cutaneous lupus ery-thematosus: a new variety? Acta Dermato-Venereologica 80(4):308–9

McCormack LS, Elgart ML, Turner ML (1984) Annular subacute cutaneous lupus erythematosus responsive to Dapsone. J Am Acad Dermatol 11:397–401

McGrath H Jr, Scopelitis E, Nesbitt LT Jr (1990) Subacute cutaneous lupus erythematosus during psoralen ultraviolet A therapy [letter]. Arthritis Rheum 33:302–303

McGrath H (1997) Prospects for UV-A1 therapy as a treatment modality in cutaneous lupus ery-thematosus and systemic LE. Lupus 6:209–217

Messenger AG, Church RE (1986) Subacute cutaneous lupus erythematosus and malabsorption. Br J Dermatol 115 (supplement 30):56–57

Meymandi S, Wiseman MC, Crawford RI (2003) Tinea faciei mimicking cutaneous lupus erythe-matosus: a histopathologic case report. J Am Acad Dermatol 48(2 Suppl): S7–8

Millard TP, McGregor JM (2001) Molecular genetics of cutaneous lupus erythematosus. Clinical and Experimental Dermatol 26:184–91

Millard TP, Kondeatis E, Cox A, Wilson AG, Grabczynska SA, Carey BS, Lewis CM, Khamashta MA, Duff GW, Hughes GR, Hawk JL, Vaughan RW, McGregor JM (2001a) A candidate gene analysis of three related photosensitivity disorders: cutaneous lupus erythematosus, polymorphic light eruption and actinic prurigo Br J Dermatol 145(2):229–36

Millard TP, Kondeatis E, Vaughan RW, Lewis CM, Khamashta MA, Hughes GR, Hawk JL, McGregor JM (2001b) Polymorphic light eruption and the HLA DRB1*0301 extended haplotype are independent risk factors for cutaneous lupus erythematosus. Lupus 10(7):473–9

Miyagawa S, Okuchi T, Shiomi Y, Sakamoto K (1989) Subacute cutaneous lupus erythematosus lesions precipitated by griseofulvin. J Am Acad Dermatol 21:343–346

Modley C, Wood D, Horn T (1989) Metastatic malignant melanoma arising from a common blue nevus in a patient with subacute cutaneous lupus erythematosus. Dermatologica 178:171–175

Molad Y, Weinberger A, David M, Garty B, Wysenbeek AJ, Pinkas J (1987) Clinical manifestations and laboratory data of subacute cutaneous lupus erythematosus. Isr J Med. Sci 23:278–280

Morgan KW, Callen JP (2001) Calcifying lupus panniculitis in a patient with subacute cutaneous lupus erythematosus: response to diltiazem and chloroquine J Rheumatol 28(9):2129–32

Mutasim DF. (2003) Severe subacute cutaneous lupus erythematosus presenting with generalized erythroderma and bullae. J Am Acad Dermatol 48(6):947–9

Neri R, Mosca M, Bernacchi E, Bombardieri S (1999) A case of SLE with acute, subacute and chronic cutaneous lesions successfully treated with Dapsone. Lupus 8:240–243

Ng PP, Tan SH, Koh ET, Tan T (2000) Epidemiology of cutaneous lupus erythematosus in a tertiary referral center in Singapore Australasian J Dermatol 41(4):229–33

Nieboer C, Tak-Diamand Z, VanLeeuwen-Wallau AG (1988) Dust-like particles: a specific direct immunofluorescence pattern in subacute cutaneous lupus erythematosus. Br J Dermatol 118:725–734

Nived O, Johansen PB, Sturfelt G (1993) Standardized ultraviolet-A exposure provokes skin reaction in systemic lupus erythematosus. Lupus 2:247–250

Norris DA (1993) Pathomechanisms of photosensitive lupus erythematosus. J Invest Dermatol 100:58S–68S

Nousari HC, Kimyai-Asadi A, Tausk FA (1998) Subacute cutaneous lupus erythematosus associated with beta interferon-1a. Lancet 352:1825–1826

Ordi-Ros J, Cortes F, Cucurull E, Mauri M, Bujan S, Vilardell M (2000) Thalidomide in the treatment of cutaneous lupus refractory to conventional therapy. Journal of Phycology 27:1429–1433

Orteu DH, Sontheimer RD, Dutz JP (2001) The pathophysiology of photosensitivity in lupus erythematosus. Photodermatol Photoimmunol Photomed 17:95–113

Pantoja L, Gonzalez-Lopez MA, Bouso M, Alija A, Ortiz-Saracho J (2002) Subacute cutaneous lupus erythematosus in a patient with rheumatoid arthritis. Scandinavian J Rheumatol 31(6):377–9

Parodi A, Romagnoli M, Rebora A (1989) Subacute cutaneous lupus erythematosus-like eruption caused by hydrochlorothiazide. Photodermatol 6(2):100–2

Parodi A, Rivara G, Guarrera M (1992) Possible naproxen-induced relapse of subacute cutaneous lupus erythematosus. JAMA 268:51–52

Parodi A, Caproni M, Cardinali C, Bernacchi E, Fuligni A, De Panfilis G, Zane C, Papini M, Veller FC, Vaccaro M, Fabbri P, Bader U, Banyai M, Boni R, Burg G, Hafner J (2000) Clinical, histological and immunopathological features of 58 patients with subacute cutaneous lupus erythematosus – A review by the Italian Group of Immunodermatology. Dermatology 200:6–10

Patri P, Nigro A, Rebora A (1985) Lupus erythematosus-like eruption from captopril. Acta Derm Venereol 65:447–448

Perrotta S, Locatelli F, La Manna A et al. (2002) Anti-CD20 monoclonal antibody (Rituximab) for life-threatening autoimmune haemolytic anaemia in a patient with systemic lupus erythematosus Br J of Haematol 116:465–7

Piette JC, Sbai A, Frances C (2002) Warning: thalidomide-related thrombotic risk potentially concerns patients with lupus Lupus 11(2):67–70

Pramatarov K, Vassileva S, Miteva L (2000) Subacute cutaneous lupus erythematosus presenting with generalized poiklioderma. J Am Acad Dermatol 42:286–288

Price P, Witt C, Allock D, et al. (1999) The genetic basis for the association of the 8.1 ancestral haplotype (A1, B8, DR3) with multiple immunopathological diseases. Immunological Reviews. 167:257–74

Prinz JC, Meurer M, Reiter C, Rieber EP, Plewig G, Riethmuller G (1996) Treatment of severe cutaneous lupus erythematosus with a chimeric CD4 monoclonal antibody, cM-T412. J Am Acad Dermatol 34:244–252

Provost TT, Talal N, Bias W, Harley JB, Reichlin M, Alexander EL (1988) Ro/SS-A positive Sjogren's/lupus erythematosus overlap patients are associated with the HLA-DR3 and/or DRW6 phenotypes. J Invest Dermatol 91:369–371

Racila DM, Sontheimer CJ, Sheffield A, Wisnieski JJ, Racila E, Sontheimer RD, (2003) Homozygous single nucleotide polmorphism of the complement C1QA gene is associated with decreased levels of C1q in patients with subacute cutaneous lupus erythematosus. Lupus 12(2):124–32

Rahman P, Gladman DD, Urowitz MB (1998) Smoking interferes with efficacy of antimalarial therapy in cutaneous lupus. J Rheumatol 25:1716–1719

Rao BK, Coldiron BM, Freeman RF, Sontheimer RD (1990) Subacute cutaneous lupus erythematosus lesions progressing to morphea. J Am Acad Dermatol 23:1019–1022

Reed BJ, Huff JC, Jones SK, Orton DW, Lee LA, Norris DA (1985) Subacute cutaneous lupus erythematosus associated with hydrochlorothiazide therapy. Ann Intern Med 103:49–51

Reichlin M (2000)ANA negative systemic lupus erythematosus sera revisited serologically Lupus 9(2):116–9

Richardson TT, Cohen PR (2000) Subacute cutaneous lupus erythematosus: report of a patient who subsequently developed a meningioma and whose skin lesions were treated with isotretinoin. Cutis 66:183–188

Rihner M, McGrath H, Jr. (1992) Fluorescent light photosensitivity in patients with systemic lupus erythematosus. Arthritis Rheum 35:949–952

Ross S, Dywer C, Ormerod AD, Herriot R, Roberts C (2002) Subacute cutaneous lupus erythematosus associated with phenytoin. Clinical & Experimental Dermatology 27:474–476

Roura M, Lopez-Gil F, Umbert P (1991) Systemic lupus erythematosus exacerbated by piroxicam. Dermatologica 182:56–58

Roustan G, Salas C, Barbadillo C, Sanchez Yus E, Mulero J, Simon A (2000) Lupus erythematosus with an erythema multiforme-like eruption Eur J Dermatol 10:459–462

Rowell NR, Swanson-Beck J, Andrson JR (1963) Lupus erythematosus and erythema multiforme-like lesions. Arch Dermatol 88:176–180

Rua-Figueroa I, Erausquin C, Naranjo A, Carretero-Hernandez G, Rodriguez-Lozano C, De la RP (1999) Pustuloderma during cutaneous lupus treatment with thalidomide [letter]. Lupus 8:248–249

Rubin, RL (2002) Drug-Induced Lupus. In Dubois' Lupus Erythematosus. D.J. Wallace and B.H. Hahn, editors. Lippincott Williams and Wilkins, Philadelphia

Rudnicka L, Szymanska E, Walecka I, Slowinska M (2000) Long-term cefuroxime axetil in subacute cutaneous lupus erythematosus: a report of three cases. Dermatology 200:129–131

Sanders CJ, Van Weelden H, Kazzaz GA, Sigurdsson V, Toonstra J, Bruijnzeel-Koomen CA (2003) Photosensitivity in patients with lupus erythematosus: a clinical and photobiological study of 100 patients using a prolonged phototest protocol. Br J Dermatol 149(1):131–7

Schanz S, Ulmer A, Rassner G, Fierlbeck G (2002) Successful treatment of subacute cutaneous lupus erythematosus with mycophenolate mofetil Br J Dermatol 147(1):174–8

Scheinman PL (1994) Acral subacute cutaneous lupus erythematosus: an unusual variant. J Am Acad Dermatol 30:800–801

Schulz EJ, Menter MA (1971) Treatment of discoid and subacute cutaneous lupus erythematosus with cyclophosphamide. Br J Dermatol 85:60–65

Sheretz EF (1988) Lichen planus following procainamide induced lupus erythematosus. Cutis 42:51–53

Siamopoulou-Mavridou A, Stefanou D, Dross AA (1989) Subacute lupus erythematosus childhood. Clin. Rheum. 8:533–7

Sonnichsen N, Meffert H, Kunzelmann V, Audring H (1993) [UV-A-1 therapy of subacute cutaneous lupus erythematosus]. [German]. Hautarzt 44:723–725

Sonntag M, Lehmann P, Megahed M, Ruzicka T, Kuhn A (2003) Papulonodular mucinosis associated with subacute cutaneous lupus erythematosus. Dermatology 206(4):326–9

Sontheimer RD, Gilliam JN (1979) A reappraisal of the relationship between subepidermal immunoglobulin deposits and DNA antibodies in systemic lupus erythematosus: a study using the Crithidia luciliae immunofluorescence anti-DNA assay. J Invest Dermatol 72:29–32

Sontheimer RD, Thomas JR, Gilliam JN (1979) Subacute cutaneous lupus erythematosus: a cutaneous marker for a distinct lupus erythematosus subset. Arch Dermatol 115:1409–1415

Sontheimer RD, Stastny P, Gilliam JN (1981) Human histocompatibility antigen associations in subacute cutaneous lupus erythematosus. J Clin Invest 67:312–316

Sontheimer RD, Maddison PJ, Reichlin M, Jordan RE, Stastny P, Gilliam JN (1982) Serologic and HLA associations in subacute cutaneous lupus erythematosus, a clinical subset of lupus erythematosus. Ann Intern Med 97:644–671

Sontheimer RD (1985) Clinical significance of subacute cutaneous lupus erythematosus skin lesions. J Dermatol 12:205–212

Sontheimer RD (1989) Subacute cutaneous lupus erythematosus: a decade's perspective. Med Clin North Am 73:1073

Sontheimer RD, Provost TT (1996) Lupus erythematosus. In Sontheimer RD, Provost TT (eds) Cutaneous Manifestations of Rheumatic Diseases. Williams and Wilkins, Baltimore, p 31

Srivastava, M, Rencic A, Diglio G, Santana H, Bonitz P, Watson R, Ha E, Anhalt GJ, Provost TT, Nousari CH (2003) Drug-induced, Ro / SSA-positive cutaneous lupus erythematosus. Arch Dermatol 139:45–49

Stege H, Budde MA, Grether-Beck S, Krutmann J (2000) Evaluation of the capacity of sunscreens to photoprotect lupus erythematosus patients by employing the photoprovocation test Photodermatol, Photoimmunol, & Photomed 16(6):256–9

Stevens RJ, Andujar C, Edwards CJ, Ames PR, Barwick AR, Khamashta MA, Hughes GR (1997) Thalidomide in the treatment of the cutaneous manifestations of lupus erythematosus: experience in sixteen consecutive patients. Br J Rheumatol 36:353–359

Tebbe B, Mansmann U, Wollina U, Auergrumbach P, Lichtmbalyohere A, Arensmeier M, Orfanos CE (1997) Markers in cutaneous lupus erythematosus indicating systemic involvement – A multicenter study on 296 patients. Acta Dermato-Venereologica 77:305–308

Tebbe B, Orfanos CE (1997) Epidemiology and socioeconomic impact of skin disease in lupus erythematosus. Lupus 6:96–104

Thivolet J, Nicolas JF, Kanitakis J, Lyonnet S, Chouvet B (1990) Recombinant interferon a2a is effective in the treatment of discoid and subacute cutaneous lupus erythematosus. Br J Dermatol 122:405–409

Ting W, Sontheimer RD (2001) Local therapy for cutaneous LE and systemic LE: Practical and theoretical consideration. Lupus 10:171–189

Toll A, Campo-Pisa P, Gonzalez-Castro J, Campo-Voegeli A, Azon A, Iranzo P, Lecha M, Herrero C (1998) Subacute cutaneous lupus erythematosus associated with cinnarizine and thiethylperazine therapy. Lupus 7:364–366

Topaloglu R, Bakkaloglu A, Slingsby JH et al. (2000) Survey of Turkish systemic lupus erythematosus patients for a particular mutation of C1Q deficiency. Clinical and Experimental Rheumatol 18:75–77

5

Trenholme GM, Carson PE (1978) Therapy and prophylaxis of malaria. JAMA 240:2293–229

Valeski JE, Kumar V, Forman AB, Beutner EH, Chorzelski TP (1992) J Am Acad Derm 27:194–198

Vasquez-Doval J, Ruiz de Erenchun F, Sanchz-Ibarrola A, Contrera F, Soto de Delas J, Quintanilla E (1992) Subacute cutaneous lupus erythematosus – clinical, histopathological and immunophe-notypical study of five cases. J Invest Allerg 2:27–32

Velthuis PJ, Kater L, Van der Tweel I, Baart de la Faille H, Van Vloten WA (1992) Immunofluores-cence microscopy of healthy skin from patients with systemic lupus erythematosus: More than just the lupus band. Ann Rheum Dis 51:720–725

Walport MJ, Davies KA, Botto M (1998) C1q and systemic lupus erythematosus. Immunobiol 199:265–85

Warren KJ, Nopper AJ, Crosby DL (1998) Thalidomide for recalcitrant discoid lesions in a patient with systemic lupus erythematosus. J Am Acad Dermatol 39:293–295

Watson RM, Talwar P, Alexander E, Bias WB, Provost TT (1991) Subacute cutaneous lupus erythe-matosus-immunogenetic associations. J Autoimmun 4:73–85

Wenzel J, Bauer R, Bieber T, Bohm I (2000) Autoantibodies in patients with lupus erythematosus: spectrum and frequencies Dermatology 201(3):282–3

Wenzel J, Bauer R, Uerlich M, Bieber T, Boehm I (2002) The value of lymphocytopenia as a marker of systemic involvement in cutaneous lupus erythematosus Br J Dermatol 146(5):869–71

Werth VP, Zhang W, Dortzbach K, Sullivan, K (2000) Association of a promoter polymorphism of tumor necrosis factor-alpha with subacute cutaneous lupus erythematosus and distinct photo-regulation of transcription. J Invest Dermatol 115:726–730

Wollina U, Barta U, Uhlemann C, Oelzner P (1999) Lupus erythematosus-associated red lunula. J Am Acad Dermatol 41:419–421

Wollina U, Schreiber G (2003) Polyglandular autoimmune syndrome type II (Schmidt's syndrome) in patients with autoimmune connective tissue disorders. J Euro Acad Derm & Venereol 17(3):371–2

Yung RL, Richardson BC (1995) Cytarabine therapy for refractory cutaneous lupus. Arthritis Rheum 38:1341–1343

Dermatomyositis

6

Ruth Ann Vleugels and Jeffrey P. Callen

Introduction

Dermatomyositis (DM), along with polymyositis (PM) and inclusion body myositis, is classified as one of the idiopathic inflammatory myopathies (IIM) (Callen, 2000; Plotz et al., 1995; Targoff, 1991). In 1975, Bohan and Peter published a landmark article in two parts that suggested a set of criteria to aid in the diagnosis and classification of DM and PM. Four of the five criteria related specifically to the muscle disease, 1) progressive proximal symmetrical weakness 2) elevated muscle enzymes, 3) an abnormal electromyogram, and 4) an abnormal muscle biopsy, while the fifth was the presence of compatible cutaneous disease. At that time, it was felt that DM differed from PM only by the presence of cutaneous disease. Studies on the pathogenesis of the myopathy, however, have been controversial, with some suggesting that the myopathies in DM and PM are pathogenetically different with DM being due to a vascular inflammation (Kuru et al., 2000) and other studies of cytokines suggesting that the processes are similar (Wanchu et al., 1999; Shimizu et al., 2000; Sugiura et al., 2000; Nyberg et al., 2000). More recently, however, there has been increasing evidence to support the concept that the pathogenetic mechanisms of the muscle disease in DM and PM differ significantly (Dalakas et al., 2003). In polymyositis, clonally expanded autoreactive CD8-positive T-cells invade myocytes expressing MHC class I antigens and cause necrosis via the perforin pathway. In dermatomyositis, autoantigens seem to activate a humoral immune process in which complement is deposited in capillaries causing capillary necrosis and ischemia.

Additional studies on the pathogenetic mechanisms involved in the myopathy have demonstrated abnormal levels of nitric oxide, elevation of circulating tumor necrosis factor receptors, elevated soluble CD40 expression, increased expression of interleukin-1-alpha within the muscle, and upregulation of type I interferon-α/β inducible genes in blood samples. Despite numerous studies focusing on the pathogenetic mechanisms of the myopathy, the pathogenesis of the cutaneous disease is poorly understood. Although the exact pathogenesis has yet to be elucidated, DM is thought to occur when varying factors, such as a malignancy, medication, or infection, trigger an immune-mediated process in a genetically predisposed individual.

Epidemiology

A study published in 1990 reported an incidence of dermatomyositis of 5.5 cases per million, with an increasing incidence noted over the two decades represented in the study period (Oddis et al., 1990). A recent population-based study from Mayo Clinic found the incidence of dermatomyositis to be 9.63 per million, with an incidence of clinically amyopathic dermatomyositis of 2.08 per million (Bendewald et al., 2010). In addition, this study also found the incidence of dermatomyositis to be 13.98 per million in women and 4.68 per million in men, supporting previous epidemiological data indicating that women are affected by dermatomyositis more often than men. The incidence of the juvenile form of dermatomyositis has been estimated to be 1.9 per million, with a female-to-male ratio of 5:1 and median age of onset of 6.8 years (Symmons et al., 1995).

Classification and Clinical Appearance

Classification

Bohan and Peter (1975) suggested five subsets of myositis: 1) DM, 2) PM, 3) myositis with cancer, 4) juvenile DM / PM (most often diagnosed before age 16), and 5) myositis overlapping with another collagen-vascular disorder. In a subsequent publication, Bohan et al. (1977) noted that cutaneous disease may precede the development of the myopathy. It was more recently recognized that another subset of patients with disease that affects only the skin (amyopathic dermatomyositis [ADM] or DM-sine myositis) may occur as well (Euwer and Sontheimer 1991, Sontheimer RD 2002, Gerami et al., 2006). A seventh subset known as inclusion body myositis (IBM) has been recognized, in which a unique pattern of weakness with prominent involvement of the wrist and finger flexors and quadriceps exists in the absence of cutaneous disease (Sayers et al., 1992). An eighth group exists in which characteristic cutaneous and / or muscle disease is drug-induced (Dourmishev and Dourmishev, 1999, Seidler AM and Gottleib AB, 2008). Sontheimer has proposed another subset that classifies patients as having hypomyopathic dermatomyositis when skin disease is present in the absence of clinical weakness but with evidence of subclinical myositis on studies. Finally, post-myopathic DM refers to those patients in whom the myositis component of the disease resolves with therapy while the skin disease remains active and often is challenging to manage (Sontheimer, 2002).

Cutaneous Manifestations

The characteristic and possibly pathognomonic cutaneous features of DM are the heliotrope rash and *Gottron's* papules. The heliotrope rash consists of a violaceous to dusky erythematous rash with or without edema in a symmetrical distribution involving periorbital skin (Fig. 1). Sometimes this sign is quite subtle and may involve only a mild discoloration

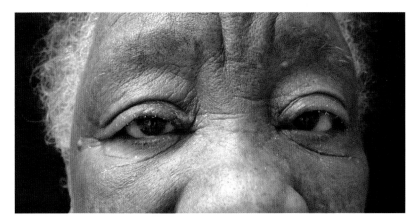

Fig. 1. Facial erythema with periorbital edema are present in this woman with dermatomyositis. The periorbital changes represent the heliotrope eruption

along the eyelid margin. A heliotrope rash is rarely observed in lupus erythematosus (LE) and scleroderma. The differential diagnosis for the heliotrope eruption often includes angioedema or dermatitis.

Gottron's papules are found over bony prominences, particularly the metacarpophalangeal (MCP) joints, the proximal interphalangeal (PIP) joints, and/or the distal interphalangeal (DIP) joints (Fig. 2). They may also be found overlying the elbows, knees, and/or feet, referred to as Gottron's sign. The lesions consist of slightly elevated, violaceous papules and plaques. There may be a slight associated scale and on some occasions there is a thick psoriasiform scale. Within the lesions, there is often telangiectasia. These lesions may be clinically confused with lesions of LE, or, at times, with papulosquamous disorders, such as psoriasis or lichen planus. Routine histopathological evaluation will aid in the differentiation from psoriasis or lichen planus, but cannot reliably distinguish the cutaneous lesions of DM from those of LE.

Several other cutaneous features are characteristic of the disease despite not being pathognomonic. They include malar erythema, poikiloderma in a photosensitive distribution, violaceous erythema on the extensor surfaces, and periungual and cuticular changes. Nailfold changes consist of periungual telangiectasia and/or a characteristic cuticular change with hypertrophy of the cuticle and small, hemorrhagic infarcts within this hypertrophic area. Periungual telangiectasia may be clinically apparent or may be appreciated only by capillary microscopy. Poikiloderma (the combination of atrophy, dyspigmentation, and telangiectasia) may occur on exposed skin such as the extensor surfaces of the arm, the 'V' of the neck (Fig. 3), or the upper back (*Shawl sign*). Patients rarely complain of photosensitivity, despite the prominent photodistribution of the rash. This photosensitive poikilodermatous eruption may be difficult to differentiate from LE. Facial erythema may also occur in DM. This change must be differentiated from LE, rosacea, seborrheic dermatitis, or atopic dermatitis. A helpful clue in distinguishing the mid-facial erythema of dermatomyositis from that of LE is that it tends to involve the nasolabial folds, whereas LE classi-

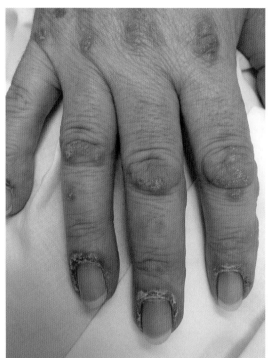

Fig. 2. Gottron's papules. Erythematous scaly plaques are present on the dorsal hands, particularly over the bony prominences (MCP, PIP, and DIP joints). There are also marked periungual telangiectasia and cuticular overgrowth

6

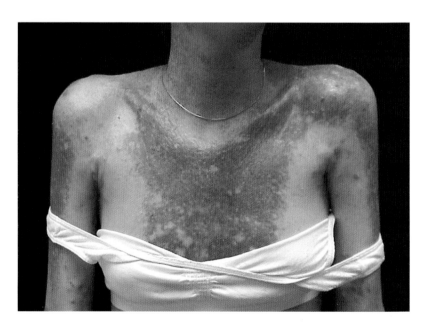

Fig. 3. Poikiloderma of the upper chest in a patient with dermatomyositis

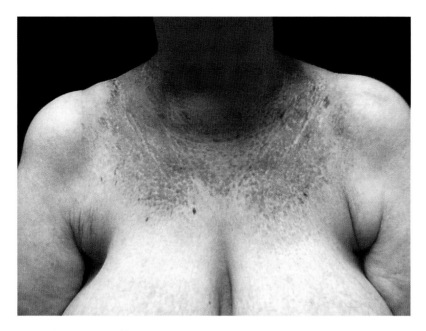

Fig. 4. Papular mucinosis-like lesions in a patient with dermatomyositis. Prominent papular lesions are present within the poikilodermatous eruption. Histopathology revealed deposition of massive amounts of mucin in the dermis

cally spares these areas. Scalp involvement in dermatomyositis is relatively common and is manifest by an erythematous to violaceous, psoriasiform dermatitis (Kasteler and Callen, 1994). Clinical distinction from seborrheic dermatitis or psoriasis is occasionally difficult, but histopathologic evaluation is helpful. Scalp pruritus can be particularly challenging to manage in patients with DM. Nonscarring alopecia may occur in some patients and often follows a flare of the systemic disease.

Rare cutaneous manifestations include vesiculobullous lesions (McCollough and Cockerell, 1998), an eruption that simulates pityriasis rubra pilaris (Requena et al., 1997), vasculitis, erosive lesions, as well as an exfoliative erythroderma (Miyagawa et al., 1992, Chander et al., 2009). In small case series it has been suggested that some of these cutaneous manifestations may be more common in patients with an associated malignancy.

A variety of other cutaneous lesions have been described in patients with DM that do not demonstrate the interface changes observed histopathologically with the pathognomonic or characteristic lesions. These include panniculitis, plaque-like mucinosis (Fig. 4) (Abernethy et al., 1996; Kaufman et al., 1998), a flagellate erythema (Nousari et al., 1999), urticaria, as well as mechanic's hands (hyperkeratosis of the lateral fingers and palms) (Vleugels and Callen, 2009).

Calcinosis is rare in adults, but affects between 23–70% of patients with juvenile DM (Dalakas, 1991, Fisler et al., 2002). In addition, reports have detailed the findings of gingival telangiectasia (Ghali et al., 1999) and angiokeratomas (Shannon and Ford, 1999) in children with DM. Finally, lipodystrophy is increasingly being recognized as a potential complication of juvenile DM as well (Heumer et al., 2001, Bingham et al., 2008).

Patients with DM can also develop the lesions of other collagen-vascular disorders as well as present with an overlap syndrome. In general, sclerodermatous cutaneous changes have been the most frequently reported in patients with overlap syndrome, however lesions of discoid lupus and rheumatoid nodules have also been reported.

Patients with DM are at times difficult to distinguish from patients with either systemic LE or subacute cutaneous lupus erythematosus (SCLE). The lesions of DM differ slightly in their distribution, occurring more over bony prominences, and they are frequently accompanied by severe pruritus; whereas LE lesions tend to occur between the knuckles and are usually asymptomatic. Routine skin biopsy is not helpful in the distinction between LE and DM. Immunofluorescence microscopy (IF) should be negative in DM and positive in LE, however, about 50% of SCLE patients have a negative IF, and IF may be falsely positive on sun-exposed skin. Serologic testing is also imperfect, since only 25% of DM patients are Mi-2 positive (which is specific for DM, but not sensitive), and on a single testing only 60–70% of SCLE patients are Ro (SS-A) antibody positive.

Pruritus is a common symptom of the skin disease of dermatomyositis and can significantly affect the patient's quality of life (Shirani et al., 2004, Hundley et al., 2006). In addition, pruritus is a feature that can occasionally help distinguish dermatomyositis from lupus erythematosus. The skin lesions of DM are also likely photoaggravated despite the lack of symptoms suggestive of photosensitivity reported by patients (Cheong et al., 1994). Clinical observations suggest that not only is the skin disease exacerbated by light, but muscle disease may **also** be worsened after sun exposure (Woo et al., 1985; Callen, 1993; Zuber et al., 1996; Callen, 1999). However, phototesting has not been able to reliably reproduce the skin lesions, thus, the wavelength of light that is responsible for the clinical manifestations (action spectrum) is not known.

Skin lesions of DM may precede the development of myopathy and may persist well after the control and quiescence of the myositis. Patients' skin lesions may flare with sun exposure, but only some of these patients will have a flare of their muscle involvement. Thus, in many instances the course of the skin lesions does not parallel that of the muscle disease.

Muscle Disease

Clinical and laboratory abnormalities suggestive of muscle disease are characteristic features of DM (Wortmann, 2000). The myopathy primarily affects the proximal muscles, is usually symmetrical and is slowly progressive over a period of weeks to months. Initial complaints including myalgias, fatigue, or weakness manifest as an inability to climb stairs, to raise the arms for actions like hair grooming or shaving, to rise from a squatting or sitting position, or a combination of these features. Tenderness upon palpation of the muscles is variable. An inability to swallow and symptoms of aspiration may reflect the involvement of striated muscle of the pharynx or upper esophagus. Dysphagia or dysphonia generally signifies a rapidly progressive course and may be associated with poor prognosis.

Systemic Features

Dermatomyositis is a multisystem disorder (Spiera and Kagen, 1998). Arthralgias and / or arthritis may be present in up to one fourth of patients with inflammatory myopathy. The usual picture is one of generalized arthralgias accompanied by morning stiffness. The small joints of the hands, wrists, and ankles may be involved with a symmetric nondeforming arthritis.

Esophageal disease as manifested by dysphagia is estimated to be present in 15% to 50% of patients with inflammatory myopathy. The dysphagia can be of two types: proximal dysphagia or distal dysphagia. Proximal dysphagia is caused by involvement of striated muscle in the pharynx or proximal esophagus. This involvement correlates well with the severity of the muscle disease and is steroid-responsive. Distal dysphagia, which often presents as reflux, is related to involvement of nonstriated muscle and appears to be more frequent in patients who have an overlap syndrome with scleroderma or another collagen vascular disorder. Dysphagia is associated with a poor prognosis and correlates with the presence of pulmonary involvement.

Pulmonary disease occurs in dermatomyositis and polymyositis in approximately 15% to 30% of patients (Marie et al., 1998). Interstitial lung disease (ILD) is a primary process observed in DM / PM. It is more frequent in patients with esophageal involvement. Lung disease may also occur as a direct complication of the muscle disease, such as hypoventilation or aspiration in patients with dysphagia, or may be a result of treatment, such as with opportunistic infections or drug-induced hypersensitivity pneumonitis. Data have suggested that patients with myositis and the presence of Jo-1 antibodies have an increased risk of ILD. In fact, ILD will develop in up to 70% of patients with Jo-1 antibodies. Antisynthetase syndrome is the constellation of ILD, myositis, polyarthritis, Raynaud's, fever, and mechanic's hands seen in patients with anti-transfer RNA autoantibodies.

In a retrospective review of 70 patients with myositis-associated interstitial lung disease seen at Mayo Clinic between 1990 and 1998, most of the patients presented with either symptoms of lung disease or symptoms of myositis alone, whereas only 15 patients presented with the involvement of both simultaneously (Douglas et al., 2001). In general, the lung disease was at first felt to be a pneumonitis that was antibiotic resistant. Biopsy of the lung revealed non-specific interstitial pneumonitis or diffuse alveolar damage in a majority of those who were biopsied. Only two patients had bronchiolitis obliterans organizing pneumonia (BOOP). It is unclear exactly how many of these patients had dermatomyositis, but perhaps between 8 and 12. Therapy included corticosteroids with or without an immunosuppressive agent, and the prognosis was poorer for this subset of patients with ILD than for unselected patients with myositis alone as demonstrated by a 5-year survival of 60.4%. Patients with Jo-1 antibodies (19 of 50 who were tested) had roughly the same features and prognosis as those who did not have this antibody.

Clinically symptomatic cardiac involvement in patients with DM or PM is uncommon, but when present it is associated with a poor prognosis (Gonzalez-Lopez et al., 1996). Various abnormalities have been described which most commonly include conduction defects and rhythm disturbances. Although congestive heart failure, pericarditis, and valvular disease may occur, they are much less frequent. Depending on the report, cardiac manifestations may occur in up to 50% of patients, but only a small proportion of these patients manifest symptoms. It is not known whether the identification of asymptomatic abnormalities has an effect on long-term outcome, or even if the findings are more prevalent in DM / PM than in an age-matched control group.

Calcinosis of the skin or muscle is unusual in adults but occurs frequently in children and adolescents with DM. Calcinosis cutis is manifested by firm, yellow-white or skin-colored nodules, which often occur over bony prominences. Occasionally, these nodules can extrude through the surface of the skin, in which case secondary infection may occur. Calcification of the muscles is often asymptomatic and may be seen only on radiological examination. In severe forms, the calcinosis can cause loss of function, and rarely, bone formation is possible.

Amyopathic Dermatomyositis

It is becoming more widely accepted that a subset of patients with dermatomyositis will have skin-limited disease, similar to patients with lupus limited to the skin rather than with systemic involvement. This is a change from the previous notion that all patients with dermatomyositis would have some degree of muscle involvement by definition if physicians simply investigated sufficiently to find it. Within current nomenclature proposed by Sontheimer, clinically amyopathic dermatomyositis includes patients with both amyopathic and hypomyopathic dermatomyositis (Sontheimer, 2002).

Amyopathic dermatomyositis, historically known as dermatomyositis siné myositis (Bohan et al., 1977; Rockerbie et al., 1989; Stonecipher, 1993; Cosnes et al., 1995), refers to the presence of biopsy-proven cutaneous manifestations of dermatomyositis in the absence of objective muscle inflammation (normal strength and normal muscle derived enzymes) for at least six months. By definition, these patients must not have received two consecutive months or more of systemic immunosuppressive therapy in the first six months after skin disease onset and must not have received medications known to cause dermatomyositis-like skin changes (Sontheimer, 2002). These cases can be referred to as provisional amyopathic dermatomyositis until two years after diagnosis, at which point they can be called confirmed amyopathic dermatomyositis. Using these criteria, 10–20% of patients with dermatomyositis seen in academic health centers have clinically amyopathic disease (Jorizzo, 2002). This percentage is as high as 40% when considering patients with dermatomyositis seen specifically by dermatologists in a referral center (Klein RQ et al., 2007).

Although amyopathic dermatomyositis presents with cutaneous disease indistinguishable from that of classic dermatomyositis, it is considered a distinct entity rather than a group of patients in which muscle abnormalities are not yet detectable. In the largest systematic review of adult-onset clinically amyopathic dermatomyositis, most patients had a normal EMG, muscle biopsy, and or muscle MRI when performed (Gerami et al., 2006).

Hypomyopathic dermatomyositis includes patients with cutaneous findings and subclinical myositis evident on laboratories, EMG, biopsy, and / or MRI, but no clinical weakness or muscle tenderness. Importantly, these findings do not reliably predict the onset of clinically significant muscle disease at a later time and should therefore not necessarily warrant more aggressive therapeutic intervention. Sontheimer reported that none of the patients with hypomyopathic dermatomyositis in the series mentioned above had developed clinically significant muscle weakness at the time of follow-up despite an average duration of skin disease of 5.4 years (Gerami et al., 2006).

Cutaneous lesions and histopathology are indistinguishable from that of classic dermatomyositis. Similar to classic dermatomyositis, there is a female predominence, a peak onset in adults in the fifth and sixth decades, and a pediatric population affected by amyopathic dermatomyositis. Finally, similar to classic dermatomyositis, amyopathic deramtomyositis has associations with both pulmonary disease and cancer, mandating that these patients be followed for manifestations of both interstitial lung disease and malignancy.

Myositis and Malignancy

The previously controversial relationship of DM and PM to malignancy has been clarified in recent years (Hill et al., 2001). Overall, the reported frequency of malignancy in dermatomyositis has varied from 6% to 60%, with most large population-based cohort studies revealing a frequency of about 20 to 25%.

Several Scandinavian studies have documented the increased frequency of malignancy in DM over the general population (Siguregeirsson et al., 1992; Chow et al., 1995; Ario et al., 1995; Hill et al., 2001). While polymyositis patients had a slight increase in cancer frequency, it was not highly significant and could be explained by a more aggressive cancer search creating a diagnostic suspicion bias. A recent study from New England, USA, also supported that malignancy is associated with dermatomyositis but not polymyositis (Antiochos et al., 2009). In this study, patients with malignancy-associated dermatomyositis were more frequently male and over the age of forty-five and were less likely to have interstitial lung disease. As mentioned above, patients with amyopathic DM may also have an associated malignancy (el-Azhary and Pakzad, 2002). In the recent population-based study from Mayo Clinic, malignancy was present in 28% of patients (Bendewald et al., 2010), strengthening the best previously existing data that 18–32% of dermatomyositis patients have or will develop a malignancy.

Malignancies may occur prior to the onset of myositis, concurrently with myositis, or after the onset of DM. In addition, the myositis may follow the course of the malignancy (a paraneoplastic course) or may follow its own course independent of the treatment of the malignancy. Studies demonstrating the benefits of cancer surgery on myositis as well as those showing no relationship of the myositis to the malignancy have been reported. In one retrospective study, independent factors associated with an underlying malignancy in dermatomyositis included age at diagnosis, rapid onset of skin and / or muscle symptoms, the presence of skin necrosis or periungal erythema, and a low baseline level of complement factor C4, whereas a low baseline lymphocyte count was a protective factor for associated malignancy (Fardet et al., 2009).

A wide variety of malignancies have been reported in patients with DM. Gynecologic malignancy, in particular ovarian carcinoma may be overrepresented in DM (Whitmore et al., 1994; Hill et al., 2001). In some Southeast Asian populations, nasopharyngeal cancer seems to be overrepresented (Peng et al., 1995, Hu et al., 1996, Huang et al., 2009). In the recent analysis of combined data from Scandinavia, Hill et al. (2001) again noted the increased association of ovarian cancer, but also noted increases in lung, pancreatic, stomach, colorectal cancer, and non-Hodgkin's lymphoma as well. Malignancy is more common in older patients (> 50 years) (Marie et al., 1998; Pautas et al., 2000), but reports of young adults with DM have appeared, suggesting that age alone should not dissuade the physician from a careful evaluation **in adult patients with DM** (see below). The site of malignancy can be predicted by the patient's age (e. g., malignancy in a young man is more often testicular cancer, whereas, in an elderly male, colon or prostate cancer would be more common). Of note, the increased risk of malignancy occurs with adult dermatomyositis, but not with the juvenile form of the disease.

In the past, there was concern about whether the use of immunosuppressive therapies would predispose the patient to an excess cancer risk. This has not proven to be the case in several studies, with most cancers being reported within the first three years following diagnosis. There have been, however, cases of Epstein-Barr virus-associated lymphomas arising in patients with rheumatic diseases, including dermatomyositis, on methotrexate, which have resolved on discontinuation of immunosuppressive therapy without requiring additional therapy.

Juvenile (Childhood) Dermatomyositis (JDMS)

DM is much more common than polymyositis in children and adolescents (Pachman, 1995). A fulminant course may be present, but most often the onset is indolent and children are first thought to have viral infections or dermatitis. Delayed diagnosis is more common in the non-white population. Children may also have amyopathic disease. There is thought to be little to no increased risk of malignancy in children with JDMS.

Often JDMS is characterized as a vasculitis, but the major difference in clinical features between JDMS and adult DM is the greater potential for calcinosis in children. A recent report detailed the chronic nature of this disease in children, with many patients requiring therapy to suppress their disease activity more than three years after diagnosis (Huber et al., 2000). Pachman et al. (2000) linked the presence of calcinosis and a prolonged course of disease with the TNF alpha-308A allele in their patients with juvenile DM.

In one study it was noted that the development of calcinosis was not related to initial therapy, but was associated with a lower score on an assessment instrument of physical function. Additional studies demonstrate that early and aggressive intervention with systemic therapy seems to decrease the risk of development of calcinosis (Fisler et al., 2002, Al-Mayouf, 2000b, Pachman et al., 1998). Early aggressive therapy is often warranted in JDMS given that another retrospective study demonstrated improved outcomes and sustained remission of disease in pediatric patients treated with this approach (Kim et al., 2009).

Children with JDMS should be followed by a pediatrician comfortable with monitoring their developmental milestones while on immunosuppressive therapy. In addition, both lipodystrophy and metabolic abnormalities (including hypertriglyceridemia and insulin resistance) have increasingly been recognized as potential complications of JDMS and should be screened for routinely (Huemer et al., 2001, Bingham et al., 2008).

Drug-Induced Dermatomyositis

The etiology of most cases of DM is unknown, however, in a small number of patients, the cutaneous manifestations are due to or exacerbated by drugs. This has been best documented for hydroxyurea in which de-challenges and re-challenges have been performed (Daoud et al., 1997, Marie et al., 2000, Dacey and Callen, 2003). In a review of 70 reported cases, 51% were from hydroxyurea (Seidler, 2008). None of the cases associated with hydroxyurea had associated mysotis, however, greater than seventy-five percent of the non-hydroxyurea cases reported myositis and several had associated pulmonary involvement.

HMG-CoA-reductase inhibitors and D-penicillamine have each also had multiple case reports. In addition, quinidine, non-steroidal anti-inflammatory drugs, gemfibrozil, omeprazole, etoposide, alfuzosin, cyclophosphamide, tegafur, phenytoin, imatinib mesylate, interferon alfa-2b, ipecac, sulfacetamide sodium ophthalmic drops, as well as the BCG vaccine have each also been linked to DM in at least one case report (Dourmishev and Dourmishev, 1999, Seidler, 2008). Notably, there have also been cases of drug-induced DM attributed to both etanercept and lenercept, a recombinant TNF receptor p55 immunoglobulin fusion protein (Flendrie et al., 2005).

Diagnosis and Evaluation of the Patient with Dermatomyositis

The diagnosis of DM is suspected in patients with clinically compatible cutaneous findings. Exclusion of other possible cutaneous conditions is aided by skin biopsy, which classically has an interface dermatitis and the presence of mucin in the dermis, however the histopathologic findings of LE can be identical. Both LE and DM can also demonstrate an interferon-α-inducible cytokine milieu, however, phenotypic profiling has also suggested some differences such as the relative lack of CD4/CXCR3-positive mononuclear cells in LE as compared to DM (Magro et al., 2009). Once the presence of cutaneous disease has been established, a systematic investigation for the presence of muscle disease, systemic disease, and/or a potentially associated malignancy should ensue.

Muscle involvement is suspected clinically. Enzymatic testing will often reveal elevations of muscle-derived enzymes, including creatine kinase (CK), aldolase, lactic dehydrogenase (LDH), alanine aminotransferase (ALT), or (aspartate aminotransferase (AST). The serum CK level seems to be the most specific and is a useful test for following response to therapy. Additional testing including electromyography (EMG), muscle biopsy, ultrasound, or MR imaging may be ordered in patients in whom other tests are inconclusive (Garcia, 2000). Muscle weakness may be caused by many other disorders including toxins, infections, metabolic abnormalities, and neurologic disorders, and these causes must be excluded (Wortmann, 2000).

Serologic tests are often ordered, but their clinical application is at best controversial. Antinuclear antibody (ANA) testing is positive in approximately two-thirds of patients with DM, however, the presence has not been shown to influence the prediction of the course of the disease or its therapy. Numerous myositis-specific autoantibodies (MSAs) have been recognized, including Jo-1, Mi-2, PL-7, PL-12, EJ, OJ, KS, MJ, PMS1, SRP, YRS, and Zo, and some correlate with certain subsets of disease (Love et al., 1991, Mimori et al., 2007, Gunawardena et al., 2009). The anti-Jo-1 antibody is predictive of pulmonary involvement, but rarely occurs in DM patients. Anti-Mi-2 occurs in roughly 25% of DM patients and although specific for DM, it is not sensitive. Targoff et al. (2000) described an antibody to a 155 kd antigen or Se antigen (90–95 kd) that appears to be a marker of amyopathic DM (16 of 18 patients studied). The anti-155 kd antibody may also be associated with juvenile DM and might predict a chronic course. Another novel autoantibody, anti-CADM-140, has been identified in clinically amyopathic dermatomyositis. Anti-p155 / 140, an antibody specific to dermatomyositis that is not yet commercially available, may also be correlated with cancer-associated DM (Madan et al., 2009). In fact, in one study, testing for the anti-155 / 140 antibody alone had 50% sensitivity and 96% specificity for detection of cancer-associated DM, with an excellent negative predictive value as well (Chinoy et al., 2007). Anti-Ro (SS-A) antibody may rarely occur in DM as well. Finally, three other autoantibodies, U1RNP, Ku, and PM-Scl, have been found in myositis-overlap syndromes. Perhaps as further studies are performed, serologic testing will become clinically useful. Until then, these tests are primarily reserved for investigation.

Once the diagnosis is confirmed, the patient should have a thorough evaluation. Evaluation has several purposes: assessment of severity, prediction of prognosis, and identification of associated disorders. The severity of the myositis often correlates with enzyme levels and degree of weakness. Patients should be assessed for esophageal, pulmonary, and cardiac involvement with tests such as a barium swallow and / or esophageal motility studies, chest x-ray and / or high resolution chest CT, pulmonary function studies including diffusion capacity, and an electrocardiogram.

An evaluation for malignancy should be considered in all adult patients with DM (Callen, 1982, Callen, 2002). The type of evaluation is selected based upon the patient's age and sex. The likelihood of malignancy increases with age and the sites vary depending on the patient's age. It has been suggested that patients should be followed in conjunction with an internist with ongoing vigilance based on thorough medical histories, review of symptoms, complete physical examinations, and screening laboratory tests (Callen, 1994). Women need to undergo mammograms, pelvic ultrasound, Papanicolao smear, and CA-125 testing; whereas men need Prostate Specific Antigen (PSA) testing. Some have advocated including CT scans of the chest (rather than relying on a chest x-ray), abdomen, and pelvis as part of the routine malignancy work-up in adult patients with DM.

Malignancy evaluation is repeated annually for at least the first three-years following diagnosis as well as with any new symptoms. The overrepresentation of cancer in these patients seemingly approaches normal levels after three-years (Hill et al., 2001), thus, age-specific malignancy screening, along with evaluation of any abnormal symptoms or findings, is recommended for following patients more than three years after the initial diagnosis.

Course and Therapy

Several general measures are helpful in treating patients with DM. Bedrest is often valuable in the individual with progressive weakness; however, this must be combined with a range-of-motion exercise program to prevent contractures. Patients who have evidence of dysphagia should have the head of their bed elevated and should avoid eating meals immediately before retiring.

All patients with muscle disease should be considered for exercise and rehabilitation programs because even in patients responding to pharmacologic interventions for myositis, a majority will develop sustained disability (Alexanderson H, 2009). Studies demonstrate that patients with inflammatory muscle disease who participate in these programs have improved muscle strength and endurance and note reduced disease activity. In addition, improvement in strength has been demonstrated even in the course of active disease, rather than inducing flares in muscle involvement (de Salles Painelli et al., 2009).

In both adults and children, attention to general health maintenance principles and osteoporosis prevention is a key element of patient management. This can be accomplished by joint longitudinal care with an internist or pediatrician.

Corticosteroids and Immunosuppressive Agents

The mainstay of therapy for DM muscle disease or systemic involvement is the use of systemic corticosteroids. Traditionally, prednisone is given at a dose of 0.5 to 1 mg / kg daily as initial therapy. The treatment should continue for at least one month after the myositis has become clinically and enzymatically inactive. At this point, the dose is slowly tapered, generally over a period lasting one and a half to two times as long as the period of active treatment. Approximately 25% of patients with dermatomyositis will not respond to systemic corticosteroids, another 25–50% will develop significant steroid-related side effects. Therefore, early intervention with steroid-sparing agents, primarily immunosuppressive agents, such as methotrexate, azathioprine, mycophenolate mofetil, high-dose intravenous immunoglobulin (IVIG), cyclophosphamide, chlorambucil, or cyclosporine may be an effective means of inducing or maintaining a remission (Sinoway and Callen, 1993; Villalba and Adams, 1996; Gelber et al., 2000; Vencovsky et al., 2000; Dalakas et al., 1993). High-dose IVIG is one of the only agents that has been evaluated in a randomized, placebo-controlled clinical trial, which demonstrated benefit in both the muscle disease and cutaneous disease of DM (Dalakaas et al., 1993). Further open-label studies have demonstrated similar results (Cherin et al., 2002).

Roughly one-half to three fourths of patients treated with an immunosuppressive agent will respond with an increase in strength, a decrease in enzyme levels, or a reduction in corticosteroid dosage. However, there are few double-blind, placebo-controlled studies that demonstrate the effectiveness of any of these agents.

Additional Therapeutic Options for Muscle and / or Systemic Involvement

Patients who fail to respond to these immunosuppressives may respond to pulse methylprednisolone therapy (Callen et al., 1994; Sawhney et al., 2000; Al-Mayouf et al., 2000a), combination immunosuppressive therapy (Villalba et al., 1998), etanercept (Saadeh, 2000), infliximab (Hengstman et al., 2000), rituximab (Levine, 2005), oral tacrolimus (Ochi et al., 2005, Mitsui et al., 2005), sirolimus (Nadiminti and Arbiser, 2005), total body irradiation (Kelly et al., 1988), or hematopoietic stem cell transplantation (HSCT, Saccardi et al., 2008, Wu et al., 2007). Notably, there have also been treatment failures reported with most of these potential therapies. Early enthusiasm for plasmapheresis and/or leukapheresis was followed by a placebo-controlled study that failed to demonstrate effectiveness (Miller et al., 1992).

Therapeutic Options for Cutaneous Disease

Even after the myositis and systemic disease of DM are controlled with corticosteroids and/or immunosuppressive therapy, the cutaneous disease often remains recalcitrant to therapy and can be particularly challenging to manage. In fact, there is known to be a discordant response to therapy between muscle and skin disease in DM (Dawkins et al., 1998). For these reasons, there are subsets of patients in which cutaneous disease becomes the primary component of disease management. This includes patients with postmyopathic dermatomyositis and those with clinically amyopathic dermatomyositis. In both of these subsets of patients, aggressive corticosteroid therapy is frequently not warranted.

Anecdotal experience supports the concept that systemic corticosteroids have varying degrees of efficacy for the cutaneous manifestations of dermatomyositis, with only a small subgroup of patients having excellent responses at doses that do not cause toxicity. In addition, many patients on toxic doses of systemic corticosteroids have little to no effect on their cutaneous disease or its associated symptoms. In sum, given the host of potential side effects of long-term systemic corticosteroid therapy as well as the refractory nature of the skin lesions in dermatomyositis, systemic corticosteroids are not considered the mainstay in therapy for cutaneous disease.

Most patients with cutaneous lesions are photosensitive; thus, the daily use of a broad-spectrum sunscreen with a high sun protective factor is recommended. Wide-brimmed hats, sun protective clothing, and behavioral modification should also be encouraged as skin manifestations are challenging to control without adequate photoprotection. Antipruritics, both topical and oral, are often necessary given the prominent pruritus that is often associated with DM. Topical therapy with an appropriately selected corticosteroid or with a calcineurin inhibitor, such as tacrolimus or pimecrolimus, may be useful adjunctive therapy (Hollar and Jorizzo, 2004).

Hydroxychloroquine HCL in dosages of 200 mg to 400 mg per day is effective in approximately 80% of patients with DM in serving as a steroid-sparing agent (Woo et al., 1984). Patients who do not respond well to hydroxychloroquine can be switched to chloroquine phosphate 250 to 500 mg per day or can have quinacrine HCL 100 mg once or twice daily added to the regimen. One published report has supported the synergistic effect of combination antimalarials in cutaneous dermatomyositis (Ang and Werth, 2005). Patients on continuous antimalarial therapy should have periodic ophthalmologic examinations and blood counts. It appears that patients with DM have a greater frequency of drug eruptions from antimalarials, thus patients should be warned about this possibility (Pelle and Callen, 2002).

Methotrexate in doses of 15–35 mg per week has been reported to be useful for skin lesions of DM (Zieglschmid et al., 1995; Kasteler and Callen, 1997). These studies, however, are uncontrolled, open-label observations. The need for routine liver biopsy in the DM patient treated with methotrexate is controversial, but patients who are obese, diabetic, or have abnormal liver function tests should potentially have periodic liver biopsies.

Only IVIG has been studied for the cutaneous disease of DM in a randomized-controlled fashion (Dalakas et al., 1993). Other immunosuppressive agents have not been systematically studied specifically for the cutaneous lesions of DM, but anecdotal reports have demonstrated benefit from mycophenolate mofetil (Tausche and Maurer, 2001, Gelber et al., 2000, Edge et al., 2006), thalidomide (Stirling, 1998), dapsone (Konohana and Kawashima, 1994, Cohen JB, 2002), adjuvant leflunomide (Boswell and Costner, 2008), antiestrogen medications (Sereda and Werth, 2006), infliximab (Dold et al., 2007), etanercept (Saddeh, 2000), efalizumab (this drug has been withdrawn from the market) (Huber et al., 2006), rituximab (Feist et al., 2008, Dinh et al., 2007), oral tacrolimus (Hassan et al., 2008, Martin Nalda et al., 2006, Yamada et al., 2004), sirolimus (Nadiminti and Arbiser, 2005), total body irradiation (Kelly et al., 1988), and HSCT (Wu et al., 2007) in some cases.

Calcinosis is a complication of DM frequently seen in children and adolescents and occasionally seen in adults. This process may be prevented by aggressive early treatment (Kim et al., 2009). The use of intravenous methylprednisolone may lessen the frequency and severity of this process (Callen et al., 1994, Pachman LM, 1994). Others have suggested that immunosuppressives may similarly reduce the chance of calcinosis (Al-Mayouf et al., 2000b). Once established, calcinosis is difficult to treat. Although possible, spontaneous regression is unusual. Individual patients have been treated with low-dose warfarin (Matsuoka et al., 1998), oral aluminum hydroxide (Wang et al., 1988), probenecid (Harel et al., 2001), alendronate (Ambler et al., 2005), infliximab (Riley et al., 2008), IVIG (Schanz et al., 2008, Penate et al., 2009), HSCT (Holzer et al., 2010), pamidronate (Slimani et al., 2010), electric shock wave lithotripsy (ESWL, Chan and Li, 2005), and/or surgical excision (Downey et al., 1988), however, no studies have documented the usefulness **of these therapies** in larger groups of patients. Reports of long-term administration of diltiazem are promising (Oliveri et al., 1996, Vinen et al., 2000, Abdallah-Lotf et al., 2005).

The prognosis of dermatomyositis varies greatly, depending on the series of patients studied. Factors that affect prognosis include the patient's age, the severity of myositis, progressive disease, the presence of dysphagia, the presence of cardiopulmonary involvement, the presence of an associated malignancy, a longer duration of symptoms prior to diagnosis and initiation of therapy, and the response to systemic corticosteroid therapy (Marie et al., 1999; Iorizzo and Jorizzo, 2008). It seems to be well established by retrospective reports that the use of systemic corticosteroids and/or immunosuppressive therapies improves the prognosis.

Summary

DM is a condition primarily of the skin and muscles, but other systemic features may occur. DM appears to be the predominant idiopathic inflammatory myopathy in children, whereas in adults, many patients lack skin disease (polymyositis or inclusion body myositis). In addition, a subset of both adult and juvenile patients with DM have cutaneous disease in the absence of myositis, referred to as amyopathic DM. These patients are still at risk for malignancy and systemic disease.

The pathogenesis of the muscle disease is becoming better understood, but the cutaneous disease mechanisms remain enigmatic. DM in adults is associated with malignancy and thus a careful evaluation of each patient should be part of their initial and follow-up assessments. Patients should also be evaluated for the presence of associated systemic disease, particularly esophageal, pulmonary, and / or cardiac disease.

Corticosteroids, immunosuppressives, biologic agents, and / or intravenous immunoglobulin are effective therapies for the myopathy of DM, whereas the skin disease is best managed with photoprotection, topical corticosteroids and / or topical calcineurin inhibitors, antimalarials, methotrexate, mycophenolate mofetil, and / or intravenous immunoglobulin. Calcinosis occurs more frequently in children with DM, and early aggressive therapy may limit the chance of this complication. Overall, the prognosis of DM is good except for patients with malignancy, those with severe and progressive weakness, and those with cardiopulmonary dysfunction.

References

Abdallah-Lotf M, Grasland A, Vinceneux P, Sigal-Grinberg M (2005) Regression of cutis calcinosis with diltiazem in adult dermatomyositis. Eur J Dermatol 15(2):102–4

Abernethy ML, Arterberry JF, Callen JP (1996)Low-dose methotrexate as an adjunctive therapy with surgery for ectropion complicating dermatomyositis. Dermatology 192(2):153–155

Alexanderson H (2009) Exercise effects in patients with adult idiopathic inflammatory myopathies. Curr Opin Rheumatol;21(2):158–63

Al-Mayouf SM, Laxer RM, Schneider R, Silverman ED, Feldman BM (2000a) Intravenous immunoglobulin therapy for juvenile dermatomyositis: efficacy and safety. J Rheumatol 27:2498–2503

Al-Mayouf S, Al-Mazyed A, Bahabri S (2000b) Efficacy of early treatment of severe juvenile dermatomyositis with intravenous methylprednisolone and methotrexate. Clin Rheumatol 19:138–141

Ambler GR, Chaitow J, Rogers M, McDonald DW, Ouvrier RA (2005) Rapid improvement of calcinosis in juvenile dermatomyositis with alendronate therapy. The Journal of rheumatology;32(9):1837–9

Ang GC, Werth VP (2005) Combination antimalarials in the treatment of cutaneous dermatomyositis: a retrospective study. Archives of dermatology;141(7):855–9

Antiochos BB, Brown LA, Li Z, Tosteson TD, Wortmann RL, Rigby WF (2009) Malignancy is associated with dermatomyositis but not polymyositis in Northern New England, USA. J Rheumatol. 36(12):2704–10

Airio A, Pukkala E, Isomäki (1995) Elevated cancer incidence in patients with dermatomyositis: A population based study. J Rheumatol 22:1300–1303

Bohan A, Peter JB (1975) Polymyositis and dermatomyositis. N Engl J Med 292:344–347 and 403–407 (two part article)

Bohan A, Peter JB, Bowman RL, Pearson CM (1977) A computer-assisted analysis of 153 patients with polymyositis and dermatomyositis. Medicine 56:255–286

Bendewald MJ, Wetter DA, Li X, Davis MD (2010) Incidence of dermatomyositis and clinically amyopathic dermatomyositis: a population-based study in Olmsted County, Minnesota. Archives of dermatology;146(1):26–30

Bingham A, Mamyrova G, Rother KI, et al. (2008) Predictors of acquired lipodystrophy in juvenile-onset dermatomyositis and a gradient of severity. Medicine;87(2):70–86

Boswell JS, Costner MI (2008) Leflunomide as adjuvant treatment of dermatomyositis. Journal of the American Academy of Dermatology;58(3):403–6

Callen JP (1982) The value of malignancy evaluation in patients with dermatomyositis. J Am Acad Dermatol 6:253–259

Callen JP (1993) Photodermatitis in a 6-year-old child. Arhthritis Rheum 36:1483–1485

Callen AM, Pachman LM, Hayford J, Chung A, Ramsey-Goldman R (1994) Intermittent high dose intravenous methylprednisolone (IV pulse) prevents calcinosis and shortens disease course in juvenile dermatomyositis (JDMS). Arth Rheum 37: R10A

Callen JP (1994) Myositis and malignancy. Curr Opin Rheumatol;6:590–4

Callen JP (1999) Photosensitivity in collagen vascular diseases. Semin Cutan Med Surg 18(4):293–296

Callen JP (2000) Dermatomyositis. Lancet 355:53–57

Callen JP (2002) When and how should the patient with dermatomyositis or amyopathic dermatomyositis be assessed for possible cancer? Arch Dermatol 138(7):969–971

Chan AY, Li E (2005) Electric shock wave lithotripsy (ESWL) as a pain control measure in dermatomyositis with calcinosis cutis – old method, new discovery. Clin Rheumatol;24:172–3

Chander R, Gupta T, Rani S, Nagia A (2009) Erythrodermic juvenile dermatomyositis. Pediatr Dermatol Mar-Apr;26(2):234–5

Cheong W-K, Hughes GRV, Norris PG, Hawk JLM (1994) Cutaneous photosensitivity in dermatomyositis. Brit J Dermatol 131:205–208

Cherin P, Pelletier S, Teixeira A, Laforet P, Genereau T, Simon A, Maisonobe T, Eymard B, Herson S (2002): Results and long-term followup of intravenous immunoglobulin infusions in chronic, refractory polymyositis. Arthritis Rheum 46:467–74

Chinoy H, Fertig N, Oddis CV, Ollier WE, Cooper RG (2007) The diagnostic utility of myositis autoantibody testing for predicting the risk of cancer-associated myositis. Ann Rheum Dis 66(10):1345–9

Chow WH, Gridley G, Mellemkjaer L, McLaughlin JK, Olsen JH, Fraumeni JF Jr (1995) Cancer risk following polymyositis and dermatomyositis: A nationwide cohort study in Denmark. Cancer Causes and Control 5:9–13

Cohen JB (2002) Cutaneous involvement of dermatomyositis can respond to Dapsone therapy. Int J Dermatol;41(3):182–4

Cosnes A, Amaudric F, Gherardi R, Verroust J, Wechsler J, Revuz J, Roujeau JC (1995) Dermatomyositis without muscle weakness. Long-term follow-up of 12 patients without systemic corticosteroids. Arch Dermatol 131:1381–1385

Dacey MJ, Callen JP (2003) Hydroxyurea-induced dermatomyositis-like eruption. J Am Acad Dermatol 48:439–441

Dalakas MC, Illa I, Dambrosia JM, Soueidan SA, Stein DP, Otero C, Dinsmore ST, McCrosky S (1993) A controlled trial of high-dose intravenous immune globulin infusions as treatment for dermatomyositis. N Engl J Med 329:1993–2000

Dalakas MC (1991) Polymyositis, dermatomyositis and inclusion-body myositis. N Engl J Med;325:1487–98

Dalakas MC (1998) Molecular immunology and genetics of inflammatory muscle diseases. Arch Neurol 54:1509–1512

Dalakas MC, Hohlfeld R (2003) Polymyositis and dermatomyositis. *Lancet* 362(9388), 971–982

Daoud MS, Gibson LE, Pittelkow MR (1997) Hydroxyurea dermopathy. A unique lichenoid eruption complicating long-term therapy with hydroxyurea. J Am Acad Dermatol 36:178–182

Dawkins MA, Jorizzo JL, Walker FO, Albertson D, Sinal SH, Hinds A (1998) Dermatomyositis: a dermatology-based case series. Journal of the American Academy of Dermatology;38(3):397–404 de Salles Painelli V, Gualano B, Artioli GG, et al. (2009) The possible role of physical exercise on the treatment of idiopathic inflammatory myopathies. Autoimmun Rev;8(5):355–9

Dinh HV, McCormack C, Hall S, Prince HM (2007) Rituximab for the treatment of the skin manifestations of dermatomyositis: a report of 3 cases. Journal of the American Academy of Dermatology;56(1):148–53

Dold S, Justiniano ME, Marquez J, Espinoza LR (2007) Treatment of early and refractory dermatomyositis with infliximab: a report of two cases. Clinical rheumatology;26(7):1186–8

Douglas WW, Tazelaar HD, Hartman TE, Hartman RP, Decker PA, Schroeder DR, Ryu JH (2001) Polymyositis-dermatomyositis-associated interstitial lung disease. Am J Respir Crit Care Med. 164:1182–5

Dourmishev AL, Dourshimev LA (1999) Dermatomyositis and drugs. Adv Exp Med Biol 445:187–191

Downey EC, Jr., Woolley MM, Hanson V (1988) Required surgical therapy in the pediatric patient with dermatomyositis. Arch Surg;123(9):1117–20

Edge JC, Outland JD, Dempsey JR, Callen JP (2006) Mycophenolate mofetil as an effective corticosteroid-sparing therapy for recalcitrant dermatomyositis. Archives of dermatology;142(1):65–9

El-Azhary RA, Pakzad SY (2002) Amyopathic dermatomyositis: retrospective review of 37 cases. J Am Acad Dermatol 46:560–565

Euwer RL, Sontheimer RD (1991) Amyopathic DM (DM siné myositis). J Am Acad Dermatol 24:959–966

Fardet L, Dupuy A, Gain M, Kettaneh A, Chérin P, Bachelez H, Dubertret L, Lebbe C, Morel P, Rybojad M (2009) Factors associated with underlying malignancy in a retrospective cohort of 121 patients with dermatomyositis. Medicine (Baltimore) 88(2):91–7

Feist E, Dorner T, Sorensen H, Burmester GR (2008) Longlasting remissions after treatment with rituximab for autoimmune myositis. The Journal of rheumatology;35(6):1230–2

Fisler RE, et al. (2002) Aggressive management of juvenile dermatomyositis results in improved outcome and decreased incidence of calcinosis. J Am Acad dermatol;47(4):505–511

Flendrie M, Vissers WH, Creemers MC, de Jong EM, van de Kerkhof PC, van Riel PL (2005) Dermatological conditions during TNF-alpha-blocking therapy in patients with rheumatoid arthritis: a prospective study. Arthritis Res Ther;7:R666–76

Garcia J (2000) MRI in inflammatory myopathies. Skeletal Radiol 29:425–438

Gelber AC, Nousari HC, Wigley FM (2000) Mycophenolate mofetil in the treatment of severe skin manifestations of dermatomyositis: a series of 4 cases. J Rheumatol 27:1542–1545

Gerami P, Schope Jm, Mcdonald L, Walling Hw, Sontheimer Rd (2006) A systematic review of adult-onset clinically amyopathic dermatomyositis (dermatomyositis sine myositis): A missing link within the spectrum of the idiopathic inflammatory myopathies. J Am Acad Dermatol 54(4), 597–613

Ghali FE, Stein LD, Fine J-D, Burkes EJ, McCauliffe DP (1999) Gingival telangiectases. An underappreciated physical sign of juvenile dermatomyositis. Arch Dermatol 135:1370–1374

Gonzalez-Lopez L, Gamez-Nava JI, Sanchez L, Rosas E, Suarez-Almazor M, Cardona-Munoz C, Ramos-Remus C (1996) Cardiac manifestations in dermato-polymyositis. Clin Exp Rheumatol 14:373–379

Gunawardena H, Betteridge ZE, McHugh NJ (2009) Myostis-specific autoantibodies: their clinical and pathogenic significance in disease expression. Rheumatology;48:607–612

Harel L, Harel G, Korenreich L, Straussberg R, Amir J (2001) Treatment of calcinosis in juvenile dermatomyositis with probenecid: the role of phosphorus metabolism in the development of calcifications. The Journal of rheumatology;28(5):1129–32

Hassan J, van der Net JJ, van Royen-Kerkhof A (2008) Treatment of refractory juvenile dermatomyositis with tacrolimus. Clinical rheumatology;27(11):1469–71

Hengstman G, van den Hoogen F, van Engelen B, Barrera P, Netea M, van den Putte L (2000) Anti-TNF-blockade with infliximab (remicade) in polymyositis and dermatomyositis. Arthritis Rheum 43: S193A

Hill CL, Zhang Y, Sigurgeirsson B, Pukkala E, Mellemkjaer L, Airio A, Evan SR, Felson DT (2001) Frequency of specific cancer types in dermatomyositis and polymyositis: A population-based study. Lancet 357:96–100

Hollar CB, Jorizzo JL (2004) Topical tacrolimus 0.1% ointment for refractory skin disease in dermatomyositis: a pilot study. J Dermatol Treat 15:35–9

Holzer U, van Royen-Kerkhof A, van der Torre P, et al. (2010) Successful autologous stem cell transplantation in two patients with juvenile dermatomyositis. Scandinavian journal of rheumatology;39(1):88–92

Hu WJ, Chen DL, Min HQ (1996) Study of 45 cases of nasopharyngeal carcinoma with dermatomyositis. Am J Clin Oncol;19:35–38

Huang YL et al. (2009) Malignancies associated with dermatomyositis and polymyositis in Taiwan: a nationwide population-based study. Br J Dermatol;161(4):854–60

Huber A, Gaffal E, Bieber T, Tuting T, Wenzel J (2006) Treatment of recalcitrant dermatomyositis with efalizumab. Acta Derm Venereol;86(3):254–5

Huber AM, Lang B, LeBlanc CM, Birdi N, Bolaria RK, Malleson P (2000) Medium- and long-term functional outcomes in a multicenter cohort of children with juvenile dermatomyositis. Arthritis Rheum 43:541–549

Huemer C, Kitson H, Malleson PN, Sanderson S, Huemer M, Cabral DA, Chanoine J-P, Petty RE (2001) Lipodystrophy in patients with juvenile dermatomyositis – evaluation of clinical and metabolic abnormalities. J Rheumatol 28:610–615

Hundley JL, Carroll CL, Lang W, Snively B, Yosipovitch G, Feldman SR, Jorizzo JL (2006) Cutaneous symptoms of dermatomyositis significantly impact patients' quality of life. J Am Acad Dermatol;54:217–20

Iorizzo LJ, 3rd, Jorizzo JL (2008) The treatment and prognosis of dermatomyositis: an updated review. Journal of the American Academy of Dermatology;59(1):99–112

Jorizzo Jl (2002) Dermatomyositis: Practical aspects. Arch Dermatol 138(1), 114–116

Kasteler JS, Callen JP (1994) Scalp involvement in dermatomyositis. Often overlooked or misdiagnosed. JAMA 272:1939–1941

Kasteler JS, Callen JP (1997) Low-dose methotrexate administered weekly in an effective corticosteroid-sparing agent for the treatment of the cutaneous manifestations of dermatomyositis. J Am Acad Dermatol 36:67–71

Kaufmann R, Greiner D, Schmidt P, Wolter M (1998) Dermatomyositis presenting as plaque-like mucinosis. Brit J Dermatol 138:889–892

Kelly JJ, Madoc-Jones H, Adelman LS, Andres PL (1988) Munsat TL. Response to total body irradiation in dermatomyositis. Muscle & nerve;11(2):120–3

Kim S, El-Hallak M, Dedeoglu F, Zurakowski D, Fuhlbrigge RC, Sundel RP (2009) Complete and sustained remission of juvenile dermatomyositis resulting from aggressive treatment. Arthritis and rheumatism;60(6):1825–30

Klein Rq, Teal V, Taylor L, Troxel Ab, Werth Vp (2007) Number, characteristics, and classification of patients with dermatomyositis seen by dermatology and rheumatology departments at a large tertiary medical center. J Am Acad Dermatol 57(6), 937–943

Konohana A, Kawashima J (1994) Successful treatment of dermatomyositis with dapsone. Clinical and experimental dermatology;19(4):367

Kuru S, Inukai A, Liang Y, Doyu M, Takano A, Sobue G (2000) Tumor necrosis factor-a expression in muscles of polymyositis and dermatomyositis. Acta Neuropathol 99:585–588

Levine TD 2005 Rituximab in the treatment of dermatomyositis: an open-label pilot study. Arthritis and rheumatism;52(2):601–7

Love LA, Leff RL, Fraser DD, Targoff IN, Dalakas M, Plotz PH, Miller FW (1991) A new approach to the classification of idiopathic inflammatory myopathy: Myositis-specific autoantibodies define useful homogeneous patient groups. Medicine 70(6):360–374

Lundberg IE, Nyberg P (1998) New developments in the role of cytokines and chemokines in inflammatory myopathies. Curr Opinion in Rheumatol 10:521–529

Madan V, Chinoy H, Griffiths CE, Cooper RG (2009) Defining cancer risk in dermatomyositis. Part II. Assessing diagnostic usefulness of myositis serology. Clin Exp Dermatol 34(5):561–5

Magro CM, Segal JP, Neil Crowson A, Chadwick P (2010) The phenotypic profile of dermatomyositis and lupus erythematosus: a comparative analysis. J Cutan Pathol 37(6):659–671

Marie I, Hatron P-Y, Hachulla E, Wallaert B, Michon-Pasturel U, Devulder B (1998) Pulmonary involvement in polymyositis and in dermatomyositis. J Rheumatol 25:1336–1343

Marie I, Hatron PY, Levesque H, Hachulla E, Hellot MF, Michon-Pasturel U, Courtois H, Devulder B (1999) Influence of age on characteristics of polymyositis and dermatomyositis in adults. Medicine 78:139–147

Marie I, Joly P, Levesque H, Heron F, Courville P, Cailleux N, Courtois H (2000) Pseudo-dermatomyositis as a complication of hydroxyurea therapy. Clin Exp Rheumatol 18:536–537

Martin Nalda A, Modesto Caballero C, Arnal Guimeral C, Boronat Rom M, Barcelo Garcia P (2006). [Efficacy of tacrolimus (FK-506) in the treatment of recalcitrant juvenile dermatomyositis: study of 6 cases]. Med Clin (Barc);127(18):697–701

Matsuoka Y, Miyajima S, Okada N (1998) A case of calcinosis universalis successfully treated with low-dose warfarin. J Dermatol;25(11):716–20

McCollough ML, Cockerell CJ (1998) Vesiculo-Bullous Dermatomyositis. Am J Dermatopathol 20:170–174

Miller FW, Leitman SF, Cronin ME, Hicks JE, Leff RL, Wesley R, Fraser DD, Dalakas M, Plotz PH (1992) Controlled trial of plasma exchange and leukapheresis in polymyositis and dermatomyositis. N Engl J Med 326:1380–1384

Mimori T, Imura Y, Nakashima R, Yoshifugi H (2007) Autoantibodies in idiopathic inflammatory myopathy: an update on clinical and pathophysiological significance. Curr Opin Reumatol;19:523–529

Mitsui T, Kuroda Y, Kunishige M, Matsumoto T (2005) Successful treatment with tacrolimus in a case of refractory dermatomyositis. Intern Med;44(11):1197–9

Miyagawa S, Okazaki A, Minowa R, Shirai T (1992) Dermatomyositis presenting as erythroderma. J Am Acad Dermatol;26(3 Pt 2):489–90

Nadiminti U, Arbiser JL (2005) Rapamycin (sirolimus) as a steroid-sparing agent in dermatomyositis. Journal of the American Academy of Dermatology;52(2 Suppl 1):17–9

Nousari HC, Ha VT, Laman SD, Provost TT, Tausk FA (1999) 'Centripetal Flagellate Erythema': A Cutaneous Manifestation Associated with Dermatomyositis. J Rheumatol 26:692–695

Nyberg P, Wikman A-L, Nennesmo I, Lundberg I (2000) Increased expression of Interleukin 1a and MHC class I in muscle tissue of patients with chronic, inactive polymyositis and dermatomyositis. J Rheumatol 27:940–948

Ochi S, Nanki T, Takada K, et al. (2005) Favorable outcomes with tacrolimus in two patients with refractory interstitial lung disease associated with polymyositis / dermatomyositis. Clinical and experimental rheumatology;23(5):707–10

Oddis CV, Conte CG, Steen VD, Medsger TA, Jr. (1990) Incidence of polymyositis-dermatomyositis: a 20-year study of hospital diagnosed cases in Allegheny County, PA 1963–1982. J Rheumatol 17(10):1329–34

Oliveri MB, Palermo R, Mautalen C, Hübscher O (1996) Regression of calcinosis during Diltiazem treatment of juvenile dermatomyositis. J Rheumatol 23:2152–2155

Pachman LM (1995) An update on juvenile dermatomyositis. Curr Opin Rheumatol 7:437–441

Pachman LM (1994) Juvenile dermatomyositis: Decreased calcinosis with intermittent high-dose intravenous methylprednisolone therapy. *Arthritis and rheumatism* 37(Suppl):429

Pachman LM, Hayford JR, Chung A, et al. (1998) Juvenile dermatomyositis at diagnosis: clinical characteristics of 79 children. The Journal of rheumatology;25(6):1198–204

Pachman LM, Liotta-Davis MR, Hong DK, Kinsella TR, Mendez EP, Kinder JM, Chen EH (2000) TNFa-308A allele in juvenile dermatomyositis. Arthritis Rheum 43:2368–2377

Pautas E, Cherin P, Piette J-C, Pelletier S, Wechsler B, Cabane J, Herson S (2000) Features of polymyositis and dermatomyositis in the elderly: A case-control study. Clin Exp Rheumatol 18:241–244

Pelle MT, Callen JP (2002) Adverse cutaneous reactions to hydroxychloroquine are more common in patients with dermatomyositis than in patients with cutaneous lupus erythematosus. Arch Dermatol 138:1231–1233

Penate Y, Guillermo N, Melwani P, Martel R, Hernandez-Machin B, Borrego L (2009) Calcinosis cutis associated with amyopathic dermatomyositis: response to intravenous immunoglobulin. Journal of the American Academy of Dermatology;60(6):1076–7

Peng J-C, Sheem T-S, Hsu M-M (1995) Nasopharyngeal carcinoma with dermatomyositis. Analysis of 12 cases. Arch Otolaryngol Head Neck Surg 121:1298–1301

Plotz PH, Rider LG, Targoff IN, Raben N, O'Hanlon TP, Miller FW (1995) Myositis: Immunologic Contributions to Understanding Cause, Pathogenesis, and Therapy. Ann Intern Med 122:715–724

Requena L, Grilli R, Soriano L, Escalonilla P, Farina C, Martin L (1997) Dermatomyositis with a pityriasis rubra pilaris-like eruption: a little-known distinctive cutaneous manifestation of dermatomyositis. Brit J Dermatol 136:768–771

Riley P, Mccann Lj, Maillard Sm, Woo P, Murray Kj, Pilkington Ca (2008) Effectiveness of infliximab in the treatment of refractory juvenile dermatomyositis with calcinosis. *Rheumatology (Oxford, England)* 47(6), 877–880

Rockerbie NR, Woo TY, Callen JP, Giustina T (1989) Cutaneous changes of dermatomyositis precede muscle weakness. J Am Acad Dermatol 20:629–632

Saadeh CK (2000) Etanercept is effective in the treatment of polymyositis/dermatomyositis which is refractory to conventional therapy including steroids and other disease modifying agents. Arhtritis Rheum 43: S193A

Saccardi R, Di Gioia M, Bosi A (2008). Haematopoietic stem cell transplantation for autoimmune disorders. Curr Opin Hematol;15(6):594–600

Sawhney S, Sidoti G, Woo P, Murray KJ (2000) Clinical characteristics and outcome of idiopathic inflammatory myositis (IIM) in childhood: A 2 year follow up. Arthritis Rheum 43: A

Sayers ME, Chou SM, Calabrese LH (1992) Inclusion body myositis: Analysis of 32 cases. J Rheumatol 19:1385–1389

Schanz S, Ulmer A, Fierlbeck G (2008) Response of dystrophic calcification to intravenous immunoglobulin. Archives of dermatology;144(5):585–7

Seidler AM, Gottlieb AB (2008) Dermatomyositis induced by drug therapy: a review of case reports. J Am Acad Dermatol;59:5:872–880

Sereda D, Werth VP (2006) Improvement in dermatomyositis rash associated with the use of anti-estrogen medication. Archives of dermatology;142(1):70–2

Shannon PL, Ford MJ (1999) Angiokeratomas in juvenile dermatomyositis. Pediatr Dermatol 16:448–451

Shimizu T, Tomita Y, Son K, Nishinarita S, Sawada S, Horie T (2000) Elevation of serum soluble tumor necrosis factor receptors in patients with polymyositis and dermatomyositis. Clin Rheumatol 19:352–359

Shirani Z, Kucenic MJ, Carroll CL, Fleischer AB Jr, Feldman SR, Yosipovitch G, Jorizzo JL (2004) Pruritus in adult dermatomyositis. Clin Exp Dermatol. 2004;29:273–6

Sontheimer RD (2002) Would a new name hasten the acceptance of amyopathic dermatomyositis (dermatomyositis sine myositis) as a distinctive subset within the idiopathic inflammatory dermatomyopathies spectrum of clinical illness? J Am Acad Dermatol 46:626–636

Spiera R, Kagen L (1998) Extramuscular manifestations in idiopathic inflammatory myopathies. Curr Opinion in Rheumatol 10:556–561

Siguregeirsson B, Lindelöf B, Edhag O, Allander E (1992) Risk of cancer in patients with dermatomyositis or polymyositis. N Engl J Med 325:363–367

Sinoway PA, Callen JP (1993) Chlorambucil: An Effective Corticosteroid-Sparing Agent for Patients with Recalcitrant Dermatomyositis. Arthritis Rheum 36:319–324

Slimani S, Abdessemed A, Haddouche A, Ladjouze-Rezig A (2010) Complete resolution of universal calcinosis in a patient with juvenile dermatomyositis using pamidronate. Joint Bone Spine 77:70–72

Sugugiura T, Kawaguchi Y, Harigai M, Takagi K, Ohta S, Fukasawa C, Hara M, Kamatani N (2000) Increased CD40 expression on muscle cells of polymyositis and dermatomyositis: Role of CD40-CD40 ligand interaction in IL-6, IL-8, IL-5, and monocyte chemoattractant protein-1 production. J Immunol 164:6593–6000

Stirling DI (1998) Thalidomide and its impact in dermatology. Semin Cutan Med Surg;17(4):231–42

Stonecipher MR, Jorizzo JL, White WL, Walker FO, Prichard E (1993) Cutaneous changes of dermatomyositis in patients with normal muscle enzymes: DM siné myositis? J Am Acad Dermatol 28:951–956

Symmons DP, Sills JA, Davis SM (1995) The incidence of juvenile dermatomyositis: results from a nation-wide study. British journal of rheumatology;34(8):732–6

Targoff IN (1991) Dermatomyositis and polymyositis. Curr Prob Dermatol 3:131–180

Targoff IN, Trieu EP, Sontheimer RD (2000) Autoantibodies to 155 kd and Se antigens in patients with clinically-amyopathic dermatomyositis. Arthritis Rheum 43: S194A

Tausche AK, Meurer M (2001) Mycophenolate mofetil for dermatomyositis. Dermatology;202(4):341–3

Vencovsky J, Jarosova K, Machacek S, Studynkova J, Kafvova J, Bartunkova J, Nemcova D, Charvat F (2000) Cyclosporine A versus methotrexate in the treatment of polymyositis and dermatomyositis. Scand J Rheumatol 29:95–102

Villalba L, Adams EM (1996) Update on therapy for refractory dermatomyositis and polymyositis. Curr Opinion Rheumatol 8:544–551

Villalba L, Hicks JE, Adams EM, Sherman JB, Gourley MF, Leff RL, Thornton BC, Burgess SH, Plotz PH, Miller FW (1998) Treatment of refractory myositis. A randomized crossover study of two new cytotoxic regimens. Arthritis Rheum 41(3):392–399

Vinen CS, Patel S, Bruckner FE (2000) Regression of calcinosis associated with adult dermatomyositis following diltiazem therapy. Rheumatology (Oxford);39(3):333–4

Vleugels RA, Callen JP (2009). Dermatomyositis: Current and Future Treatments. Expert Review of Dermatology CME;4(6):581–94

Wanchu A, Khullar M, Sud A, Bambery P (1999) Nitric oxide production is increased in patient with inflammatory myositis. Nitric Oxide 3:454–458

Wang WJ, Lo WL, Wong CK (1988) Calcinosis cutis in juvenile dermatomyositis: remarkable response to aluminum hydroxide therapy. Archives of dermatology;124(11):1721–2

Whitmore SE, Rosenshein NB, Provost TT (1994) Ovarian cancer in patients with dermatomyositis. Medicine 73:153–160

Woo TY, Callen JP, Voorhees JJ, Bickers DR, Hanno R, Hawkins C (1984) Cutaneous lesions of dermatomyositis are improved by hydroxychloroquine. J Am Acad Dermatol 10:592–600

Woo TR, Rasmussen J, Callen JP (1985) Recurrent photosensitive dermatitis preceding juvenile dermatomyositis. Pediatr Dermatol 2:207–212

Wortmann RL (2001) Idiopathic Inflammatory diseases of muscle. In Treatment of the Rheumatic Diseases. Weisman ML, Weinblatt ME, Louie JS (eds) W. B. Saunders Co. pp 390–402

Wu FQ, Luan Z, Lai JM, et al. (2007) [Treatment of refractory rheumatism among preschool children with autologous peripheral blood hematopoietic stem cell transplantation]. Zhonghua Er Ke Za Zhi;45(11):809–13

Yamada A, Ohshima Y, Omata N, Yasutomi M, Mayumi M (2004). Steroid-sparing effect of tacrolimus in a patient with juvenile dermatomyositis presenting poor bioavailability of cyclosporine A. Eur J Pediatr;163(9):561–2

Zieglschmid-Adams ME, Pandya AG, Cohen SB, Sontheimer RD (1995) Treatment of dermato-
    myositis with methotrexate. J Am Acad Dermatol 32:754–757
Zuber M, John S, Pfreundschuh M, Gause A (1996) A young woman with a photosensitive pruritic
    rash on her face and upper trunk. Arthritis Rheum 39:1419–1422

Mixed Connective Tissue Disease

7

Reiji Kasukawa

Introduction

Since Klemperer proposed a concept on diffuse collagen disease in 1942, diseases occurring in the connective tissue have been understood to reveal their clinical symptoms in various tissues and organs with a variety of findings. This concept consequently allowed us to believe in the presence of a disease appearing between two established diseases or being an overlapped or mixed form of two diseases.

Sharp had recognized a group of patients who have mixed clinical features of systemic lupus erythematosus (SLE), systemic sclerosis (SSc) and polymyositis (PM). All such patients had high titers of anti-extractable nuclear antigen (ENA) antibody and a good prognosis. In 1972, Sharp et al. published a group of these conditions as a new disease entity: mixed connective tissue disease (MCTD).

The independent feature of the clinical entity of MCTD, however, was criticized by several investigators including Reichlin et al. (1976), LeRoy et al. (1980) and Nimelstein et al. (1980) on the following two points. The clinical features of MCTD do not differ from those of anti-snRNP antibody-positive SLE patients and most MCTD patients progress to scleroderma during the observation period.

Nevertheless, MCTD has been a recognized disease all over the world having characteristic mixed clinical features of several connective tissue diseases and autoantibody to U1snRNP.

Etiopathogenesis

Anti-U1snRNP Autoantibodies

The etiopathogenesis of MCTD is not clear, a fact true of other connective tissue diseases. However, the function of U1snRNP to which anti-U1snRNP antibody reacts was clarified by Lerner and Steitz (1979) to be a splicing of the precursor of mRNA. The mechanism underlying the production and pathogenic significance of anti-U1snRNP antibody has been studied by many investigators and clarified in part. Query et al. (1987) described a fact of molecular mimicry between RNP antigen and retroviral p30gag antigen. They demonstrated that 11 of 25 or 12 of 24 amino acids of the 70 kDa RNP antigen are homologous to those of Molony MuLV p30gag protein, and further observed that heteroimmune anti-p30gag antibody reacted to 70 kDa protein of RNP. Alarcon-Segovia et al. (1978) presented the attractive phenomenon of sufficient penetration of the anti-U1snRNP antibody but little penetration of anti-DNA antibody into the living cells. In their recent publication (Alarcon-Segovia et al., 1996), they demonstrated that anti-U1snRNP antibody penetrated into human mononuclear cells and induced apoptosis of the autoreactive lymphocytes at a higher frequency of 7.70% than control IgG at 1.21%, with the higher frequency believed to induce subsequently autoimmune disease.

Other Autoantibodies

In addition to anti-U1snRNP antibody (Burdt et al., 1999), several autoantibodies have been found in patients with MCTD. These autoantibodies and their frequencies in the sera of MCTD patients were presented in Table 1. The pathogenic and clinical significance of these autoantibodies, however, remains unclear, in the same manner as anti-U1snRNP antibody. Mairesse et al. (1993) tested serum samples from 18 patients with MCTD against human constitutive HSP 73 kDa protein and found a positive reaction with higher titers in all 18 patients, in contrast to the negative reaction of the sera of patients with rheumatoid arthritis (RA), SLE, SSc and PM. They concluded that anti-HSP 70kDa antibody could become a new diagnostic marker for MCTD. Anti-casein kinase II (CKII) antibody was found in 15% (8/52) of patients with MCTD, but in none of 52 healthy donors (Wiemann et al., 1993). The epitope of CKII was identified to be present in a subunit of the CKII molecule. However, they could not find any correlation between the occurrence of anti-casein kinase II antibody and anti-U1snRNP antibody. Anti-endotheial cell (EC) antibody was found in serum samples of 57% of patients with MCTD, and these antibody-positive patients were found to have higher levels of serum endothelin-1 at 7.3 ± 1.5 pg/ml ($n = 12$) by Filep et al. (1995). Both anti-EC antibody and endothelin-1 have been considered to participate in the process of vascular damage in MCTD patients. The antibody to spliceosome (A2/hn RNP) was first described by Hassfeld et al. (1995) in the sera of 38% of patients with MCTD, and this antibody was considered to interact with other hnRNP proteins. This antibody to heterogeneous nuclear ribonucleoprotein complex (hn RNP-A2) was found at almost an equivalent frequency in the sera of patients with RA and SLE. However, in recent studies, an epitope difference between anti-A3/RA33 antibody in MCTD and those in RA or SLE was reported (Steiner et al., 1996; Skriner et al., 1997).

Anti-human endogenous retrovirus (HERV) p30gag antibody was detected in the sera of MCTD patients at a frequency of 33%, and also found at a similar frequency in the sera of SLE (48.3%) and Sjogren's syndrome (35.0%) patients (Hishikawa et al., 1997). Antiphospholipid antibodies were found in MCTD patients at 15% (7/48) with low titers and none of these antibody-positive patients demonstrated vascular lesions due to thromboembolisms including pulmonary embolism. This findings differed from the reported thromboembolism of antibody-positive SLE patients (Komarireddy et al., 1997). However, anticardiolipin antibody has been reported to be associated with pulmonary hypertension

Table 1. Immunological Aberrations of Patients with Mixed Connective Tissue Disease

A. Autoantibodies to		Frequency	Reference
U1snRNP		100%	Burdt et al., 1999
73 kDa HSP		100%	Mairesse et al., 1993
Casein kinase		15%	Wiemann et al., 1993
Endothelial cells		57%	Filep et al., 1995
Spliceosome (A2/hn RNP)		38%	Hassfeld et al., 1995
Human endogenous retrovirus p30gag		33%	Hishikawa et al., 1997
Phospholipid		15%	Komatireddy et al., 1997
Fibrillin-1		34%	Tan et al., 1999
Nuclear matrix		100%	Sato et al., 2000
B. T cell characteristics			
CD4 + CD45 + RA		increased ($p < 0.01$)	Becker et al., 1992
TCR Vβ8 / Vβ11 / Cβ		decreased ($p = 0.029$)	Ikaeheimo et al., 1994
TCR Vβ1, 3, 4, 5.2, 14, 16		frequently used	Okubo et al., 1994
TCR AV CDR3 (common motif)		highly conserved ($p < 0.03$)	Talken et al., 1999
C. HLA class II specificity			
DR4	in American	increased	Hoffmann et al., 1990
DR4 (B15, DR4)	in Finnish	increased ($p < 0.05$)	Ruuska et al., 1992
DR2 or DR4	in English (UCTD)	increased ($p = 0.007$)	Gendi et al., 1995
DRB4* 0101,	in Japanese	increased	Dong et al., 1993
DQB1* 0501 ($p = 0.0051$)	in Mexican	increased	Weckmann et al., 1999

U1snRNP: U1 small nuclear ribonucleoprotein, HSP: heat shock protein, hnRNP: heterogenous nuclear ribonucleoprotein, TCR: T cell receptor, Vβ: variable region of β-chain, AV: variable region of α-chain, CDR: complementary determining region, UCTD: undifferentiated connective tissue disease

in patients with MCTD (Miyata et al., 1992, 1993). Anti-fibrillin-1 antibody was found by Tan et al. (1999) in the sera of 38% of MCTD patients. The fibrillin-1 is the major structural glycoprotein of connective tissue microfibrils, especially of elastic fibers. This antibody was similarly found in the sera of patients with diffuse SSc (37%) and CREST syndrome (51%). Similar results have been reported by Lundberg et al. (2000) on anti-fibrillin-1 antibody in MCTD and CREST syndrome. Recently, Sato et al. (2000) reported the presence of anti-nuclear matrix antibody in the sera of patients with anti-U1RNP antibody at a frequency of 100%. Higher titers of this antibody were detected in MCTD and SSc patients, and lower titers in SLE and undifferentiated connective tissue disease (UCTD) patients. They considered this antibody to be potentially useful in distinguishing MCTD or SSc from SLE or UCTD. This antibody to the nuclear matrix, a relatively insoluble component of the cell nucleus, was originally reported by Fritzler et al. (1984).

Additional Immune Phenomena

The T cell population of MCTD patients has been characterized by several investigators. Becker et al. (1992) reported an increased percentage of CD4+ CD29+ T cells in MCTD patients compared with controls ($p < 0.01$ and $p < 0.001$, respectively). They considered this imbalance of the T cell population to likely enhance autoimmunity. A haplotype of TCR Vβ8/Vβ11/Cβ was reported to be reduced in Finnish MCTD patients ($p < 0.029$) compared to controls (Ikaeheimo, 1994). On the other hand, an increased frequency of TCR Vβ, 3, 4, 5.2, 14 and 16 in Japanese MCTD patients was reported by Okubo et al. (1994). Holyst et al. (1997) reported that T cells in MCTD patients responding to 70 kDa, B or D protein of RNP antigen produced a higher level of IL-4 and IFN-γ, but a lower level of IL-2 and IL-6. Talkin et al. (1999) reported that the T cell receptor reactive to U1 70 kDa snRNP has hold a highly conserved common motif in the CDR 3 region of the α chain of the receptor.

The specificity of HLA class II antigen in MCTD patients has been investigated in several studies. An increased frequency of HLA-DR4 has been found in North American patients (Hoffman et al., 1990). Similarly, an increased frequency of DR4 (B15, DR4) was found in Finnish patients compared with controls ($p < 0.05$) (Ruuska et al., 1992), and an increased association with DR2 or DR4 was found in the undifferentiated type of MCTD in English patients (p = 0.007, Gendi et al., 1995). An increased frequency of DRB4*0101 and DQA1*03 was observed in Japanese MCTD patients compared with SLE patients (RR = 2.47 and 2.25, respectively, Dong et al., 1993). Finally, an increased frequency of DQB1*0501 was found in Mexican patients (p = 0.0051, Weckmann et al., 1999).

Increased serum levels of several proteins are present in MCTD patients. Filep et al. (1995) reported an increased level of serum endothelin-1. Moreover, patients with MCTD complicated by pulmonary hypertension showed increased serum levels of angiotensin converting enzymes (Ozawa et al., 1995), IL-1 and IL-6 (Okawa et al., 1994), and IL-6 and IgG anticardiolipin antibody (Nishimaki et al., 1999).

Clinical Appearance

The clinical features of patients with MCTD vary and include those found in SLE, SSc, PM and occasionally RA. The frequency of each clinical findings differs slightly depending on the race of the patients studied and on the diagnostic criteria used. The frequencies of each findings observed in a multi-institutional study including 284 MCTD patients in Japan (Miyawaki et al., 1988) and those of a study involving 47 MCTD patients in the USA

Table 2. Clinical Findings of Patients with Mixed Connective Tissue Disease

	Japanese patients (Miyawaki et al., 1988) 284 cases	US patients (Burdt et al., 1999) 47 cases
Raynaud's phenomenon	97.9%	96%*
Swollen fingers or hands	73.9	66
Anti-U1snRNP antibody positive	96.6	100
Arthritis	69.5	96 (arthralgia)
Sclerodactyly	50.2	49
Reduced diffusion capacity	48.5	66 (pulmonary)
Pulmonary fibrosis	40.1	dysfunction
Restrictive changes of lung	33.5	
Pulmonary hypertension	4.5	23
Muscle weakness	39.3	51 (myositis)
Myogenic pattern on EMG	35.4	
Elevated muscle enzymes	31.0	
Leukocytopenia	37.7	53 (leukopenia /
Thrombocytopenia	8.9	lymphopenia)
Lymphoadenopathy	29.2	–
Esophageal hypomotility or dilatation	27.7	66
Facial erythema	19.5	53 (skin rash)
Pleuritis	6.5	43 (pericarditis)
Pericarditis	5.7	
Anti-Sm antibody	11.5	22
Diffuse sclerosis	11.6	19
Proteinuria	7.8	11 (renal disease)
Urinary casts	1.8	

* Cumulative findings

(Burdt et al., 1999) are presented in Table 2. As seen in this table, the findings observed at the highest frequency in both groups of patients were Raynaud's phenomenon, polyarthritis/arthralgia, swollen hands, sclerodactyly, pulmonary lesions and muscle symptoms. The second tier of the frequently observed findings include esophageal dysfunction, leukocytopenia or thrombocytopenia and pleuritis and pericarditis. Rarely found clinical findings were alterations of the nervous system, renal lesions and diffuse sclerosis in both groups. One of the characteristic features of MCTD patients is swollen fingers or hands, a symptom referred to "sausage-like fingers" (Fig. 1). No significant differences between MCTD and SLE in the features of facial erythema have been described. In Fig. 2, a photograph of

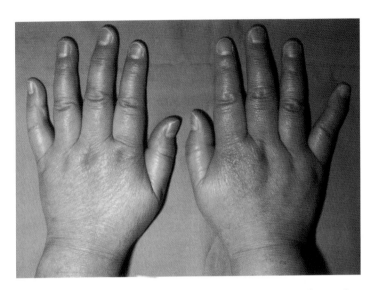

Fig. 1. Swollen fingers and hands of a 58-year-old woman with mixed connective tissue disease

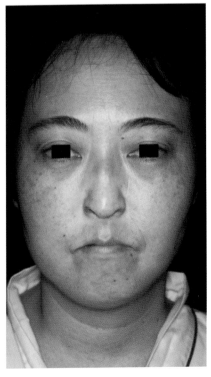

Fig. 2. Face of a 32-year-old woman with mixed connective tissue disease. Discrete facial erythema and slightly sclerotic skin at the nose and around the mouth

the face of a MCTD patient with faded erythema and acrosclerosis is presented. Among these findings in MCTD patients, some show a tendency to diminish while others persist or increase during the observation period. A similar change in the clinical features of the patients during the observation period has been reported in several studies. The results of two studies done in Japan (Miyawaki et al., 1988) on 284 patients followed for a mean period of 6 years, and those of a study in the USA (Burdt et al., 1999) on 47 patients followed for a mean period of 15 years were very similar. Diminished symptoms included myositis, arthritis, facial erythema, pleuritis/pericarditis in both studies. On the other hand, persistent or increased symptoms were pulmonary lesions, scleroderma and esophageal dysfunction. Raynaud's phenomenon remained almost unchanged in both groups.

Pulmonary hypertension in MCTD patients had been recognized in the early 1980's by Esther et al. (1981), Graziano et al. (1983) and Sullivan et al. (1984). The prevalence of pulmonary hypertension in MCTD patients was reported to be 4% by Esther et al. (1981) and 3.9% by Miyawaki et al. (1988). Sharp stressed the clinical importance of pulmonary hypertension and included it in his diagnostic criteria as one of major symptoms (Sharp, 1987). Pulmonary hypertension is the most critical symptom related to the prognosis of MCTD patients. Sawai et al. (1997) reported that the most frequent cause of death in MCTD patients is pulmonary hypertension, accounting for 11 of 32 (34%) autopsy cases with MCTD. In a comparison between MCTD patients and those with SLE and SSc, we reported that pulmonary hypertension in MCTD occurred more quickly and carried a shorter survival period than in other diseases (Kasukawa et al., 1990). Characteristic histopathological findings of pulmonary hypertension in MCTD patients include a marked internal thickening of the pulmonary arteries especially in the distal portion, and the hypertensive pulmonary vascular change with plexiform lesions accompanied by or without pulmonary fibrosis (Hosoda et al., 1994; Sawai et al., 1997). The five-year survival rate of MCTD patients was reported to be 96.5% (Tojo et al., 1991).

Diagnosis

Since Sharp reported MCTD to be a distinct disease entity in 1972, criticism has been raised over its supposed independent nature. The main thrust of the criticism can be summarized as follows: the first is the difficulty in distinguishing patients whose symptoms could simultaneously satisfy two criteria for MCTD and other connective tissue diseases such as SLE (Reichlin, 1976) or SSc and the second is the shifting of clinical features of MCTD to those of other connective tissue diseases such as SSc or SLE during the observation period (LeRoy et al., 1980, Nimelstein et al., 1980; Black et al., 1992; van den Hoogen et al., 1994).

To address these problems, a classification criteria for MCTD was eagerly pursued. To date, three criteria for MCTD have been proposed: Alarcon-Segovia's criteria (1976; revised in 1987), Sharp's criteria (1987) and the criteria of The Research Committee of the Japanese Ministry of Health and Welfare for MCTD (JMHW, Kasukawa et al., 1987). The three sets of criteria for MCTD arranged by Smolen and Steiner (1998) are presented in Table 3. The reliability of the diagnostic criteria depends on their sensitivity and specificity when tested

Table 3. Characteristics of 3 Sets of Criteria for the Classification of Mixed Connective Tissue Disease*

Reference	Criteria	Requirements for diagnosis

Alarcon-Segovia and Villarreal (1987)	A. Serologic
	
	  1. Anti-RNP at a hemagglutination titer of $\geq$ 1:1600
	
	B. Clinical
	
	  1. Edema in the hands
	
	  2. Synovitis
	
	  3. Myositis
	
	  4. Raynaud's phenomenon
	
	  5. Acrosclerosis
		Serological criterion plus at least 3 clinical criteria, including either synovitis or myositis.

Kasukawa et al. (1987)	A. Common symptoms
	
	  1. Raynaud's phenomenon
	
	  2. Swollen fingers or hands
	
	B. Anti-snRNP antibody positive
	
	C. Mixed symptoms
	
	  1. SLE-like findings
	
	    a. Polyarthritis
	
	    b. Lymphadenopathy
	
	    c. Facial erythema
	
	    d. Pericarditis or pleuritis
	
	    e. Leuko- or thrombocytopenia
	
	  2. SSc-like findings
	
	    a. Sclerodactyly
	
	    b. Pulmonary fibrosis, restrictive changes of lung, or reduced diffusion capacity
	
	    c. Hypomotility or dilatation of esophagus
	
	  3. PM-like findings
	
	    a. Muscle weakness
	
	    b. Elevated serum levels of muscle enzymes (CPK)
	
	    c. Myogenic pattern on EMG
		At least 1 of the 2 common symptoms plus positive for anti-snRNP plus 1 or more of the mixed symptoms in at
		
		least 2 of the 3 disease categories.

Sharp (1987)	A. Major At least 4 major criteria plus anti-U1 RNP titer of at least	

Table 3. (continued) Characteristics of 3 Sets of Criteria for the Classification of Mixed Connective Tissue Disease*

Reference	Criteria	Requirements for diagnosis
	1. Myositis, severe	1:4000 (exclusion criterion: positivity for anti-Sm);
	2. Pulmonary involvement	Or, 2 major criteria from among criteria 1, 2, and 3 plus
	a. Diffusion capacity < 70% of normal values	2 minor criteria plus anti-U1 RNP titer of at least 1:1000
	b. Pulmonary hypertension	
	c. Proliferative vascular lesions on lung biopsy	
	3. Raynaud's phenomenon or esophageal hypomotility	
	4. Swollen hands or sclerodactyly	
	5. Anti-ENA ≥ 1:10,000 and anti-U1 RNP positive and anti-Sm negative	
	B. Minor	
	1. Alopecia	
	2. Leukopenia	
	3. Anemia	
	4. Pleuritis	
	5. Pericarditis	
	6. Arthritis	
	7. Trigeminal neuropathy	
	8. Malar rash	
	9. Thrombocytopenia	
	10. Mild myositis	
	11. History of swollen hands	

* snRNP = small nuclear RNP; SLE = systemic lupus erythematosus; SSc = systemic sclerosis; PM = polymyositis; CPK = creatine phosphokinase; EMG = electromyogram; ENA = extractable nuclear antigen (Smolen and Steiner: Arthritis Rheum 1998)

on patients with objective disease and control diseases. Few studies have been performed to test the sensitivity and specificity of the proposed criteria for MCTD. The results of the five reported studies are listed chronologically in Table 4 (Kasukawa et al., 1987; Alarcon-Segovia et al., 1989; Doria et al., 1991; Amigues et al., 1996; Smolen and Steiner, 1998). The sensitivity and specificity of these three criteria were found to be satisfactorily high except for the study of Amigues et al. (1996). In general, the criteria of Alarcon-Segovia are simple

Table 4. Sensitivity and Specificity of Three Sets of Criteria for Mixed Connective Tissue Disease

Criteria of							
Investigators	Year studied	Objective disease (OD) and Control disease (CD)	No. of patients studied	Sensitivity and Specificity	Alarcon-Segovia and Villarreal 1987	Sharp 1987	JMHW(22) 987
Kasukawa et al.	1987	OD: MCTD CD: SLE/SSc/PM/DM	81 261	Sensi: Speci:			88% 87%
Alarcon-Segovia and Cardiel	1989	OD: MCTD CD: SLE/SSc/RA PM/DM/SS	80 518	Sensi: Speci:	100% 99–100%	100% 55–100%	96% 99–100%
Doria et al.	1991	OD: MCTD CD: SLE/SSc/PM	32 75	Speci: Sensi:			87% 94%
Amigues et al.	1996	OD: aRNP positive pts including control pts CD: RA/SLE/SSc/Ov	45 25	Sensi: Speci:	62.5% 86.2%	100% 38%	56.2% 65.5%
Smolen and Steiner	1998	OD: MCTD	26	Sensi:	100%	70%	92%

JMHW: Japanese Ministry of Health and Welfare, MCTD: mixed connective tissue disease, SLE: systemic lupus erythematosus,
SSc: systemic sclerosis, PM: polymyositis, DM: dermatomyositis, RA: rheumatoid arthritis,
SS: Sjoegren's syndrome, aRNP: anti-U1snRNP antibody, pts: patients, Ov: overlap syndrome

and suitable for screening MCTD from various connective tissue diseases, whereas the criteria of Sharp and JMHW are suitable not only for classifying MCTD as a connective tissue disease but also for analyzing each of the clinical features of MCTD patients.

Therapy

Therapeutic regimens for treating MCTD patients are similar to those used for patients with SLE, SSc or PM. The main therapeutic approach is the administration of systemic corticosteroids. Nonsteroidal anti-inflammatory drugs (NSAID) and vasodilatators are often used, and immunosuppressants are occasionally used. In our multi-institutional study done in Japan (Miyawaki et al., 1988) on 284 patients with MCTD, the therapeutic methods used were as follows: corticosteroids in 230 cases (81.0%), vasodilatators in 123 (43.3%), NSAID in 109 (38.4%), prostaglandin or prostacyclin derivatives in 37 (13.0%), and immunosuppressants in 16 (5.6%). In the above study, the correlation between doses of prednisolone and prognosis was analyzed. Administration of 30 mg or more of prednisolone per day induced a better prognosis of MCTD patients ($p < 0.05$) than doses of less than 30 mg of prednisolone per day according to Radit and Mann-Whitney tests (Table 5, Miyawaki et al., 1988). Aside from these drugs, several other therapeutic methods have been used for MCTD patients, including anticoagulants, plasma exchange and O_2 inhalation.

Table 5. Correlation between Doses of Prednisolone used for 284 Patients with Mixed Connective Tissue Disease and their Prognosis for 6 Years at Mean (Miyawaki et al., 1988)

		No. of patients who revealed the prognosis of					
		Remission 125 (45.0%)	Unchanged 124 (43.7%)	Worse 12 (4.2%)	Deceased 16 (5.6%)	Unknown 4 (1.4%)	
Not used	69	15 (21.7)	48 (69.6)	3 (4.3)	2772 (2.9)	1 (1.4)	
							**
Used	215	113 (52.6)	76 (35.3)	9 (4.2)	14 (6.5)	3 (1.4)	
Less than 20 mg	54	22 (40.7)	28 (51.9)	1 (1.9)	2 (3.7)	1 (1.9)	
							ns
More than 20 mg	161	91 (56.5)	48 (29.8)	8 (5.0)	12 (7.5)	2 (1.2)	
Less than 30 mg	88	36 (40.9)	46 (52.3)	1 (1.1)	3 (3.4)	2 (2.3)	
							*
More than 30 mg	127	77 (60.6)	30 (23.6)	8 (6.3)	11 (8.7)	1 (0.8)	

* $p < 0.05$, ** $p < 0.01$, ns: not significant

Summary

Pulmonary hypertension in MCTD patients is the most critical factor affecting the prognosis of MCTD patients. Corticosteroids are occasionally effective during the early stage of the disease. Anticoagulants (warfarin potassium), antiplatelets (ticlopidine hydrochloride), and vasodilatators (prostaglandin or prostacyclin derivatives, calcium antagonists) are used for the progressive stage of pulmonary hypertension. Digitalis products and diuretics are used to treat heart failure in the advanced stage of pulmonary hypertension. A combination of cyclophosphamide and cyclosporin A was reported to be effective against the pulmonary hypertension in MCTD patients (Dahl et al., 1992). However, to date no promising therapeutic methods have been established for both primary and secondary type of the pulmonary hypertension. Inhalation of NO in addition to O_2 is effective against pulmonary hypertension (Pepke-Zaba, 1991).

References

Alarcon-Segovia D (1976) Symptomatic Sjoegren's syndrome in mixed connective tissue disease. J Rheumatol 3:191–195

Alarcon-Segovia D, Villarreal M (1987) Classification and diagnostic criteria for mixed connective tissue disease. In: Kasukawa R, Sharp GC (eds) Mixed Connective Tissue Disease and Antinuclear Antibodies. Elsevier, Amsterdam, pp 33–40

Alarcon-Segovia D, Cardiel MH (1989) Comparison between three diagnostic criteria for mixed connective tissue disease. Studies of 593 patients. J Rheumatol 16:328–334

Amigues JM, Cantagrel A, Abbal M, Mazieres B, and the Autoimmunity Group of the Hospitals of Toulouse (1996) Comparative study of 4 diagnosis criteria sets in mixed connective tissue disease in patients with anti-RNP antibodies. J Rheumatol 23:2055–2062 (see comments)

Becker H, Langrock A, Federlin K (1992) Imbalance of CD4+ lymphocyte subsets in patients with mixed connective tissue disease. Clin Exp Immunol 88:91–95

Black C, Isenberg DA (1992) Mixed connective tissue disease – goodbye to all that. Br J Rheumatol 31:695–700 (see comments)

Burdt MA, Hoffman RW, Dertscher SL, Wang GS, Johnson JC, Sharp GC (1999) Long-term outcome in mixed connective tissue disease: longitudinal clinical and serological findings. Arthritis Rheum 42:899–909

Dahl M, Chalmers A, Wade J, Calverley D, Munt B (1992) Ten year survival of a patient with advanced hypertension and mixed connective tissue disease treated with immunosuppressive therapy. J Rheumatol 19:1807–1809

Dong RP, Kimura A, Hashimoto H, Akizuki M, Nishimura Y, Sasazuki T (1993) Difference in HLA-linked genetic background between mixed connective tissue disease and systemic lupus erythematosus. Tissue Antigens 41:21–25

Doria A, Ghirardello A, de Zambiasi P, Ruffatti A, Gambari PF (1992) Japanese diagnostic criteria for mixed connective tissue disease in Caucasian patients. J Rheumatol 19:259–264

Esther JH, Sharp GC, Agia G, Hurst DJ, Maricq HR (1981) Pulmonary hypertension in a patient with connective tissue disease and antibody to nuclear ribonucleoprotein. Arthritis Rheum 24:2105

Filep JG, Bodolay E, Sipka S, Gyimesi E, Csipoe I, Szegedi G (1995) Plasma endothelin correlate with antiendothelial antibodies in patients with mixed connective tissue disease. Circulation 92:2969–2974

Fritzler MJ, Ali R, Tan EM (1984) Antibodies from patients with mixed connective tissue disease react with heterogeneous nuclear ribonucleoprotein or ribonucleic acid (hn RNP/RNA) of the nuclear matrix. J Immunol 132:1216–1222

Gendi NS, Welsh KI, van Venrooij WJ, Vancheeswaran R, Girloy J, Black CM (1995) HLA type as a predictor of mixed connective tissue disease differentiation: ten-year clinical and immunologic follow up of 46 patients. Arthritis Rheum 38:259–266

Graziano FM, Friedman LCV, Grossmaen J (1983) Pulmonary hypertension in a patient with mixed connective tissue disease. Clin Exp Rheumatol 1:251–255

Hassfeld W, Steiner G, Studinicka-Benke A, Skriner K, Graninger W, Fisher I, Smolen JS (1995) Autoimmune response to the spliceosome: an immunologic link between rheumatoid arthritis, mixed connective tissue disease, and systemic lupus erythematosus. Arthritis Rheum 38:777–785

Hishikawa T, Ogasawara H, Kaneko H, Shirasawa T, Matsuura Y, Sekigawa I, Takasaki Y, Hashimoto H, Hirose S, Handa S, Nagasawa R, Maruyama N (1997) Detection of autoantibodies to a recombinant gag protein derived from human endogenous retrovirus clone 4-1 in autoimmune diseases. Viral Immunol 10:137–147

Hoffman RW, Rettenmaier LJ, Takeda Y, Hewette JE, Pettersson I, Nyman U, Luger AM, Sharp GC (1990) Human autoantibodies against the 70-kd polypeptide of U1 small nuclear RNP are associated with HLA-DR 4 among connective tissue disease patients. Arthritis Rheum 33:666–673

Holyst MM, Hill DL, Hoch SO, Hoffman RW (1997) Analysis of human T cell and B cell response against U small nuclear ribonucreoprotein 70-kd, B, and D polypeptides among patients with systemic lupus erythematosus and mixed connective tissue disease. Arthritis Rheum 40:1493–1503

Hosoda Y (1994) Pathology of pulmonary hypertension: A human and experimental study. Pathol Int 44:241–267

Ikaeheimo H, Tiilikainen AS, Hameenkorpi R, Silvennoinen-Kassinen SH (1994) Different distribution of T cell receptor beta-chain haplotypes in mixed connective tissue disease and systemic lupus erythematosus. Ann Med 26:129–132

Kasukawa R, Tojo T, Miyawaki S, Yoshida H, Tanimoto K, Nobunaga M, Suzuki T, Takasaki Y, Tamura T (1987) Preliminary diagnostic criteria for classification of mixed connective tissue disease: In: Kasukawa R, Sharp GC (eds) Mixed Connective Tissue Disease and Antinuclear Antibodies. Elsevier, Amsterdam, pp 41–47

Kasukawa R, Nishimaki T, Takagi T, Miyawaki S, Yokohari R, Tsunematsu T (1990) Pulmonary hypertension in connective tissue disease. Clinical study of sixty patients in multi-institutional study. Clin Rheum 9:56–62

Klemperer P, Pollack AD, Baehr G (1942) Diffuse collagen diseases, acute disseminated lupus erythematosus and diffuse scleroderma. JAMA 119:331–332

Komatireddy GR, Wang GS, Sharp GC, Hoffman RW (1997) Antiphospholipid antibodies among anti-U1-70 kda autoantibody positive patients with mixed connective tissue disease. J Rheumatol 24:319–322 (see comments)

Le Roy EC, Maricq HR, Kahaleh MB (1980) Undifferentiated connective tissue syndromes. Arthritis Rheum 23:341–343

Lerner MR, Steitz JA (1979) Antibodies to small nuclear RNAs complexed with proteins are produced by patients with systemic lupus erythematosus. Proc Natl Acad Sci USA 76:5495–5499

Lundberg I, Antohi S, Takeuki K, Arnett F, Steiner G, Brumeanu TD, Klareskog L, Bona C (2000) Kinetics of anti-fibrillin-1 autoantibodies in MCTD and CREST syndrome. J Autoimmun 14:267–274

Mairesse N, Kahn MF, Appelboom T (1993) Antibodies to the constitutive 73-kd heat shock protein: A new marker for mixed connective tissue disease? Am J Med 95:595–600

Miyata M, Kida S, Kanno T, Suzuki K, Watanabe H, Kaise S, Nishimaki T, Hosoda Y, Kasukawa R (1992) Pulmonary hypertension in MCTD: Report of two cases with anticardiolipin antibody. Clin Rheumatol 11:195–201

Miyata M, Suzuki K, Sakuma F, Watanabe H, Kaise S, Nishimaki T, Kasukawa R (1993) Anticardiolipin antibodies are associated with pulmonary hypertension in patients with mixed connective tissue disease or systemic lupus erythemotosus. Int Arch Allergy Immunol 100:351–354

Miyawaki S, Kasukawa R, Nishimaki T, Onodera H (1988) Treatment and prognosis of patients with mixed connective tissue disease. A multi-center co-operative study. In: Kasukawa R (ed) 1987 Annual Report of The Research Committee of Japanese Ministry of Health and Welfare for Mixed Connective Tissue Disease pp 31–41 (in Japanese, Abstract in English)

Nimelstein SH, Brody S, Mc Shane D, Holman HR (1980) Mixed connective tissue disease: a subsequent evaluation of the original 25 patients. Medicine (Baltimore) 59:239–248

Nishimaki T, Aotsuka S,Kondo H, Yamamoto K, Takasaki Y, Sumiya M, Yokohari R (1999) Immunological analysis of pulmonary hypertension in connective tissue disease. J Rheumatol 26:2357–2362

Okawa-Takatsuji M, Aotsuka S, Uwatoko M, Sumiya M, Yokohari R (1994) Enhanced synthesis of cytokines by peripheral blood monocytes cultured in the presence of autoantibodies against U1-ribonucreoprotein and/or negatively charged molecules: implication in the pathogenesis of pulmonary hypertension in mixed connective tissue disease (MCTD). Clin Exp Immunol 98:427–433

Okubo M, Kurokawa M, Ohto H, Nishimaki T, Nishioka K, Kasukawa R, Yamamoto K (1994) Clonotype analysis of peripheral blood T cells and autoantigen-reactive T cells from patients with mixed connective tissue disease. J Immunol 153:3784–3790

Ozawa T, Ninomiya Y, Honma T, Kikuchi M, Sato T, Nakano M, Arakawa M (1995) Increased serum angiotensin-1 converting enzyme activity in patients with mixed connective tissue disease and pulmonary hypertension. Scand J Rheumatol 24:38–43

Pepke-Zaba J, Higenbottam TW, Dinh-Xuan AT, Stone D, Wallwork J (1991) Inhaled nitric oxide as a cause of selective pulmonary vasodilatation in pulmonary hypertension. Lancet 338:1173–1174

Query CC, Keene JD (1987) A human autoimmune protein associated with U1 RNA contains a region of homology that is cross reactive with retroviral p30gag antigen. Cell 51:211–220

Reichlin M (1976) Problems in differentiating SLE and mixed connective tissue disease. N Engl J Med 295:1194–1195

Ruuska P, Hameenkorpi R, Forsberg S, Julkunen H, Maekitalo R, Ilonen J, Tilikainen A (1992) Differences in HLA antigens between patients with mixed connective tissue disease and systemic lupus erythematosus. Ann Rheum Dis 51:52–55

Sato S, Hasegawa M, Ihn H, Kikuchi K, Takehara K (2000) Clinical significance of antinuclear matrix antibody in serum from patients with anti-U1 RNP antibody. Arch Dermatol Res 292:55–59

Sawai T, Murakami K, Kasukawa R, Kyogoku M (1997) Histopathological study of mixed connective tissue disease for 32 autopsy cases in Japan. Jpn J Rheumatol 7:279–292

Sharp GC, Irvin WS, Tan EM, Gould RG, Holman HR (1972) Mixed connective tissue disease: an apparently distinct rheumatic disease syndrome associated with a specific antibody to an extractable nuclear antigen (ENA). Am J Med 52:148–159

Sharp GC (1987) Diagnostic criteria for classification of MCTD. In: Kasukawa R, Sharp GC (eds) Mixed Connective Tissue Disease and Antinuclear Autoantibodies. Elsevier, Amsterdam, pp 23–32

Skriner K, Sommergruber WH, Tremmel V, Fischer I, Barta A, Smolen JS, Steiner G (1997) Anti-A2/RA33 autoantibodies are directed to the RNA binding region of A2 protein of the heterogeneous nuclear ribonucleoprotein complex: differential epitope recognition in rheumatoid arthritis, systemic lupus erythematosus and mixed connective tissue disease. J Clin Invest 100:127–135

Smolen JS, Steiner G (1998) Mixed connective tissue disease. To be or not to be? Arthritis Rheum 41:768–777

Steiner G, Skriner K, Smolen JS (1996) Autoantibodies to the A/B proteins of the heterogeneous nuclear ribonucleoprotein complex: Novel tools for the diagnosis of rheumatic diseases. Int Arch Allergy Immunol 111:314–319

Sullivan WD, Hurst DJ, Harmon CE, Esther JH, Agia GA, Maltby JD, Lillard SB, Held CN, Wolfe JF, Sunderrajan EV, Maricq HR, Sharp GC (1984) Prospective evaluation emphasizing pulmonary involvement in patients with mixed connective tissue disease. Medicine 63:92–107

Talken BL, Lee DR, Caldwell CW, Quinn TP, Schaefermeyer KR, Hoffman RW (1999) Analysis of T cell receptors specific for U1-70 kD small nuclear ribonucleoprotein autoantigen: The alpha chain complementary determining region three is highly conserved among connective tissue disease patients. Human Immunol 60:200–208

Tan FK, Arnett FC, Antohi S, Saito S, Mirarchi A, Spiera H, Sasaki T, Shoichi O, Takeuchi K, Pandy JP, Silver RM, LeRoy C, Postlethwaite AE, Bona CA (1999) Autoantibodies to the extracellular matrix microfibrillar protein, fibrillin-1, in patients with scleroderma and other connective tissue diseases. J Immunol 163:1066–1072

Tojo T, Ogasawara T, Aotsuka S, Yokohari R (1991) Major causes of death and five year survival rates in mixed connective tissue disease. In: Yokohari R (ed) 1999 Annual Report of The Research Committee of Japanese Ministry of Health and Welfare for Mixed Connective Tissue Disease. pp 10–13 (in Japanese, Abstract in English)

van den Hoogen FH, Spronk PE, Boerbooms AM, Bootsma H, de Rooij DJ, Kallenberg CG, van de Putte LB (1994) Long-term follow up of 46 patients with anti-(U1) sn RNP antibodies. Br J Rheumatol 33:1117–1120

Weckmann AL, Granados J, Cardiel MH, Andrede F, Vargas-Alarcon G, Alcocer-Varela J, Alarcon-Segovia D (1999) Immunogenetics of mixed connective tissue disease in Mexican Mestizo population. Clin Exp Rheumatol 17:91–94

Wiemann C, Bodenbach L, Pyerin W (1993) Antibodies to casein kinase II in sera of patients with mixed connective tissue disease: Evaluation with recombinant protein. Clin Chem 39:2492–2494

Sjögren's Syndrome

8

Robert I. Fox and Carla M. Fox

Introduction

Sjögren's syndrome (**SS**) is an autoimmune disorder characterized by dry eyes (kerato-conjuctivitis sicca) and dry mouth due to lymphocytic infiltrates of lacrimal and salivary glands. The symptoms of dryness result from glandular destruction and the dysfunction in residual glands due to local production of cytokines and metalloproteinases. When the condition occurs without association with other autoimmune diseases, it is classified as *primary Sjögren's syndrome ("1° SS")*. However, SS is often found in conjunction with other autoimmune disorders such as rheumatoid arthritis (RA), systemic lupus erythematosus (SLE), dermatomyositis, scleroderma (progressive systemic sclerosis, PSS), and primary biliary cirrhosis, and in these cases is termed secondary SS (2° SS).

The dermatologist and rheumatologist should be aware that although many clinical and laboratory features in 1°SS patients are similar to SLE patients, due to the low recognition of SS as a clinical entity among referring primary MDs who note a positive ANA and label the patient as SLE, many patients (especially among the older patients) who are labeled as SLE would better fulfill criteria for SS than for SLE (discussed below).

There are overlaps of SS with other autoimmune diseases such as scleroderma (progressive systemic sclerosis, or PSS), dermatomyositis, and rheumatoid arthritis. There is also a significant overlap with patients who have "fibromyalgia", a poorly defined disorder characterized by fatigue and a centralized pain syndrome.

This chapter will concentrate on dermatologic manifestations of primary SS with emphasis on the ocular surface, oral manifestations, and cutaneous findings.

Therapies will be reviewed, and we will concentrate on *four basic areas*:

a) **methods to improve lubrication** of local manifestations of dryness involving the eye and mouth;

b) **recognition of associated problems of xeropthalmia and xerostomia**, such as oral yeast infections, ocular blepharitis and gastro-tracheal reflux;

c) **recognition and treatment of systemic manifestations of SS** including vasculitis and lymphoproliferative features;

d) **assessment and therapy of fatigue and vague cognitive symptoms** that are not clearly the result of a systemic autoimmune process, but are similar to symptoms of "fibromyalgia" patients.

Background

The first description of SS is generally credited to Johann Mikulicz, who in 1892, described a 42-year-old farmer with bilateral parotid and lacrimal gland enlargement associated with a small round cell infiltrate (Mikulicz, 1892). Because the term "Mikulicz's Syndrome" could encompass so many different entities including tuberculosis, other infections, sarcoidosis, and lymphoma, the term "Mikulicz Syndrome" fell into disuse because it did not provide sufficient prognostic or therapeutic information (Daniels and Fox, 1992). The term is still occasionally used to describe the histologic appearance of focal lymphocytic infiltrates on salivary gland biopsies.

In 1933, the Swedish ophthalmologist Henrik Sjögren described clinical and histologic findings in 19 women, 13 of whom had probable rheumatoid arthritis, with dry mouth and dry eyes. Sjogren introduced the term "keratoconjunctivitis sicca" (KCS) for this syndrome to distinguish it from dry eyes caused by lack of vitamin A ("xerophthalmia").

In 1953, Morgan and Castleman presented a case study of a patient with Sjögren's Syndrome in a clinical pathologic conference and rekindled interest in the condition originally known as "Mikulicz's Disease," and subsequently these patients have been termed "SS," while the term Mikulitz is still occasionally used to refer to the lymphoepithelial islands seen on glandular biopsy (Morgan and Castleman, 1953).

The clinical features of the disease as we currently recognize SS in its florid form were outlined in 1956 by Bloch et al. (Bloch et al., 1956). There has been considerable debate about the classification criteria of milder forms of SS that are discussed below.

Primary SS is a systemic autoimmune disorder with a prevalence of about 0.5% in the general population, with a female preponderance of 9:1, which is roughly similar to SLE (Bowman et al., 2004; Fox, Tornwall, and Michelson, 1999). This would make SS one of the three most frequent autoimmune disorders (Pillemer et al., 2001), although it has received far less research and therapeutic attention than SLE or PSS.

There are two age peaks of primary SS, with the first peak after menarche during 20's to 30's and the second peak incidence after menopause in the mid-50-year age range. In a multicenter study, 40 cases of SS with onset prior to age 16 were identified based on parotid gland swelling and characteristic autoantibodies at presentation and a mild course during 7-year follow-up (Cimaz et al., 2003).

Criteria for Diagnosis

There is relatively little disagreement among rheumatologists regarding the clinical diagnosis of SS in a patient with:
- florid physical exam findings of keratoconjunctivitis on ocular exam
- dry mouth (xerostomia) and parotid swelling;
- positive ANA and anti-SS-A/SS-B antibodies.

Until recently, there were multiple sets of diagnostic criteria for primary SS including those by American (Daniels and Fox, 1992; Fox, Robinson et al., 1986) and European (EEC) groups (Vitali, Moutsopoulos, and Bombardieri, 1994) that were so significantly different, diagnoses of "SS" rendered by European physicians were almost ten-fold when utilizing the EEC criteria than in two different US criteria (Fox, 1997). This discrepancy in diagnostic criteria led to confusion in the research and clinical trial literature.

The criteria in current use is the European-American Consensus Group Modification of the European Community Criteria for SS (Vitali, 2003) (Table I). There are 6 criteria under this classification:

1) Symptoms of dry eye
2) Signs of dry eye (Schirmer or Rose Bengal test, see below)
3) Symptoms of dry mouth
4) Salivary gland function test (scintigram, sialogram, abnormal flow)
5) Minor salivary gland biopsy
6) SS-A or SS-B autoantibodies

For a diagnosis of primary SS, patients must fulfill 4 criteria, one of them being either:
- positive salivary gland biopsy (focus score > 1, see below); or
- positive SS-A or SS-B autoantibody.

Several points about autoantibodies associated with SS are worth reviewing. Some authors use the terms SS-A or B (Sjögren Associated Antigen A or B) and some use the terms Ro and La (named after the patients sera that were initially used for identification of these antigens (Chan et al., 1989). The SS-A antigen was found identical to the Ro antigen. Gene cloning has identified that the SS-A antigen contains a 60 kd and a 52 kd molecule that associate with a tRNA like structure (called hYRNA) that serves a function in mRNA processing. Also, a 48 kd molecule termed SS-B is associated with the SS-A/hYRNA complex(Chan et al., 1989; Ben-Chetrit, Fox, and Tan, 1990).

The presence or absence of antibody to SS-A/SS-B has been found to be closely associated with specific HLA-DR loci. In Caucasian populations, the association is with the extended HLA-DR3 locus that also includes specific DQ and complement C4 alleles (Harley et al., 1986). In populations such as Chinese and Japanese where DR3 is infrequent, a different extended HLA-DR haplotype is associated with these autoantibodies (Fei et al., 1991). As will be discussed below, a functional role for these antibodies (that bind to hYRNA in immune complexes) in pathogenesis has recently been identified.

About 60% of 1° SS patients have anti-SS-A antibody and about half of the anti-SS-A patients have anti-SS antibody. It is very uncommon to have anti-SS-B in the absence of anti-SS-A antibody (Harley et al., 1986; Hamilton et al., 1988; Rader et al., 1989; Gaither et al., 1987; Sestak et al., 1987).

Diagnosis of secondary SS has not yet been addressed by the American European Consensus Group. However, in practice we usually require the patient to fulfill the criteria for 1° SS and to additionally fulfill American College of Rheumatology (ACR) criteria for an established connective-tissue disease such as RA, SLE, dermatomyositis or myositis, PSS, or biliary cirrhosis. For ease of comparison, the diagnostic criteria for SLE and PSS are provided in Tables II and III.

Table 1. International Consensus Criteria for Sjögren's Syndrome

I.	**Primary SS**

A. Ocular symptoms (at least 1 present)

   1. Daily, persistent, troublesome dry eyes for more than 3 months

   2. Recurrent sensation of sand or gravel in the eyes

   3. Use of a tear substitute more than 3 times a day

B. Oral symptoms (at least 1 present)

   1. Daily feeling of dry mouth for at least 3 months

   2. Recurrent feeling of swollen salivary glands as an adult

   3. Need to drink liquids to aid in washing down dry foods

C. Objective evidence of dry eyes (at least 1 present)

   1. Schirmer I test

   2. Rose Bengal

   3. Lacrimal gland biopsy with focus score ≥ 1

D. Objective evidence of salivary gland involvement (at least 1 present)

   1. Salivary gland scintigraphy

   2. Parotid sialography

   3. Unstimulated whole sialometry (≤ 1.5 ml per 15 minutes)

E. Laboratory Abnormality (at least 1 present)

   1. Anti-SS A or anti-SS B antibody

   2. Antinuclear antibody (ANA)

   3. IgM rheumatoid factor (anti-IgG Fc)

- Diagnosis of primary Sjogren's syndrome requires 4 of 6 criteria, including a positive minor salivary gland biopsy or antibody to SS-A/SS-B.
- Exclusions include previous radiation to the head and neck lymphoma, Sarcoidosis, hepatitis C infection, AIDS, graft-versus-host disease, and medications that can cause dryness.
- Diagnosis of secondary SS requires an established connective tissue disease and one sicca symptom plus 2 objective tests for dry mouth and dry eyes at the time of their clinical entry into study cohort.
- Diagnosis of SS can be made in patients who have no sicca symptoms if objective tests of ocular and oral dryness are fulfilled including either a minor salivary gland biopsy or anti-SS A/SS-B antibody.

Exclusions to the diagnosis of 1° SS include previous radiotherapy to the head and neck, lymphoma, sarcoidosis, graft-versus-host disease, infection with Hepatitis C virus, human T-lymphotropic virus type I, or HIV. Measurements of tear and saliva flow must be made in the absence of drugs that have anticholinergic side-effects.

Table 2. Diagnostic Criteria of SLE

Criterion Definition:
A. Malar Rash
B. Rash over the cheeks
C. Discoid Rash
D. Red raised patches
E. Photosensitivity
F. Reaction to sunlight, resulting in the development of or increase in skin rash
G. Oral Ulcers
H. Ulcers in the nose or mouth, usually painless
I. Arthritis
J. Nonerosive arthritis involving two or more peripheral joints (arthritis in which the bones around the joints do not become destroyed)
K. Serositis
L. Pleuritis or pericarditis
M. Renal Disorder
N. Excessive protein in the urine (greater than 0.5 gm/day or 3+ on test sticks) and/or cellular casts (abnormal elements the urine, derived from red and/or white cells and/or kidney tubule cells)
O. Neurologic
P. Seizures
Q. (convulsions) and/or psychosis in the absence of drugs or metabolic disturbances which are known to cause such effects
R. Hematologic
S. Hemolytic anemia or leukopenia (white bloodcount below 4,000 cells per cubic millimeter) or lymphopenia (less than 1,500 lymphocytes per cubic millimeter) or thrombocytopenia (less than 100,000 platelets per cubic millimeter). The leukopenia and lymphopenia must be detected on two or more occasions. The thrombocytopenia must be detected in the absence of drugs known to induce it.
T. Immunologic
U. Positive LE prep test, positive anti-DNA test positive anti-Sm test or false positive syphilis test (VDRL).
V. Positive test for antinuclear antibodies in the absence of drugs known to induce it.

Although 1 SS patients are at increased risk for lymphoma, patients with pre-existing lymphoma are typically excluded from studies to ensure entry of a relatively homogeneous group into studies of therapy and prognosis.

Table 3. Diagnostic Criteria of Progressive Systemic Sclerosis (Scleroderma)

The American College of Rheumatology (ACR) criteria for the classification of scleroderma require *one major criterion* or *two minor criteria*, which are as follows:
Major criterion
Proximal scleroderma is characterized by symmetric thickening, tightening, and induration of the skin of the fingers and the skin that is proximal to the metacarpophalangeal or metatarsophalangeal joints. These changes may affect the entire extremity, face, neck, and trunk (thorax and abdomen;
Minor criteria
Sclerodactyly includes the above major criterion characteristics but is limited to only the fingers.
Digital pitting scars or a loss of substance from the finger pad: As a result of ischemia, depressed areas of the fingertips or a loss of digital pad tissue occurs.
Bibasilar pulmonary fibrosis includes a bilateral reticular pattern of linear or lineonodular densities most pronounced in basilar portions of the lungs on standard chest roentgenograms. These densities may assume the appearance of diffuse mottling or a honeycomb lung and are not attributable to primary lung disease.

Pitfalls in Diagnosis and Methodology

There are two common areas of confusion in clinical diagnosis regarding the specificity/sensitivity of the ANA and of the minor salivary gland biopsy.

The ANA frequently is used as a "screening" test in patients with rheumatic disease symptoms. However, Tan et al. (Tan et al., 1997) reported that the frequency in "normal individuals" of a positive ANA titer using Hep 2 cells at titer 1:40 was 31.7% of individual, at 1:80 was 13%, at 1:160 was 5%, and at 1:320 was 3.3%.

Using a Bayesian analysis, Lightfoot et al. found similar results and calculated that the risk of an individual with an ANA 1:320 developing SLE or SS during a 10-year follow-up period was less than 5% (Lightfoot, 1997).

The high incidence of ANA in the "normal population" is not commonly understood by either patients or primary care MDs who make the diagnosis of SLE or SS based on the finding of an abnormal autoantibody test result, but in the absence of characteristic clinical findings.

The dermatologist may be asked to help confirm the diagnosis of SS with a minor salivary gland biopsy (Daniels, 1992). The method of obtaining the biopsy is important to obtain an adequate sample and to avoid injuring the nerve that innervates the lip. The biopsy should not be taken from a region of the buccal mucosa where there is inflammation, as this can give false positive results (Fox, Robinson et al., 1986; Fox and Howell, 1986; Bone et al., 1985).

The biopsy is generally taken from the lower lip to the side of midline, as this site has less nonspecific fibrotic change. The minor salivary gland biopsy is performed on the inner lower lip mucosa after local anesthesia. A vertical incision is made, and minor salivary

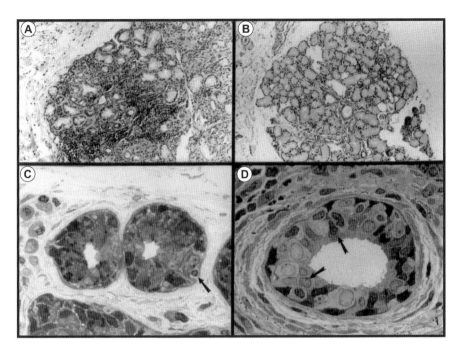

Fig. 1. Minor salivary gland biopsy from patients with Sjogren's syndrome (**A**) and (**B**) from a patient with fibromyalgia (a histologically normal biopsy). Higher power views of the Sjogren's biopsy are shown in **C** and **D**

glands exposed. Five glands are excised with scissors. The wound is sutured in the usual fashion (silk sutures can be used, which would be removed in one week, or alternatively, absorbable sutures can be used). The incision is closed with sutures that can be removed by the dermatologist or the rheumatologist. By undermining the mucosa, the nerves that run just below the surface will not be injured by the procedure and the patient will not suffer from a numb lip region as a result of the biopsy.

An example of a salivary gland biopsy from a SS patient (Fig 1, Frame A) and from a normal individual (Fig 1, Frame B) is shown. The key features in reading the minor salivary gland biopsy include an adequate number of valuable lobules (at least 4) and the determination of an average *focus* score (a "focus" refers to a cluster of at least 50 lymphocytes) based on survey of at least 4 lobules. Lobules that have been ruptured due to non-immune mechanisms (called "sialidentis" due to rupture of ducts that release mucus) need to be discarded from the quantization of the focus score (Daniels, 1984; Daniels and Wu, 2000).

Non-specific sialidentis including focal infiltrates, was a relatively frequent finding in minor salivary gland biopsies taken in a "control population" studied at National Institutes of Health (Radfar et al., 2002). However, most pathologists are not experienced in reading these samples. In one recent report, almost 50% of biopsies labeled as SS were reclassified when examined by a pathologist experienced in SS (Vivino, Gala, and Hermann, 2002).

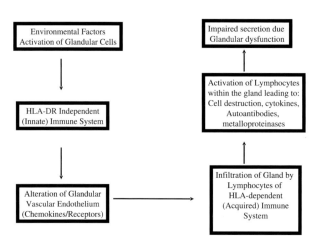

Fig. 2 Pathogenetic events in Sjogren's syndrome

Overview of Pathogenesis and Correlation with Clinical Symptoms

In spite of extensive effort spent in studying the underlying cause of SS, the pathogenesis remains obscure.

In broad terms, SS can be considered a multifactor complex disease in which environmental factors are thought to trigger inflammation in individuals with a genetic predisposition for the disease. In comparison to many other organ-specific autoimmune disorders, the relative ease of minor salivary gland biopsy in SS provides researchers an opportunity to study the interaction of the immune system and the neuro-endocrine system. The pathogenesis results from the continued mutual stimulation of the "acquired" (HLA-DR dependent) response and the "innate" (HLA-DR independent) arm of the immune system.

The pathogenesis of SS includes multiple different steps that are schematically shown in Fig. 2:

a) The initial steps in pathogenesis probably involve intrinsic defects in the glandular epithelial cells or their underlying stromal/dendritic cells (Tapinos et al., 1999). These cells would normally undergo a normal cycle of apoptosis but mutant mice with abnormal glandular apoptotic pathways develop a SS like disease. In animal models of SS (the NOD.SCID mouse), apoptotic changes of epithelial cells and local endothelial venules occur in the absence of functional lymphocytes (Robinson et al., 1996).

b) Environmental triggers may include a viral infection of the glands or any intercurrent infection that stimulates dendritic or glandular cells to activate the HLA-independent "innate immune system." The innate immune system utilizes Toll and Toll-like receptors that recognize conserved molecular patterns (pathogen-associated molecular patterns), which are shared by large groups of microorganisms and apoptotic products (Takeda, Kaisho, and Akira, 2003).

c) Continued migration of lymphocytes and dendritic cells to the gland in response to chemokines, adhesion to specific vascular adhesion molecules and later retention of T- and B-lymphocytes.(Jonsson, Gordon, and Konttinen, 2003).

Activation of T-lymphocytes and B-lymphocytes within the glands and in extraglandular sites occurs as a result of HLA-DR restricted antigen presenting cells in the presence of co-stimulatory molecules. This is called the "acquired immune system" that perpetuates immune response with memory lymphocytes and autoantibodies (Sawalha et al., 2003).

d) Extraglandular manifestations occur as a result of lymphocytic infiltration into other tissues or generation of pathogenetic autoantibodies. The anti-SS-A and SS-B antibodies form a complex with hYRNA that are involved in splicing functions (Scofield et al., 1999). This protein/RNA complex exposes both single- and double-strand RNA components and the complex traffics to the blebs on apoptotic cells where they can trigger the innate immune system (as described below(McClain et al., 2005; Sawalha et al., 2003; Heinlen et al., 2003; Arbuckle et al., 2003; Kaufman et al., 2001; Scofield et al., 1999).

e) The innate and acquired immune systems can be mutually co-stimulatory (Santiago-Raber et al., 2003). Studies on cytokine production in the salivary gland biopsies using gene profiling suggest an important role for Type I and Type II interferons in this perpetuation of the immune response (Jonsson, Gordon, and Konttinen, 2003; Ogawa et al., 2002). Plasmacytic dendritic cells and glandular epithelial cells can be potent sources of Type I IFN in the salivary gland. These cells express a series of Toll receptors that bind to conserved epitopes associated with infection (such as lipopolysacharide) or products of apoptotic cells.

f) Glandular destruction may occur by perforin/granzyme-A methods as well as Fas/Fas Ligand mechanisms (Bolstad et al., 2003). However, only partial destruction of the gland is noted in most patients, and it is likely that local production of cytokines, autoantibodies and metalloproteinases leads to dysfunction of the residual glandular tissue (Konttinen et al., 1992; Konttinen and Kasna-Ronkainen, 2002).

g) The sensation of "dryness" depends on a functional circuit that starts at the mucosal surface (i. e., unmyelinated nerves of corneal membrane or oral mucosa) that send afferent nerves to specific areas of the mid-brain (Stern et al., 1998; Fox and Stern, 2002). The midbrain (salivatory and lacrimatory nuclei) then send efferent adrenergic and cholinergic nerves back to the glands to regulate secretion. This may help explain the high prevalence of sicca symptoms in non-SS patients including Alzheimer's disease and fibromyalgia.

In summary, it is now possible to propose a mechanism that includes the findings of genetic association (HLA-DR), autoantibody production, immunohistrology, the results of gene expression profiling in the gland, and clinical symptoms of dryness.

The organ distribution is determined by the homing pattern of the lymphocytes and dendritic cells. The tendency to lymphoma results from the chronic stimulation of the B-lymphocytes in non-lymphoid organs where they are not down-regulated as efficiently as in lymphoid structures. In addition to these cellular features of SS, the patients continue to exhibit the antibody/complement-mediated features that they share in common with SLE patients.

Ocular Symptoms and Signs in the SS Patient

The characteristic ophthalmologic finding in SS is keratoconjunctivitis sicca, due to destruction of the lacrimal glands, leading to decreased lacrimal secretions. Patients may complain of dry eyes, irritation, soreness, foreign body sensation, pain, or photophobia. In severe cases, patients may have strings of mucous filaments attached to the cornea.

When evaluating the patient with a complaint of dry eyes, it is important to determine whether the objective signs of dry eyes are commensurate with the patient's symptoms.

Methods to measure the integrity of the corneal surface, tear film, and tear production include *Rose-Bengal*, fluorescein, and lissamine green dye staining, and the *Schirmer's test*.

Rose Bengal dye can detect punctate epithelial erosions of the cornea, and attached mucous and devitalized cells.

In the Schirmer's test, a Whatman paper wick is folded over the lower eyelid, and the migration of tear fluid is measured over 5 minutes. Some ophthalmology texts mention that the latter test may be unreliable. A referral to the ophthalmologist is warranted for complete evaluation, as ocular complications can include corneal ulceration or perforation.

Ocular processes that mimic KCS include blepharitis (irritation and low grade infection of the Meibomian glands in the lids), herpetic keratitis (usually with ophthalmic distribution of shingles), conjunctivitis (both viral and bacterial), blepharospasm (uncontrolled blinking due to an increased local neural reflex circuit), sarcoidosis, and anterior uveitis (usually associated with marked photosensitivity). More commonly, modest dry eye symptoms and signs are exacerbated by anxiety, depression or medications (Pflugfelder, 1996)

Oral Symptoms and Signs in the SS Patient

Xerostomia is caused by destruction of the major and minor salivary glands. Dryness of the mouth can make it difficult to swallow food or even to talk, due to dryness of the buccal mucosa. Patients may have difficulty wearing dentures, mucosal surfaces in advanced dryness may become dry and wrinkled, and saliva can become thick and stringy. As saliva also functions to protect the mouth from infection due to antimicrobial properties and mechanical flushing, SS patients are at risk for tooth decay, periodontal disease, and mucosal infections, such as candidiasis.

Because a dry mouth is not necessarily a painful mouth, the sudden development of pain should stimulate a search for signs of angular cheilitis or oral candidiasis, including under dentures (Daniels, 2000). Salivary glands may become enlarged.

Saliva flow can be measured by sialometry, which measures saliva flow into a calibrated tube for 15 minutes. Parotid sialography can demonstrate distortion of normal ductules, and salivary gland scintigraphy can demonstrate decreased uptake and release of tracer. Salivary gland biopsy was mentioned previously.

Health impact questionnaires specific for SS demonstrate the impact on social interactions among women (who use meals as a significant source of socialization) as well as the expense of dental restorations in SS patients (Allison, Locker, and Feine, 1999). Physicians (Soto-Rojas and Kraus, 2002) do not generally recognize the contribution of oral symptoms to the patient's quality of life.

Dryness of the mouth cannot simply be attributed to the total destruction of the gland in the majority of SS biopsies. The residual glandular elements in the salivary gland (Fig. 1) appear dysfunctional even though they maintain their neural innervation (Konttinen et al., 1992) and upregulation of their muscarinic receptors (Beroukas et al., 2002). The normal innervation of the gland is shown schematically in Fig. 3. The gland has an excess of receptors beyond the number of neural synapses noted on electron microscopy, providing a target for the therapeutic use of secretagogues such as pilocarpine or cevimeline. (Fox, Konttinen, and Fisher, 2001). The optimal glandular secretion is obtained when both M1 and M3 receptors are stimulated.

Dryness of the oral mucosa stimulates unmyelinated nerves that go to the midbrain, which also receives input from higher cortical centers. If a net signal for secretion is needed, adrenergic nerves are sent to the glandular blood vessels while cholinergic nerves go to the gland (Stern et al., 1998).

In patients with SS, the local environment of the inflamed gland leads to dysfunction of the residual glandular units due to release of cytokines, metalloproteinases, and autoantibodies.

Dryness in patients with Alzheimer's disease and multiple sclerosis have been proposed to result from dysfunction of the subcortical white matter that signals the lacrimatory/salivatory nuclei (Fisher et al., 1996). Symptoms of dry burning mouth have been associated with depression and anxiety (Bergdahl and Bergdahl, 2001), presumably reflecting the contribution of cortical factors on "functional" circuitry that regulates glandular function and/or the cortical sensation of dryness.

The sudden swelling of a unilateral gland suggests infection, while presence of swollen glands and/or lymphadenopathy raises the possibility of lymphoma, a process, which is markedly more frequent in SS patients. Both high resolution CAT scans and MRI imaging are helpful (Yousem, Kraut, and Chalian, 2000). Recent advances in MRI imaging have indicated that studies using gadolinium imaging with fat subtraction views (called MRI contrast sialography) may allow excellent identification of the ductal structures as well as cystic changes or lymphoma (Tonami et al., 2001).

Another alternative is parotid ultrasound, particularly in centers where the radiologist has experience with this technique (Salaffi et al., 2000).

An additional important factor in the oropharynx of SS patients is gastro-tracheal reflux (Belafsky and Postma, 2003). Since saliva has elevated pH that normally neutralizes gastric acid reflux, the SS patient may be predisposed to not only gastro-esophageal reflux, but also reflux into the trachea that can mimic upper respiratory tract infection. Decreased mucous secretions can also lead to dryness of the pharynx and trachea. Application of rigorous methods to prevent and treat reflux may dramatically change our management of these recurrent problems. (Belafsky and Postma, 2003)

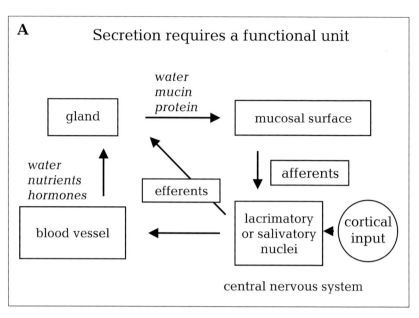

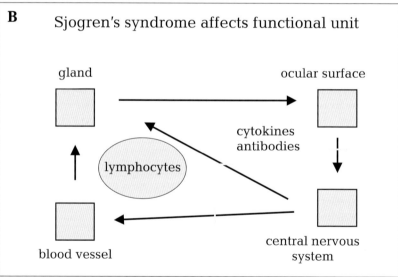

Fig. 3. A. "Circuit" that controls normal tear flow or salivation and interruption of the circuit in patients with Sjögren's syndrome. The stimulation of the ocular or oral mucosal surface leads to afferent nerve signals that reach the lacrimatory or salivatory nuclei in the medulla. Efferent neural signals stimulate both blood vessels and glandular epithelial cells. The medullary signal may be affected by cortical inputs that reflect stimuli such as taste, smell, anxiety, or depression. The efferent neural signal to the gland is mediated by acetylcholine. The gland contains receptors for acetylcholine of the muscarinic class, particularly M3 receptors (shown by arrow). **B.** In Sjögren's syndrome, lymphocytic infiltrates in the gland secrete cytokines that inhibit the release of neurotransmitters and the response of receptors that initiate glandular secretion

Cutaneous Symptoms and Signs in the SS Patient

Cutaneous manifestations of SS include:
- *Dry skin (xerosis)*
- *Vasospastic disorders ranging from Raynaud's to acrocyanosis*
- *Macular, papular and vesicular rashes*
- *Infections such as varicella zoster*
- *Palpable and non-palpable purpura due vasculitis, and*
- *Embolic lesions and thrombotic lesions*
- *Acute or chronic thrombosis with lymphedema*
- *Other associated skin conditions including urticaria or allergic skin eruptions*

Complaints of dry skin occur in about 50% of SS patients (Bloch et al., 1956; Alexander and Provost, 1983; Ito et al., 1999). It is unclear whether or not the xerosis is due to infiltrate of the eccrine or sebaceous glands, or dysfunctional response of the residual glands (Tapinos et al., 1999). In many biopsies from SS patients, dryness of the skin has been associated with lymphocytic infiltrates in the eccrine glands (Sais et al., 1998). Similar to SLE patients, antibody and complement fixation is often detected clinically "normal" skin.

However, the extent of dryness of the skin and the clinical appearance termed "xerosis" is often more severe than that expected for the degree of lymphocytic infiltration (and glandular destruction).

A common finding on deeper skin biopsy is "non-specific perivascular lymphocytic infiltrates." Immuno-histologic studies have also indicated an increase in peri-vascular dendritic cells of both the mesenchymal and Plasmacytoid types. These histologic findings on SS skin biopsy are so common that the pathologist may often only mentions them "in passing," while they emphasize that no leukocytoclastic vasculitic changes were present. But these "perivascular" lymphocytic (and dendritic) cell infiltrates may be the crucial factor in xerosis of SS.

It has been proposed that cytokines, neural or vasoconstrive factors may be released from these peri-vascular lymphocytic and monocytic infiltrates, and may impair the normal function capacity of capillaries or sweat glands. This explanation of skin dryness would be analogous to the severe xerostomia in SS patients whose lip biopsy continues to show significant numbers of glandular acini and ducts between the focal lymphocytic infiltrates on minor salivary gland biopsy.

The skin findings of SS include hyper-gammaglobulinemic purpura, and often occur on the legs in a symmetric fashion. The rash may exhibit palpable or non-palpable purpura. It is common to have onset after prolonged standing or after a long airplane ride (perhaps due to the lower atmospheric pressure at altitude).

In comparison, *among a large cohort of patients with hyperglobulinemic purpura without prior diagnosis of SS – about 50% were subsequently found to have SS* (Kyle et al., 1971). The skin lesions are non-palpable and often associated with rheumatoid factor (especially IgM- kappa monoclonal rheumatoid factor) containing VKIIIb subclass of light chains (Fox, Carson et al., 1986; Fox, Chen et al., 1986). This is commonly associated with a type II mixed cryoglobulin. The differential diagnosis should immediately include unrecognized hepatitis C virus infection.

Skin biopsies generally show ruptured blood vessels and deposition of complement. It has been assumed that immune complexes become trapped at the bifurcation of small blood vessels, leading to complement activation by the immune complex.

In one report, **cutaneous vasculitis** *was found in 52 out of 558 (9%) of patients with primary SS* (Ramos-Casals et al., 1998) appearing as purpura, urticarial lesions, and maculopapules.

Within the vasculitis group, 27% had *cryoglobulinemic vasculitis*, and 21% had urticarial vasculits.

- Most patients had small vessel vasculitis (leukocytoclastic), and only 2 had medium-size vessel involvement-
- Compared to the patients without vasculitis, affected patients had a higher prevalence of systemic involvement, positive ANA, anti-Ro/SS-A antibodies, and rheumatoid factor.

Cryoglobulinemia was associated with worse outcome.

Features of cryoglobulinemia:
- Cryoglobulins are immunoglobulins that precipitate from serum under laboratory conditions of cold.
- *False-negative results in testing for cryoglobulins are common.*
- Sensitive testing for cryoglobulins requires an experienced laboratory that is set up to perform the collection in proper condition.
- While the patient is fasting (lipids can interfere with the assay), at least 20ml of blood should be drawn into a tube that has not been treated with anti-coagulant.
- The tube should be transported and centrifuged at 37 C, then kept for 72 hours at 4° C.

Cryoglobulinemia is divided into three clinical subsets: Types I, II, and III.

This classification is based on *two features:*
(1) the clonality of the IgM component; and
(2) the presence of rheumatoid factor activity.
- In its clinical manifestations, **Type I cryoglobulinemia** is usually quite distinct from types II and III.
- In contrast, substantial clinical overlap exists between Types II and III.

Type I cryoglobulinemia is associated with a monoclonal component and is often associated with a hematopoietic malignancy.

The *symptoms of hyperviscosity are more common with Type I* and increased chance that symptoms such as neuropathy may be related to amyloid.

Type II and III cryoglobulinemia are often termed "mixed" cryoglobulinemias, as they are comprised of both IgG and IgM components. A low complement C4 (either as a C4 null patient) or due to complement consumption are common, so disproportionate decrease in C4 levels are commonly found.

In contrast to lupus glomerulonephritis, membranoproliferative glomerulonephritis due to cryoglobulenimia is usually a "later" presentation.

Vasculitis associated with mixed cryoglobulinemia involves both small- and medium-sized blood vessels. Small-vessel disease is more common than medium vessel disease.

Vasculitis associated with mixed cryoglobulinemia may be caused by hepatitis C virus (HCV) infections and the diagnosis of SS does not rule out co-existent HCV.

- It is also worth remembering that treatment with interferon alpha (either standard form or pegylated), the cornerstone of HCV infection, may exacerbate Type II mixed cryoglobulins in their cutaneous or other manifestations.

Virtually, all patients with Type II mixed cryoglobulinemia are rheumatoid factor positive. SS patients with monoclonal RF and type II mixed cryoglobulinemia have higher frequency of developing non-Hodgkin's lymphoma.

Peripheral nerve involvement is common in patients with cryoglobulenmic vasculitis, occurring in up to 80%. The most common type is a distal symmetric polyneuropathy with predilection for lower extremities. Mononeuritis multiplex may occur but is less common.

For the *treatment of cryoglobulinemia*, please refer to Fox's chapter on THERAPY OF EXTRAGLANDULAR MANIFESTATIONS.

Other authors have reported vasculitis in 30% of both primary and secondary SS patients (Bernacchi et al., 2004). *Palpable purpura* is also found in SS patients (Alexander and Provost, 1987) with biopsies showing leukocytoclastic vasculitis (Ramos-Casals et al., 1998) and may be associated with central nervous system involvement (Provost, Watson, and Simmons, 1997) or pulmonary involvement (Konishi et al., 1997).

Urticarial vasculitis *has been reported in association with SS(O'Donnell and Black, 1995).* Urticarial vasculitis somewhat resembles urticaria, but lesions last typically for 3–4 days, and can be painful. This type of vasculitis has also been reported in SLE patients.

Histopathology of SS vasculitis lesions has demonstrated classic leukocytoclastic vasculitis with neutrophilic destruction of small vessel walls with fibrinoid necrosis, and also a separate pattern of lymphocytic infiltrate of the vessel wall (Provost, Watson, and Simmons-O'Brien, 1997; Provost and Watson, 1992).

Patients with anti-neutrophil cytoplasmic antibodies (ANCA) are relatively uncommon in primary SS and when present are usually p-ANCA (perinuclear) antibodies. Caution must be used in interpreting the ANCA in SS patients since false positive results may result from the presence of other anti-nuclear antibodies (Merkel et al., 1997; Merkel et al., 1996).

Antibodies against endothelial cells have been found in a subset of SS patients, but are also detected in many other autoimmune disorders, and are not closely associated with skin vasculitis (Navarro et al., 1997). Anticardiolipin antibodies are found in a subset of SS patients and are generally IgA isotype, with lower incidence of thrombosis than found in SLE patients (Asherson et al., 1992).

Additional reported *non-vasculitic cutaneous manifestations* of SS include *vitiligo, anetoderma, alopecia, and cutaneous lymphomas* (Roguedas et al., 2004). The presence of anetoderma has been associated with B-Cell lymphomas (Jubert et al., 1993).

Additional cutaneous features include subcutaneous amyloid (Pablos et al., 1993) (Yoneyama et al., 2005). Erythema multi-forme-like, erythema perstans-like, and erythema-nodosum-like lesions (Yamamoto, Katayama, and Nishioka, 1998) have been reported along with Sweet's syndrome (Roguedas et al., 2004; Ramos-Casals et al., 2004; Bernacchi et al., 2004; Foster et al., 2005).

Raynaud's has been reported in 30% of patients with primary SS, although the severe vasomotor instability should suggest the diagnosis of co-existent PSS (usually characterized by telangiectasis and calcinosis) or cryoglobulinemia (Pirildar et al., 2005; Ramos-Casals et al., 2004; Manoussakis et al., 2004; Tektonidou et al., 1999).

Closely related digital skin lesions (which often exhibit T-cell infiltrates on biopsy of the nail beds) with vasospasm induced by cold exposure are termed "chilblains" or "perniosis," where there is a close association with anti-SS A antibody, and the lesions may precede either SS or SLE by up to 10 years (Franceschini et al., 1999; Millard and Rowell, 1978; Rustin et al., 1989).

Attention to potential problems such as bland (atherosclerotic) or septic emboli, digital vasculopathy in smokers (Buerger's disease), and mono-neuritis multiplex must be considered in the patient with cold cyanotic extremity. Severe ischemic or gangrenous changes, ulcerating dystrophic calcification with purulent or ulcerative changes, should suggest systemic sclerosis, deep tissue plane infection and may constitute a medical/surgery emergency.

A sub-epidermal blistering *dermatosis* similar to bullous SLE, with antibodies to Type VII collagen, has been reported in a patient with primary SS who did not fulfill the SLE criteria of the American Rheumatism Association at the time (Gyulai et al., 2002).

Among Asian SS patients, a specific cutaneous finding – annular erythema – of Sjögren's syndrome (AE-SS) has been reported in a relatively high proportion of patients (Ruzicka et al., 1991; Mori et al., 2005; Watanabe et al., 1996; Watanabe et al., 1997; Katayama and Kohriyama, 2001; Katayama et al., 1994), including those with childhood onset (Miyagawa et al., 1995). Although this eruption appears similar to SCLE, histologically, it is distinguishable by coat-sleeve-like infiltration of lymphocytes around the appendages, similar to gyrate erythema. A Caucasian female with SS was reported to have AE-SS (Haimowitz et al., 2000). Many of these patients have antibody to the 60kd epitope of SS-A.

Because many SS patients are often taking multiple medications, the differential diagnosis of cutaneous eruptions always includes drug eruption. Patients can also have infectious processes, especially if they are immuno-suppressed due to treatment. A skin biopsy with direct immunofluorescence can be very helpful in distinguishing these latter two entities from vasculitis or other dermatoses associated with SS.

Systemic Findings in the SS Patient

Extraglandular disease manifestations (Table 4) are subdivided into nonvisceral (skin, arthralgia, myalgia) and visceral (lung, heart, kidney, gastrointestinal, endocrine, central and peripheral nervous system). Cutaneous manifestations are discussed above. There is often a close overlap in the symptoms/signs between SLE and SS patients (Manoussakis et al., 2004). Particular attention below is paid to conditions more common in SS patients.

The symmetric distribution and appearance of *arthralgia/arthritis* generally are similar to either RA or SLE (Manoussakis et al., 2004; Pease et al., 1993); also, patients may show a pattern termed "erosive" osteoarthritis (Fox, 2000). The emergence of an asymmetric swollen joint should suggest an additional process such as crystalline or infectious arthropathy.

Myalgia and symptoms of weakness also occur frequently (Lindvall et al., 2002). Poly-myositis may be associated with sicca symptoms. Other processes including polymyalgia rheumatica, inclusion body myositis, and myopathy due to medications (including statins and steroids) must be considered. Also, neurological problems including vasculitis, throm-botic and paraneoplastic processes may present with weakness. Elevation of acute phase re-actants, muscle enzymes, electromyogram or even muscle biopsy may be required. Myalgia attributed to associated fibromyalgia is common (Bonafede, Downey, and Bennett, 1995).

Interstitial pneumonitis and tracheobronchial sicca are the most common presenta-tion of pulmonary involvement in SS (Quismorio, 1996). The classification of interstitial pneumonitis is undergoing change (Battista et al., 2003) with recognition of subsets in-cluding lymphocytic interstitial pneumonitis (LIP), "usual interstitial pneumonitis (UIP)," bronchiolitis obliterans, and organizing pneumonia (BOOP), and non-specific pneumoni-tis. Also, SS patients may have MALT or other types of lymphoma of the lung (Constan-topoulos, Tsianos, and Moutsopoulos, 1992). Other causes include hypersensitivity lung and drug toxicity (including methotrexate or alkylating agents) as well as opportunistic in-fections in patients receiving immunosuppressive medications must be considered (Kim et al., 2002). Of potential importance are reports of pneumonitis in patients receiving inf-liximab (Chatterjee, 2004) and rituximab (Swords et al., 2004).

Pericarditis and pulmonary hypertension can occur in SS patients (Gyongyosi et al., 1996). Cardiovascular tests suggestive of autonomic neuropathy such as response of blood pressure to sustained hand grip, valsalva maneuver, heart rate response to deep breathing, and heart rate and blood pressure response to standing may be increased in SS patients (Andonopoulos et al., 1998). There is an increased incidence of congenital heart block in mothers bearing anti-SS antibody (Press et al., 1996), although other autoantibodies have also been suggested as causative agents in this condition (Li, Horsfall, and Maini, 1995; Borda et al., 1999),

Renal manifestations include interstitial nephritis, (which is common in SS on provoc-ative testing (Gamron et al., 2000). Some patients may present with hypokalemic paralysis (Siamopoulos, Elisaf, and Moutsopoulos, 1994), renal calculi, or osteomalacia (Fulop and Mackay, 2004). Deterioration in renal status should focus attention to medications includ-ing nonsteroidal anti-inflammatory agents. Also, recently, a role for Chinese herbs in exac-erbating renal disease has been recognized (Nishimagi et al., 2001). SS patients may develop glomerulonephritis (that is negative for anti-ds DNA antibodies) and this suggests the need to consider amyloidsisis, immune complex disorder, or unappreciated SLE with error in lab testing (Dabadghao et al., 1995). Interstitial cystitis symptoms are more common in SS pa-tients (Leppilahti et al., 2003) and may be severe (Shibata et al., 2004). SS patients' bladder symptoms may be exacerbated by their large fluid intake, and the antibodies to muscarinic cholinergic receptors found on bladder epithelial cells (Beroukas et al., 2001).

Gastrointestinal manifestations include dysphagia that is partly due to xerostomia, but also may be due to esophageal dysfunction (Feist et al., 1999). In SS patients, mild atrophic changes in the antrum were more common than in control patients, but severe mucosal at-rophy was rare (Collin, Karvonen et al., 1997). The patient with gastritis should be exam-ined for helicobacter pylori, especially as this agent has been associated with MALT lym-phomas in SS patients (Raderer et al., 2001). An association of sicca symptoms and pri-mary biliary cirrhosis (PBC) has been noted (Invernizzi et al., 1998), but the difference in autoantibody profiles suggests that these are distinct processes in most patients (Tishler et al., 1995). In patients with PBC, treatment with ursodeoxycholic acid may be helpful (Zukowski et al., 1998). Celiac sprue has also been reported in association with SS (Sheikh and Shaw-Stiffel, 1995) and it is important to identify these patients that present with mild or atypical symptoms (Collin, Reunala et al., 1997).

Hypothyroidism appears commonly in SS patients (D'Arbonneau et al., 2003; Perez et al., 1995). Also among patients with autoimmune thyroid disease, SS may be present in about 10% of patients with autoimmune thyroid disease (Tektonidou et al., 2004). Although SS patients may exhibit immune responses to pancreatic antigens, the incidence of clinically significant pancreatic disease is low (Nishimori et al., 1993). SS patients have a blunted pituitary and adrenal response to test with corticotropin releasing factor (Johnson et al., 1998).

Lymphoproliferative disease is a particular concern in SS patients since there is a *40-fold* increased risk of lymphoma (Kassan et al., 1978). The types of lymphomas have been reviewed in a multicenter European study (Voulgarelis et al., 1999). In a recent series, most lymphomas in patients with SS were marginal zone B-Cell neoplasms, arose in diverse extranodal and nodal sites, and generally were not associated with viruses (Royer et al., 1997). However, there have been case reports of the association of SS with infectious agents such as Helicobacter pylori (Nishimura, Miyajima, and Okada, 2000), HHV-6 (Josephs et al., 1988), HTLV-1 (Nakamura et al., 2000) and EBV (Kamel et al., 1993). The emergence of lymphoma may be signaled by persistently enlarged parotid glands, regional or generalized lymphadenopathy, hepatosplenomegaly, pulmonary infiltrates, vasculitis, and hypergammaglobulinemia. None of these are specific, but should raise the index of suspicion for, particularly if accompanied by serologic features such as a falling hematocrit, high sedimentation rate, or the presence of monoclonal cryoglobulins. Further investigation might include biopsy of lymph node, bone marrow, or salivary gland, or imaging studies such as abdominal CT scanning.

Neurologic manifestations are reported in about 20% of SS patients (Delalande et al., 2004) and may include central nervous system involvement, cranial neuropathies (Urban et al., 2001), myelopathy and peripheral neuropathies (Barendregt et al., 2001). Sensory neuropathies are most common, and epineural inflammatory changes have been found on nerve biopsy (Grant et al., 1997). The onset of an asymmetric motor and sensory neuropathy may signal small or medium sized vessel vasculitis (Ramos-Casals et al., 2004). Ischemic neuropathies including optic atrophy may be associated with demyelinating and thromboembolic processes (Rosler et al., 1995). A syndrome of multiple sclerosis associated with cutaneous vasculitis was initially reported to occur in a very high frequency in SS patients at one medical center (Alexander et al., 1986) although a longer-term follow-up did not confirm the initial results (Simmons-O'Brien et al., 1995). The frequency of central demyelinating disease appears similar to SLE patients (Pender, 1999) with abnormal oligoclonal bands on lumbar puncture and abnormal brain MRI. However, it also important to point out that patients with multiple sclerosis (de Seze et al., 2001) and with Alzheimer's disease have increased frequency of sicca complaints, probably as a result of abnormalities in the central outflow of cholinergic nerve fibers (Fisher, 1999).

Psychiatric disorders including depression and anxiety have been described in many patients with SS, and the increased frequency suggests that this may be part of the underlying process (rather than simply a response to the stress of an autoimmune disorder)(Utset et al., 1994). In both SS and SLE patients, these symptoms often precede the diagnosis of autoimmune disease (van Dam et al., 1994). Abnormalities in neuropsychimetric testing (mainly frontal lobe and memory loss) and abnormalities in PET scanning in the brain have been reported in SS patients (Lass et al., 2000; Belin et al., 1999). Although initial studies suggested a potential role for anti-ribosomal P antibodies, subsequent studies in SS did not confirm this result (Spezialetti et al., 1993). The subtlest are changes in cognitive function, with poor memory and concentration. Although infrequently mentioned by patients, these changes can be confirmed on formal cognitive testing.

Complaints of *fatigue and myalgia often termed "fibromyalgia"* are common. The *Medical Outcomes Study Short-Form General Health Survey* (SF-36) and *VAS* shows frequent symptoms of fatigue in both SS and non-SS patients complaining of sicca symptoms (Tensing et al., 2001; Lwin et al., 2003). In SS patients, neither hemoglobin, ESR or CRP predicted fatigue. Sleep disturbances were a common cause of fatigue (Tishler et al., 1997).

Neonatal lupus may be found in the children of mothers with SS, SLE, and in a proportion of mothers bearing antibodies against SS-A and SS-B antigens but lacking clinical SS (Buyon et al., 1996). Neonatal lupus has been associated with anti-SS-A (anti-Ro) antibodies to the 52kD protein.

Table 4. Disease Manifestations and Therapy

Manifestation	Therapy
Ocular	Artificial tears- preserved/nonpreserved
Xerophthalmia	Punctual occlusion
Blepharitis	Topical cyclosporine
Iritis/uveitis	Topical androgen (in trial)
	Topical purinogenic receptor agonist (in trial)
	Topical (nonpreserved) steroids
	Autologous serum tears
	Lid scrubs for blepharitis
	Bandage contact lens
Dental	
Xerostomia	Mechanical Stimulation
Periodontal	
Gingitivis	Regular Oral hygiene
Oral candida	Topical fluoride
	Artificial saliva and lubricants
	Secretagogues including
	Pilocarpine
	Cevimeline
	Sailor
	Anhydrous maltose lozenge
	Interferon-alpha (in trial)
	Oral candida therapy
	Diet Modification
	Gene therapies (pre-clinical)

Table 4. (*continued*) Disease Manifestations and Therapy

Manifestation	Therapy
Joint/Muscle Arthralgia/myalgia Arthritis/myositis	NSAIDs Antimalarials
	DMARDs including Methotrexate azathioprine Leflunomide TNF inhibitors Anti-CD20 (in trial)
Cutaneous	
Raynaud's Hyperglobulinemia purpura Mixed cryoglobulinemia	Corticosteroids (topical and systemic) Tacrolimus (topical) Antimalarials
E. multipforme E. annulare Necrotizing vasculitis	DMARDs for vasculitis Cytotoxic agents
Vitiligo, xerosis, alopeccia Amyloid anetoderma	
Embolic and thrombotic lesions due to pro-coagulants	
<u>Ears, Nose, Throat</u> Sinusitis Esophageal Reflux Tracheal Reflux Parotid/Submandibular Swelling Hearing Loss	Moisturing Agents Antibiotics/Antifungal Proton pump inhibitors Gastric motility agents Diet Modification Steroids and DMARDs
Cardiovascular Pericarditis Cardiomyopathy Pulmonary hypertension Accelerated atherosclerosis Pro-coagulants	Corticosteroids DMARDs including Cyclophosphamide Mycophenolic Acid Rituximab corticosteroids ACE and IRB inhibitor Calcium channel Blockers

Table 4. (*continued*) Disease Manifestations and Therapy

Manifestation	Therapy
Pulmonary Interstitial pneumonitis	Steroids DMARDS and
Pseudolymphoma and lymphoma Pleurisal effusions Pulmonary emboli	Cytotoxic agents Endothelin receptor antgonist (bosantin)
Pulmonary hypertension	
Gastrointestinal Atrophic gastritis	Proton pump inhibitors H2 blockers Motility agents
Biliary cirrhosis Sclerosising cholangitis Pancreatitis Celiac sprue	Diet modification Bile salt chelation
Hematolologic Anemia	Corticosteroids
Leukopenia thrombocytopenia Pro-coagulants	DMARDs Rituximab (in trial) Anti-coagulation
Lymphoproliferative Monoclonal gammopathy Lymphadenopathy Pseudolymphoma Lymphoma (MALT and non-MALT)	Corticosteroids DMARDs including Anti-malarials Chemotherapy Rituximab (in trial)
Renal Interstitial nephritis (type I and type II) Hypokalemia (periodic paralysis) Renal Calculi	Bicarbonate Corticosteroids Avoid NSAIDs DMARD
Glomerulonephritis (in absence of anti-DNA antibodies) Nephrogenic diabestes Amyloid	Choice of anti-hypertensive (lacking anti-cholinergic activity)
Renal artery vasculitis and thrombosis	

Table 4. (*continued*) Disease Manifestations and Therapy

Manifestation	Therapy
Endocrine	Hormonal replacement
Thyroid (hyper and hypo)	Replacement of gluco- and mineralocorticoids
Autonomic neuropathy	
Pancreatitis	
Blunted hypothalamic-adrenal axis response	
Central Nervous System	
Demyelinating	DMARDs including
(brain including optic atrophy and spinal cord)	Cyclophosphamide
	Corticosteroids
Seizures	Anticoagulants
Toxi-metabolic encephalopathy	
Vasculitic stroke	
Thrombotic stroke	
Cranial neuropathy	
(Trigeminal, Facial, Cochlear)	
Autonomic neuropathy	
Peripheral Neuropathy	
Sensory	Corticosteroids and DMARDs
Symmetrical	
Axonal sensori-motor	
Asymmetric Motor	
Mononeuritis multiplex	
Fatigue	
(Not due to Inflammatory or endocrine cause)	Hypnotics for sleep SSRI s and SNSRIs
Depression	
Fibromyalgia	

Differential Diagnosis

When approaching a patient with possible SS, it is important to rule out other causes of keratoconjunctivitis sicca, xerostomia, and parotid gland enlargement (reviewed in Kassan and Moutsopoulos '04). Dry eyes can be caused by sarcoidosis, amyloidosis, medications, trauma or scarring, infection, inflammatory conditions such as blepharitis or pemphigoid, neurologic conditions impairing eyelid or lacrimal gland function, or hypovitaminosis A. Dry mouth can be caused by medications (antihypertensive, parasympatholytic, psychotropic), amyloidosis, sarcoidosis, diabetes mellitus, infections, trauma, irradiation, or could be psychogenic. Endocrine disorders can affect the parotid gland, along with infections such as mumps, Hepatitis C or HIV. Pancreatitis, diabetes, cirrhosis, lymphoma, and lipid abnormalities can also lead to gland enlargement. Neurologic disorders associated with dryness include multiple sclerosis.

It may also be crucial to differentiate SS from other rheumatologic autoimmune disorders, especially when treatment decisions need to be made. The most common area of diagnostic confusion is between Sjögren's and SLE. It is important to recognize that the group of patients we currently "lump" as SLE really comprise at least 3 subsets that have distinct patterns of HLA-DR associations, autoantibody profiles, and clinical features. One subset of the SLE patients lack glomerulonephritis and have arthritis and rash. This subset frequently has HLA-DR3, antibody to SS-A, and has great similarity to Sjögren's syndrome. There are several ways to look at the relationship between 1° SS and SLE. One easy method is that SS is "SLE with only 4 of the 5 required criteria." However, another distinction is the slight difference in underlying pathogenesis.

SLE is generally characterized by antibody and complement mediated tissue damage (immune complex glomerulonephritis, pleural and pericardial effusion, thrombocytopenia and hemolytic anemia. Although these features may be present in SS patients, the characteristic feature of these SS patients is their lymphoproliferative tendency. At the most basic level, the salivary and lacrimal glands are supposed to lack focal lymphoid infiltrates. Their presence as a characteristic of SS indicates the presence of homing receptors and dendritic cell architecture in extra glandular tissues that form the pathologic basis for their sicca symptoms. From a clinical standpoint, 1° SS patients specifically require attention to manifestations of lymphocytic infiltration into different tissues. This abnormality can result in interstitial nephritis, interstitial pneumonitis, as well as an increased risk of lymphoproliferative disease, such as lymphoma.

The clinical overlap with PSS patients also may be considerable with variation in their patterns of autoantibodies, histocompatibility associations, and tissue biopsies. Some PSS patients have a fibrotic pattern on their lip biopsies while others have lymphocytic infiltrates (suggesting more of an overlap syndrome "termed mixed connective tissue disease).

Although RA is the most "common" autoimmune disorder associated with SS, the clinical features (of RA) (ocular dryness more than oral dryness), difference in pattern of ANA (rare occurrence of anti-SS A antibody) and different histocompatibility antigen suggest that these disorders (i. e., RA plus SS) are much less closely related to 1°SS than is SLE with 2° SS.

The initial evaluation needs to determine if the patient presents with evidence suggestive of an objective autoimmune disease, not just a positive ANA, and this will involve specific autoantibody profiles, ophthalmologic studies, salivary flow studies, and/or minor lip biopsies. The patient may have the SS secondary to another autoimmune condition (RA, systemic sclerosis, etc) or as part of an overlap syndrome with another autoimmune condition. Other conditions that mimic SS need to be evaluated. In addition to the ocular and oral evaluation, the workup for SS can also include complete history and physical, CBC, ESR, comprehensive metabolic panel (including liver and renal evaluation), serum immunoglogulins, TSH, urinalysis, CXR, lymph node or marrow biopsy, complement, ACE, and serologies for Hep B, Hep C, EBV, and HIV. Autoantibody serologies as discussed include ANA, anti-SS-A, anti-SS-B, anti-SM/RNP, anti-ds-DNA, and RF.

Treatment

A. Cutaneous Therapy

Local treatment for cutaneous symptoms of Sjogren's syndrome focuses on dry skin. If a patient suffers from more serious skin findings such as *vasculitis*, their disease may warrant systemic management. Treatment needs to be aggressive and may require higher dose corticosteroids or even cyclophosphamide.

Treatment of dry skin in Sjogren's syndrome is similar to managing xerosis in other conditions. The patient should moisturize with a fragrance-free cream moisturizer once or twice a day. Moisturizing is performed immediately after bathing or showering, while the skin is still damp, to prevent further evaporation from the skin. Sometimes in cases of extreme dryness, an ointment is suggested, for its barrier and protective properties (such as petrolatum jelly or Aquaphor). If this is used, then application should be onto damp skin, as the ointment itself does not contain water. Excess greasiness can be blotted with a towel. Sometimes a moisturizing cream with beta or alpha hydroxy acid, or urea, can add extra moisture, but in cases of cracks in the skin, will sting and irritate. Excess, long, hot showers or baths should be avoided, in addition to heavily fragranced cleansers. The usual recommendation is to cleanse with a moisturizing soap such as Dove fragrance-free bar, or a soap-free cleanser such as Cetaphil gentle cleanser or Aquanil cleanser.

If the xerosis leads to pruritis, then safe anti-pruritic topical treatments are recommended. Over-the-counter lotions containing menthol, camphor (Sarna Anti-Itch Lotion), 2% lidocaine (Neutrogena Norwegian Formula Soothing Relief, Anti-Itch Moisturizer), and pramoxine (Aveeno Anti-Itch Concentrated Lotion) are readily available. Oral antihistamines should be used with caution because of their anticholinergic effects. Sometimes topical corticosteroids are used for pruritis, but their use should be limited due to long-term side effects such as skin atrophy, tachyphylaxis, and absorption. We generally do not like to use topical corticosteroids for more than a couple of weeks at a time, especially the ultra-potent ones, but even the mid-potency ones. In the case of inflammatory skin findings, local treatment with potent topical steroids can augment systemic treatments.

We always suggest constant daily sun protection for patients with autoimmune conditions. Because the wavelength of light causing sun sensitivity in autoimmune conditions may not be in the UVB spectrum (290–320 nm), patients should use a broad spectrum sunscreen. SPF factors refer to UVB protection only, so patients cannot count on simply the SPF factor. Most sunscreens available now have added UVA protection (290–320 nm), commonly from chemical UVA absorbing compounds, such as Parsol, 1789 (avobenzone). However, we prefer physical sun blocks, since wavelengths outside of both UVB and UVA may affect the patient with autoimmune disease. Physical sunblocks contain titanium dioxide or zinc oxide, which reflect rays. One commonly available sun block is Neutrogena Sensitive Skin Sun Block SPF-30, which uses purely titanium dioxide as its active ingredient. The most effective protection is sun protective clothing, since it will not wear off as sunscreens do. Obviously, avoiding excess sun contact altogether is prudent, such as trying to stay indoors during the intense sunlight hours of 10 AM to 2–4 PM.

B. Ocular Therapy

Symptoms of *dryness* result from the increased friction as the upper eyelid moves over the surface of the eye. This movement is facilitated by the tear film that consists of a mixture of aqueous secretions and mucins produced by the lacrimal gland, and that contains a variety of proteins and nutrients derived not only from the lacrimal glands but also from the sera (transported into the tears by the lacrimal glands). The tear film is stabilized by a lipid layer to prevent evaporation, and these lipids are made by Meibomian glands located at the edge of the lower lid; inflammation of these glands leads to blepharitis, which is a common problem in dry eye patients.

Artificial lubricants: Patients can use over-the-counter preservative-free artificial tears, lubricating ointments, and methylcellulose. The latter two are usually used at night since they are viscous. Preservatives can lead to topical irritation, especially in the dry eye, where the concentration can become high. Other prescription ophthalmologic drops (such as antibiotics and glaucoma drops) may still have irritating preservatives.

Various measures are employed to conserve the tear film for as long as possible:

- *Side shields* (e. g., Moist Eye Moisture Panels, Eagle Vision Inc., Memphis TN) can be fitted into eyeglass frames, reducing the evaporation rate of normal or artificial tears.
- *Ski or swim goggles* are very effective at reducing evaporation, but social considerations limit their use.
- *Wrap-around sunglasses* are somewhat more acceptable socially.
- Other general measures to minimize the loss of tears include use of *humidifiers*, particularly in rooms in which a lot of time is spent such as a bedroom, and the occasional use of a moist washcloth over the eyes.

Punctal occlusion

If frequent installation of artificial tears is inadequate or impractical, punctal occlusion is the treatment of choice. It is a highly effective method for maximizing the preservation of tears. This technique involves sealing of the lacrimal puncta, through which the tears normally drain away to the nose; 90 percent of drainage occurs through the inferior punctum. Several different types of punctual plugs are available and plugs (called intra-cannicular plugs) that do not protrude onto the corneal surface seem to be preferred (Hamano, 2005). However, it should be noted that local infections and even pyoderma-like reactions have been reported around the plugs(Musadiq, Mukherji, and Sandramouli, 2005; Kim, Osmanovic, and Edward, 2005).

Some ophthalmologists begin with preliminary temporary plugs to ensure that punctal occlusion does not result in excess tear accumulation. However, temporary plugs often do not adequately block the puncta. Thus, failure to improve comfort with these temporary devices does not preclude the use of permanent punctal occlusion. Also, temporary plugs might be used to avoid a permanent change in patients who might regain near-normal lacrimal function with appropriate therapy. The availability of intra-cannicular plugs (that do not protrude into the ocular surface) has the added advantage that they can be removed non-surgically. When indicated, laser or hand-held thermal cautery can be used for a permanent closure. It is important to realize that punctal occlusion is a tear preservation strategy; as a result, it is of little benefit, unless supplemented with artificial lubricants, in those with minimal to no tear production.

Recognition of certain environments that exacerbate dry eyes should lead to increased use of methods to prevent ocular complications. It may take 2 or 3 days to build (heal) the tear film but only 2–3 hours in a dry environment for it to be disturbed. For example:

- *Travel to areas with low humidity* and dry winds are obvious.
- Many large offices that *use central heating/air conditioning* are extremely dry.
- *Trips in automobiles* not only use dry heating and air conditioning, but also present additional problems of pollution from the road.
- There has been recent recognition that the blink rate goes down dramatically among patients who *sit at computer terminals for prolonged periods.*
- Another important environment for complications including corneal abrasions is *the operating room*, where the humidity is very low, and particularly in the post-operative recovery room, where the patient frequently has non-humidified oxygen delivered by a face mask.

The increased frequency of use of artificial tears in these environments may help to prevent complications, and should even be started prophylactically.

Topical cyclosporine

The United States Food and Drug Administration approved the use of a cyclosporine ophthalmic emulsion (0.05 percent) based upon four studies that compared this agent to a castor oil-based vehicle in 1200 patients (Pflugfelder, 2004). One of the studies presented in abstract form noted a decrease of 38 percent in infiltrating CD3 positive T-Cells in the conjunctival biopsies of 293 subjects receiving cyclosporine, versus a 15 percent increase in those receiving the vehicle alone (Sall et al., 2000).

Among 877 patients randomly assigned to receive twice-daily instillation of cyclosporine (0.05 percent, 0.1 percent) or vehicle alone, there was increased wetting on Schirmer testing in 15 percent of patients receiving the active drug (Strong et al., 2005). The most common adverse effect was a burning sensation in the eyes after administration; less frequent side effects were red eye, epiphoria, foreign body sensation, itching, and blurred vision.

A recent study (Tatlipinar and Akpek, 2005) examined cyclosporine 0.1% emulsion to evaluate cyclosporine 0.1% ophthalmic emulsion over a 1- to 3-year period in moderate to severe dry eye disease patients. Four hundred twelve patients previously dosed for 6 to 12 months with cyclosporine 0.05% or 0.1% in prior Phase III trials were enrolled. Corneal staining, Schirmer tests, and symptom severity assessments were conducted during the first 12-month extension, with a patient survey during the second 12-month extension. Mean duration of treatment was 19.8 months.

Improvements in objective and subjective measures of dry eye disease were modest, probably because of prior treatment with cyclosporine. Most survey respondents said their symptoms began to resolve in the first 3 months of cyclosporine treatment during the previous Phase III clinical trials. No serious treatment-related adverse events occurred. The results supplement the safety record of the commercially available cyclosporine 0.05% ophthalmic emulsion.

Topical Tacrolimus

Bourdoulay et al. (Berdoulay, English, and Nadelstein, 2005) reported the use of 0.02% tacrolimus in aqueous suspension on tear production in dogs with keratoconjunctivitis sicca (KCS). They suggest that this agent (which is water soluble, in contrast to relatively insoluble cyclosporin) may be a promising alternative to topical CsA for treatment of KCS and may be beneficial in patients with less than optimal response to topical CsA.

Topical nonsteroidal eye drops (such as indomethacin) have been found to provide symptomatic relief, but they should be used with caution and under close monitoring, and the treatment should be promptly discontinued if corneal epithelial defects develop or worsen during treatment (Aragona et al., 2005). Similarly, chronic use of topical cortisones has to managed carefully by the ophthalmologist, because of risk of glaucoma, cataracts, sclera melting, and infections.

Blepharitis management

Blepharitis commonly occurs with dry eyes, and detection and management can aid SS symptoms. The source of lipids in the tear film is the Meiobian glands that are predominately located in the margin of the eyelids near the eyelashes. In SS patients, inflammation of the lower glands is common and may be caused by "plugging" by viscous secretions (including the overuse of ocular lubricants and ointments). Application of warm compresses followed by eyelid scrubs comprise the most critical elements of effective blepharitis control. This therapy removes the eyelid debris (which can be colonized by bacteria), and stabilizes the tear film by releasing oily secretions from the meibomian glands, thus reducing tear evaporation

Scrubs can be performed with dilute baby shampoo or commercially available cleansing products (OCuSOFT Lid Scrubs or Novartis Eye-Scrub).

C. Oral Therapy

One of the most important consequences of oral dryness is the loss of teeth. Saliva has multiple functions within the oral cavity that include:
- *lubrication of the mucosa* so that the tongue can help with cleaning out residual food that leads to dental plaque and bacteria;
- *buffering of acids* that reabsorb calcium from teeth; as well as
- *the ability to modulate viral, bacterial, and fungal populations* in the mouth.

It is extremely important that the SS patient regularly floss their teeth after meals, receive regular professional dental hygiene treatments including fluoride treatments (discussed below) at frequent intervals such as every 3 months (Papas et al., 1993), and recognize the role of dietary factors with respect to the correlation between sucrose intake and caries(Papas, Joshi, Belanger et al., 1995; Papas, Joshi, Palmer et al., 1995). Although frequently grouped together, it is important to consider dental caries as distinct from periodontal disease.

The loss of teeth in SS patients results from a combination of low oral pH that facilitates loss of dental calcium and the alterations of oral flora that lead to accelerated decay(Suzuki et al., 2005; Soto-Rojas and Kraus, 2002; Christensen et al., 2001; Schiodt et al., 2001; Isidor et al., 1999; Robinson et al., 1997; Yamamoto et al., 1997).

These problems have been recently reviewed by Wu et al. (Wu and Fox, 1994; Wu, 2003). For individuals with very low to no salivary production, the amount of phosphate and calcium ions available for incorporation onto the tooth surface and enhancement of the remineralization process may be limited. These individuals could possibly benefit from the exogenous addition of calcium phosphate ions commercially available as a toothpaste, in specialized chewing gums, and as a solution.

A double-blind clinical trial examined the efficacy of a dentifrice containing calcium phosphate and found modest benefit in the prevention of root caries, but no benefit on coronal caries was noted (Wu, 2003). These findings are consistent with the observation that individuals with salivary dysfunction are prone to root and incisal caries, rather than coronal caries.

Another clinical trial examined the caries preventive effect of a mouth rinse containing casein derivatives coupled to calcium phosphate in patients with Sjögren's syndrome and dry mouth secondary to radiation therapy (Hay and Morton, 2003). The mouthwash failed to show complete efficacy (Wu, 2003). The majority of studies supporting the addition of calcium and phosphate as an aid to remineralization have been primarily short-term studies in animals and humans. There is currently no agreed-upon formulation/concentration of calcium phosphate or consensus on how often exposure should occur which could influence the results of any clinical trial. Definitive proof would require large long-term clinical trials, which are notoriously difficult and expensive(Hay and Morton, 2003; Hay and Thomson, 2002).

Artificial sweeteners that are not fermentable by acid-producing bacteria have also been implicated in the promotion of the remineralization process(Pers, d'Arbonneau et al., 2005). Convincing data primarily from studies done with children has shown that certain natural sweeteners such as xylitol and sorbitol (usually in a chewing gum formulation) have a significant anti-caries effect. There has been some suggestion that the caries-preventative effect of xylitol/sorbitol is due to the effect of chewing alone, via the production of saliva(Wu and Fox, 1994; Wu, 2003). But other mechanisms have been suggested including: the growth inhibition of caries-inducing bacteria, the selection of xylitol-resistant strains with a resultant shift to less virulent and cariogenic strains, and the binding of xylitol to surface receptors on Strep. mutans species modulating their function(Pers, d'Arbonneau et al., 2005; Pers, Daridon et al., 2005).

The mainstay in the prevention of dental caries remains *fluoride* (Daniels and Wu, 2000). A high dose 5% sodium fluoride varnish is currently available in the United States, but apparently not as widely used in the United States as in Europe where it was developed and tested primarily in children.

Two mechanisms by which topical fluoride promotes remineralization include:

1) the development of a crystalline protective veneer (varnish) at the site of demineralization; and,
2) inhibition of bacterial metabolism and thus reduction of their acid production.

The theoretical advantage of using the **varnish** is not only in the higher level of fluoride but also in the sustained release delivery system. One *in-vitro* study determined that a single application of the varnish could release fluoride for up to 6 months (Wu, 2003). Varnish application is fast and easy and does not necessarily require professional prophylaxis prior to application, and can be applied directly to the root and incisal surfaces that are most vulnerable to decay in the SS patient population(Castillo and Milgrom, 2004; Castillo et al., 2001).

Chlorhexidine (CHX) is a topical antimicrobial agent that is used to decrease the intraoral bacterial load thought to contribute to periodontal disease and caries(Banting et al., 2000). In addition, CHX has an antifungal effect that is relevant to the SS population. In our experience, the available CHX oral rinses have not been well tolerated by the SS patient group. Chlorhexidine is now being developed in the varnish format and as a chlorhexidine-fluoride combination varnish that may be more acceptable to the SS population.

Oral Candidiasis is treated with Nystatin or clotrimazole troches or oral suspensions. Dentures should be cleansed regularly.

Saliva substitutes are generally not tolerated by patients.

Medications that increase oral dryness such as antihistamines and diuretics should be avoided if possible.

D. Secretagogues

Two muscarinic agonists – **pilocarpine** and **cevimeline** – have recently been approved as secretagogues for the treatment of symptoms of xerostomia in Sjogren's syndrome (SS) (Papas et al., 1998). These agents stimulate the M1 and M3 receptors present on salivary glands, leading to increased secretory function.

Pilocarpine was initially used for treatment of radiation xerostomia and subsequently for SS (Katelaris, 2005; Wall, Magarity, and Jundt, 2002; Fox, Konttinen, and Fisher, 2001).

In our experience, pilocarpine has a shorter onset of action but also a shorter duration of action with suggesting dosing 4 times a day. This leads to a narrow window between efficacy and side effects of sweating.

Cevimeline (also known in neuropharmacology literature as AF102) was originally developed for treatment of Alzheimer's disease (where M1 agonist activity is neuroprotective) and found to increase salivation through its M1 and M3 agonist activities (Fox, Konttinen, and Fisher, 2001). It was subsequently shown effective in increasing saliva flow and symptom improvement in SS (Petrone et al., 2002).

Cevimeline is generally used three times a day. However, we recommend gradually increasing the dose and taking about 30 minutes before meals. Initially, patients may have some increased symptoms of gastric acidity (also stimulated by the muscarinic receptors) and this can be minimized by use of a proton pump inhibitor while initiating therapy.

E. Systemic Therapy for Extraglandular manifestations of SS

Nonvisceral manifestations such as *arthralgia* and *myalgia* are generally treated with salicy-
lates, nonsteroidal agents and often hydroxychloroquine. As in SLE patients, corticosteroids
are effective but limited by their usual side effects including osteoporosis, diabetes, cardio-
vascular and mood disruption. In addition, SS patients have increased problems with corticosteroids including acceleration of their periodontal disease and oral candidiasis. Another
problem in the SS patient is decreased tolerance of NSAIDs due to dysphagia secondary to
decreased salivary flow and esophageal motility (Belafsky and Postma, 2003) as well as the
increased frequency of GERD noted above. In terms of NSAIDs for the treatment of arthralgias in the SS patient, generic NSAIDS can be prepared as a topical cream or as a rectal sup-
pository by a "compounding pharmacy" for the patient with difficulty swallowing tablets.

Among the "slow-acting" drugs, antimalarials (hydroxychloroquine) have proven useful in decreasing the arthralgia, myalgia and lymphadenopathy in SS patients (Fox et al.,
1988; Fox et al., 1996), similar to its benefit in some SLE patients (Wallace, 1994). We have
used hydroxychloroquine (6–8 mg / kg / day) in SS patients where there is elevation of
erythrocyte sedimentation rate (ESR) and polyclonal hyperglobulinemia. In a European
study, Kruize et al. (Kruize et al., 1993) also found that hydroxychloroquine improved ESR
but did not increase tear flow volumes. When taken at the proper dose (6–8 mg / kg / day),
hydroxychloroquine has a very good safety record, although there remains a remote possibility (probably less than 1/1,000) (Bernstein, 1991) of significant build-up in the eye. For
this reason, periodic eye checks (generally every 6–12 months) are recommended so that
the medicine can be discontinued if there is any significant build-up.

For visceral involvement including vasculitic skin lesions, pneumonitis, neuropathy
and nephritis, corticosteroids are used in a manner similar to SLE patients. Drugs such as
hydroxychloroquine, azathioprine and methotrexate are used to help taper the corticosteroids (Deheinzelin et al., 1996). Methotrexate appeared more useful than azathioprine in SS
(Skopouli et al., 1996; Price et al., 1998). It is likely that leflunomide will prove useful in
selected SS patients (Wallace, 2002) similar to its role in SLE patients. In some SS patients,
cyclosporine may be used (Dalavanga et al., 1990) but the tendency towards interstitial nephritis in many Sjögren's patients limits the usefulness of the drug. For patients with sicca
symptoms and PBC, the use of urosedeoycholic acid is important (Zukowski et al., 1998).

For life-threatening illness, cyclophosphamide is occasionally required (Fox, 2000).
However, the increased frequency of lymphoma in SS patients requires caution in the use
of cyclophosphamide and has suggested its use as a "pulse therapy" rather than daily administration. Because of side effects, the use of mycophenolic mofetil is currently being explored as an alternative to cyclophosphamide in treatment of vasculitis (Gross, 1999).

One pilot study suggested that one tumor necrosis factor inhibitor (infliximab) might
be beneficial (Steinfeld et al., 2001), but subsequent multicenter trials failed to confirm
these results (Marriette, 2003). Similarly, double-blind studies have not shown significant
benefit with etanercept (Zandbelt et al., 2004; Sankar et al., 2004). As in other autoimmune
disorders, there is increasing interest in B-Cell depletion through the use of monoclonal
anti-CD20 antibody (rituximab) (Cohen, Polliack, and Nagler, 2003).

Outcome measures in SS are important and have been the subject of recent confer-
ences (Bowman, 2002), with assessment subdivided into:

a) exocrine (including sicca symptoms and signs) and-nonexocrine disease activity and systemic symptoms (objective evidence of extraglandular activity and damage (present for over 6 months);

b) health-related and generic quality of life (including fatigue); c) standard approaches to adverse events/toxicity; and d) health economic aspects. The use of biomarkers similar to SLE (Illei et al., 2004) including autoantibodies, chemokines and cytokines may supplement clinical measurements.

Summary

Cutaneous manifestations of Sjogren's syndrome (SS) include:
- *Dry skin (xerosis)*
- *Vasospastic disorders ranging from Raynaud's to acrocyanosis*
- *Macular, papular and vesicular rashes*
- *Infections such as varicella zoster*
- *Palpable and non-palpable purpura due vasculitis, and*
- *Embolic lesions and thrombotic lesions*
- *Acute or chronic thrombosis with lymphedema*
- *Other associated skin conditions including urticaria or allergic skin eruptions*

Complaints of dry skin occur in about 50% of SS patients. It is unclear whether or not the xerosis is due to infiltrate of the eccrine or sebaceous glands, or dysfunctional response of the residual glands. In many biopsies from SS patients, dryness of the skin has been associated with lymphocytic infiltrates in the eccrine glands. Similar to SLE patients, antibody and complement fixation is often detected clinically "normal" skin.

However, the extent of dryness of the skin and the clinical appearance termed "xerosis" is often more severe than that expected for the degree of lymphocytic infiltration (and glandular destruction).

A common finding on deeper skin biopsy is "non-specific perivascular lymphocytic infiltrates." Immuno-histologic studies have also indicated an increase in peri-vascular dendritic cells of both the mesenchymal and Plasmacytoid types. These histologic findings on SS skin biopsy are so common that the pathologist may often only mentions them "in passing," while they emphasize that no leukocytoclastic vasculitic changes were present. But these "perivascular" lymphocytic (and dendritic) cell infiltrates may be the crucial factor in xerosis of SS.

Treatment of SS is generally symptomatic, with most patients requiring treatment only for dryness. Adequate explanation is essential; many subjects, for example, may not realize that their central heating or air conditioning creates a drying environment or that a windy day is likely to make their eyes dryer. Simple measures such as humidifiers, sips of water, chewing gums, and simple replacement tears will be adequate in the majority of subjects. The rest should be told of the wide range of artificial fluids available and encouraged to try several different formulations.

Treatment of other manifestations of SS has been influenced by our treatment of other connective tissue diseases. The most serious (and fortunately rare) complications such as vasculitis and neurologic disease probably require immunosuppression with drugs such as cyclophosphamide, as in systemic lupus erythematosus.

Because many lupus symptoms mimic other illnesses, are sometimes vague and may come and go, lupus can be difficult to diagnose. Diagnosis is usually made by a careful review of a person's entire medical history coupled with an analysis of the results obtained in routine laboratory tests and some specialized tests related to immune status. Currently, there is no single laboratory test that can determine whether a person has lupus or not. To assist the physician in the diagnosis of lupus, the American Rheumatism Association issued a list of 11 symptoms or signs that help distinguish lupus from other diseases. A person should have four or more of these symptoms to suspect lupus. The symptoms do not all have to occur at the same time

8

References

Alexander, E.L., T.T. Provost (1983) Cutaneous manifestations of primary Sjögren's syndrome: a reflection of vasculitis and association with anti-Ro (SSA) antibodies. *J. Invest. Dermatol.* 80:386–91

Alexander, E.L., K. Malinow, J.E. Lejewski, M.S. Jerdan, T.T. Provost, and G.E. Alexander. (1986) Primary Sjögren's syndrome with central nervous system disease mimicking multiple sclerosis. *Annals of Internal Medicine* 104:323–30

Alexander, E., T.T. Provost (1987) Sjögren's syndrome. Association of cutaneous vasculitis with central nervous system disease. *Arch. Dermatol.* 123:801–10

Allison, P. J., D. Locker, J. S. Feine (1999) The relationship between dental status and health-related quality of life in upper aerodigestive tract cancer patients. *Oral Oncol* 35 (2):138–43

Andonopoulos, A. P., J. Christodoulou, C. Ballas, A. Bounas, D. Alexopoulos (1998) Autonomic cardiovascular neuropathy in Sjogren's syndrome. A controlled study. *J Rheumatol* 25 (12):2385–8

Aragona, P., A. Stilo, F. Ferreri, M. Mobrici (2005) Effects of the topical treatment with NSAIDs on corneal sensitivity and ocular surface of Sjogren's syndrome patients. *Eye* 19 (5):535–9

Arbuckle, M. R., M. T. McClain, M. V. Rubertone, R. H. Scofield, G. J. Dennis, J. A. James, J. B. Harley (2003) Development of autoantibodies before the clinical onset of systemic lupus erythematosus. *N Engl J Med* 349 (16):1526–33

Asherson, R.A., H.M. Fei, H.L. Staub, M.A. Khamashta, G.R.V. Hughes, R.I. Fox (1992) Antiphospholipid antibodies and HLA associations in primary Sjögren's syndrome. *Ann Rheum Dis* 51:495–8

Banting, D. W., A. Papas, D. C. Clark, H. M. Proskin, M. Schultz, R. Perry (2000) The effectiveness of 10% chlorhexidine varnish treatment on dental caries incidence in adults with dry mouth. *Gerodontology* 17 (2):67–76

Barendregt, P. J., M. J. van Den Bent, V. J. van Raaij-Van Den Aarssen, A. H. van Den Meiracker, C. J. Vecht, G. L. van Der Heijde, H. M. Markusse (2001) Involvement of the peripheral nervous system in primary Sjogren's syndrome. *Ann Rheum Dis* 60 (9):876–81

Battista, G., M. Zompatori, V. Poletti, R. Canini (2003) Thoracic manifestations of the less common collagen diseases. A pictorial essay. *Radiol Med (Torino)* 106 (5–6):445–51; quiz 52–3

Belafsky, P. C., G. N. Postma (2003) The laryngeal and esophageal manifestations of Sjogren's syndrome. *Curr Rheumatol Rep* 5 (4):297–303

Belin, C., C. Moroni, N. Caillat-Vigneron, M. Debray, M. Baudin, J. L. Dumas, J. L. Moretti, P. Delaporte, L. Guillevin (1999) Central nervous system involvement in Sjogren's syndrome: evidence from neuropsychological testing and HMPAO-SPECT [In Process Citation]. *Ann Med Interne (Paris)* 150 (8):598–604

Ben-Chetrit, E., R.I. Fox, E.M. Tan (1990) Dissociation of immune responses to the SS-A (Ro) 52-kd and 60-kd polypeptides in systemic lupus erythematosus and Sjögren's syndrome. *Arthritis & Rheum.* 33:349–55

Berdoulay, A., R. V. English, B. Nadelstein (2005) Effect of topical 0.02% tacrolimus aqueous suspension on tear production in dogs with keratoconjunctivitis sicca. *Vet Ophthalmol* 8 (4):225–32

Bergdahl, J., M. Bergdahl (2001) Environmental illness: evaluation of salivary flow, symptoms, diseases, medications, and psychological factors. *Acta Odontol Scand* 59 (2):104–10

Bernacchi, E., L. Amato, A. Parodi, F. Cottoni, P. Rubegni, O. De Pita, M. Papini, A. Rebora, S. Bombardieri, P. Fabbri (2004) Sjogren's syndrome: a retrospective review of the cutaneous features of 93 patients by the Italian Group of Immunodermatology. *Clin Exp Rheumatol* 22 (1):55–62

Bernstein, H.N (1991) Ocular safety of hydroxychloroquine. *Annals Ophthalmol* 23:292–6

Beroukas, D., R. Goodfellow, J. Hiscock, R. Jonsson, T. P. Gordon, S. A. Waterman (2002) Up-regulation of M3-muscarinic receptors in labial salivary gland acini in primary Sjogren's syndrome. *Lab Invest* 82 (2):203–10

Beroukas, D., J. Hiscock, R. Jonsson, S. A. Waterman, T. P. Gordon (2001) Subcellular distribution of aquaporin 5 in salivary glands in primary Sjogren's syndrome. *Lancet* 358 (9296):1875–6

Bloch, K.J., W.W. Buchanan, M.J. Wohl, J.J. Bunim (1956) Sjögren's syndrome: A clinical, pathological and serological study of 62 cases. *Medicine (Baltimore)* 44:187–231

Bolstad, A. I., H. G. Eiken, B. Rosenlund, M. E. Alarcon-Riquelme, R. Jonsson (2003) Increased salivary gland tissue expression of Fas, Fas ligand, cytotoxic T lymphocyte-associated antigen 4, and programmed cell death 1 in primary Sjogren's syndrome. *Arthritis Rheum* 48 (1):174–85

Bonafede, R. P., D. C. Downey, R. M. Bennett (1995) An association of fibromyalgia with primary Sjogren's syndrome: a prospective study of 72 patients. *J Rheumatol* 22 (1):133–6

Bone, R C, R I Fox, F V Howell, R Fantozzi (1985) Sjögren's syndrome: New immunologic assessments for a persistent clinical problem. *Laryngoscope* 95:295–9

Borda, E., C. P. Leiros, S. Bacman, A. Berra, L. Sterin-Borda (1999) Sjogren autoantibodies modify neonatal cardiac function via M1 muscarinic acetylcholine receptor activation. *Int J Cardiol* 70 (1):23–32

Bowman, S. J (2002) Collaborative research into outcome measures in Sjogren's syndrome. Update on disease assessment. *Scand J Rheumatol Suppl* (116):23–7

Bowman, S. J., G. H. Ibrahim, G. Holmes, J. Hamburger, J. R. Ainsworth (2004) Estimating the prevalence among Caucasian women of primary Sjogren's syndrome in two general practices in Birmingham, UK. *Scandinavian J Rheumatol* 33 (1):39–43

Castillo, J. L. and P. Milgrom (2004) Fluoride release from varnishes in two in vitro protocols. *J Am Dent Assoc* 135 (12):1696–9

Castillo, J. L., P. Milgrom, E. Kharasch, K. Izutsu, M. Fey (2001) Evaluation of fluoride release from commercially available fluoride varnishes. *J Am Dent Assoc* 132 (10):1389–92; 459–60

Chan, E K L, K F Sullivan, R I Fox, E M Tan (1989) Sjögren's syndrome nuclear antigen B (La): cDNA cloning, structural domains, and autoepitopes. *J Autoimmun* 2:321–7

Chatterjee, S (2004) Severe interstitial pneumonitis associated with infliximab therapy. *Scand J Rheumatol* 33 (4):276–7

Christensen, L. B., P. E. Petersen, J. J. Thorn, M. Schiodt (2001) Dental caries and dental health behavior of patients with primary Sjogren syndrome. *Acta Odontol Scand* 59 (3):116–20

Cimaz, R., A. Casadei, C. Rose, J. Bartunkova, A. Sediva, F. Falcini, P. Picco, M. Taglietti, F. Zulian, R. Ten Cate, F. R. Sztajnbok, P. V. Voulgari, A. A. Drosos (2003) Primary Sjogren syndrome in the paediatric age: a multicentre survey. *Eur J Pediatr* 162 (10):661–5

Cohen, Y., A. Polliack, and A. Nagler (2003) Treatment of Refractory Autoimmune Diseases with Ablative Immunotherapy Using Monoclonal Antibodies and/or High Dose Chemotherapy with Hematopoietic Stem Cell Support. *Curr Pharm Des* 9 (3):279–88

Collin, P., A. L. Karvonen, M. Korpela, P. Laippala, and H. Helin (1997) Gastritis classified in accordance with the Sydney system in patients with primary Sjogren's syndrome. *Scand J Gastroenterol* 32 (2):108–11

Collin, P., T. Reunala, M. Rasmussen, S. Kyronpalo, E. Pehkonen, P. Laippala, and M. Maki (1997) High incidence and prevalence of adult coeliac disease. Augmented diagnostic approach. *Scand J Gastroenterol* 32 (11):1129–33

Constantopoulos, S. H., E. V. Tsianos, H. M. Moutsopoulos (1992) Pulmonary and gastrointestinal manifestations of Sjogren's syndrome. *Rheum Dis Clin North Am* 18 (3):617–35

D'Arbonneau, F., S. Ansart, R. Le Berre, M. Dueymes, P. Youinou, and Y. L. Pennec (2003) Thyroid dysfunction in primary Sjogren's syndrome: a long-term followup study. *Arthritis Rheum* 49 (6):804–9

Dabadghao, S., A. Aggarwal, P. Arora, R. Pandey, R. Misra (1995) Glomerulonephritis leading to end stage renal disease in a patient with primary Sjogren syndrome. *Clin Exp Rheumatol* 13 (4):509–11

Dalavanga, Y.A., B. Detrick, J.J. Hooks, A.A. Drosos, H.M. Moutsopoulos (1990) Effect of cyclosporin A (CyA) on the immunopathological lesion of the minor salivary glands from patients with Sjögren's syndrome. *Annals of the Rheu. Diseases* 46:89–92

Daniels, T.E.(1984) Labial salivary gland biopsy in Sjögren's syndrome. *Arthritis Rheum.* 27:147–56

Daniels, T, Fox, PC (1992) Salivary and Oral Components of Sjogren's Syndrome. *Rheum Clinics NA* 18:571–83

Daniels, T. E., P. C. Fox (1992) Salivary and oral components of Sjogren's syndrome. *Rheum Dis Clin North Am* 18 (3):571–89

Daniels, T. E (2000) Evaluation, differential diagnosis, and treatment of xerostomia. *J Rheumatol Suppl* 61:6–10

Daniels, T. E., A. J. Wu (2000) Xerostomia – clinical evaluation and treatment in general practice. *J Calif Dent Assoc* 28 (12):933–41

de Seze, J., D. Devos, G. Castelnovo, P. Labauge, S. Dubucquoi, T. Stojkovic, D. Ferriby, P. Vermersch (2001) The prevalence of Sjogren syndrome in patients with primary progressive multiple sclerosis. *Neurology* 57 (8):1359–63

Deheinzelin, D., V. L. Capelozzi, R. A. Kairalla, J. V. Barbas Filho, P. H. Saldiva, C. R. de Carvalho (1996) Interstitial lung disease in primary Sjogren's syndrome. Clinical- pathological evaluation and response to treatment [see comments]. *Am J Respir Crit Care Med* 154 (3 Pt 1):794–9

Delalande, S., J. de Seze, A. L. Fauchais, E. Hachulla, T. Stojkovic, D. Ferriby, S. Dubucquoi, J. P. Pruvo, P. Vermersch, P. Y. Hatron (2004) Neurologic manifestations in primary Sjogren syndrome: a study of 82 patients. *Medicine (Baltimore)* 83 (5):280–91

Fei, H.M., H.-I. Kang, S. Scharf, H. Erlich, C. Peebles, R.I. Fox (1991) Specific HLA-DQA and HLA-DRB1 alleles confer susceptibility to Sjögren's syndrome and autoantibody SS-B production. *J. Clin. Lab. Analysis* 5:382–91

Feist, E., U. Kuckelkorn, T. Dorner, H. Donitz, S. Scheffler, F. Hiepe, P. M. Kloetzel, G. R. Burmester (1999) Autoantibodies in primary Sjogren's syndrome are directed against proteasomal subunits of the alpha and beta type. *Arthritis Rheum* 42 (4):697–702

Fisher, A. 1999. Muscarinic Receptor Agonists in Alzheimer's Disease. *CNS Drugs* 12:197–214

Fisher, A., E. Heldman, D. Gurwitz, R. Haring, Y. Karton, H. Meshulam, Z. Pittel, D. Marciano, R. Brandeis, E. Sadot, Y. Barg, R. Pinkas-Kramarski, Z. Vogel, I. Ginzburg, T. A. Treves, R. Verchovsky, S. Klimowsky, A. D. Korczyn (1996) M1 agonists for the treatment of Alzheimer's disease. Novel properties and clinical update. *Ann N Y Acad Sci* 777 (2):189–96

Foster, E. N., K. K. Nguyen, R. A. Sheikh, T. P. Prindiville (2005) Crohn's disease associated with Sweet's syndrome and Sjogren's syndrome treated with Infliximab. *Clin Dev Immunol* 12 (2):145–9

Fox, R I, D A Carson, P Chen, S Fong (1986) Characterization of a cross reactive idiotype in Sjögren's syndrome. *Scandinavian journal of rheumatology* 561:83–8

Fox, R I, P P Chen, D A Carson, S Fong (1986) Expression of a cross reactive idiotype on rheumatoid factor in patients with Sjögren's syndrome. *J Immunol* 136:477–83

Fox, R I, C Robinson, J Curd, P Michelson, R Bone, F V Howell (1986) First international symposium on Sjögren's syndrome: Suggested criteria for classification. *Scandinavian journal of rheumatology* 562:28–30

Fox, R. I., F. V. Howell (1986) Oral problems in patients with Sjögren's syndrome. *Scandinavian journal of rheumatology* S61:194–200

Fox, R I, E Chan, L Benton, S Fong, M Friedlaender, F V Howell (1988) Treatment of primary Sjögren's syndrome with hydroxychloroquine. *Amer J Med* 85:62–7

Fox, R. I., R. Dixon, V. Guarrasi, S. Krubel (1996) Treatment of primary Sjögren's syndrome with hydroxychloroquine: a retrospective, open-label study. *Lupus* 5 Suppl 1:S31–6

Fox, R (1997) Sjogren's syndrome: Progress and controversies. *Med Clin NA* 17:441–34

Fox, R. I., J. Tornwall, P. Michelson (1999) Current issues in the diagnosis and treatment of Sjögren's syndrome. *Curr Opin Rheumatol* 11 (5):364–71

Fox, R. I (2000) Sjogren's syndrome: current therapies remain inadequate for a common disease. *Expert Opin Investig Drugs* 9 (9):2007–16

Fox, R. I., Y. Konttinen, A. Fisher (2001) Use of muscarinic agonists in the treatment of Sjogren's syndrome. *Clin Immunol* 101 (3):249–63

Fox, R. I., M. Stern (2002) Sjogren's syndrome: mechanisms of pathogenesis involve interaction of immune and neurosecretory systems. *Scand J Rheumatol Suppl* (116):3–13

Franceschini, F., P. Calzavara-Pinton, M. Quinzanini, I. Cavazzana, L. Bettoni, C. Zane, F. Facchetti, P. Airo, D. P. McCauliffe, R. Cattaneo (1999) Chilblain lupus erythematosus is associated with antibodies to SSA/Ro. *Lupus* 8 (3):215

Fulop, M., M. Mackay (2004) Renal tubular acidosis, Sjogren syndrome, and bone disease. *Arch Intern Med* 164 (8):905–9

Gaither, K.K., O.W. Fox, H. Yamagata, M.J. Mamula, M. Reichlin, J.B. Harley (1987) Implications of anti-Ro/Sjögren's syndrome A antigen autoantibody in normal sera for autoimmunity. *J. Clin. Invest.* 79:841–6

Gamron, S., G. Barberis, C. M. Onetti, I. Strusberg, E. Hliba, G. Martellotto, H. G. Jara, A. M. Sesin (2000) Mesangial nephropathy in Sjögren's syndrome. *Scandinavian journal of rheumatology* 29 (1):65–7

Grant, I. A., G. G. Hunder, H. A. Homburger, P. J. Dyck (1997) Peripheral neuropathy associated with sicca complex. *Neurology* 48 (4):855–62

Gross, W. L (1999) New concepts in treatment protocols for severe systemic vasculitis. *Curr Opin Rheumatol* 11 (1):41–6

Gyongyosi, M., G. Pokorny, Z. Jambrik, L. Kovacs, A. Kovacs, E. Makula, M. Csanady (1996) Cardiac manifestations in primary Sjogren's syndrome. *Ann Rheum Dis* 55 (7):450–4

Gyulai, R., M. Kiss, M. Mehravaran, L. Kovacs, G. Pokorny, S. Husz, A. Dobozy (2002) Atypical autoimmune blistering dermatosis associated with Sjögren's syndrome. *Acta Derm Venereol* 82 (6):462–4

Haimowitz, J. E., D. P. McCauliffe, J. Seykora, V. P. Werth (2000) Annular erythema of Sjögren's syndrome in a white woman. *J Am Acad Dermatol* 42 (6):1069–72

Hamano, T (2005) Lacrimal duct occlusion for the treatment of dry eye. *Semin Ophthalmol* 20 (2):71–4

Hamilton, R.G., J.B. Harley, W. B. Bias, al et (1988) Two Ro (SS-A) autoantibody responses in systemic lupus erythematous. *Arthritis Rheum.* 31:446–505

Harley, J.B., E.L. Alexander, W.B. Bias, O.F. Fox, T.T. Provost, M. Richlin, H. Yanagata, F.C. Arnett (1986) Anti-Ro (SS-A) and Anti-La (SS-B) in patients with Sjögren's syndrome. *Arthritis Rheum* 29:196–206

Hay, K. D, R. P. Morton (2003) The efficacy of casein phosphoprotein-calcium phosphate complex (DC-CP) [Dentacal] as a mouth moistener in patients with severe xerostomia. *N Z Dent J* 99 (2):46–8

Hay, K. D., W. M. Thomson (2002) A clinical trial of the anticaries efficacy of casein derivatives complexed with calcium phosphate in patients with salivary gland dysfunction. *Oral Surg Oral Med Oral Pathol Oral Radiol Endod* 93 (3):271–5

Heinlen, L. D., M. T. McClain, X. Kim, D. R. Quintero, J. A. James, J. B. Harley, R. H. Scofield (2003) Anti-Ro and anti-nRNP response in unaffected family members of SLE patients. *Lupus* 12 (4):335–7

Illei, G. G., E. Tackey, L. Lapteva, P. E. Lipsky (2004) Biomarkers in systemic lupus erythematosus: II. Markers of disease activity. *Arthritis Rheum* 50 (7):2048–65

Invernizzi, P., P. M. Battezzati, A. Crosignani, P. Zermiani, M. Bignotto, N. Del Papa, M. Zuin, M. Podda (1998) Antibody to carbonic anhydrase II is present in primary biliary cirrhosis (PBC) irrespective of antimitochondrial antibody status. *Clin Exp Immunol* 114 (3):448–54

Isidor, F., K. Brondum, H. J. Hansen, J. Jensen, S. Sindet-Pedersen (1999) Outcome of treatment with implant-retained dental prostheses in patients with Sjogren syndrome. *Int J Oral Maxillofac Implants* 14 (5):736–43

Ito, Y., N. Kanda, H. Mitsui, T. Watanabe, S. Kobayashi, S. Murayama, K. Tamaki (1999) Cutaneous manifestations of Sjogren's syndrome associated with myasthenia gravis [letter]. *Br J Dermatol* 141 (2):362–3

Johnson, E. O., P. G. Vlachoyiannopoulos, F. N. Skopouli, A. G. Tzioufas, H. M. Moutsopoulos (1998) Hypofunction of the stress axis in Sjogren's syndrome. *J Rheumatol* 25 (8):1508–14

Jonsson, R., T. P. Gordon, Y. T. Konttinen (2003) Recent advances in understanding molecular mechanisms in the pathogenesis and antibody profile of Sjogren's syndrome. *Curr Rheumatol Rep* 5 (4):311–6

Josephs, S.F., A. Buchbinder, H.Z. Streicher, D.V. Ablashi, S.Z. Salahuddin, H.G. Guo, R.F. Krueger, R.I. Fox, R.C. Gallo (1988) Detection of human B-lymphotropic virus (human herpesvirus 6) sequences in B-cell lymphoma tissues of three patients. *Leukemia* 2:132–5

Jubert, C., A. Cosnes, T. Clerici, P. Gaulard, P. Andre, J. Revuz, M. Bagot (1993) Sjogren's syndrome and cutaneous B cell lymphoma revealed by anetoderma. *Arthritis Rheum* 36 (1):133–4

Kamel, O. W., M. van de Rijn, L. M. Weiss, G. J. Del Zoppo, P. K. Hench, B. A. Robbins, P. G. Montgomery, R. A. Warnke, R. F. Dorfman (1993) Brief report: reversible lymphomas associated with Epstein-Barr virus occurring during methotrexate therapy for rheumatoid arthritis and dermatomyositis. *N Engl J Med* 328 (18):1317–21

Kassan, S.S., T.L. Thomas, H.M. Moutsopoulos, R. Hoover, R.P. Kimberly, D.R. Budman, J. Costa, J.L. Decker, T.M. Chused (1978) Increased risk of lymphoma in sicca syndrome. *Ann. Intern. Med.* 89:888–92

Katayama, I., T. Yamamoto, K. Otoyama, T. Matsunaga, K. Nishioka (1994) Clinical and immunological analysis of annular erythema associated with Sjogren syndrome. *Dermatology* 189 Suppl 1:14–7

Katayama, Y., K. Kohriyama (2001) Telomerase activity in peripheral blood mononuclear cells of systemic connective tissue diseases. *J Rheumatol* 28 (2):288–91

Katelaris, C. H. (2005) Pilocarpine for Dry Mouth and Dry Eye in Sjogren's Syndrome. *Curr Allergy Asthma Rep* 5 (4):321

Kaufman, K. M., M. Y. Kirby, M. T. McClain, J. B. Harley, J. A. James (2001) Lupus autoantibodies recognize the product of an alternative open reading frame of SmB/B'. *Biochem Biophys Res Commun* 285 (5):1206–12

Kim, B. M., S. S. Osmanovic, D. P. Edward (2005) Pyogenic granulomas after silicone punctal plugs: a clinical and histopathologic study. *Am J Ophthalmol* 139 (4):678–84

Kim, E. A., K. S. Lee, T. Johkoh, T. S. Kim, G. Y. Suh, O. J. Kwon, J. Han (2002) Interstitial lung diseases associated with collagen vascular diseases: radiologic and histopathologic findings. *Radiographics* 22 Spec No:S151–65

Konishi, M., Y. Ohosone, M. Matsumura, Y. Oyamada, K. Yamaguchi, Y. Kawahara, T. Mimori, Y. Ikeda (1997) Mixed-cryoglobulinemia associated with cutaneous vasculitis and pulmonary symptoms. *Intern Med* 36 (1):62–7

Konttinen, Y. T., L. Kasna-Ronkainen (2002) Sjogren's syndrome: viewpoint on pathogenesis. One of the reasons I was never asked to write a textbook chapter on it. *Scand J Rheumatol Suppl* (116):15–22

Konttinen, Y.T., M. Hukkanen, P. Kemppinen, M. Segerberg, al. et. (1992) Peptide-containing nerves in labial salivary glands in Sjogren's syndrome. *Arthritis Rheum* 35:815–20

Kruize, A., R. Hene, C. Kallenberg, O. van Bijsterveld, A. van der Heide, L. Kater, J. Bijlsma (1993) Hydroxychloroquine treatment for primary Sjögren's syndrome: a two year double blind cross-over trial. *Ann Rheum Dis* 52:360–4

Kyle, R., G. Gleich, E. Baynd, and et a. (1971) Benign hyperglobuliemic purpura of Waldenstrom. *Medicine (Baltimore)* 50:113–23

Lass, P., J. Krajka-Lauer, M. Homziuk, B. Iwaszkiewicz-Bilikiewicz, M. Koseda, M. Hebanowski, P. Lyczak (2000) Cerebral blood flow in Sjogren's syndrome using 99Tcm-HMPAO brain SPET. *Nucl Med Commun* 21 (1):31–5

Leppilahti, M., T. L. Tammela, H. Huhtala, P. Kiilholma, K. Leppilahti, A. Auvinen (2003) Interstitial cystitis-like urinary symptoms among patients with Sjogren's syndrome: a population-based study in Finland. *Am J Med* 115 (1):62–5

Li, J. M., A. C. Horsfall, R. N. Maini (1995) Anti-La (SS-B) but not anti-Ro52 (SS-A) antibodies cross-react with laminin – a role in the pathogenesis of congenital heart block? *Clin Exp Immunol* 99 (3):316–24

Lightfoot, R. (1997) Cost Effective use of Laboratory Tests in Rheumatology. *Bul Rheum Dis* 46:1–3

Lindvall, B., A. Bengtsson, J. Ernerudh, P. Eriksson (2002) Subclinical myositis is common in primary Sjogren's syndrome and is not related to muscle pain. *J Rheumatol* 29 (4):717–25

Lwin, C. T., M. Bishay, R. G. Platts, D. A. Booth, S. J. Bowman (2003) The assessment of fatigue in primary Sjogren's syndrome. *Scandinavian journal of rheumatology* 32 (1):33–7

Manoussakis, M. N., C. Georgopoulou, E. Zintzaras, M. Spyropoulou, A. Stavropoulou, F. N. Skopouli, H. M. Moutsopoulos (2004) Sjogren's syndrome associated with systemic lupus erythematosus: clinical and laboratory profiles and comparison with primary Sjogren's syndrome. *Arthritis Rheum* 50 (3):882–91

Marriette, X. (2003) Lack of benefit of Infliximab in Sjogren's Syndrome. *Arth Rhem* abstract S19

McClain, M. T., L. D. Heinlen, G. J. Dennis, J. Roebuck, J. B. Harley, J. A. James (2005) Early events in lupus humoral autoimmunity suggest initiation through molecular mimicry. *Nat Med* 11 (1):85–9

Merkel, P. A., Y. Chang, S. S. Pierangeli, K. Convery, E. N. Harris, R. P. Polisson (1996) The prevalence and clinical associations of anticardiolipin antibodies in a large inception cohort of patients with connective tissue diseases. *Am J Med* 101 (6):576–83

Merkel, P. A., R. P. Polisson, Y. Chang, S. J. Skates, J. L. Niles (1997) Prevalence of antineutrophil cytoplasmic antibodies in a large inception cohort of patients with connective tissue disease. *Ann Intern Med* 126 (11):866–73

Mikulicz, J.H. (1892) Uber eine eigenartige symmetrische Erkrankung der Tranen- und Mundspeicheldrusen. In *Beitr. Chir. Fortschr.*, edited by G. T. Billroth. Stuttgart

Millard, L. G., N. R. Rowell (1978) Chilblain lupus erythematosus (Hutchinson) A CLINICAL AND LABORATORY STUDY OF 17 PATIENTS. *British Journal of Dermatology* 98 (5):497–506

Miyagawa, S., T. Iida, T. Fukumoto, T. Matsunaga, A. Yoshioka, T. Shirai (1995) Anti-Ro/SSA-associated annular erythema in childhood. *Br J Dermatol* 133 (5):779–82

Morgan, W., B Castleman (1953) A clinicopathologic study of Mikulicz'a disease. *Am J Pathol* 29:471–503

Mori, K., M. Iijima, H. Koike, N. Hattori, F. Tanaka, H. Watanabe, M. Katsuno, A. Fujita, I. Aiba, A. Ogata, T. Saito, K. Asakura, M. Yoshida, M. Hirayama, G. Sobue (2005) The wide spectrum of clinical manifestations in Sjogren's syndrome-associated neuropathy. *Brain* 128 (Pt 11):2518–34

Musadiq, M., S. Mukherji, S. Sandramouli (2005) Pyogenic granuloma following silicone punctal plugs: report of two cases. *Orbit* 24 (2):149–51

Nakamura, H., A. Kawakami, M. Tominaga, A. Hida, S. Yamasaki, K. Migita, Y. Kawabe, T. Nakamura, K. Eguchi (2000) Relationship between Sjogren's syndrome and human T-lymphotropic virus type I infection: follow-up study of 83 patients [In Process Citation]. *J Lab Clin Med* 135 (2):139–44

Navarro, M., R. Cervera, J. Font, J. C. Reverter, J. Monteagudo, G. Escolar, A. Lopez-Soto, A. Ordinas, M. Ingelmo (1997) Anti-endothelial cell antibodies in systemic autoimmune diseases: prevalence and clinical significance. *Lupus* 6 (6):521–6

Nishimagi, E., Y. Kawaguchi, C. Terai, H. Kajiyama, M. Hara, N. Kamatani (2001) Progressive interstitial renal fibrosis due to Chinese herbs in a patient with calcinosis Raynaud esophageal sclerodactyly telangiectasia (CREST) syndrome. *Intern Med* 40 (10):1059–63

Nishimori, I., K. Okazaki, Y. Yamamoto, M. Morita, S. Tamura, Y. Yamamoto (1993) Specific cellular immune responses to pancreatic antigen in chronic pancreatitis and Sjögren's syndrome. *J Clin Immunol* 13 (4):265–71

Nishimura, M., S. Miyajima, N. Okada (2000) Salivary gland MALT lymphoma associated with Helicobacter pylori infection in a patient with Sjogren's Syndrome [In Process Citation]. *J Dermatol* 27 (7):450–2

O'Donnell, B., A. K. Black (1995) Urticarial vasculitis. *Int Angiol* 14 (2):166–74

Ogawa, N., L. Ping, L. Zhenjun, Y. Takada, S. Sugai (2002) Involvement of the interferon-gamma-induced T cell-attracting chemokines, interferon-gamma-inducible 10-kd protein (CXCL10) and monokine induced by interferon-gamma (CXCL9), in the salivary gland lesions of patients with Sjogren's syndrome. *Arthritis Rheum* 46 (10):2730–41

Pablos, J. L., V. Cogolludo, F. Pinedo, P. E. Carreira (1993) Subcutaneous nodular amyloidosis in Sjögren's syndrome. *Scandinavian journal of rheumatology* 22:250–1

Papas, A. S., A. Joshi, S. L. MacDonald, L. Maravelis-Splagounias, P. Pretara-Spanedda, F. A. Curro (1993) Caries prevalence in xerostomic individuals. *J Can Dent Assoc* 59 (2):171–4, 7–9

Papas, A. S., A. Joshi, A. J. Belanger, R. L. Kent, Jr., C. A. Palmer, P. F. DePaola (1995) Dietary models for root caries. *Am J Clin Nutr* 61 (2):417S–22S

Papas, A. S., A. Joshi, C. A. Palmer, J. L. Giunta, J. T. Dwyer (1995) Relationship of diet to root caries. *Am J Clin Nutr* 61 (2):423S–9S

Papas, A. S., M. M. Fernandez, R. A. Castano, S. C. Gallagher, M. Trivedi, R. C. Shrotriya (1998) Oral pilocarpine for symptomatic relief of dry mouth and dry eyes in patients with Sjogrens syndrome. *Adv Exp Med Biol* 438:973–8

Pease, C. T., W. Shattles, N. K. Barrett, R. N. Maini (1993) The arthropathy of Sjogren's syndrome. *Br J Rheumatol* 32 (7):609–13

Pender, M. P. (1999) Recent progress in the diagnosis and treatment of multiple sclerosis. *J Clin Neurosci* 6 (5):367–72

Perez, B., A. Kraus, G. Lopez, M. Cifuentes, D. Alarcon-Segovia (1995) Autoimmune thyroid disease in primary Sjogren's syndrome. *Am J Med* 99 (5):480–4

Pers, J. O., F. d'Arbonneau, V. Devauchelle-Pensec, A. Saraux, Y. L. Pennec, P. Youinou (2005) Is periodontal disease mediated by salivary baff in sjogren's syndrome? *Arthritis Rheum* 52 (8):2411–4

Pers, J. O., C. Daridon, V. Devauchelle, S. Jousse, A. Saraux, C. Jamin, P. Youinou (2005) BAFF Overexpression Is Associated with Autoantibody Production in Autoimmune Diseases. *Ann N Y Acad Sci* 1050:34–9

Petrone, D., J. J. Condemi, R. Fife, O. Gluck, S. Cohen, P. Dalgin (2002) A double-blind, randomized, placebo-controlled study of cevimeline in Sjogren's syndrome patients with xerostomia and keratoconjunctivitis sicca. *Arthritis Rheum* 46 (3):748–54

Pflugfelder, S. C. (1996) Differential diagnosis of dry eye conditions. *Adv Dent Res* 10 (1):9–12

Pflugfelder, S. C. (2004) Antiinflammatory therapy for dry eye. *Am J Ophthalmol* 137 (2):337–42

Pillemer, S. R., E. L. Matteson, L. T. Jacobsson, P. B. Martens, L. J. Melton, 3rd, W. M. O'Fallon, P. C. Fox (2001) Incidence of physician-diagnosed primary Sjogren syndrome in residents of Olmsted County, Minnesota. *Mayo Clin Proc* 76 (6):593–9

Pirildar, T., C. Tikiz, S. Ozkaya, S. Tarhan, O. Utuk, H. Tikiz, U. K. Tezcan (2005) Endothelial dysfunction in patients with primary Sjogren's syndrome. *Rheumatology international* 25 (7):536–9

Press, J., Y. Uziel, R. M. Laxer, L. Luy, R. M. Hamilton, E. D. Silverman (1996) Long-term outcome of mothers of children with complete congenital heart block. *Am J Med* 100 (3):328–32

Price, E. J., S. P. Rigby, U. Clancy, P. J. Venables (1998) A double blind placebo controlled trial of azathioprine in the treatment of primary Sjogren's syndrome. *J Rheumatol* 25 (5):896–9

Provost, T. T., R. Watson (1992) Cutaneous manifestations of Sjogren's syndrome. *Rheum Dis Clin North Am* 18 (3):609–16

Provost, T. T., R. Watson, O. Brien E. Simmons (1997) Anti-Ro(SS-A) antibody positive Sjogren's/lupus erythematosus overlap syndrome. *Lupus* 6 (2):105–11

Provost, T. T., R. Watson, E. Simmons-O'Brien (1997) Anti-Ro(SS-A) antibody positive Sjogren's/lupus erythematosus overlap syndrome. *Lupus* 6 (2):105–11

Quismorio, F. P., Jr. (1996) Pulmonary involvement in primary Sjogren's syndrome. *Curr Opin Pulm Med* 2 (5):424–8

Rader, M.D., C. O'Brien, Y. Liu, J.B. Harley, M. Reichlin (1989) Heterogeneity of the Ro/SSA antigen. *J. Clin. Invest.* 83:1293–8

Raderer, M., C. Osterreicher, K. Machold, M. Formanek, W. Fiebiger, M. Penz, B. Dragosics, A. Chott (2001) Impaired response of gastric MALT-lymphoma to Helicobacter pylori eradication in patients with autoimmune disease. *Ann Oncol* 12 (7):937–9

Radfar, L., D. E. Kleiner, P. C. Fox, S. R. Pillemer (2002) Prevalence and clinical significance of lymphocytic foci in minor salivary glands of healthy volunteers. *Arthritis Rheum* 47 (5):520–4

Ramos-Casals, M., J. M. Anaya, M. Garcia-Carrasco, J. Rosas, A. Bove, G. Claver, L. A. Diaz, C. Herrero, J. Font (2004) Cutaneous vasculitis in primary Sjogren syndrome: classification and clinical significance of 52 patients. *Medicine (Baltimore)* 83 (2):96–106

Ramos-Casals, M., R. Cervera, J. Yague, M. Garcia-Carrasco, O. Trejo, S. Jimenez, R. M. Morla, J. Font, M. Ingelmo (1998) Cryoglobulinemia in primary Sjogren's syndrome: prevalence and clinical characteristics in a series of 115 patients. *Semin Arthritis Rheum* 28 (3):200–5

Robinson, C. P., H. Yamamoto, A. B. Peck, M. G. Humphreys-Beher (1996) Genetically programmed development of salivary gland abnormalities in the NOD (nonobese diabetic)-scid mouse in the absence of detectable lymphocytic infiltration: a potential trigger for sialoadenitis of NOD mice. *Clin Immunol Immunopathol* 79 (1):50–9

Robinson, C., S. Yamciuka, C. Alford, C. Cooper, E. Pichardo, N. Shah, M. Peck, M. Humphrey-Beher (1997) Elevated levels of cysteine protease activity in saliva and salivary glands of NOD mouse model for Sjogren's syndrome. *Proc Nat Acad Sci* 94:5767–71

Roguedas, A. M., L. Misery, B. Sassolas, G. Le Masson, Y. L. Pennec, P. Youinou (2004) Cutaneous manifestations of primary Sjogren's syndrome are underestimated. *Clin Exp Rheumatol* 22 (5):632–6

Rosler, D. H., M. D. Conway, J. M. Anaya, J. F. Molina, R. F. Carr, A. E. Gharavi, W. A. Wilson (1995) Ischemic optic neuropathy and high-level anticardiolipin antibodies in primary Sjogren's syndrome. *Lupus* 4 (2):155–7

Royer, B., D. Cazals-Hatem, J. Sibilia, F. Agbalika, J. M. Cayuela, T. Soussi, F. Maloisel, J. P. Clauvel, J. C. Brouet, X. Mariette (1997) Lymphomas in patients with Sjogren's syndrome are marginal zone B-cell neoplasms, arise in diverse extranodal and nodal sites, and are not associated with viruses. *Blood* 90 (2):766–75

Rustin, M. H. A., J. A. Newton, N. P. Smith, P. M. Dowd (1989) The treatment of chilblains with nifedipine: the results of a pilot study, a double-blind placebo-controlled randomized study and a long-term open trial. *British Journal of Dermatology* 120 (2):267–75

Ruzicka, T., J. Faes, T. Bergner, R. U. Peter, O. Braun-Falco (1991) Annular erythema associated with Sjogren's syndrome: a variant of systemic lupus erythematosus. *J Am Acad Dermatol* 25 (3):557–60

Sais, G., C. Admella, M. J. Fantova, J. C. Montero (1998) Lymphocytic autoimmune hidradenitis, cutaneous leucocytoclastic vasculitis and primary Sjogren's syndrome. *Br J Dermatol* 139 (6):1073–6

Salaffi, F., G. Argalia, M. Carotti, F. B. Giannini, C. Palombi (2000) Salivary gland ultrasonography in the evaluation of primary Sjogren's syndrome. Comparison with minor salivary gland biopsy. *J Rheumatol* 27 (5):1229–36

Sall, K, OD Stevenson, TK Mundorf, BL Reis (2000) Two multicenter, randomized studies of the efficacy and safety of cyclosporine ophthalmic emulsion in moderate to severe dry eye disease. CsA Phase 3 Study Group. *Ophthalmology* 107 (4):631

Sankar, V., M. T. Brennan, M. R. Kok, R. A. Leakan, J. A. Smith, J. Manny, B. J. Baum, S. R. Pillemer (2004) Etanercept in Sjogren's syndrome: a twelve-week randomized, double-blind, placebo-controlled pilot clinical trial. *Arthritis Rheum* 50 (7):2240–5

Santiago-Raber, M. L., R. Baccala, K. M. Haraldsson, D. Choubey, T. A. Stewart, D. H. Kono, A. N. Theofilopoulos (2003) Type-I interferon receptor deficiency reduces lupus-like disease in NZB mice. *J Exp Med* 197 (6):777–88

Sawalha, A. H., R. Potts, W. R. Schmid, R. H. Scofield, J. B. Harley (2003) The genetics of primary Sjogren's syndrome. *Curr Rheumatol Rep* 5 (4):324–32

Schiodt, M., L. B. Christensen, P. E. Petersen, J. J. Thorn (2001) Periodontal disease in primary Sjogren's syndrome. *Oral Dis* 7 (2):106–8

Scofield, R. H., B. T. Kurien, F. Zhang, P. Mehta, K. Kaufman, T. Gross, M. Bachmann, T. Gordon, J. B. Harley (1999) Protein-protein interaction of the Ro-ribonucleoprotein particle using multiple antigenic peptides [In Process Citation]. *Mol Immunol* 36 (15–16):1093–106

Sestak, A.L., J.B. Harley, S. Yoshida, M. Reichlin (1987) Lupus/Sjögren's autoantibody specificities in sera with paraproteins. *J. Clin. Invest.* 80:138–44

Sheikh, S. H., T. A. Shaw-Stiffel (1995) The gastrointestinal manifestations of Sjogren's syndrome. *Am J Gastroenterol* 90 (1):9–14

Shibata, S., Y. Ubara, N. Sawa, T. Tagami, J. Hosino, M. Yokota, H. Katori, F. Takemoto, S. Hara, K. Takaichi, A. Fujii, H. Murata, T. Nishi (2004) Severe interstitial cystitis associated with Sjogren's syndrome. *Intern Med* 43 (3):248–52

Siamopoulos, K. C., M. Elisaf, H. M. Moutsopoulos (1994) Hypokalaemic paralysis as the presenting manifestation of primary Sjogren's syndrome. *Nephrol Dial Transplant* 9 (8):1176–8

Simmons-O'Brien, E., S. Chen, R. Watson, C. Antoni, M. Petri, M. Hochberg, M. B. Stevens, T. T. Provost (1995) One hundred anti-Ro (SS-A) antibody positive patients: a 10-year follow-up. *Medicine (Baltimore)* 74 (3):109–30

Skopouli, F. N., P. Jagiello, N. Tsifetaki, H. M. Moutsopoulos (1996) Methotrexate in primary Sjogren's syndrome. *Clin Exp Rheumatol* 14 (5):555–8

Soto-Rojas, A. E., A. Kraus (2002) The oral side of sjogren syndrome. Diagnosis and treatment. A review. *Arch Med Res* 33 (2):95–106

Spezialetti, R., H. G. Bluestein, J. B. Peter, E. L. Alexander (1993) Neuropsychiatric disease in Sjogren's syndrome: anti-ribosomal P and anti-neuronal antibodies. *Am J Med* 95 (2):153–60

Steinfeld, S. D., P. Demols, I. Salmon, R. Kiss, T. Appelboom (2001) Infliximab in patients with primary Sjogren's syndrome: a pilot study. *Arthritis Rheum* 44 (10):2371–5

Stern, M. E., R. W. Beuerman, R. I. Fox, J. Gao, A. K. Mircheff, S. C. Pflugfelder (1998) A unified theory of the role of the ocular surface in dry eye. *Adv Exp Med Biol* 438:643–51

Strong, B., W. Farley, M. E. Stern, S. C. Pflugfelder (2005) Topical cyclosporine inhibits conjunctival epithelial apoptosis in experimental murine keratoconjunctivitis sicca. *Cornea* 24 (1):80–5

Suzuki, K., M. Matsumoto, M. Nakashima, K. Takada, T. Nakanishi, M. Okada, F. Ohsuzu (2005) Effect of cevimeline on salivary components in patients with Sjogren syndrome. *Pharmacology* 74 (2):100–5

Swords, R., D. Power, M. Fay, R. O'Donnell, P. T. Murphy (2004) Interstitial pneumonitis following rituximab therapy for immune thrombocytopenic purpura (ITP). *Am J Hematol* 77 (1):103–4

Takeda, K., T. Kaisho, S. Akira (2003) Toll-like receptors. *Annu Rev Immunol* 21:335–76

Tan, E. M., T. E. Feltkamp, J. S. Smolen, B. Butcher, R. Dawkins, M. J. Fritzler, T. Gordon, J. A. Hardin, J. R. Kalden, R. G. Lahita, R. N. Maini, J. S. McDougal, N. F. Rothfield, R. J. Smeenk, Y. Takasaki, A. Wiik, M. R. Wilson, J. A. Koziol (1997) Range of antinuclear antibodies in "healthy" individuals. *Arthritis Rheum* 40 (9):1601–11

Tapinos, N. I., M. Polihronis, A. G. Tzioufas, H. M. Moutsopoulos (1999) Sjogren's syndrome. Autoimmune epithelitis. *Adv Exp Med Biol* 455:127–34

Tatlipinar, S., E. K. Akpek (2005) Topical ciclosporin in the treatment of ocular surface disorders. *Br J Ophthalmol* 89 (10):1363–7

Tektonidou, M. G., M. Anapliotou, P. Vlachoyiannopoulos, H. M. Moutsopoulos (2004) Presence of systemic autoimmune disorders in patients with autoimmune thyroid diseases. *Ann Rheum Dis* 63 (9):1159–61

Tektonidou, M., E. Kaskani, F. N. Skopouli, H. M. Moutsopoulos (1999) Microvascular abnormalities in Sjogren's syndrome: nailfold capillaroscopy. *Rheumatology (Oxford)* 38 (9):826–30

Tensing, E. K., S. A. Solovieva, T. Tervahartiala, D. C. Nordstrom, M. Laine, S. Niissalo, Y. T. Konttinen (2001) Fatigue and health profile in sicca syndrome of Sjogren's and non-Sjogren's syndrome origin. *Clin Exp Rheumatol* 19 (3):313–6

Tishler, M., I. Alosachie, N. Barka, H. C. Lin, M. E. Gershwin, J. B. Peter, Y. Shoenfeld (1995) Primary Sjogren's syndrome and primary biliary cirrhosis: differences and similarities in the autoantibody profile. *Clin Exp Rheumatol* 13 (4):497–500

Tishler, M., Y. Barak, D. Paran, M. Yaron (1997) Sleep disturbances, fibromyalgia and primary Sjogren's syndrome. *Clin Exp Rheumatol* 15 (1):71–4

Tonami, H., K. Higashi, K. Matoba, H. Yokota, I. Yamamoto, S. Sugai (2001) A comparative study between MR sialography and salivary gland scintigraphy in the diagnosis of Sjogren syndrome. *J Comput Assist Tomogr* 25 (2):262–8

Urban, P. P., A. Keilmann, E. M. Teichmann, H. C. Hopf (2001) Sensory neuropathy of the trigeminal, glossopharyngeal, and vagal nerves in Sjogren's syndrome. *J Neurol Sci* 186 (1–2):59–63

Utset, T. O., M. Golden, G. Siberry, N. Kiri, R. M. Crum, M. Petri (1994) Depressive symptoms in patients with systemic lupus erythematosus: association with central nervous system lupus and Sjogren's syndrome. *J Rheumatol* 21 (11):2039–45

van Dam, A. P., E. M. Wekking, J. A. Callewaert, A. J. Schipperijn, H. A. Oomen, J. de Jong, A. J. Swaak, R. J. Smeenk, T. E. Feltkamp (1994) Psychiatric symptoms before systemic lupus erythematosus is diagnosed. *Rheumatology international* 14 (2):57–62

Vitali, C. (2003) Classification criteria for Sjogren's syndrome. *Ann Rheum Dis* 62 (1):94–5; author reply 5

Vitali, C., H. M. Moutsopoulos, S. Bombardieri (1994) The European Community Study Group on diagnostic criteria for Sjogren's syndrome. Sensitivity and specificity of tests for ocular and oral involvement in Sjogren's syndrome. *Ann Rheum Dis* 53 (10):637–47

Vivino, F. B., I. Gala, G. A. Hermann (2002) Change in final diagnosis on second evaluation of labial minor salivary gland biopsies. *J Rheumatol* 29 (5):938–44

Voulgarelis, M., U. G. Dafni, D. A. Isenberg, H. M. Moutsopoulos (1999) Malignant lymphoma in primary Sjogren's syndrome: a multicenter, retrospective, clinical study by the European Concerted Action on Sjogren's Syndrome. *Arthritis Rheum* 42 (8):1765–72

Wall, G. C., M. L. Magarity, J. W. Jundt (2002) Pharmacotherapy of xerostomia in primary Sjogren's syndrome. *Pharmacotherapy* 22 (5):621–9

Wallace, D. (1994) Antimalarial agents and lupus. *Rheum Dis Clinics NA* 20:243–63

Wallace, D. J. 2002. Management of lupus erythematosus: recent insights. *Curr Opin Rheumatol* 14 (3):212–9

Watanabe, T., T. Tsuchida, M. Furue, S. Yoshinoya (1996) Annular erythema, dermatomyositis, and Sjogren's syndrome. *Int J Dermatol* 35 (4):285–7

Watanabe, T., T. Tsuchida, Y. Ito, N. Kanda, Y. Ueda, K. Tamaki (1997) Annular erythema associated with lupus erythematosus/Sjogren's syndrome. *J Am Acad Dermatol* 36:214–8

Wu, A. J. (2003) The oral component of Sjogren's syndrome: pass the scalpel and check the water. *Curr Rheumatol Rep* 5 (4):304–10

Wu, A. J., P. C. Fox (1994) Sjogren's syndrome. *Semin Dermatol* 13 (2):138–43

Yamamoto, H., K. Ishibashi, Y. Nakagawa, N. Maeda, T. Zeng, C. P. Robinson, G. E. Oxford, N. Chegini, M. G. Humphreys-Beher (1997) Detection of alterations in the levels of neuropeptides and salivary gland responses in the non-obese diabetic mouse model for autoimmune sialoadenitis. *Scand J Immunol* 45 (1):55–61

Yamamoto, T., I. Katayama, K. Nishioka (1998) Analysis of T cell receptor Vbeta repertoires of annular erythema associated with Sjogren's syndrome. *Eur J Dermatol* 8 (4):248–51

Yoneyama, K., N. Tochigi, A. Oikawa, H. Shinkai, A. Utani (2005) Primary localized cutaneous nodular amyloidosis in a patient with Sjogren's syndrome: a review of the literature. *J Dermatol* 32 (2):120–3

Yousem, D. M., M. A. Kraut, A. A. Chalian (2000) Major salivary gland imaging. *Radiology* 216 (1):19–29

Zandbelt, M. M., P. de Wilde, P. van Damme, C. B. Hoyng, L. van de Putte, F. van den Hoogen (2004) Etanercept in the treatment of patients with primary Sjogren's syndrome: a pilot study. *J Rheumatol* 31 (1):96–101

Zukowski, T. H., R. A. Jorgensen, E. R. Dickson, K. D. Lindor (1998) Autoimmune conditions associated with primary biliary cirrhosis: response to ursodeoxycholic acid therapy. *Am J Gastroenterol* 93 (6):958–61

8

Psoriasis Vulgaris and Arthopathica

9

Arnd Jacobi and Jörg Christoph Prinz

Introduction

Psoriasis vulgaris is an HLA-associated inflammatory disorder, which affects ~ 2% of the Caucasian population. It presents with a characteristic type of skin lesions which appear as sharply demarcated reddish plaques of variant size covered with intensive silvery scaling. In a significant proportion of patients psoriasis also involves the joints, sometimes leading to severe arthritis.

Psoriasis has been documented already in ancient times. The earliest descriptions are attributed to Celsus (25 a.c. to 50 p.c.) (Dirckx, 1983) and to the 3rd Book of Moses in the Book of Leviticus, chapter 13, of the Old Testament (Glickman, 1986). Here, psoriasis is assumed behind the term "zaraath". In 1801 psoriasis was clearly distinguished from leprosy by Robert Willan (1757–1812) (Leach and Beckwith, 1999). Since then, pathophysiology and therapy of psoriasis have remained an intellectual challenge.

Epidemiology and genetics of psoriasis

The true incidence of psoriasis is difficult to determine. The prevalence varies in different parts of the world between 0.1% to 3%. In Western industrialized nations it is estimated to affect 1.5–2% of the population, with worldwide approximately 100 million affected individuals.

Psoriasis has a strong hereditary background. The concordance in monozygotic twins is 65 to 70% (Brandrup et al., 1982; Farber et al., 1974), compared to 15 to 20% in dizygotic twins. The risk of first-degree relatives to acquire psoriasis ranges from 8 to 23%. The inherited predisposition involves various gene loci. Many of them are related to inflammation and immunity. They include PSORS1 (psoriasis susceptibility locus) on chromosome 6p21.3, PSORS2 on 17q24-q25, PSORS3 on 4qter, PSORS4 on 1cen-q21, PSORS5 on 3q21, PSORS6 on 19p13, PSORS71p35-p34, PSORS8 on 16q12-q13, and PSORS9 on 4q31 (http://www.ncbi.nlm.nih.gov/Omim). Potential other psoriasis gene loci are 16q und 20p (Nair et al., 1997). Some of these gene loci are identical to gene loci of atopic childhood eczema (20p, PSORS2, PSORS4) (Cookson et al., 2001). A strong association has been observed with single nucleotide polymorphisms in the *IL12B* and *IL23R* genes. Interestingly, these genetic associations are shared between psoriasis and Crohn's disease, a chronic immune-mediated inflammatory bowel disease (Tsunemi et al., 2002, Cargill et al., 2007). Psoriasis susceptibility is furthermore influenced by polymorphisms in various cytokine alleles (IL-1, IL-6, IL-10, IL12, TNF-α) (Tsunemi et al., 2002; Reich et al., 2002; Asadullah et al., 2001; Arias et al., 1997). Copy number variations with multiplication of genes coding for proinflammatory anti-microbial peptides may enhance the risk for acquiring psoriasis further (Hollox et al., 2008). Recent observations point to a role of gene deletions related to epidermal barrier function (de Cid R et al., 2009). PSORS1 contributes approximately 30–50% to the genetic predisposition (Trembath et al., 1997). It reflects the association of psoriasis with HLA-Cw6 that was identified as the first correlate of the genetic predisposition (Russel et al., 1972). In northern Europe and the U.S.A. two thirds of the psoriasis patients are HLA-Cw6 positive (Elder et al., 2001). Experimental results suggest that the association of psoriasis with HLA-Cw6 might reflect a select capacity of this HLA-allele to present particular skin-selective proteins as autoantigens to T cells, which may subsequently become activated in an autoimmune response (Besgen et al., 2010). Approximately 10% of the HLA-Cw6 positive individuals acquire psoriasis. Because of this relative association it still remains uncertain whether HLA-Cw6 itself or a closely adjoining gene polymorphism represents the actual risk allele (Nair et al., 2000). HLA-Cw6 is inherited as a conserved set of genes (extended haplotype, EH57.1/I) that involves the HLA molecules Cw6-B57-DRB1*0701-DQA1*0201-DQB1*0303 and particular alleles of corneodesmosin, MICA (class I major histocompatibility complex chain-related gene A), and HCR (Schmitt Egenolf et al., 1996; Tazi Ahnini et al., 1999; Jenisch et al., 1999; Asumalahti et al., 2002; Gonzalez et al., 1999). Each of these alleles has single nucleotide polymorphisms (SNP) that are associated with psoriasis and make them potential candidates for risk alleles.

For PSORS2 on 17q24-q25 the situation is much better defined. It carries a particular psoriasis-associated SNP that is located between *SLC9A3R1* (EBP50/ERM-binding phosphoprotein 50 kDA or NHERF1) and *NAT9* (Helms et al., 2003). The SNP affects a binding site for the transcription factor, RUNX1, and, at least experimentally, ablates RUNX1 binding and RUNX1-regulated expression of *SLC9A3R1*. *SLC9A3R1* codes for a linker protein that binds members of the ezrin-radixin-moesin family via a PDZ domain (Reczek et al., 1997). It is involved in both, epithelial membrane function and the formation of the immunologic synapse, and it mediates inhibitory signals during T cell activation (Itoh et al., 2002). Since *SLC9A3R1* is expressed in the upper epidermal layers and in resting T cells ablation of RUNX1 binding may contribute to both epidermal dysregulation and exaggerated T-cell activation of psoriatic skin lesions. An altered RUNX-mediated gene expression has also been suggested for lupus erythematosus and rheumatoid arthritis, making RUNX-related immune dysregulation a potential mechanism of autoimmunity (Tokuhiro et al., 2003; Prokunina et al., 2002).

HLA-Cw6 and psoriasis-subtypes

The biologic role of the HLA-Cw6 in psoriasis is still unknown. Yet, HLA-Cw6 as the major risk allele defines several clinical aspects of psoriasis. Acute-exanthematic, socalled gutatte psoriasis shows a high prevalence for HLA-Cw6 (Mallon et al., 2000). Homzygosity for HLA-Cw6 confers a higher risk for psoriasis than heterozygosity (Gudjonsson et al., 2003). HLA-Cw6 is furthermore associated with an early onset of the disease and a positive family history for psoriasis (Queiro et al., 2003).

Two subtypes of non-pustular psoriasis have been defined by the age of disease onset, HLA-expression and family history (Christophers and Henseler, 1985). Type 1 represents approximately two thirds of the psoriasis patients. It is characterized by the presence of HLA-Cw6, a positive family history for psoriasis, and an early disease manifestation usually before the age of 40 years, with a maximum of onset at the age of 16 (females) or 22 (males) years. Type 2 psoriasis is characterized by a late onset with a maximum at the age of 60 (females) or 57 (males) years, and by an overrepresentation of HLA-Cw2. Other HLA-alleles found more frequently in non-pustular psoriasis are A2, A24, B13, B27, B37, Cw7, Cw8 and Cw11 (Henseler, 1998). Unlike type 2 psoriasis, type 1 psoriasis is selectively associated with streptococcal throat infection as major environmental trigger of psoriasis onset (Weisenseel et al., 2002).

Histopathology

The histopathologic picture of psoriasis depends on stage and localisation of the lesion. Early lesions display quite unspecific changes with dilatation of the papillary capillaries, oedema and a mononuclear infiltrate, from which fewer cells exocytose into the lower epidermis (Braun-Falco and Christophers, 1974). Only then, epidermal changes develop with parakeratosis (incomplete cornification) and disappearance of the granular layer. At this stage the phenomenon of the "squirting papillae" occurs, with release of neutrophilic granulocytes (Pinkus and Mehregan, 1966) from the dermal capillaries. They accumulate as Munro microabscesses within the parakeratotic layer or, intermingled with epidermal cells (Ragaz and Ackerman, 1979), as spongiform pustules of Kogoj beneath the parakeratotic stratum corneum (Gordon and Johnson, 1967). Increased numbers of mast cells are observed in the dermis.

The fully developed lesions are characterized by acanthosis (thickening of the epidermis), elongated rete ridges with often club-shaped dermal papillae and thinning of the suprapapillary layers of the epidermis (Fig. 1). The granular layer is absent. Parakeratosis may be accompanied by ortho-hyperkeratosis. Only the intra-epidermal pustules or microabscesses, however, represent fully pathognomonic features of psoriasis. They become predominant in pustular psoriasis, with spongiform macropustules in a degenerated epidermis (Shelley and Kirschbaum, 1961).

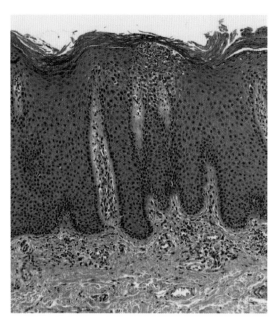

Fig. 1. Histopathology with acanthosis, parakeratosis, loss of granular cell layer

Gene expression analysis

Large scale gene expression analysis of affected and unaffected psoriatic skin as well as skin from healthy individuals demonstrated that more than 1300 genes are differentially expressed in psoriatic inflammation. These genes are particularly relevant for wound healing and epidermal regeneration, inflammation and immunity, epidermal proliferation and differentiation, the JAK-STAT-signalling cascade, neurogenesis, melanogenesis, and the pathogen defence. They reflect the different compartments involved in the pathogenic cascade (Bowcock et al., 2001; Zhou et al., 2003). Interestingly, gene expression revealed no difference between type 1 and type 2 psoriasis patients.

Environmental factors

Throat infections with group A ß-haemolytic streptococci are the most frequent trigger of psoriasis onset, but may also induce relapses. Reports on the incidence of streptococcal throat infection preceding first psoriasis onset range from 56 to 97% (Norrlind, 1954; Tervaert and Esseveld, 1970). Elevated serum antibody titres against streptococcal antigens (Streptolysin O, DNAse B) are found in ~ 50% of patients with chronic plaque psoriasis. Other triggering factors are drugs (mainly lithium, ß-adrenergic blocking agents, anti-malaria agents, IFN-α, Interleukin-2), withdrawal of steroids, alcohol, emotional stress and hypocalcaemia, to name the most frequent ones. These factors somehow seem to act on the genetic predisposition to turn the latent state into the full psoriatic phenotype.

Immune mechanisms in the pathogenesis of psoriasis

Several fully reversible features shape the clinical appearance of psoriasis. They include a strong increase in keratinocyte proliferation and epidermal turnover, accumulation of neutrophilic granulocytes, inflammatory changes with elongation of the papillary capillaries, and a mononuclear infiltrate with activated T cells.

Accordingly, the cause of psoriasis has been assumed in a disturbed growth regulation of keratinocytes, abnormal function and chemotaxis of neutrophilic granulocytes, or in defects in the cAMP-cascade or arachidonic acid metabolism, to name some of the former approaches. Intensive analysis of these compartments, however, did not reveal clues to explain the pathogenesis of psoriasis.

T cell activation in psoriasis

Recent progress in the understanding of psoriasis vulgaris has suggested that activation of the specific cellular immune system, particularly T cells, in the skin is an essential step in disease manifestation, and that it is responsible for all the different lesional psoriatic changes including the increased keratinocyte proliferation (Fig. 2) (Valdimarsson et al., 1986, Nickoloff and Nestle, 2004). This role was first suggested in 1976 by the ability of cyclosporine A to clear psoriasis (Mueller and Hermann, 1976), but in order to convince of the pivotal position of T cells in the realisation of a genetic predisposition which includes HLA-association and – less stringently – other gene loci (Henseler, 1997; Trembath et al., 1997; Tomfohrde et al., 1994), further observations were necessary. They were based mainly on the therapeutic efficacy of other immunosuppressive regimens such as FK506 (Michel et al., 1996), monoclonal CD3 and CD4 antibodies (Weinshenker et al., 1989; Prinz et al., 1991; Nicolas et al., 1991), or a T cell-selective toxin, $DAB_{389}IL$-2 (Gottlieb et al., 1995), but also of immunomodulatory cytokines such as IL-10 (Asadullah et al., 1998).

The T cells accused for mediating psoriasis constitute a dense inflammatory infiltrate in the papillary dermis and, to a much lesser degree, in the epidermis. The majority of the dermal T cells are CD4+, while CD8+ T cells represent the majority of the epidermal T cell infiltrate (Bos et al., 1983). According to the expression of the low molecular isoform of the tyrosine-phosphatase CD45 (CD45RO) the lesional psoriatic T cells are memory T cells (Bos et al., 1989). Accumulation of these T cells within the psoriatic skin lesions is mediated by the interaction of various glycoprotein ligands and chemokine receptors on the T cell surface (cutaneous lymphocyte-associated antigen / CLA, intracellular adhesion molecule-1 / ICAM-1, CD11a / LFA-1, chemokine receptor / CCR10) with various adhesion molecules on the vascular endothelium of the papillary venules (P-selectin, E-selec-

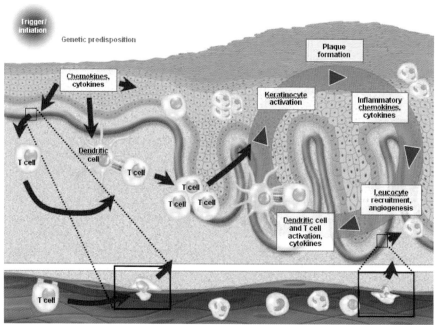

Adapted from: Nickoloff BJ, Nestle FO. J Clin Invest. 2004; 113: 1664-1675.

Fig. 2. Immunopathogenesis of psoriasis

tin, ICAM-1, chemokine CCL27) (Prinz, 2003). CLA and CCR10 characterize T lymphocytes of inflammatory skin diseases. They mediate binding of T cells to the endothelium of the postcapillary venules and thus promote extravasation and migration into the dermal extracellular matrix.

Functional analysis of T cells isolated and cloned from these infiltrates revealed that a substantial proportion was capable of stimulating the proliferation of keratinocyte by the secretion of mediators (Prinz et al., 1994; Bata-Csorgo et al., 1995). Whether a particular hyperresponsiveness of psoriatic keratinocytes to growth promoting signals from T cells is involved in this effect is still a matter of investigation. Studies on cytokine secretion furthermore suggested, that the lesional T cells represent a particular regulatory T cell subset. They produce a particular cytokine pattern that by its biological activities should be able to mediate the features of psoriasis (Vollmer et al., 1994; Kagi et al., 1994). Today, these T cells are being identified as Th17 or Th22 cells. They develop under the influence of IL-23. IL-23 is a heterodimeric cytokine, which consists of two protein chains, IL-23p19 and IL-12p40, which it shares with another cytokine, IL-12. IL-23 promotes the differentiation of naïve T cells into Th17 cells. The cytokine pattern of Th17 cells is dominated by IL-17, IL22, IFN-γ and TNF-α. These cytokines mediate epidermal hyperplasia, acanthosis, hyperparakeratosis and orthohyperkeratosis (Nestle et al., 2009). An over-expression of IL-23p19 and IL-12p40 (precursors of IL-23) has been seen at the mRNA level in psoriatic skin lesions, compared to uninvolved skin (Lee et al., 2004). IL-23 is produced by tissue-resident and / or recruited immune cells, such as dendritic cells and possibly keratinocytes. The pathogenic role of IL-23 and of Th17 cells in psoriasis is supported by the genetic association with polymorphisms in the genes for IL23 and its receptor, and by the clinical findings that therapeutic p40 antibodies (ustekinumab, briakinumab), which neutralize the biologic activity of IL-12 and IL-23 are highly efficient psoriasis treatment. anti-TNF-α agents can reduce IL-23p19 and IL-12p40 mRNA levels, and a reduction of IL-23 levels by cyclosporin A, UV-therapy and biological agents correlates to clinical improvements in psoriasis patients (Nestle et al., 2009). The role of IL-23 and TH17 cells in the psoriatic inflammation may be considered as a functional correlate of the genetic association with the IL12B and IL23R genes.

Regulatory T (Treg) cells are characterized by their ability to suppress the activation and proliferation of CD4+ and CD8+ effector T cells via mechanisms that either require direct contact with antigen presenting cells or by releasing IL-10 or transforming growth factor beta 1 (TGF-b1). Treg cells express CD4, CD25 and the specific transcription factor Foxp3. They account for between 1–5% of the total population of peripheral CD4+ cells. Dysfunction of Treg cells has been implicated in the pathogenesis of autoimmune diseases such as multiple sclerosis, rheumatoid arthritis and autoimmune polyglandular syndrome type II. In psoriasis, Treg function and proliferation are both defective (Nestle et al., 2009). This combination may result in a failure to constrain the activation and proliferation of pathogenic T cells, contributing to the ongoing inflammation seen in psoriasis. Hence strategies that correct Treg function or increase the Treg: pathogenic T cell ratio may be potential treatments for psoriasis.

Molecular analysis of TCR usage in psoriatic skin lesions has provided strong evidence in favour of an antigen-driven lesional T cell response. The TCR usage within psoriatic skin lesions appears highly restricted, with repetitive TCR rearrangements being reflected by the presence of clonally expanded T cell populations (Chang et al., 1994; Menssen et al., 1995). The same clonally expanded T cell populations were associated with the lesional psoriatic immune response over prolonged periods of time and in relapsing disease (Chang et al., 1997; Menssen et al., 1995). Extensive cloning and sequencing of TCR rearrangements of several BV gene families in repetitive biopsies from the same patients indicated that the lesional T cell receptor usage is quite stable in general, with hardly any variations in the selected TCR rearrangements over time. These results emphasize that the psoriatic immune response involves a restricted subset of clonally expanded T cells. It is apparently induced against antigens, which are continuously present within the psoriatic skin lesions, and it shows no signs of epitope spreading. Instead, identification of a conserved T cell receptor ß-chain (TCRB) CDR3-motif within multiple lesions from different patients suggested that the psoriatic immune response is not only preserved within individual patients but that a common psoriatic antigen may be driving responses in different patients (Prinz et al., 1999). Potential autoantigens were identified by molecular mimicry with antigens from *Streptococcus pyogenes*, which is the main infectious trigger of psoriasis. They include keratin 6, keratin 17, ezrin, maspin, peroxiredoxin 2 and hsp27. (Gudmundsdottir et al., 1999., Besgen et al., 2010). Identical T-cell clones in psoriatic skin lesions and tonsils of patients with streptococcal-driven psoriasis as well as the improvement of psoriasis following tonsillectomy in these patients support that T cells may represent a cellular link between streptococcal infection and psoriatic immune activation (Diluvio et al., 2006) Thus, at least in a subset of patients psoriasis may be driven by a cross-reactive T-cell mediated streptococcal-driven immune response.

Clinical manifestations of psoriasis

Acute guttate and chronic plaque psoriasis

Psoriasis presents with two major clinical forms of manifestation, acute guttate psoriasis and chronic plaque psoriasis, as well as several less frequent clinical variants, mainly pustular psoriasis, erythrodermic psoriasis, and psoriasis arthritis (Fig. 3).

The classical psoriatic skin lesion is a well-defined sharply demarcated plaque of salmon pink colour covered with a variable amount of silvery scales (erythemato-squamous plaques). It is characteristic of chronic plaque psoriasis. Scratching off the scaling reveals a glossy, red, dry membrane that upon further removal develops small bleeding points from the elongated papillary capillaries (Auspitz sign). Chronic psoriatic plaques show mostly uniform appearance. They are usually symmetrically distributed with a preference for certain predilection sites: extensor side of joints (particularly knees and elbows), umbilicus, anal cleft, genital region, ears, and scalp. The extend may vary from a few small lesions to extensive confluent plaques that cover large areas of the body.

Acute guttate psoriasis shows small pinpoint lesions with often only little scaling that are tightly scattered over trunk and limbs, less frequently also on face and scalp. It develops as acute, exanthematic form particularly after streptococcal throat infections in first onset psoriasis, but also in acute psoriasis relapses.

Modification by site

The *scalp* is often involved with inflammation and scaling that extends approximately 1 cm onto the forehead. Taenia amiantacea can be considered as the most severe form of shell-like, firmly adherent scales. Although hair loss is not a prevailing sign of scalp psoriasis, a diffuse reversible inflammatory effluvium may develop.

Fingernails and toenails may be affected in two different ways: psoriasis of nailbed and hyponychium leads to subungual hyperkeratosis, onycholysis, and yellow discoloration (oil drop). Small indentations (pitting), grooves and ridges of the nail result from psoriatic involvement of the nail matrix.

In *flexual psoriasis* skin lesions show an "inverse" distribution pattern. They affect mainly axillae, groins, and submammary folds. Due to maceration scaling is usually absent.

Psoriasis of palms and soles is characterized by scaling, hyperkeratotic erythemata or intra-epidermal yellow, later on brown pustules.

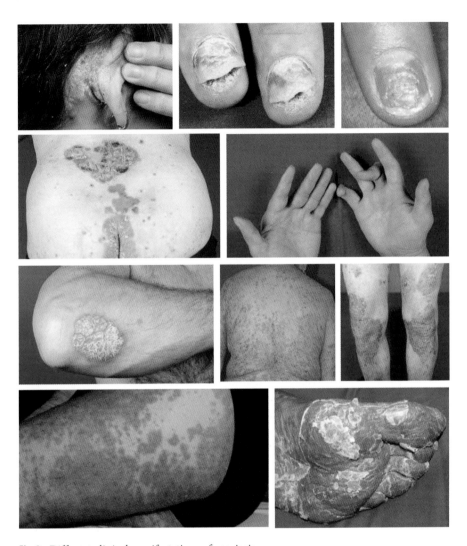

Fig. 3. Different clinical manifestations of psoriasis

Clinical variants

Accumulation of neutrophilic granulocytes in small intra-epidermal microabscesses is a pathognomonic feature of psoriatic skin lesions. If this aspect becomes more pronounced macroscopic visible sterile pustules develop on the skin, leading to pustular psoriasis. Two main forms are distinguished: psoriasis of early onset may develop into pustular psoriasis under certain circumstances such as withdrawal of internal steroids or external irritation or high eruption pressure (*psoriasis cum pustulatione, generalized pustular psoriasis von Zumbusch*). The second group of pustular psoriasis usually develops later in life, often shows an atypical (flexural, acral = inverse) distribution and may display pustulation from onset on (*palmoplantar pustular psoriasis of the Barber Type, acrodermatitis continua suppurativa of Hallopeau, annular pustular psoriasis, generalized pustular psoriasis von Zumbusch*). In both groups localized or generalized forms are distinguished.

In erythrodermic psoriasis psoriatic inflammation has become generalized with highly inflammatory, exfoliative erythema and profuse scaling of the whole skin. Together with generalized pustular psoriasis it represents the most severe form of psoriasis and may become live-threatening.

Psoriatic arthritis is defined as the association of psoriasis with peripheral or spinal arthropathy and negative serological tests for rheumatoid arthritis. The incidence of arthritis in psoriasis patients ranges from ~ 5 to 40%, depending on the diagnostic criteria included. In 65% of psoriatic arthritis patients psoriatic skin lesions preceded arthritis, in 16% joint and skin affection appeared simultaneously, and in 19% skin lesions developed after arthritis onset. HLA-B27, but also HLA-A2, B38, and DR4 confer an increased risk for psoriatic arthritis. Psoriatic arthritis affects men and women almost equally. The average age at onset in most studies is 36–40 years. Psoriatic arthritis affects both peripheral joints and the axial skeleton.

The classification of Wright and Moll distinguishes five subgroups of psoriatic arthritis (Moll and Wright, 1973). *Peripheral asymmetric mono- or oligoarthritis* is most common (~ 70%). It preferentially affects single interphalangeal joints and usually is accompanied by a sausage-like digital swelling. *Distal interphalangeal arthritis* (~ 5–10%) involves the distal interphalangeal joints. In *mutilating psoriatic arthritis (arthritis mutilans,* ~ 5%) multiple interphalangeal joints and adjacent bone are destroyed by osteolysis with subsequent telescope-like shortening of the fingers, ankylosis and arthrogenic contractures. *Symmetric psoriatic polyarthritis* (~ 15%) is similar to rheumatoid arthritis, but usually less severe and rheumatoid factor-negative. *Psoriatic spondylarthritis* (~ 5%) is clinically similar to spondylitis ancylopoetica and affects spine and / or sacroiliac joints. As additional type *pustular arthro-osteitis* is characterized by psoriasis pustulosa palmoplantaris and osteoarthritis of the sternocostoclavicular joints (Edlund et al., 1988).

The peripheral arthritis generally presents as an inflammatory arthritis, manifesting with pain and tenderness over the affected joints, with or without swelling. The distribution of affected joints is often in a "ray" pattern, involving all three joints of an affected digit, whereas other digits are spared. This is in contradistinction to rheumatoid arthritis, where the joints at the same level tend to get involved, leading to a symmetric distribution. A typical feature of psoriatic arthritis is the reddish discoloration over the inflamed joint. Morning stiffness, a feature of inflammatory arthritis is only detected in 50% of patients with psoriatic arthritis. Dactylitis, or sausage digit, is also a typical feature of psoriatic arthritis, which may occur in about half the patients. Dactylitis results from inflammation of both the joints and tendons, leading to swelling and tenderness of the whole digit. It is associated with a higher rate of erosions in the affected digits. Psoriatic arthritis patients also suffer from tendonitis or tendosynovitis which may affect the flexor tendons of the fingers, the wrist as well as the Achilles tendon and the plantar fascia. Enthesitis, or inflammation at the site of tendon insertion into bone, particularly at these latter sites, is also common (Ritchlin et al., 2009).

Spondylitis, which includes sacroiliac and apophyseal joint involvement, may present with inflammatory back pain, which usually occurs at rest and immobility and improves with activity and exercise. It often wakes the patient up at night and responds to walking around or taking a shower. It is associated with prolonged morning stiffness. But spondylitis in psoriatic arthritis may be also totally asymptomatic. The sacroiliac changes may be asymmetrical in psoriatic arthritis and is often less severe than that seen in ankylosing spondylitis (Taylor et al., 2006).

The understanding of psoriatic arthritis has significantly improved recently. It is now being considered as a complex inflammatory disorder of the joints, bone, soft and connective tissue. As distinct features, psoriatic arthritis may comprise synovialitis with new bone formation and bone destruction, tenosynovitis, ostitis and periostitis, and enthesitis. Enthesitis may represent the primary lesion of psoriatic arthritis. The Classification of Psoriatic Arthritis (CASPAR) group, which includes 30 international centers, studied 588 patients with psoriatic arthritis and 536 patients with other forms of inflammatory arthritis to derive classification criteria for psoriatic arthritis (Taylor et al., 2006). Based on logistic regression analyses, classification and regression tree analyses, classification criteria were derived. In order to apply the criteria, a patient must suffer from an inflammatory musculoskeletal disease including peripheral arthritis, spondylitis or enthesitis. Once the presence of a musculoskeletal inflammatory condition is established, if the patient accumulates three or more points of the following, they can be classified as psoriatic arthritis with over 90% certainty. The criteria include the presence of psoriasis, which, if current, provides two points. If not current, either a history of psoriasis or a family history of psoriasis may be counted as one point. The presence of nail lesions provides a point, as does the presence of dactylitis, either current or documented by a rheumatologist. A negative rheumatoid factor provides one point, as does the presence of fluffy periostitis adjacent to joints. Although the criteria were derived from patients with long-standing disease, they have recently been confirmed both in an early psoriatic arthritis clinic and in a family medicine clinic, both providing high sensitivity and specificity, thus suggesting that they may be used as diagnostic criteria (Gladman, 2009).

There are common extra-articular features in psoriatic arthritis. The major feature is psoriasis. Nail lesions occur in much higher frequency among patients with psoriatic arthritis than in those with uncomplicated psoriasis. Although it had been thought that patients with psoriatic arthritis have more severe psoriasis, recent studies demonstrate that there is no direct relationship between the extent and severity of psoriasis and joint manifestations. Other extra-articular manifestations include ocular involvement, which may present as conjunctivitis or iritis. It occurs in 7–33% of patients with psoriatic arthritis. Aortic incompetence was reported in less than 4% of patients with psoriatic arthritis and usually develops late in the course of the disease. These extra-articular manifestations are similar to those observed in other spondyloarthropathies (Gladman, 2009).

Course of psoriasis

The course of psoriasis is unpredictable. After onset, approximately 60% of the patients suffer from chronic persistent or recurring psoriasis with frequent relapses. In the remaining 40% of patients complete and prolonged remission may develop.

Diagnosis

The diagnosis of psoriasis is usually made on clinical grounds by the combination of erythematous plaques, affected predelection sites, nail changes, and a positive familiar history. Diagnostic difficulties of atypical manifestation such as in seborrhoic or flexural psoriasis as well as in palmoplantar psoriasis may require histopathological support.

Comorbidities

A landmark study based on a cohort of almost 3000 patients found an association between psoriasis and diabetes mellitus, obesity, heart failure and hypertension (Henseler and Christophers, 1995). The metabolic syndrome which compromises abdominal obesity, arterial hypertension, abnormal oral glucose tolerance and abnormal blood lipids is the most important comorbidity of psoriasis (Griffiths and Barker, 2007). Other comorbidities include Crohn's disease and ulcerative colitis, depression and cancer. Patients with psoriasis have a fivefold increase in risk of developing type 2 diabetes and double the risk of myocardial infarction. Psoriasis is associated with an independent risk for cardio-vascular morbidity and increased mortality (Mallbris et al., 2004, Gelfand et al., 2006). A large, population based study found that life expectancy was about four years shorter in patients with severe psoriasis than in healthy controls (Gelfand et al., 2007). Pathophysiologically the increased cardiovascular mortality of patients with psoriasis seems to be a consequence of the "psoriatic march" (Boehncke et al., 2007, Boehncke et al., 2009). Psoriasis and its comorbidities produce a systemic inflammatory burden. Systemic inflammation in turn causes insulin resistance, a state in which the equilibrium between proatherogenic and antiatherogenic effects of insulin is shifted towards proatherogenic effects. This shift expedites endothelial dysfunction, which leads to atherosclerosis and eventually myocardial infarction if coronary arteries are involved. Several cross sectional studies have independently described a correlation between psoriasis severity and the patients` blood levels of adipokines, soluble mediators interfering with insulin functions. The mechanisms outlined here suggest a metabolic state comparable to that in patients developing type 2 diabetes mellitus (Davidovici et al., 2010). Treatment decisions of patients with psoriasis should take into account patients' comorbidities to identify contraindications and comedication to avoid drug interactions.

Management of psoriasis

Therapy should take into consideration that psoriasis often is a life long recurring but not life threatening disease. Due to the large clinical variability of psoriasis, therapy has to be adapted individually. The mode of therapy has to consider the individual extend, localisation, acutity and duration of psoriasis, sex and age of the patient, social and private aspects, and patient compliance. Fore a more detailed information evidence-based guide-lines for the treatment of psoriasis have recently become available (Nast et al., 2006, Pathirana et al., 2009).

General measures:

Patients should occasionally be examined for inflammatory foci (oto-laryngologic, dental) that may serve as constant triggers of relapses. Streptococcal throat infection should be treated antibiotically. Tonsillectomy may be beneficial particularly in early psoriasis triggered by streptococcal sore throat. Triggering drugs and alcohol should be avoided, whenever possible. The influence of diet is unclear. It might be advisory in severe and refractory psoriasis to avoid meet and sausages from cattle and pig because of the fat-content in precursors of arachidonic acid that may fuel psoriatic inflammation unspecifically (Adam, 1995).

Therapy should address the different aspects of psoriatic skin lesions: it should suppress keratinocyte proliferation, be anti-inflammatory and immunosuppressive.

Topical therapy

Dithranol (anthralin) was introduced into psoriasis therapy by Unna and Galewsky in 1916 (Farber, 1992). It replaced chrysarobin, a natural tree-bark extract that was not available any more during the 1st world war. Dithranol still represents a kind of gold standard. Its mode of action involves a cytostatic effect. It may be used in combination with UVB light (Ingram regimen) or as short contact application. Since it is highly irritative it is used in low concentrations that during the course of treatment are cautiously increased. Dithranol formulations have to be protected from oxidation by the addition of salicylic acid. As a disadvantage, dithranol stains the skin as well as cloth with a brownish discoloration.

Coal tars have been known for their antipsoriatic effects since long. They probably act cytostatically. Tars are mainly used as creams or ointments and as bath in combination with UV light (Goeckerman regimen). In experienced hands they represent an effective, although by now old-fashioned approach particularly for chronic plaque psoriasis. Because of the high content in potentially carcinogenic polycyclic aromatic hydrocarbons and occasional reports on the occurrence of skin cancer in tar-treated areas, tar should be used with care. It definitely is not the first line of treatment anymore.

Topical steroids are effective in clearing psoriatic skin lesions. The mode of action involves anti-inflammatory and immunosuppressive effects. In addition to the disadvantages of long-term use (atrophy, systemic resorption etc.), steroid treatment induces rebounds that are usually more recalcitrant to further treatment. In order to reduce side effects and enhance efficiency, steroids should be used in combination with other treatment modalities, such as topical vitamin D or A analogues.

Vitamin D analogues (calcipotriol, tacalcitol) inhibit proliferation and enhance differention of epithelial cells via binding to vitamin D-receptors. Furthermore, they suppress T cell activation. They are quite effective in reducing psoriasis activity, but may leave a residual erythema. Advantages are ease of application and the absence of staining. Because of the potential of calcium mobilization from bone their use should be restricted to a certain amount used for a certain area in a certain interval according to the manufacturers' advice. Efficacy is enhanced when combined with topical steroids, tazarotene, or phototherapy.

A topical vitamin A analogue is tazarotene. It is a retinoic acid receptor-specific acetylenic retinoid, which is effective for the topical treatment of patients with stable plaque psoriasis. The low systemic absorption and rapid systemic elimination of tazarotene results in limited systemic exposure. Topical application may produce reversible skin irritation. The efficacy of monotherapy can be greatly increased when combined with topical steroids, vitamin D analogues, UVB or photochemotherapy.

Topical calcineurin inhibitors have not yet been approved for the treatment of psoriasis vulgaris. Their use in psoriasis vulgaris however is based on the results of clinical studies which demonstrated efficacy especially under occlusion for tacrolimus and pimecrolimus. Subsequent investigations demonstrated the efficacy of topical calcineurin inhibitors in the treatment of psoriasis lesions in intertriginous areas and facial psoriasis (Jacobi et al., 2008).

Phototherapy and photochemotherapy

Basically, two different modes of UV-light therapy are used in psoriasis treatment: UV-B therapy, and UV-A photochemotherapy. Both can be applied as partial or whole body therapy. A natural form of phototherapy is helio-/thalasso-therapy (climate therapy) in the Dead Sea area, which, however, seems to produce shorter remissions than office based UV-therapy (Koo and Lebwohl, 1999).

The most effective therapeutic UV-B spectrum for psoriasis lies between a wavelength of 304 and 314 nm. A lamp emitting a narrow UVB band at 311 nm is available. Narrow band UV-B is superior to broadband UV-B in terms of efficacy and reduced carcinogenicity. UV-B efficacy is increased by combination with dithranol (Ingram regimen), vitamin D or A analogues.

Psoralen and UV-A (PUVA) therapy, also termed photochemotherapy, is mainly used as a combination of 8-methoxypsoralen (8-MOP) with subsequent UV-A-radiation. 8-MOP, while formerly given systemically, is now largely applied topically either as bath or as cream. Following photoactivation by UV-A in the skin 8-MOP induces crosslinking of DNA-strands and thus inhibits DNA-replication and RNA-transcription. Various studies demonstrated a tendency for PUVA being superior to narrowband UV-B. Because of the higher degree of cutaneous immunosuppression and long-term carcinogenic hazard, however, PUVA should be applied with caution. It remains the mainstay for psoriasis patients with high PASI scores who do not respond or that cannot be controlled adequately by narrowband UV-B. A history of skin cancer, exposure to treatment with arsenic or cyclosporine A are relative contraindications (Morison et al., 1998; Halpern et al., 2000).

According to a large survey of the literature by Koo and Lebwohl (Koo and Lebwohl, 1999), PUVA and Ingram-regimen seem to induce the longest remissions of all treatment modalities.

Systemic therapy

Systemic therapy is indicated particularly in patients with moderate to severe psoriasis. Rotation of available therapies should always be considered to minimize long-term toxicity and allow effective treatments to be maintained for many years.

Four drugs are mainly used in systemic therapy: Methotrexate, acitretin, cyclosporine A, and fumaric acid esters. Rarely used are hydroxyurea and 6-thioguanine. Mycophenolate mofetil, a novel lymphocyte-selective immunosuppressant, seems to be less potent than initially expected. Further studies are necessary to decide whether it is a therapeutic alternative for patients with psoriatic arthritis. FK506, although effective, has not yet gained a place in psoriasis therapy.

Methotrexate represents an efficient anti-psoriatic drug. It is a dihydrofolate reductase inhibitor and has anti-proliferative and immunosuppressive effects. It usually is given as bolus therapy once a week. When liver function is carefully monitored and additional hepatotoxic hazards are avoided (alcohol) methotrexate appears save even in long-term usage (Roenigk, Jr. et al., 1998).

Acitretin is the active metabolite of the retinoid etretinate. It replaced etretinate because of its decreased lipophilicity and shorter elimination half life (50h versus 80 days). Yet, a minor fraction of acitretin is metabolised back into etretinate. Because of the teratogenic hazards of retinoids and the long-term storage of etretinate in subcutaneous fat, women have to avoid pregnancy for two years after acitretin therapy. Although acitretin has beneficial effects on psoriasis as monotherapy, its main domain is the combination with UV-B or PUVA therapy (Re-UVB, Re-PUVA). In particular when started before onset of phototherapy, it can significantly enhance the efficiency of both UV-B and PUVA. Furthermore, it is often effective in stabilizing pustular psoriasis and acrodermatitis continua suppurativa Hallopeau. It may furthermore enhance the efficacy of TNF-α antagonists in these conditions (Brenner et al., 2009).

A 75 year old female patient with severe pustular psoriasis von Zumbusch (Fig. 4A) was treated with acitretin, initially 50mg per day and 0.1 % triamcinolone ointment. After two weeks she showed a significant improvement of her skin lesions with a disappearance of pustules and erythema (Fig. 4B) and the treatment was reduced to acitretin 30 mg per day with topically applied bland emollients. This stable skin condition is ongoing during this treatment.

Cyclosporine A can efficiently improve psoriasis, probably by its immunosuppressive effects on T cells, but also antigen-presenting cells such as dendritic cells or mast cells. Its use is limited by nephrotoxic side effects and subsequent arterial hypertension. Furthermore, it increases the risk of cutaneous malignancies in patients with previous extensive phototherapy. Short-term usage for a few months in order to induce remission in recalcitrant and severe psoriasis appears as the main indication of this drug (Lebwohl et al., 1998).

Fumaric acid esters were introduced into psoriasis therapy nearly 30 years ago. They have proved to be safe and effective in patients with severe chronic plaque psoriasis. At the moment it is licensed in Germany. It seems to act as immunomodulator that induces a Th1-Th2 shift, and it inhibits the formation of proinflammatory cytokines by blocking NFκB-mediating pathways. Former reports on renal toxicity ask for a close monitoring of renal function. Lymphopenia usually develops without clinical signs of immunosuppression. In

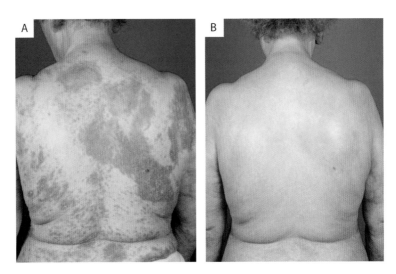

Fig. 4. A 75 year old female patient with severe pustular psioriasis von Zumbusch before (Fig. 4A) and two weeks after treatment with acitretin (Fig. 4B)

some patients severe flushing and diarrhoea may impede further usage. No data are available on the use of fumaric acid esters in combination regimens (Mrowietz et al., 1999).

Biologics. Novel anti-psoriatic drugs have recently been developed on the basis of genetically engineered monoclonal antibodies or recombinant fusion proteins. Due to their efficacy and select biologic activity they have revolutionized the treatment of psoriasis. Biologics aim mainly at the exaggerated lesional psoriatic immune response and offer novel, efficient approaches for the treatment of psoriasis and psoriatic arthritis. Among others they involve:

- monoclonal antibodies against TNF-α (such as infliximab, adalimumab and golimumab) or soluble TNF-α-antagonists (etanercept) (Jacobi et al., 2006);
- monoclonal antibodies to IL-12 and IL-23 (ustekinumab and ABT-874) (Rozenblit and Lebwohl, 2009);
- an antibody against LFA-1 / CD11a (efalizumab) which has been withdrawn due to adverse events in Europe but is still available in the U.S.A.;
- a genetically engineered recombinant fusion protein that interferes with T cell activation (alefacept) (Chaarani and Lebwohl, 2010);

In addition, clinical trials of certolizumab pegol, a PEGylated Fab`fragment of an anti-TNFα monoclonal antibody, show promising results for treating rheumatoid arthritis and suggest that it may be applicable for treating psoriasis and psoriatic arthritis in the future (Rozenblit and Lebwohl, 2009).

It is beyond the purpose of this chapter to review these drugs in more detail. It needs to be stressed, however, that these approaches have different efficiencies in controlling psoriatic inflammation. As compared to the established psoriasis treatment modalities they offer as a particular advantage a lack of organ toxicity and drug interference, and, from the current point of view, they have a good safety profile. By interfering at select steps of the psoriatic inflammatory cascade, they have clarified the pathogenesis of psoriasis much better, and they represent a revolution in the ability to control the disease in high need patients. Of course, they should be active also in mild to moderate psoriasis, but according to the high costs of treatment their use will probably be limited to more severe indications.

The advent of targeted biologic therapies for psoriasis has also changed the management of psoriatic arthritis. TNF-α antagonists may improve joint inflammation and prevent joint destruction as demonstrated by their blocking radiographic progression of joint disease.

Psychological aspects

A major aspect in psoriasis is the reduction in health related quality of life with reduction in physical and mental functioning. It is comparable to that seen in other severe diseases such as cancer, arthritis, hypertension, heart disease, diabetes, and depression (Rapp et al., 1999). Therefore, psychological intervention and support may be necessary in patients that are emotionally and socially handicapped.

Summary

Psoriasis affects ~2% of the Caucasian population. It presents with a characteristic type of skin lesions which appear as sharply demarcated reddish plaques covered with silvery scaling. Psoriasis has only recently gained acceptance as T cell mediated disorder. Therefore, its presentation in a book on autoimmunity may still raise objections. On closer sight, however, psoriasis fulfils many criteria of an autoimmune disease: it has a hereditary background with a strong HLA-class I-association; microbial infections contribute to disease onset; and T cells apparently play an essential role in disease manifestation. Especially Th17 and Th22 cells are important in psoriasis pathogenesis. The cytokine pattern of Th17 cells is dominated by IL-17, IL22, IFN-γ and TNF-α. These cytokines mediate epidermal hyperplasia, acanthosis, hyperparakeratosis and orthohyperkeratosis in psoriasis. Yet, only the identification of the putative autoantigens will finally prove its autoimmune nature.

Psoriasis presents with two major clinical forms of manifestation, acute guttate psoriasis and chronic plaque psoriasis, as well as several comorbidities including psoriasis arthritis. The metabolic syndrome is the most important one. Furthermore psoriasis is associated with an independent risk for cardio-vascular morbidity and increased mortality. Therapy should address the different aspects of psoriasis and its comorbidities. Therefore, it is important that patients with psoriasis and psoriasis arthritis are diagnosed early and treated sufficiently at the onset of the disease to control the inflammatory process and to prevent joint destruction and disability. Newer therapies especially the biologics may be more effective than the older drugs, but will likely demonstrate the same need for early institution to prevent disease progression.

References

Abbas AK, Murphy KM, and Sher A (1996) Functional diversity of helper T lymphocytes. Nature, 383:787–793.

Adam O (1995) Anti-inflammatory diet in rheumatic diseases. Eur J Clin Nutr, 49:703–717.

Arias A, Giles B, Eiermann T, Sterry W, and Pandey J (1997) Tumor necrosis factor-alpha gene polymorphism in psoriasis. Exp Clin Immunogenet, 14:118–122.

Asadullah K, Sterry W, Stephanek K, Jasulaitis D, Leupold M, Audring H, Volk HD, and Docke WD (1998) IL-10 is a key cytokine in psoriasis. Proof of principle by IL-10 therapy: a new therapeutic approach. J Clin Invest, 101:783–794.

Asadullah K, Eskdale J, Wiese A, Gallagher G, Friedrich M, and Sterry W (2001) Interleukin-10 promoter polymorphism in psoriasis. J Invest Dermatol, 116:975–978.

Asumalahti K, Veal C, Laitinen T, Suomela S, Allen M, Elomaa O, Moser M, de Cid R, Ripatti S, Vorechovsky I, Marcusson J, Nakagawa H, Lazaro C, Estivill X, Capon F, Novelli G, Saarialho Kere U, Barker J, Trembath R, and Kere J (2002) Coding haplotype analysis supports HCR as the putative susceptibility gene for psoriasis at the MHC PSORS1 locus. Hum Mol Genet, 11:589–597.

Baker BS, Bolith S, Powles AV, Valdimarsson H, and Fry L (1992) Streptococcal antigen-specific T lymphocytes in skin lesions of guttate psoriasis. J Invest Dermatol, 98:535–538.

Baker BS, Powles AV, Malkani AK, Lewis H, Valdimarsson H, and Fry L (1991) Altered cell-mediated immunity to group A haemolytic streptococcal antigens in chronic plaque psoriasis. Br J Dermatol, 125:38–42.

Bata-Csorgo Z, Hammerberg C, Voorhees JJ, and Cooper KD (1995) Kinetics and regulation of human keratinocyte stem cell growth in short-term primary ex vivo culture. Cooperative growth factors from psoriatic lesional T lymphocytes stimulate proliferation among psoriatic uninvolved, but not normal, stem keratinocytes. J Clin Invest, 95:317–327.

Besgen P, Trommler P, Vollmer S, Prinz JC (2010) Ezrin, maspin, peroxiredoxin 2, and Hsp27: Potential targets of a streptococcal-induced autoimmune response in psoriasis. J Immunol, 184:5392–5402

Boehncke S, Thaci D, Beschmann H, Ludwig RJ, Ackermann H, Badenhoop K, Boehncke WH (2007) Psoriasis patients show signs of insulin resistance. Br J Dermatol, 157:1249–1251

Boehncke WH, Buerger C, Boehncke S (2009) Co-morbidities in psoriasis vulgaris. Hautarzt, 60:116–121

Bos JD, Hagenaars C, Das PK, Krieg SR, Voorn WJ, and Kapsenberg ML (1989) Predominance of "memory" T cells (CD4+, CDw29+) over "naive" T cells (CD4+, CD45R+) in both normal and diseased human skin. Arch Dermatol Res, 281:24–30.

Bos JD, Hulsebosch HJ, Krieg SR, Bakker PM, and Cormane RH (1983) Immunocompetent cells in psoriasis. In situ immunophenotyping by monoclonal antibodies. Arch Dermatol Res, 275:181–189.

Bowcock A, Shannon W, Du F, Duncan J, Cao K, Aftergut K, Catier J, Fernandez Vina M, and Menter A (2001) Insights into psoriasis and other inflammatory diseases from large-scale gene expression studies. Hum Mol Genet, 10:1793–1805.

Brandrup F, Holm N, Grunnet N, Henningsen K, and Hansen HE (1982) Psoriasis in monozygotic twins: variations in expression in individuals with identical genetic constitution. Acta Derm Venereol, 62:229–236.

Braun-Falco O and Christophers E (1974) Structural aspects of initial psoriatic lesions. Arch Dermatol Forsch, 251:95–110.

Brenner M, Molin S, Ruebsam K, Weisenseel P, Ruzicka T, Prinz JC (2009) Generalized pustular psoriasis induced by systemic glucocorticosteroids: four cases and recommendations for treatment. Br J Dermatol, 161:964–966

Cargill M, Schrodi SJ, Chang M, Garcia VE, Brandon R, Callis KP, Matsunami N, Ardlie KG, Civello D, Catanese JJ, Leong DU, Panko JM, McAllister LB, Hansen CB, Papenfuss J, Prescott SM, White TJ, Leppert MF, Krueger GG, Begovich AB (2007) A large-scale genetic association study confirms IL12B and leads to the identification of IL23R as psoriasis-risk genes. Am J Hum Genet, 80:273–290.

Chaarani J, Lebwohl M (2010). Alefacept: where it stands today. Expert Opin Drug Metab Toxicol, 6:355–361

Chang JC, Smith LR, Froning KJ, Kurland HH, Schwabe BJ, Blumeyer KK, Karasek MA, Wilkinson DI, Farber EM, Carlo DJ, and Brostoff SW (1997) Persistence of T-cell clones in psoriatic lesions. Arch Dermatol, 133:703–708.

Chang JCC, Smith LR, Froning KJ, Schwabe BJ, Laxer JA, Caralli LL, Kurland HH, Karasek MA, Wilkinson DI, Carlo DJ, and Brostoff SW (1994) CD8+ T cells in psoriatic lesions preferentially use T-cell receptor V?3 and/orV?13.1 genes. Proc Natl Acad Sci USA, 91:9282–9286.

Christophers E and Henseler T (1985) Characterization of disease patterns in nonpustular psoriasis. Semin Dermatol, 4:271–275.

Cookson W, Ubhi B, Lawrence R, Abecasis G, Walley A, Cox H, Coleman R, Leaves N, Trembath R, Moffatt M, and Harper J (2001) Genetic linkage of childhood atopic dermatitis to psoriasis susceptibility loci. Nat Genet, 27:372–373.

Davidovici BB, Sattar N, Prinz JC, Puig L, Emery P, Barker JN, van de Kerkhof P, Ståhle M, Nestle FO, Girolomoni G, Krueger JG (2010) Psoriasis and Systemic Inflammatory Diseases: Potential Mechanistic Links between Skin Disease and Co-Morbid Conditions. J Invest Dermatol [Epub ahead of print]

de Cid R, Riveira-Munoz E, Zeeuwen PL, Robarge J, Liao W, Dannhauser EN, Giardina E, Stuart PE, Nair R, Helms C, Escaramís G, Ballana E, Martín-Ezquerra G, den Heijer M, Kamsteeg M, Joosten I, Eichler EE, Lázaro C, Pujol RM, Armengol L, Abecasis G, Elder JT, Novelli G, Armour JA, Kwok PY, Bowcock A, Schalkwijk J, Estivill X (2009) Deletion of the late cornified envelope LCE3B and LCE3C genes as a susceptibility factor for psoriasis. Nat Genet, 41:211–215

Diluvio L, Vollmer S, Besgen P, Ellwart JW, Chimenti S, Prinz JC (2006) Identical TCR beta-chain rearrangements in streptococcal angina and skin lesions of patients with psoriasis vulgaris. J. Immunol, 176:7104–7111

Dirckx JH (1983) Dermatologic terms in the De Medicina of Celsus. Am J Dermatopathol, 5:363–369.

Edlund E, Johnsson U, Lidgren L, Pettersson H, Sturfelt G, Svensson B, Theander J, and Willen H (1988) Palmoplantar pustulosis and sternocostoclavicular arthro-osteitis. Ann Rheum Dis, 47:809–815.

Elder J, Nair R, Henseler T, Jenisch S, Stuart P, Chia N, Christophers E, and Voorhees J (2001) The genetics of psoriasis 2001: the odyssey continues. Arch Dermatol, 137:1447–1454.

Farber EM (1992) History of the treatment of psoriasis. J Am Acad Dermatol, 27:640–645.

Farber EM, Nall ML, and Watson W (1974) Natural history of psoriasis in 61 twin pairs. Arch Dermatol, 109:207–211.

Fujinami RS and Oldstone MB (1985) Amino acid homology between the encephalitogenic site of myelin basic protein and virus: mechanism for autoimmunity. Science, 230:1043–1045.

Gelfand JM, Neimann AL, Shin DB, Wang X, Margolis DJ, Troxel AB (2006) Risk of myocardial infarction in patients with psoriasis. JAMA, 296:1735–1741

Gelfand JM, Troxel AB, Lewis JD, Kurd SK, Shin DB, Wang X, Margolis DJ, Strom BL (2007). The risk of mortality in patients with psoriasis: results from a population-based study. Arch Dermatol, 143:1493–1499

Gladman DD (2009) Psoriatic arthritis. Dermatol Ther, 22:40–55

Glickman FS (1986) Lepra, psora, psoriasis. J Am Acad Dermatol, 14:863–866.

Gonzalez S, Martinez Borra J, Torre Alonso J, Gonzalez Roces S, Sanchez del Rio J, Rodriguez Perez A, Brautbar C, and Lopez Larrea C (1999) The MICA-A9 triplet repeat polymorphism in the transmembrane region confers additional susceptibility to the development of psoriatic arthritis and is independent of the association of Cw*0602 in psoriasis. Arthritis Rheum, 42:1010–1016.

Gordon M and Johnson WC (1967) Histopathology and histochemistry of psoriasis. I. The active lesion and clinically normal skin. Arch Dermatol, 95:402–407.

Gottlieb SL, Gilleaudeau P, Johnson R, Estes L, Woodworth TG, Gottlieb AB, and Krueger JG (1995) Response of psoriasis to a lymphocyte-selective toxin (DAB$_{389}$IL-2) suggests a primary immune, but not keratinocyte, pathogenic basis. Nature Med, 1:442–447.

Griffiths CE, Barker JN (2007). Pathogenesis and clinical features of psoriasis. Lancet., 21; 370:263–271

Gudjonsson J, Karason A, Antonsdottir A, Runarsdottir E, Hauksson V, Upmanyu R, Gulcher J, Stefansson K, and Valdimarsson H (2003) Psoriasis patients who are homozygous for the HLA-Cw*0602 allele have a 2.5-fold increased risk of developing psoriasis compared with Cw6 heterozygotes. Br J Dermatol, 148:233–235.

Gudmundsdottir AS, Sigmundsdottir H, Sigurgeirsson B, Good MF, Valdimarsson H, and Jonsdottir I (1999) Is an epitope on keratin 17 a major target for autoreactive T lymphocytes in psoriasis? Clin Exp Immunol, 117:580–586.

Halpern SM, Anstey AV, Dawe RS, Diffey BL, Farr PM, Ferguson J, Hawk JL, Ibbotson S, McGregor JM, Murphy GM, Thomas SE, and Rhodes LE (2000) Guidelines for topical PUVA: a report of a workshop of the British photodermatology group. Br J Dermatol, 142:22–31.

Harder J, Bartels J, Christophers E, and Schroder JM (1997) A peptide antibiotic from human skin. Nature, 387:861

Harvima IT, Naukkarinen A, Harvima RJ, and Horsmanheimo M (1989) Enzyme- and immunohistochemical localization of mast cell tryptase in psoriatic skin. Arch Dermatol Res, 281:387–391.

Helms C, Cao L, Krueger JG, Wijsman EM, Chamian F, Gordon D, Heffernan M, Daw JAW, Robarge J, Ott J, Kwok P-Y, Menter A, and Bowcock AM (2003) A putative RUNX1 binding site variant between *SLC9A3R1* and *NAT9* is associated with susceptibility to psoriasis. Nat Genet, 35:349–356.

Henseler T, Christophers E (1995). Disease concomitance in psoriasis. J Am Acad Dermatol, 32:982–986

Henseler T (1997) The genetics of psoriasis. J Am Acad Dermatol, 37: S1–11.

Henseler T (1998) Genetics of psoriasis. Arch Dermatol Res, 290:463–476.

Hollox EJ, Huffmeier U, Zeeuwen PL, Palla R, Lascorz J, Rodijk-Olthuis D, van de Kerkhof PC, Traupe H, de Jongh G, den Heijer M, Reis A, Armour JA, Schalkwijk J. (2008) Psoriasis is associated with increased beta-defensin genomic copy number. Nat Genet, 40:23–25

Homey B, Alenius H, Muller A, Soto H, Bowman E, Yuan W, McEvoy L, Lauerma A, Assmann T, Bunemann E, Lehto M, Wolff H, Yen D, Marxhausen H, To W, Sedgwick J, Ruzicka T, Lehmann P, and Zlotnik A (2002) CCL27-CCR10 interactions regulate T cell-mediated skin inflammation. Nat Med, 8:157–165.

Itoh K, Sakakibara M, Yamasaki S, Takeuchi A, Arase H, Miyazaki M, Nakajima N, Okada M, and Saito T (2002) Cutting edge: negative regulation of immune synapse formation by anchoring lipid raft to cytoskeleton through Cbp-EBP50-ERM assembly. J Immunol, 168:541–544.

Jacobi A, Braeutigam M, Mahler V, Schultz E, Hertl M (2008). Pimecrolimus 1% cream in the treatment of facial psoriasis: a 16-week open-label study. Dermatology, 216:133–136

Jacobi A, Mahler V, Schuler G, Hertl M (2006). Treatment of inflammatory dermatoses by tumour necrosis factor antagonists. J Eur Acad Dermatol Venereol, 20:1171–1187

Jenisch S, Koch S, Henseler T, Nair RP, Elder JT, Watts CE, Westphal E, Voorhees JJ, Christophers E, and Kronke M (1999) Corneodesmosin gene polymorphism demonstrates strong linkage disequilibrium with HLA and association with psoriasis vulgaris. Tissue Antigens, 54:439–449.

Kagi MK, Wüthrich B, Montano E, Baradun J, Blaser K, and Walker C (1994) Differential cytokine profiles in peripheral blood lymphocyte supernatants and skin biopsies from patients with different forms of atopic dermatitis, psoriasis and normal individuals. Int Arch Allergy Immunol, 103:332–340.

Koo J and Lebwohl M (1999) Duration of remission of psoriasis therapies. J Am Acad Dermatol, 41:51–59.

Leach D and Beckwith J (1999) The founders of dermatology: Robert Willan and Thomas Bateman. J R Coll Physicians Lond, 33:580–582.

Lebwohl M, Ellis C, Gottlieb A, Koo J, Krueger G, Linden K, Shupack J, and Weinstein G (1998) Cyclosporine consensus conference: with emphasis on the treatment of psoriasis. J Am Acad Dermatol, 39:464–475.

Lee E, Trepicchio WL, Oestreicher JL, Pittman D, Wang F, Chamian F, Dhodapkar M, Krueger JG (2004) Increased expression of interleukin 23 p19 and p40 in lesional skin of patients with psoriasis vulgaris. J Exp Med, 199:125–130

Mallbris L, Akre O, Granath F, Yin L, Lindelöf B, Ekbom A, Ståhle-Bäckdahl M (2004) Increased risk for cardiovascular mortality in psoriasis inpatients but not in outpatients. Eur J Epidemiol, 19:225–230

Mallon E, Bunce M, Savoie H, Rowe A, Newson R, Gotch F, and Bunker C (2000) HLA-C and guttate psoriasis. Br J Dermatol, 143:1177–1182.

McCarty, M. (1973) Host-parasite relations in bacterial diseases: Davis, B. D., Dulbecco, R., Eisen, H. N., Ginsberg, H. S., Wood, W. B., and McCarty, M. v. 2nd, (22):p. 627–665. Microbiology. Harper & Row: Hagerstown, New York, Evanstown, San Francisco, London.

Menssen A, Trommler P, Vollmer S, Schendel D, Albert E, Gürtler L, Riethmüller G, and Prinz JC (1995) Evidence for an antigen-specific cellular immune response in skin lesions of patients with psoriasis vulgaris. J Immunol, 155:4078–4083.

Michel G, Kemény L, Homey B, and Ruzicka T (1996) FK506 in the treatment of inflammatory skin disease: promises and perspectives. Immunol Today, 17:106–108.

Moll JM and Wright V (1973) Psoriatic arthritis. Semin Arthritis Rheum, 3:55–78.

Morison WL, Baughman RD, Day RM, Forbes PD, Hoenigsmann H, Krueger GG, Lebwohl M, Lew R, Naldi L, Parrish JA, Piepkorn M, Stern RS, Weinstein GD, and Whitmore SE (1998) Consensus workshop on the toxic effects of long-term PUVA therapy. Arch Dermatol, 134:595–598.

Mrowietz U, Christophers E, and Altmeyer P (1999) Treatment of severe psoriasis with fumaric acid esters: scientific background and guidelines for therapeutic use. The German Fumaric Acid Ester Consensus Conference. Br J Dermatol, 141:424–429.

Mueller W and Hermann B (1976) Cyclosporin A for psoriasis. N Engl J Med, 301:355

Nair RP, Henseler T, Jenisch S, Stuart P, Bichakjian CK, Lenk W, Westphal E, Guo SW, Christophers E, Voorhees JJ, and Elder JT (1997) Evidence for two psoriasis susceptibility loci (HLA and 17q) and two novel candidate regions (16q and 20p) by genome-wide scan. Hum Mol Genet, 6:1349–1356.

Nair RP, Stuart P, Henseler T, Jenisch S, Chia NV, Westphal E, Schork NJ, Kim J, Lim HW, Christophers E, Voorhees JJ, and Elder JT (2000) Localization of psoriasis-susceptibility locus PSORS1 to a 60-kb interval telomeric to HLA-C. Am J Hum Genet, 66:1833–1844.

Nast, I. Kopp, M. Augustin, K.B. Banditt, W.-H. Boehncke, M. Follmann, M. Friedrich, M. Huber, C. Kahl, J. Klaus, J. Koza, I. Kreiselmaier, J. Mohr, U. Mrowietz, H.M. Ockenfels, H.D. Orzechowski, J C. Prinz, K. Reich, T. Rosenbach, S. Rosumeck, M. Schlaeger, G. Schmid-Ott, M. Sebastian, V. Streit, T. Weberschock, B. Rzany (2006) Evidence-based (S3) guidelines for the treatment of psoriasis vulgaris. J. Dtsch. Dermatol, 4, Suppl. 2:1–121

Nestle FO, Kaplan DH, Barker J (2009). Psoriasis. N Engl J Med, 361:496–509

Nickoloff BJ, Karabin GD, and Barker JNWN (1991) Localization of IL-8 and its inducer TNF-α in psoriasis. Am J Pathol, 138:129–140.

Nickoloff BJ, Nestle FO (2004). Recent insights into the immunopathogenesis of psoriasis provide new therapeutic opportunities. J Clin Invest, 113:1664–1675

Nicolas JF, Chamchick N, Thivolet J, Wijdenes J, Morel P, and Revillard P (1991) CD4 antibody treatment of severe psoriasis. Lancet, 338:321

Norrlind R (1954) Significance of infections in origination of psoriasis. Acta Rheum Scand, 1:135–140.

Oldstone MB (1987) Molecular mimicry and autoimmune disease. Cell, 50:819–820.

Pathirana D, Ormerod AD, Saiag P, Smith C, Spuls PI, Nast A, Barker J, Bos JD, Burmester GR, Chimenti S, Dubertret L, Eberlein B, Erdmann R, Ferguson J, Girolomoni G, Gisondi P, Giunta A, Griffiths C, Hönigsmann H, Hussain M, Jobling R, Karvonen SL, Kemeny L, Kopp I, Leonardi C, Maccarone M, Menter A, Mrowietz U, Naldi L, Nijsten T, Ortonne JP, Orzechowski HD, Rantanen T, Reich K, Reytan N, Richards H, Thio HB, van de Kerkhof P, Rzany B (2009) European S3-guidelines on the systemic treatment of psoriasis vulgaris. J Eur Acad Dermatol Venereol, 23 Suppl 2:1–70

Pinkus H and Mehregan AH (1966) The primary histologic lesion of seborrheic dermatitis and psoriasis. J Invest Dermatol, 46:109–116.

Prinz JC, Braun-Falco O, Meurer M, Daddona P, Reiter C, Rieber EP, and Riethmüller G (1991) Chimeric CD4 monoclonal antibody in the treatment of generalized pustular psoriasis. Lancet, 338:320–321.

Prinz JC, Gross B, Vollmer S, Trommler P, Strobel I, Meurer M, and Plewig G (1994) T cell clones from psoriasis skin lesions can promote keratinocyte proliferation in vitro. Eur J Immunol, 24:593–598.

Prinz JC, Vollmer S, Boehncke W-H, Menssen A, Laisney I, and Trommler P (1999) Selection of conserved TCR-VDJ-rearrangements in chronic psoriatic plaques indicates a common antigen in psoriasis vulgaris. Eur J Immunol, 29:3360–3368.

Prinz JC (2003) The role of T cells in psoriasis. J Eur Ac Derm Venerol, 17:257–270.

Prinz JC (2004) Disease mimicry: A pathogenetic concept for T cell-mediated autoimmune disorders triggered by molecular mimicry? Autoimmun Rev, 3:10–15.

Prodeus AP, Zhou X, Maurer M, Galli SJ, and Carroll MC (1997) Impaired mast cell-dependent natural immunity in complement C3-deficient mice. Nature, 390:172–175.

Prokunina L, Castillejo Lopez C, Oberg F, Gunnarsson I, Berg L, Magnusson V, Brookes A, Tentler D, Kristjansdottir H, Grondal G, Bolstad A, Svenungsson E, Lundberg I, Sturfelt G, Jonssen A, Truedsson L, Lima G, Alcocer Varela J, Jonsson R, Gyllensten U, Harley J, Alarcon Segovia D, Steinsson K, and Alarcon Riquelme M (2002) A regulatory polymorphism in PDCD1 is associated with susceptibility to systemic lupus erythematosus in humans. Nat Genet, 32:666–669.

Queiro R, Torre J, Gonzalez S, Lopez Larrea C, Tinture T, and Lopez Lagunas I (2003) HLA antigens may influence the age of onset of psoriasis and psoriatic arthritis. J Rheumatol, 30:505–507.

Ragaz A and Ackerman AB (1979) Evolution, maturation, and regression of lesions of psoriasis. New observations and correlation of clinical and histologic findings. Am J Dermatopathol, 1:199–214.

Rapp SR, Feldman SR, Exum ML, Fleischer AB, Jr., and Reboussin DM (1999) Psoriasis causes as much disability as other major medical diseases. J Am Acad Dermatol, 41:401–407.

Reczek D, Berryman M, and Bretscher A (1997) Identification of EBP50: A PDZ-containing phosphoprotein that associates with members of the ezrin-radixin-moesin family. J Cell Biol, 139:169–179.

Reich K, Mossner R, Konig I, Westphal G, Ziegler A, and Neumann C (2002) Promoter polymorphisms of the genes encoding tumor necrosis factor-alpha and interleukin-1beta are associated with different subtypes of psoriasis characterized by early and late disease onset. J Invest Dermatol, 118:155–163.

Ritchlin CT, Kavanaugh A, Gladman DD, Mease PJ, Helliwell P, Boehncke WH, de Vlam K, Fiorentino D, Fitzgerald O, Gottlieb AB, McHugh NJ, Nash P, Qureshi AA, Soriano ER, Taylor WJ; Group for Research and Assessment of Psoriasis and Psoriatic Arthritis (GRAPPA) (2009) Treatment recommendations for psoriatic arthritis. Ann Rheum Dis, 68:1387–1394

Robinson JH and Kehoe MA (1992) Group A streptococcal M proteins: virulence factors and protective antigens. Immunol Today, 13:362–367.

Roenigk HH, Jr., Auerbach R, Maibach H, Weinstein G, and Lebwohl M (1998) Methotrexate in psoriasis: consensus conference. J Am Acad Dermatol, 38:478–485.

Rozenblit M, Lebwohl M (2009). New biologics for psoriasis and psoriatic arthritis. Dermatol Ther, 22:56–60

Russel TJ, Schultes LM, and Kuban DJ (1972) Histocompatibility (HL-A) antigens associated with psoriasis. N Engl J Med, 287:738–740.

Schaible UE, Collins HL, and Kaufmann SH (1999) Confrontation between intracellular bacteria and the immune system. Adv Immunol, 71:267–377.

Schmitt Egenolf M, Eiermann TH, Boehncke WH, Stander M, and Sterry W (1996) Familial juvenile onset psoriasis is associated with the human leukocyte antigen (HLA) class I side of the extended haplotype Cw6-B57-DRB1*0701-DQA1*0201-DQB1*0303: a population- and family-based study. J Invest Dermatol, 106:711–714.

Schroder JM and Harder J (1999) Human beta-defensin-2. Int J Biochem Cell Biol, 31:645–651.

Shelley WB and Kirschbaum JO (1961) Generalized pustular psoriasis. Arch Dermatol, 84:73–78.

Sigmundsdottir H, Sigurgeirsson B, Troye Blomberg M, Good MF, Valdimarsson H, and Jonsdottir I (1997) Circulating T cells of patients with active psoriasis respond to streptococcal M-peptides sharing sequences with human epidermal keratins. Scand J Immunol, 45:688–697.

Taylor W, Gladman D, Helliwell P, Marchesoni A, Mease P, Mielants H; CASPAR Study Group (2006). Classification criteria for psoriatic arthritis: development of new criteria from a large international study. Arthritis Rheum, 54:2665–2673

Tazi Ahnini R, Camp NJ, Cork MJ, Mee JB, Keohane SG, Duff GW, and di Giovine FS (1999) Novel genetic association between the corneodesmosin (MHC S) gene and susceptibility to psoriasis. Hum Mol Genet, 8:1135–1140.

Tervaert WC and Esseveld H (1970) A study of the incidence of haemolytic streptococci in the throat in patients with psoriasis vulgaris, with reference to their role in the pathogenesis of this disease. Dermatologica, 140:282–290.

Tokuhiro A, Yamada R, Chang X, Suzuki A, Kochi Y, Sawada T, Suzuki M, Nagasaki M, Ohtsuki M, Ono M, Furukawa H, Nagashima M, Yoshino S, Mabuchi A, Sekine A, Saito S, Takahashi A, Tsunoda T, Nakamura Y, and Yamamoto K (2003) An intronic SNP in a RUNX1 binding site of SLC22A4, encoding an organic cation transporter, is associated with rheumatoid arthritis. Nat Genet, 35:341–348.

Tomfohrde J, Silverman A, Barnes R, Fernandez Vina MA, Young M, Lory D, Morris L, Wuepper KD, Stastny P, Menter A, and et al. (1994) Gene for familial psoriasis susceptibility mapped to the distal end of human chromosome 17q. Science, 264:1141–1145.

Trembath RC, Clough RL, Rosbotham JL, Jones AB, Camp RD, Frodsham A, Browne J, Barber R, Terwilliger J, Lathrop GM, and Barker JN (1997) Identification of a major susceptibility locus on chromosome 6p and evidence for further disease loci revealed by a two stage genome-wide search in psoriasis. Hum Mol Genet, 6:813–820.

Tsunemi Y, Saeki H, Nakamura K, Sekiya T, Hirai K, Fujita H, Asano N, Kishimoto M, Tanida Y, Kakinuma T, Mitsui H, Tada Y, Wakugawa M, Torii H, Komine M, Asahina A, and Tamaki K (2002) Interleukin-12 p40 gene (IL12B) 3'-untranslated region polymorphism is associated with susceptibility to atopic dermatitis and psoriasis vulgaris. J Dermatol Sci, 30:161–166.

Valdimarsson H, Baker BS, Jonsdottir I, and Fry L (1986) Psoriasis: a disease of abnormal keratinocyte proliferation induced by T lymphocytes. Immunol Today, 7:256–259.

Valdimarsson H, Sigmundsdottir H, and Jonsdottir I (1997) Is psoriasis induced by streptococcal superantigens and maintained by M-protein-specific T cells that cross-react with keratin? Clin Exp Immunol, 107 Suppl 1:21–24.

Vollmer S, Menssen A, Trommler P, Schendel D, and Prinz JC (1994) T lymphocytes derived from skin lesions of patients with psoriasis vulgaris express a novel cytokine pattern that is distinct from that of T helper type 1 and T helper type 2 cells. Eur J Immunol, 24:2377–2382.

Weinshenker BG, Bass BH, Ebers GC, and Rice GP (1989) Remission of psoriatic lesions with muromonab-CD3 (orthoclone OKT3) treatment. J Am Acad Dermatol, 20:1132–1133.

Weisenseel P, Laumbacher B, Besgen P, Ludolph-Hauser D, Herzinger T, Roecken M, Wank R, and Prinz JC (2002) Streptococcal infection distinguishes different types of psoriasis. J Med Genet, 39:767–768.

Zhou X, Krueger J, Kao M, Lee E, Du F, Menter A, Wong W, and Bowcock A (2003) Novel mechanisms of T-cell and dendritic cell activation revealed by profiling of psoriasis on the 63,100-element oligonucleotide array. Physiol Genomics, 13:69–78.

9

Chronic Urticaria as an Autoimmune Disease

10

Clive Grattan, Michihiro Hide, and Malcolm W. Greaves

Introduction

Urticaria is conventionally classified as acute, intermittent or chronic (Greaves, 2000a). The cause of acute urticaria is often recognized by the patient if it is due to an IgE-mediated hypersensitive reaction, and will not be considered further. Intermittent urticaria – frequent bouts of unexplained urticaria at intervals of weeks or months – will be discussed here on the same basis as the ordinary presentation of chronic urticaria but may have a definable external trigger, such as food or drug intolerance. The latter is conventionally defined as the occurrence of daily or almost daily whealing for at least six weeks with or without angioedema. The etiology of chronic urticaria has conventionally been regarded as obscure and hence the term idiopathic is often applied. However, there is increasing evidence that up to 50% of patients with 'idiopathic' chronic urticaria have autoimmune chronic urticaria. The diagnosis is important since it carries conceptual, prognostic and therapeutic implications. Contact urticaria and angioedema without wheals will not be dealt with in this account.

Classification of Chronic Urticaria

Chronic urticaria is defined in this chapter as any pattern of urticaria showing continuous activity for 6 weeks or more. In the latest European consensus classification of urticaria chronic urticaria the inducible urticarias (physical and cholinergic) are excluded from the definition of chronic disease (Zuberbier, 2009). The clinical subtypes of chronic urticaria are illustrated in the pie chart of Fig. 1. The frequency of these subtypes is based upon the authors' experience at the St John's Institute of Dermatology in UK. Whilst there may well be minor differences, it is likely that the frequency distribution of these subtypes will be essentially similar in most centres in Europe and North America (Greaves, 1995, 2000b). However, our experience suggests that the incidence of angioedema, especially that complicated by ordinary chronic urticaria is substantially lower in Japan and south Asian countries (Tanaka et al., 2006 and MWG unpublished observation).

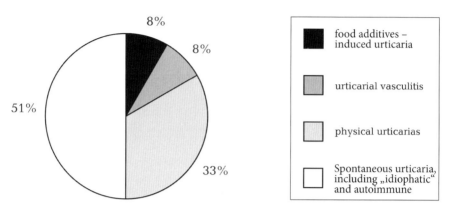

Fig. 1. Chronic urticaria. Frequency of different subtypes in the authors' practices. The proportions are probably not very different elsewhere

Physical Urticarias

These comprise about one third to one fourth of all urticaria patients seen in the authors' services. The diagnosis is mainly made by careful history taking, appropriate clinical examination and is confirmed by positive physical challenge testing. Updated guidelines for physical challenge protocols have been published recently (Magerl, 2009). It is important to identify patients in whom a physical urticaria is the main, if not the only, cause of the patient's symptoms. In this case, further investigation is not indicated, with rare exceptions (see below). Almost invariably, patients with this diagnosis are over-investigated by the time they are referred to the urticaria clinic. Skin prick testing, ImmunoCAP™ tests (previously known as RAST: radioallergosorbent tests), food exclusion diets, etc, are not normally indicated in patients with a physical urticaria with the exception of food-dependent exercise-induced urticaria, a rare variety of urticaria, which develops following exercise after food ingestion.

It is also important to appreciate that different physical urticarias can occur concurrently in the same patient; cold and cholinergic urticarias represent a well recognised example. Furthermore, chronic spontaneous urticaria is often associated with dermographism or delayed pressure urticaria. The investigation and management of chronic urticaria should be influenced by establishing the relative contributions of coexisting forms of chronic urticaria to the patient's overall disability.

Symptomatic Dermographism

This common physical urticaria presents mainly in teenagers or adults of either sex. Like most physical urticarias, individual itchy wheals, produced by gentle stroking or rubbing of the skin, last less than 30 minutes before fading (Fig. 2). Angioedema and mucosal whealing do not occur but pruritus is troublesome and there are no systemic symptoms. The eti-

Fig. 2. Symptomatic Dermographism. Upper left hand panel: use of a graduated dermographometer to test for sensitivity to a dermographic stimulus. Upper right hand panel: graded wheal and flare response to a range of pressures. Lower panel: gentle stroking by the round end of a pen with the gentle pressure may readily disclose abnormal reaction of patients

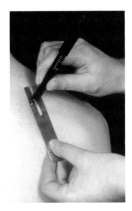
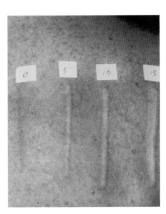
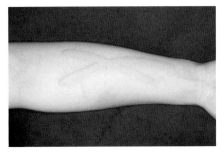

ology is unknown although skin reactivity can be passively transferred to non-human primates by intracutaneous injection of donor serum from a dermographic patient (Murphy et al., 1987). As with the majority of physical urticarias, investigations are pointless and any role for food items has not been substantiated. The prognosis is for eventual improvement in two to three years in most patients. Low sedation antihistamines such as loratadine 10 mg, cetirizine 10 mg or fexofenadine 180 mg are usually effective in relieving the itch, although additional treatment by a sedative antihistamine, such as hydroxyzine 25 mg at night, may also be useful. Up-dosing non-sedating second generation H1 antihistamines and using combinations of H_1- and H_2-antihistamines may be useful. A small open study of patients responding poorly to fexofenadine showed a benefit on pruritus and whealing from narrow-band ultraviolet B phototherapy that lasted for 6 to 12 weeks from stopping treatment (Borzova, 2008).

Cholinergic Urticaria

Cholinergic urticaria is common in children and young adults, although rare in the elderly. Historically, this type of urticaria has been classified as a physical urticaria. However, the consensus report on "definition, classification, and diagnosis of urticaria" (Zuberbier et al., 2009) classifies this urticaria as a special type of urticaria, apart from physical urticarias on

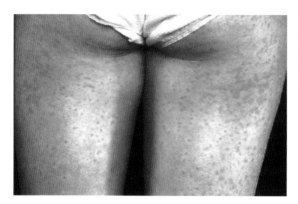

Fig. 3. Cholinergic Urticaria. Typical monomorphic symmetrical maculopapular eruption evoked by heat or exertion or stress

the grounds that the etiology involves sweating, for which the commonest stimulus is raising the body core temperature rather than the application of an external physical stimulus. Symptoms of cholinergic urticaria, typically widespread pruritic monomorphic maculopapular lesions, develop in conditions causing sweating, such as exercise, hot bath taking, or emotional stimuli (Hirschmann et al., 1987) (Fig. 3). If the patient rests, cools off or relaxes, the eruption subsides in 15–45 minutes. Typical areas of predilection include the face, neck, fronts of elbows, wrists and popliteal fossae, although almost any area of the body can be involved. It may be accompanied by angioedema and systemic symptoms include wheezing or, rarely, symptoms of non-allergic anaphylaxis. Cholinergic urticaria can be disabling, especially when provoked by occupational or emotional triggers. The diagnosis is established by appropriate challenge testing (Commens et al., 1978) (exercise, a hot bath or difficult mental arithmetic) and/or skin test with acetylcholine. No further investigations are indicated.

Clinical variants include persistent cholinergic erythema (Murphy et al., 1983), in which the rash is evident even at rest, and exercise-induced cholinergic urticaria with angioedema (Lawrence et al., 1981). Cholinergic urticaria can be distinguished from exercise-induced angioedema or anaphylaxis because the latter cannot be induced by passive heating in a hot shower or bath.

The pathomechanisms are incompletely understood. The local wheals can be blocked by atropinisation of the skin indicating involvement of acetylcholine, and histamine release has also been confirmed – presumably derived from mast cells (Herxheimer, 1956). Wheal and flare reaction to autologous sweat and histamine release from their basophils have been demonstrated in some populations of patients with cholinergic urticaria (Adachi et al., 1994, Takahagi et al., 2009). These reactions appear to be mediated by specific IgE, but the antigen in human sweat has not been identified yet. Fukunaga et al. (2005) proposed that cholinergic urticaria should be classified into two distinct subtypes; the first (non-follicular) subtype shows strong skin test reactions to autologous sweat but not autologous serum and the second (follicular pattern) shows weak positive reactions to sweat but positive reactions to autologous serum although the significance of these findings remains unclear. Cholinergic urticaria is not currently thought to have an autoimmune etiology.

The prognosis is for gradual improvement over the course of months or years in most patients, although the authors have several patients in whom cholinergic urticaria remains unremitting. The condition normally responds reasonably well to avoidance of provoking factors, together with regular daily treatment by an H_1-antihistamine, especially in children. Some patients can achieve a degree of exercise tolerance by taking light exercise to bring out a minor exacerbation of symptoms several hours before undertaking more vigorous exercise or sport. Other drugs that may be beneficial when taken in conjunction with an H1 antihistamine include montelukast (Feinberg, 2008), hysocine butyl bromide (Ujiie et al., 2006), propranolol (Pachor, 1987) or danazol (Wong, 1987).

Cold Urticaria

This less common physical urticaria occurs in children and adults. Whealing is rapidly provoked by exposure to cold fluids or cold surfaces (Fig. 4). Angioedema of the oropharynx is a potential risk, e. g. after sucking an iced lolly but is not often a problem. Systemic symptoms are common and may be severe – especially when provoked by extensive body immersion, as in sea-bathing. Cold urticaria is due to histamine release (Keahey et al., 1980), and cold-reactivity can be passively transferred to non-human primates by donor serum from affected individuals (Misch et al., 1983). The transferable factor has been variously attributed to IgE or IgM. Rarely cryoglobulins can be identified in sufferers' serum. These are usually sought routinely but positive results are exceptional. No other routine investigations are worthwhile.

In adults cold urticaria may be highly disabling especially in outdoor workers. It responds rather poorly to antihistamine treatment in all but the mildest cases and in children. Cold tolerance treatment (repeated cold exposure to induce a temporary refractory

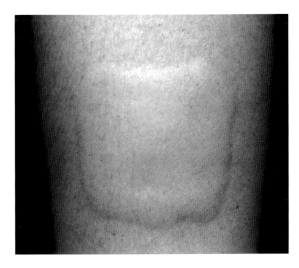

Fig. 4. Cold Urticaria. Local whealing response to application of an ice cube for 10 min

state) is effective but requires a highly motivated patient (Bentley-Phillips et al., 1976). Some remain crippled by cold sensitivity despite all these measures.

Delayed Pressure Urticaria

This common and disabling physical urticaria may resemble angioedema in that the wheals are characteristically deep and of more than 24 hours' duration (Lawlor et al., 1989a). As its name suggests, whealing occurs following a latent period of 2–4 hours after application of pressure perpendicular to the skin. Common examples of triggering factors include a tight waistband, tight footwear and golf club, tennis racquet, or steering wheel grips. Pain is more characteristic than itch although both may occur, and there is no angioedema and no mucosal involvement. A skin biopsy reveals an inflammatory infiltrate in which eosinophils are prominent but there is no vasculitis. Mild systemic symptoms are common including arthralgia and fatigue. The pathomechanisms in delayed pressure urticaria are unknown. Up to 40 per cent of patients with chronic 'spontaneous' urticaria in Caucasian populations, but possibly less population of Japan and Asian countries, have accompanying delayed pressure urticaria (Sabroe et al., 1999a, Morioke et al., 2010), and it is doubtful if it ever occurs as an isolated clinical entity.

Treatment is very difficult. Early claims of the value of the antihistamine cetirizine have not been substantiated and antihistamines are usually poorly effective. Non-steroid anti-inflammatory agents are also usually disappointing and in severely disabled patients substantial dosage with oral steroids (e.g. prednisone 30–40 mg daily) may be necessary to control symptoms. Sulphasalazine and anti-leukotrienes may be effective for patients with predominant delayed pressure urticaria who are not sensitive to non-steroidal anti-inflammatories (Engler, 1995).

Other Physical Urticarias

These are rare, and include solar urticaria (Ramsay, 1977), aquagenic urticaria (Sibbald et al., 1981), vibratory angioedema (Lawlor et al., 1989b) and heat contact urticaria (Koro et al., 1986). Although it may be useful to determine the action spectrum needed to evoke solar urticaria, generally no further investigations are needed beyond establishing the diagnosis by appropriate challenge tests. Antihistamine therapy is helpful to varying degrees in members of this group, which will not be discussed further. The reader is referred to more detailed accounts of these physical urticarias published elsewhere (Black, 2004)

Food Additive-Evoked Chronic Urticaria

Many patients with chronic urticaria believe they have an 'allergy' to food items but this is probably never the case in adults with continuous spontaneous wheals. The rare exception is young children where food allergy is said occasionally to present as chronic urticaria. The relationship between food intolerance (also known as pseudoallergy) and chronic urticaria has been investigated in several recent studies (Magerl, 2010, Bunselmeyer, 2009).

Although dietary pseudoallergens may worsen chronic spontaneous urticaria in up to 30% of patients (Magerl, 2010) it is probably a cause in less than 10% as evidenced by exclusion followed by positive open rechallenge (Bunselmeyer, 2009). The gold standard for diagnosis should be placebo-controlled double-blinded challenge testing (Pastorello, 1995; May, 1985) and in our urticaria clinics chronic urticaria can be demonstrably attributable to a food additive in no more than eight per cent of patients.

Urticarial Vasculitis

Urticarial vasculitis is included in some classifications of urticaria (Grattan, 2007) because the clinical presentation overlaps considerably with chronic spontaneous urticaria even though it is also included in classifications of small vessel vasculitis. The defining feature is the finding of small vessel vasculitis on lesional skin biopsy. A full description of the etiology, pathomechanisms, clinical presentation, investigation and treatment is outside the scope of this article. However, the subject has been comprehensively reviewed (O'Donnell and Black, 1995).

Etiology

In the majority of patients, no cause is evident but recognised etiological factors include virus infections (hepatitis B and C and HIV) and paraproteinaemia. Urticarial vasculitis may also be the first, or very early, clinical manifestation of autoimmune disease (lupus, Sjögren's syndrome), ulcerative colitis or Crohn's disease. Drug hypersensitivity may also be an occasional cause.

Clinical Presentation and Investigation

In contrast with chronic spontaneous urticaria, individual wheals are typically of duration greater than 24 hours. Itching is variable and may be less prominent than painful tenderness. Some staining of the skin may be evident due to purpura and wheals may show a predilection for pressure-bearing areas, such as the waistband. There may be associated systemic symptoms of which arthralgia is especially common. Angioedema may be seen. Urticarial vasculitis tends to pursue a chronic unremitting course.

Treatment

Urticarial vasculitis responds poorly to H_1-antihistamines. Other drug treatments include dapsone, antimalarials and colchicine although the evidence for these is mainly anecdotal. Systemic steroids may be effective but, given the frequently prolonged duration of the disease, systemic complications are almost inevitable. Other measures worth considering in selected patients include intravenous immunoglobulin, parenteral gold injections, omalizumab, rituximab and plasmapheresis.

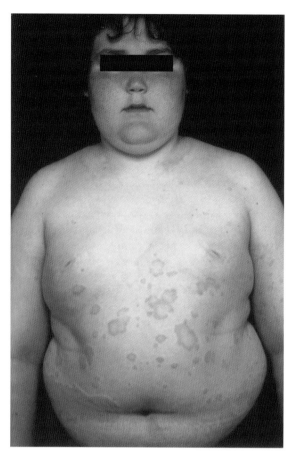

Fig. 5. Chronic Spontaneous Urticaria. This 11 year-old child was treated elsewhere with a prolonged course of systemic steroids. The child is clearly Cushingoid, and still has widespread urticaria

10

Chronic Spontaneous Urticaria (Ordinary Urticaria)

This is conventionally defined as the daily, or almost daily, occurrence of wheals and itching for 6 weeks or more (Greaves, 1995) (Fig. 5). The difference between acute urticaria that appears daily for more than a few days and chronic spontaneous urticaria with disease duration for just a few months is not clear, in terms of pathomechanism but it is likely that autoimmune urticaria more often presents as chronic than acute disease. Average duration of chronic spontaneous urticaria is two–three years, but most patients eventually move into remission.

Etiology

If the small subgroup of patients substantiated to be reactive to a food additives or other dietary pseudoallergens is discounted, then, at least until recently, the cause in the remainder was unknown (idiopathic). There have been several reports implicating local and/or systemic infections of viruses, bacteria, and fungi, such as hepatitic C virus (Kanazawa et al., 1996), *Helicobacter pylori* (H.pylori) (Wedi et al., 1998; Schnyder et al., 1999), and candida (Henz BM et al., 1998). However, they are either anecdotal or may be exacerbatory rather than causative for some populations of patients. In a study reported by one of us (MWG), although upwards 40 per cent of chronic urticaria patients had evidence of H.pylori infection, treatment of this produced no higher remission rate than when the same treatment was given to chronic urticaria patients who did not have evidence of H.pylori (Burova et al., 1998). Parasite infestation is not a cause in industrialized countries, but may be important in some developing countries (Wolfrom et al., 1995). Aspirin is a recognized cause of exacerbations of established chronic urticaria in around 25% of patients (Grattan, 2003) and may induce acute or intermittent urticaria in others but is probably never a cause of chronic disease. The observation that histamine releasing activity could be demonstrated in the serum of some patients with chronic idiopathic urticaria (Grattan et al., 1986) eventually led to the recognition of autoimmune urticaria as an important subset of patients with this condition (Grattan, 1991, Hide et al., 1993) (see below).

Pathomechanisms

Histamine is clearly implicated in the pathogenesis of the wheals and itch. Although histamine, derived from dermal mast cells, is a major contributor to the itch, its role in the wheals, which last several hours and may be relatively poorly responsive to H_1-antihistamines, is less clear. Probably mast cell-derived cytokines, proteases and eicosanoids are also involved. Blood basophils and eosinophils are also present in skin biopsy material from wheals of all ages and may also be a source of vasoactive mediators (Sabroe et al., 1999b; Ying et al., 2002; Caproni et al., 2003).

Clinical Features and Investigation

Characteristically the wheals are intensely itchy, of less than 24 hours' duration individually and clear without marking the skin. Angioedema occurs in up to 50 per cent and affects skin and/or mucous membranes. Systemic symptoms are minimal in the majority but can be disabling for severely affected patients. Delayed pressure urticaria occurs concurrently in up to 40 per cent of patients (Sabroe et al., 1999a). When delayed pressure urticaria is an accompanying feature, it is important to establish whether this physical urticaria or the accompanying spontaneous wheals and angioedema are the principal causes of the patient's disability, since no further investigations are worth while for pure delayed pressure urticaria. The incidence of chronic spontaneous urticaria complicated by angioedema and delayed pressure urticaria, appears not so high in Japan and Asian countries according to the authors' experiences (Tanaka et al., 2006, Morioke et al., 2010).

Chronic spontaneous urticaria may be a seriously disabling condition, causing occupational, social and personal disability of the same order as those consequent upon severe coronary artery disease (O'Donnell et al., 1997).

Patients with chronic urticaria are almost invariably over-investigated. No laboratory investigations are normally indicated in the first instance for anti-histamine responsive disease. Efforts should be directed at excluding urticarial vasculitis (by skin biopsy) and a differential white blood cell count (for eosinophilia) in areas where parasite infestation is endemic. Checking thyroid function and autoantibodies can be rewarding to detect patients with associated thyroid autoimmunity. In severely affected patients, poorly responsive to H_1-antihistamines, referral to a specialised unit for investigation for autoimmune chronic urticaria should be considered (see below).

Treatment

General measures are important including a cool work and domestic environment, avoidance of alcohol indulgence, taking non-steroidal anti-inflammatory drugs including aspirin, and wearing tight clothes. Although almost inevitably associated with modern living, stress, fatigue and intercurrent virus infections should at least be recognised by patients as the probable causes of occasional flare-ups of chronic urticaria.

H_1-antihistamines are the mainstay of drug treatment. It is important to establish the diurnal periodicity of symptoms (itch occurs predominantly in the evening and at night) in timing the dose. Most patients require a daily morning dose of a low sedation antihistamine. Up-dosing second generation antihistamines to four-fold above licence has been recommended for non-responders (Zuberbier, 2009) and this recommendation has been supported recently by well-conducted clinical studies for cold urticaria (Siebenhaar, 2009) and chronic spontaneous urticaria (Staevska, 2010). It has been proposed that H_1-antihistamines may exert an 'anti-allergic' action independently of H_1 receptors (Hayashi and Hashimoto, 1999). This consists of down-regulation of adhesion molecule expression leading to reduced eosinophil and neutrophil migration and possibly a mast cell 'stabilising' effect. However, such actions of H_1-antihistamines may occur only with regimens involving well above the licensed dosages.

If a sedating H1 antihistamine is prescribed at night, it is important to draw the patient's attention to the possibility of significant impairment of cognitive function the next morning (Pirisi, 2000). Topical application of 1% menthol in aqueous cream may be appreciated by patients by providing rapid but temporary relief from pruritus.

H_2-antihistamines (e.g. ranitidine or cimetidine) have a small statistically significant additive effect when combined with H_1-antihistamines but may be clinically useful for some patients. Cysteinyl leukotriene receptor antagonists may be effective in some patients especially those with delayed pressure urticaria. The efficacy of montelukast by itself or in combination with H_1-antihistamine has been shown by controlled trials (Pacor, 2001; Erbagci, 2002). On the other hand, others have proved negative (Reimers, 2002). Aggravation of urticaria by aspirin in combination with other leukotriene antagonists has been reported (Ohnishi-Inoue et al., 1998).

Oral steroids in short tapering courses can be useful in emergencies when rapid control is necessary. However, they are not recommended as a routine treatment of chronic urticaria, due to concern about side effects from long term administration (Fig. 5).

Autoimmune Chronic Urticaria

Between 30 and 50 per cent of patient with chronic spontaneous urticaria have biologically functional autoantibodies against the high affinity IgE receptor on mast cells and basophils or less commonly against IgE itself (Niimi et al., 1996). In these cases the antibody is deemed to be the cause of the disease. These patients are described as having autoimmune chronic urticaria (Grattan, 1991, Hide et al., 1993; Hide et al., 1994).

Etiology

The reason why these autoantibodies are present and causative in some patients with chronic urticaria and not others is unclear. Genetic factors are probably important. Chronic urticaria patients whose sera were positive for anti-FcεRI or anti-IgE autoantibodies showed a highly significantly increased frequency of HLA DRB1*04 (DR4) alleles (O'Donnell et al., 1999). There is also a positive association with other autoimmune diseases, notably autoimmune thyroid disease in patients with autoimmune urticaria (Leznoff et al., 1983; Leznoff and Sussman, 1989). One of us (MWG) has previously suggested that H.pylori infection could lead to development of anti-FcεRIα autoantibodies by molecular mimicry (Greaves, 2001).

Pathomechanisms

Most patients with autoimmune chronic urticaria have IgG autoantibodies directed against the α chain of the high affinity IgE receptors (FcεRIα) expressed on dermal mast cells or blood basophils (Niimi et al., 1996). Histamine release evoked by these antibodies from basophil leucocytes of healthy donors can be inhibited by prior incubation with human recombinant α chain. Some of them bind to FcεRIα, regardless of the binding of IgE. However, the binding of most of these types of autoantibodies are interfered with competitively by IgE to various degrees (Hide et al., 1995). Removal of IgE (by lactic acid stripping) enables the autoantibody to release histamine but reconstituting the IgE on the surface of the basophils inhibits release (Niimi et al., 1996). Precise epitope mapping on FcεRIα has not yet been carried out. In about nine per cent of patients with chronic spontaneous urticaria, the IgG autoantibody reacts with the Fc portion of IgE itself. Studies looking at binding of monoclonal antibodies to the IgE heavy chain suggest that these functional anti-IgE autoantibodies probably bind to the 4th constant domain (Grattan and Francis, 1999). For histamine release to occur, either anti-FcεRIα or anti-IgE autoantibodies normally cross-link adjacent high affinity IgE receptors through the α chain or IgE respectively (Fig. 6).

The role of complement activation is controversial. Our own data, which indicated that the histamine-releasing activity of anti-FcεRIα autoantibodies was heat-stable in basophil assays, argues against complement involvement. The heat-resistance of histamine releasing activity in sera of patients with chronic urticaria has been also observed by other authors (Zweiman et al., 1996; Tong et al., 1997). However, other authors, using specific in-

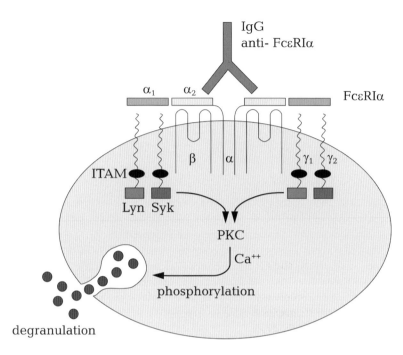

Fig. 6. Autoimmune Chronic Urticaria: Pathomechanisms. Schematic representation of a dermal mast cell. The high affinity IgE receptor (FcεRI) is represented by γ1 and γ2, β and α chains. The α chain possesses two domains (α1 and α2). In this instance IgG anti-FceRI binds to, and cross-links via α2 domain. ITAM = Immunoreceptor Tyrosine Kinase Activation Motif. Lyn, Syk = protein kinases. PKC = protein kinase C

hibitors of complement components, decomplemented sera and/or the reconstitution with C5, have reported evidence that in some circumstances the reaction between anti-FcεRIα autoantibodies and dermal mast cells may be complement-dependent (Fiebiger et al., 1998; Fagiolo et al., 2000; Kikuchi and Kaplan, 2002). Kikuchi and Kaplan (2001) showed the histamine release activity of serum IgG from 2 out of 6 patients was substantially enhanced by serum with complement, whereas that from the other 4 patients was not, suggesting a heterogeneity of anti-FcεRI autoantibodies in terms of the complement dependency for histamine release. The population density of FcεRI on the surface of dermal mast cells and basophils, and/or the binding avidity of autoantibodies may be crucial – a low population density and a moderate binding avidity may allow monovalent binding of the autoantibodies with complement activation. The subclasses of IgG in autoimmune urticaria are predominantly IgG$_1$ and IgG$_3$, which may readily activate complement (Fiebiger et al., 1998).

Subsequent intracellular events involve the activation of protein tyrosine kinases *lyn* and *syk* via immunoreceptor tyrosine kinase activation motifs located on the intracellular portions of the β and γ chains of FcεRI (Rivera J, 2002).

Table 1. Functional Properties of Anti-FcεRIα and Anti-IgE Autoantibodies

1. Cause whealing in human skin following intradermal injection
   (see autologous serum skin test) (Sabroe et al., 1999c)

2. Release histamine from dermal mast cells and blood basophils (Niimi et al., 1996)

3. Reduce numbers of circulating blood basophils

4. Serum levels are proportional to disease activity (Grattan et al., 1992, 2000; Zweiman B et al., 1996; O'Donnell BF et al., 1998)

5. Removal by plasmapheresis results in remission of chronic urticaria in autoantibody positive patients (Grattan et al., 1992)

6. Effectiveness of other immunomodulative therapies, such as ciclosporin and intravenous immunoglobulin (Grattan et al., 2000, O'Donnell BF et al., 1998) and Omalizumab that reduces both IgE and subsequently FcεRI (Kaplan et al., 2008)

That these anti-FcεRI and anti-IgE autoantibodies are functional is indicated by evidence listed in Table 1.

Can autoimmune chronic urticaria be regarded as an autoimmune disease? Removal of the antibodies by plasmapheresis leads to temporary remission of the urticaria (Grattan et al., 1992). The antibody also reproduces the urticarial wheal when introduced as an autologous serum injection into human skin, and causes histamine release from dermal mast cells and blood basophils (Niimi et al., 1996). Reproduction of urticaria in an animal model by sensitisation to the α chain of FcεRI has not yet been carried out even with a transgenic mouse expressing human FcεRIα (Fung-Leung, 1996). However, it should be noted that urticarial eruptions are not apparently observed even in the systemic anaphylactic reactions induced by antigen in animals, such as rodent and guinea-pigs.

Increased histamine releasability from dermal mast cells and basophils is an important additional factor in the pathogenesis (Sabroe et al., 1998). Numerous previously published reports have shown that although mast cell numbers and histamine content of skin are essentially normal in chronic urticaria, various chemical histamine-releasing agents (codeine, compound 48/80) cause exaggerated whealing when injected into uninvolved skin of patients with chronic urticaria (Juhlin and Michaelsson, 1969, Smith CH et al., 1992). This enhanced histamine releasability is possibly due to the action of cytokines or neurokines released locally. These cytokines also cause up-regulation of adhesion molecule expression, leading to the substantial leucocyte infiltrate characteristic of the histological appearances of autoimmune urticaria.

The organ selectivity of anti-FcεRIα autoantibodies is puzzling. Human lung mast cells express FcεRIα, but patients with anti-FcεRI autoantibodies get urticaria without pulmonary symptoms. If complement is involved in evoked histamine release by anti-FcεRIα autoantibodies, then this anomaly is explicable since dermal but not lung mast cells express complement receptors. Alternatively, local cytokine and micro-circulatory differences between lung and skin may restrict access of the autoantibodies to tissue mast cells in the lungs. There is also functional heterogeneity between dermal and lung mast cells (Lowman et al., 1988).

Clinical and Histological Features

Detailed comparative reviews of the symptoms, clinical presentation and natural history of autoimmune and the other spontaneous chronic urticaria has failed to reveal differences sufficiently distinctive to be of diagnostic value (Sabroe et al., 1999a). However, the disease does tend to run a more aggressive and protracted course in patients who possess anti-FcεRI autoantibodies than those without an autoimmune etiology. Patients with autoimmune urticaria also tend to be less responsive to routine antihistamine treatment than other spontaneous, non-autoimmune urticaria patients. Again, the difference is not so conspicuous as to be useful as a discriminating marker for an autoimmune etiology on its own.

Sabroe et al. reported that the peripheral blood basophil leucocyte count is greatly reduced in patients with anti-FcεRIα autoantibodies compared with patients who did not have these antibodies (Sabroe et al., 1998). This is not an original observation; Rorsman (1961) noted almost 45 years' ago that chronic urticaria was associated with basopenia in some patients with chronic 'idiopathic' (but not physical) urticaria. The fate of the cells is of interest; degranulation or destruction in the peripheral blood is an obvious possibility. Indeed, Kaplan's group found the increase of basophils in skin of chronic idiopathic urticaria with or without autoantibodies as well as T cells, eosinophils and neutrophils (Ying et al., 2002). The alternative of redistribution into the lesional skin of chronic urticaria may account for the basopenia.

Sabroe (1999b) carried out a detailed histological study of skin biopsy material from patients with autoimmune and other spontaneous urticaria. No significant differences were found apart from reduced numbers of activated eosinophils (EG2+) in lesional skin of autoimmune patients in which the wheal biopsied was more than 12 hours' old. There is no vasculitis in autoimmune urticaria. More recently Kaplan's group also found no difference in either the numbers of inflammatory cells or the pattern of cytokine expressions between patients with and without autoantibody (Ying et al., 2002).

Diagnosis

As pointed out above, there are no clinical or histological features that can be used as a paradigm in diagnosis (Sabroe et al., 1999a). The cornerstone of diagnosis is clearly detection of functional anti-FcεRIα or anti-IgE autoantibodies in serum of patients with chronic urticaria. The autologous serum skin test is a useful screening procedure with a very high negative predictive value for functional autoantibodies (Konstantinou et al., 2009). This test is based upon the original finding by Grattan (1986) that the serum of some patients with chronic 'idiopathic' urticaria would cause a red wheal upon autologous injection into the patient's uninvolved skin. This test has now been optimised for sensitivity and specificity of *in vitro* basophil histamine release (Sabroe et al., 1999c).

Autologous serum, collected during exacerbation of the chronic urticaria, is injected into uninvolved skin of the forearm in volume 0.05 ml. An equal volume of normal saline acts as a vehicle control. The local response is measured at 30 minutes and is deemed positive if the wheal is red in colour and the diameter is at least 1.5 mm diameter greater than the saline control (Fig. 7). This autologous serum skin test (ASST) is positive in about 40

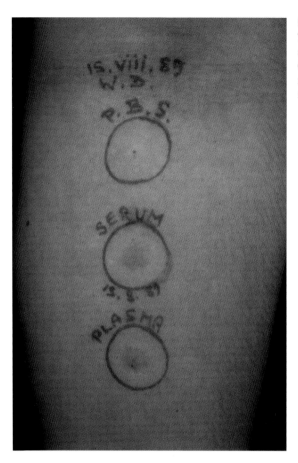

Fig. 7. Autologous Serum Skin Test. PBS = Phosphate-buffered saline; serum: undiluted 0.05 ml. Both serum and heparinized plasma show positive results at 30 min

per cent of patients with chronic spontaneous urticaria (Table 2). In this test, false negative reactions are rare, but false positives may occasionally occur and some of the sera probably contain other wheal-producing mediators including a 'mast cell specific' factor. This non-immunoglobulin mediator retained by 30 KD ultrafiltration membranes was reported by us (Kermani et al., 1995) and appears to be present in about eight per cent of patients with chronic spontaneous urticaria. It requires further characterisation. There is one study that showed no correlation between ASST and clinical features in chronic spontaneous urticaria, except for the frequency of complication with angioedema (Nettis et al., 2002). However, ASST shows a reasonable concordance with *in vitro* measurements of serum anti-FcεRI or anti-IgE autoantibodies, which also significantly correlated with clinical severities (Sabroe et al., 1999a; Zweiman et al., 1996).

A positive autologous serum skin screening test requires confirmation by *in vitro* analysis for anti-FcεRIα and anti-IgE autoantibodies. The current gold standard consists of demonstration by bioassay that either blood basophils or dermal mast cells release histamine or other mediators upon incubation with the patient's serum. Low IgE healthy donor basophils predominantly detect anti-FcεRI autoantibodies, whereas high IgE basophils detect anti-IgE autoantibodies and anti-FcεRI autoantibodies that are non-competitive with IgE. Low IgE basophils may be directly obtained from low IgE (1 IU/mml) donors or prepared by lactic acid treatment of ordinary donors' leukocytes. To distinguish between the two types of autoantibody, it is desirable to carry out inhibition experiments utilising human recombinant α-chain and monoclonal IgE. However, for practical purposes, this is usually unnecessary. In our hands, 25 per cent of chronic spontaneous urticaria sera can be confirmed to contain anti-FcεRIα autoantibodies, whereas about nine percent have anti-IgE autoantibodies (Niimi et al., 1996, Sabroe et al., 1999a).

As high as 76 per cent of chronic sponaneous urticaria patients were found to have anti-FcεRIα autoantibodies by Kaplan's group using a rat basophilic leukaemia cell line expressing α-chain of human FcεRI, which integrates chimeric FcεRI with endogenous rat β and γ chains of the receptor and using release of β-hexosaminidase as an indicator of cell degranulation (RBL-48) (Tong et al., 1997). This figure is even higher than that they observed by human basophils (52%). In our hands, however, the sensitivities of RBL-48 cell and other cell lines expressing human FcεRIα for anti-FcεRIα antibodies are not as high as human basophils obtained from healthy donors (unpublished observation). Further studies with a standardized condition may be necessary to establish the usability of RBL cells expressing human FcεRIα.

Some investigators have used immunoassays (immunoblotting, ELISA, immunoprecipitation) (Fiebiger et al., 1995, 1998; Sabroe et al., 1998; Kikuchi and Kaplan, 2001). These assays measure immunoreactive FcεRIα autoantibodies and show false positives when compared with bioassays. False positives are particularly prone to occur in autoimmune diseases including Sjögren's syndrome, dermatomyositis, pemphigus and pemphigoid (Fiebiger et al., 1998). However, unlike the anti-FcεRIα autoantibodies in urticaria, which are of subtype IgG1 and IgG3, these antibodies are predominantly of the IgG2 and IgG4 subtypes. More important, they are non-functional, being inactive (non-histamine-releasing) against basophil leucocytes. Kikuchi and Kaplan (2001) showed no correlation between positive histamine release activity and immunoblotting in sera of patients with chronic urticaria. The ELISA, though initially promising, has not yet confirmed expectations in terms of specificity and demonstration of linearity between level of antibody and immunoreactivity. Horn et al. (1999) detected substantial amount of anti-FcεRIα antibodies in sera from healthy donors and demonstrated that these antibodies are cross-reactive with tetanus toxoid by ELISA. He used recombinant protein consisting of two moieties of the extracellular part of human FcεRIα flanking one moiety of human serum albumin. Although the affinities of such autoantibodies against the recombinant FcεRIα were low (3.4×10^{-6} and 7.1×10^{-7} M), healthy donor sera containing these autoantibodies showed histamine release activity as well as sera of patients with chronic spontaneous urticaria, using basophils treated with IL-3. They recently cloned anti-FcεRIα autoantibodies from healthy donors and patients with chronic spontaneous urticaria. Both autoantibodies had the same amino acid sequence and showed the activity of histamine release from basophils that were not occupied by IgE (Pachlopnik et al., 2004). On the other hand, immunoreactivity against FcεRIα in ELISA studied by Fiebiger et al. (1998) and that in immunoblotting by the authors (Sabroe et al., 2002) were significantly correlated with basophil histamine release activities ($p<0.0001$, x^2; data were re-calculated by the authors). Moreover, studies of IgE and FcεRI revealed that cross linkage between FcεRI and FcγRII may inhibit histamine release from human mast cells and basophils (Tam et al., 2004) and binding of certain types of monomeric IgE could activate FcεRI by itself (Pandey et al., 2004). It is feasible that autoantibodies against FcεRI could mimic either of such functions. Taken together, the over all assessment of functional autoantibodies with histamine releasing assay with human basophils, or possibly mast cells, should be the gold standard for the detection of pathological autoantibodies.

Published literature on anti-FcεRIα autoantibodies incidences and positive reactions in autologous serum skin test in chronic urticaria is listed in Table 2.

Treatment of Autoimmune Urticaria

The routine treatment of autoimmune chronic urticaria is essentially the same as that for non-autoimmune urticaria. All patients with chronic urticaria should receive antihistamines commencing with a low-sedation antihistamine such as loratadine 10 mg, cetirizine 10 mg, ebastine 10 mg or fexofenadine 120 to 180 mg, (in Japan, fexofenadine is licensed for 120 mg; 60 mg each in morning and evening) usually administered in the morning. Since pruritus is mainly a problem in the evening and at night, it is useful to give a second dose of the same antihistamine in the evening or before retiring for the night. This represents a total daily dosage in excess of the licensed recommended dosage. In patients troubled by severe nocturnal pruritus, a sedative antihistamine such as hydroxyzine 25 mg may be indicated. However, patients should be warned that impairment of cognitive function may be a problem the following morning (Pirisi, 2000).

Patients with autoimmune chronic urticaria may respond poorly to the above antihistamine regime. Systemic steroids are unsuitable as long term treatment for chronic urticaria although short tapering courses may be useful to meet specific contingencies. In patients with recalcitrant autoimmune chronic urticaria, which is causing significant disability, ciclosporin may be effective (Grattan et al., 2000). The dosage for an adult is 3–4 mg / kg / day for three to four months on a tapering schedule. There is rarely a rebound withdrawal. About one-third of patients remain in remission after ciclosporin has been withdrawn; one-third relapse but only mildly and one-third relapse to their former pre-treatment level of disease activity and may have to be recontinued on ciclosporin. Authors' experiences suggest that patients with functional autoantibodies are more likely to respond well than those without. Chronic autoimmune urticaria is not a licensed indication for ciclosporin and the usual precautions regarding renal function, blood pressure monitoring and unwanted interactions with other concurrently administered drugs metabolised via the cytochrome P450 enzyme pathway have to be considered.

We have previously reported positive results using more aggressive forms of immunotherapy including intravenous immunoglobulin (O'Donnell et al., 1998) and plasmapheresis (Grattan et al., 1992) in selected patients with autoimmune urticaria. We ought to emphasise that these treatment modalities are temporary symptom-relieving rather than curative. Nevertheless, it is noteworthy that histamine releasing activity of treated patients decreased or diminished in accordance with urticarial symptoms after the treatments, endorsing the pathological role of autoantibodies and rationales for immunotherapies for chronic autoimmune urticaria.

Table 2. Prevalence of Anti-FcεRI Autoantibodies in Chronic Idiopathic Urticaria

Authors	Skin test	Immunoassay	Bioassay	
Grattan et al. (1991)	ASST[1] 20/25 (80%)		HBHR[6]	14/25 (56%)
Fiebiger et al. (1995)		Western blot (sFcεRIα) 12/32 (37%)		
Niimi et al. (1996)	ASST[2] 98/163 (60%)		HBHR[6]	47/163 (29%) anti-FcεRIα 38 (23%) anti-IgE 9 (6%)
Zweiman et al. (1996)			HBHR[6]	21/70 (30%) anti-FcεRIα 12/13 anti-IgE 1/13
Tong et al. (1997)			HBHR[6] RBL cells[7]	26/50 (52%) 38/50 (76%)
Fiebiger et al. (1998)		ELISA (sFcεRIα) 106/281 (38%)	HBHR (IL-3+)[6]	39/86 (45%) 33/50 (66%) of autoAb+ 6/36 (17%) of autoAb-
Ferrer et al. (1998)		Western blot (sFcεRIα) 34/53 (64%)	HBHR[6] foreskin-MC HR[8]	31/68 (48%) 28/65 (46%)
Sabroe et al. (1999)	ASST[3] 55/155 (35%)		HBHR[6]	54/155 (35%)
Horn et al. (1999)		ELISA (sFcεRIα) 21/21 (100%) 5/21 (9.5%)[9]	HBHR (IL-3+)[6]	1/21 (4.7%)[9]
Asero et al. (2001)	ASST[4] 205/306 (67%)		HBHR[6]	20/121 (17%) 19/87 (22%) of ASST+
Kikuchi and Kaplan (2001)		Western blot (sFcεRIα) 122/260 (47%)	HBHR[6]	111/260 (43%)

10

Table 2. (continued) Prevalence of Anti-FcεRI Autoantibodies in Chronic Idiopathic Urticaria

Authors	Skin test	Immunoassay	Bioassay
Nettis et al. (2002)	ASST[3] 42/102 (41.2%)		
Sabroe et al. (2002)	ASST[4] 27/78 (35%)	Western blot (sFcεRIα) 32/78 (41%) HR+ 20 HR- 12	HBHR[6] 27/78 (35%) skin slice-MC 31/78 (40%) HR[10]
Hide et al. (unpublished result)	ASST[5] 81/180 (45%)		HBHR[6] 15/25 (60%) of ASST+ anti-FcεRIα 11/25 anti-IgE 4/25

1) Determined as positive if wheal volume $\geq 10\,\text{mm}^3$ than saline control at 60 min.

2) Determined as positive if diameter of wheal with flare is $\geq 2\,\text{mm}$ than saline control at 30 min.

3) Determined as positive if diameter of wheal plus redness is $\geq 1.5\,\text{mm}$ than saline control at 30 min. The condition was determined to obtain the optimal sensitivity and specificity for the identification of patients with histamine-releasing activity.

4) Determined as positive if wheal-and-flare area is $\geq 50\%$ of the reaction induced by a prick test with $10\,\text{mg}/\text{ml}$ histamine at 15 and 40 min.

5) Determined as positive if flare diameter is $\geq 5\,\text{mm}$ than saline control OR serum-induced flare is larger than the flare induced by intradermal injection of $20\,\mu\text{l}$ of $10\,\mu\text{g}/\text{ml}$ histamine at 30 min.

6) Human basophil histamine release in the presence (if noted) or absence of IL-3.

7) β-hexosaminidase release from rat basophilic leukemia cell line transfected with human FcεRIα.

8) Histamine release from isolated foreskin mast cells.

9) When criteria for "positive" was set so as to exclude all data of all healthy controls.

10) Histamine release from skin slices.

More selective immunotherapeutic strategies might include administration of blocking humanized structure-based peptides recognizing the antibody-binding sites on the α-chain. Down regulation of the εRI population density on mast cells can be achieved by administration of anti-IgE antibodies reactive with the C_3 domain of the IgE heavy chain (MacGlashan et al., 1987) so it is of considerable interest that there have increasing number of reports of the effectiveness of omalizumab (anti-IgE) for both spontaneous and physical urticarias. Understanding the mechanism of action of omalizumab in urticaria should provide further insights into the pathogenesis of the disease.

References

Adachi J, Aoki T, Yamatodani A (1994) Demonstration of sweat allergy in cholinergic urticaria. J Dermatol Sci 7:142–149

Adams DD (1988) Long-acting thyroid stimulator: how receptor autoimmunity was discovered. J Autoimmunity 1:3–9

Asero R, Tedeschi A, Lorini M, Salimbeni R, Zanoletti T, Miadonna A (2001) Chronic urticaria: novel clinical and serological aspects. Clin Exp Allergy 31:1105–1110

Bentley-Phillips CB, Black AK, Greaves MW (1976) Induced tolerance in cold urticaria caused by cold-evoked histamine release. Lancet ii:63–66

Black AK, Lawlor F, Greaves MW (1996) Consensus meeting on the definition of physical urticarias and urticarial vasculitis. Clin Exp Dermatol 21:424–426

Black AK (2004) Physical and Cholinergic Urticarias. In: Urticaria and Angioedema. Eds Malcolm W Greaves, Allen P Kaplan. Marcel Dekker, New York, (2004) chapter 8, pp 171–214

Borzova E, Rutherford A, Konstatninou K, Leslie K, Grattan CEH (2008) Narrow-band ultraviolet B phototherapy is beneficial in antihistamine-resistant symptomatic dermographism. J Am Acad Dermatol 59:752–757

Bunselmeyer B, Laubach HJ, Schiller M, Stanke M, Luger TA, Brehler R (2009) Incremental build-up food challenge – a new diagnostic approach to evaluate pseudoallergic reactions in chronic urticaria: a pilot study: stepwise food challenge in chronic Clin Exp Allergy39:116–26

Burova GP, Mallet AI, Greaves MW (1998) Is Helicobacter pylori a cause of chronic urticaria? Br J Dermatol 139 (Suppl):42

Caproni M, Volpi W, Macchia D, Giomi B, Manfredi M, Campi P, Cardinali C, D'Agata A, Fabbri P. (2003) Infiltrating cells and related cytokines in lesional skin of patients with chronic idiopathic urticaria and positive autologous serum skin test. Exp Dermatol 2:621–628

Commens CA, Greaves MW (1978) Tests to establish the diagnosis in cholinergic urticaria. Br J Dermatol 98:47–51

Engler RJM, Squire E, Benson P (1995) Chronic sulphasalazine therapy in the treatment of delayed pressure urticaria and angioedema. Ann Allergy Asthma Immunol 74:155–159

Erbagci Z (2002) The leukotriene receptor antagonist montelukast in the treatment of chronic idiopathic urticaria: a single-blind, placebo-controlled, crossover clinical study. J Allergy Clin Immunol 110:484–848

Fagiolo U, Kricek F, Ruf C, Peserico A, Amadori A, Cancian M (2000) Effects of complement inactivation and IgG depletion on skin reactivity to autologous serum in chronic idiopathic urticaria. J Allergy Clin Immunol 106:567–572

Ferrer M, Kinet JP, Kaplan AP (1998) Comparative studies of functional and binding assays for IgG anti-FcεRIαh (α-subunit) in chronic urticaria. J Allergy Clin Immunol 101:672–676

Fiebiger E, Maurer D, Holubar H, Reininger B, Hartmann G, Woisetschlager M, Stingl G (1995) Serum IgG autoantibodies directed against the alpha chain of FcεRI: a selective marker and pathogenetic factor for a distinct subset of chronic urticaria patients. J Clin Invest 96:2606–2612

Fiebiger E, Hammerschmid F, Stingl G, Maurer D (1998) Anti- FcεRIα autoantibodies in autoimmune-mediated disorders. J Clin Invest 101:243–261

Feinberg JH, Toner CB (2008) Successful treatment of disabling cholinergic urticaria. Mil Med 173:217–20

Fukunaga A, Bito T, Tsuru K, Oohashi A, Yu X, Ichihashi M, Nishigori C, Horikawa T (2005) Responsiveness to autologous sweat and serum in cholinergic urticaria classifies its clinical subtypes. J Allergy Clin Immunol 116:3970402

Fung-Leung W-P, Sousa-Hitzien JD, Ishaque A (1996) Transgenic mice expressing the human high affinity immunoglobulin (Ig)E receptor α chain, respond to human IgE in mast cell degranulation and allergic reactions. J Exp Med 183:49–56

Grattan CEH, Wallington TB, Warin RP (1986) A serological mediator in chronic idiopathic urticaria: a clinical immunological and histological evaluation. Br J Dermatol 114:583–590

Grattan CEH, Francis DM, Hide M, Greaves MW (1991) Detection of circulating histamine releasing autoantibodies with functional properties of anti-IgE in chronic urticaria. Clin Exp Allergy 21:695–704

Grattan CEH, Francis DM, Slater NGP, Greaves MW (1992) Plasmapheresis for severe unremitting chronic urticaria. Lancet 339:1078–1080

Grattan CEH, Francis DM (1999) Autoimmune urticaria. Advances Dermatol 15, 311–340

Grattan CEH, O'Donnell BF, Francis DM, Niimi N, Barlow RJ, Seed PT, Black AK, Greaves MW (2000) Randomised double blind study of cyclosporin in chronic idiopathic urticaria. Br J Dermatol 143:365–372

Grattan CEH (2003) Aspirin sensitivity and urticaria. Clin Exp Dermatol 28:123–127

Grattan CEH, Humphreys F (2007) Guidelines for evaluation and management of urticaria in adults and children. Br J Dermatol 157:1116–23

Greaves MW (1995) Current concepts in chronic urticaria. New Eng J Med 332:1767–1772

Greaves MW (2000a) Management of urticaria. Hosp Med 61:463–469

Greaves MW (2000b) Chronic urticaria. J Allergy Clin Immunol 105:664–672

Greaves MW (2001) Chronic idiopathic urticaria (CIU) and Helicobacter pylori – not directly causative, but could there be a link? Allergy Clin Immunol Internat 13:23–26

Hayashi S Hashimoto S (1999) Anti-inflammatory actions of new antihistamines. Clin Exp Allergy 29:1593–1596

Henz BM, Zuberbier T (1998) Causes of urticaria. pp 20–38. in Urtcaria eds Henz BM, Zuberbier T, Grabbe J, Monroe E. Springer, Verlag Berlin Heidelberg

Herxheimer A (1956) The nervous pathway mediating cholinergic urticaria. Clin Sci 15:195–205

Hide M, Francis DM, Grattan CH, Greaves MW (1993) Autoantibodies against the high affinity IgE receptor as a cause for histamine release in chronic urticaria. New Eng J Med 328:1599–1604

Hide M, Francis DM, Grattan CEH, Barr RM, Winkelmann RK, Greaves MW (1994) The pathogenesis of chronic urticaria: new evidence suggests an autoimmune basis and implications for treatment. Clin Exp Allergy 24:624–627

Hide M, Francis DM, Barr RM and Greaves MW (1995) Skin mast cell activation by autoantibodies in urticaria and therapeutic implications. in Biological and Molecular Aspects of Mast Cell and Basophil Differentiation and Function. eds. Kitamura Y, Yamamoto S, Galli SJ, Greaves MW. pp 183–192, Raven Press, New York

Hirschmann JV, Lawlor F, English SJC, Lowback JB, Winkelmann RK, Greaves MW (1987) Cholinergic urticaria. Arch Dermatol 123:462–467

Holgate ST Bradding P Sampson AP (1996) Leukotriene antagonists and synthesis inhibitors: new directions in asthma therapy. J Allergy Clin Immunol 98:1–13

Horn MP, Gerster T, Ochensberger B, Derer T, Kricek F, Jouvin MH, Kinet JP, Tschernig T, Vogel M, Stadler BM, Miescher SM (1999) Human anti-FcepsilonRIalpha autoantibodies isolated from healthy donors cross-react with tetanus toxoid. Eur J Immunol 29:1139–1148

Juhlin L, Michaelsson G (1969) Cutaneous reactions to kallikrein, bradykinin and histamine in healthy subjects and in patients with urticaria. Acta Derm Venereol (Stockh) 49:26–36

Kanazawa K, Yaoita H, Tsuda F, Okamoto H. (1996) Hepatitis C virus infection in patients with urticaria. J Am Acad Dermatol 35:195–198

Kaplan AP, et al. 2008 Treatment of chronic autoimmune urticaria with Omalizumab. J Allergy Clin Immnol; 122:569–573

Keahey TM, Greaves MW (1980) Cold urticaria: dissociation of cold-evoked histamine release and urticaria following cold challenge. Arch Dermatol 116:174–177

Kermani F, Niimi N, Francis DM, Barr RM, Black AK, Greaves MW (1995) Characterisation of a novel mast cell-specific histamine-releasing activity in chronic idiopathic urticaria. J Invest Dermatol 105:452

Kikuchi Y, Kaplan AP (2001) Mechanisms of autoimmune activation of basophils in chronic urticaria. J Allergy Clin Immunol 107:1056–1062

Kikuchi Y, Kaplan AP (2002) A role for C5a in augmenting IgG-dependent histamine release from basophils in chronic urticaria. J Allergy Clin Immunol 109:114–118

Konstantinou GN, Asero R, Maurer M, Sabroe RA, Schmid-Grendelmeier P, Grattan CE (2009) EAACI/GA(2)LEN task force consensus report: the autologous serum skin test in urticaria. Allergy 64:1256–68

Koro O, Dover JS, Francis DM, Black AK, Kelly RW, Barr RM, Greaves MW (1986) Release of prostaglandin D^2 and histamine in a case of localised heat urticaria, and effect of treatment. Br J Dermatol 115:721–728

Lawlor F, Black AK, Milford Ward A, Morris R, Greaves MW (1989a) Delayed pressure urticaria: objective evaluation of a variable disease using a dermographometer and assessment of treatment using colchicine. Br J Dermatol 120:403–408

Lawlor F, Black AK, Breathnach AS, Greaves MW (1989b) Vibratory angioedema: lesion induction, clinical features, ultrastructural findings and response to therapy. Br J Dermatol 120:93–99

Lawrence CM, Jorizzo JL, Black AK, Coutts A, Greaves MW (1981) Cholinergic urticaria associated with angioedema. Br J Dermatol 105:543–550

Leznoff A, Josse RG, Denburg J, Dolovich J (1983) Association of chronic urticaria and angioedema with thyroid autoimmunity. Arch Dermatol 119:636–640

Leznoff A, Sussman GL (1989) Syndrome of idiopathic chronic urticaria and angioedema with thyroid autoimmunity – a study of 90 patients. J Allergy Clin Immunol 84:66–71

Lowman MA, Rees PH, Benyon RC (1988) Human mast cell heterogeneity. Histamine release from mast cells dispersed from skin, lung, adenoids, tonsils and colon in response to IgE-dependent and non-immunological stimuli. J Allergy Clin Immunol 81:590–597

MacGlashan DW, Bochner BS, Adelman DC (1987) Down regulation of FcεRI expression on human basophils during in vivo treatment of atopic human patients with anti-IgE antibody. J Immunol 158:1438–1445

Magerl M, Pisarevskaja D, Scheufele R, Zuberbier T, Maurer M (2010) Effects of a pseudoallergen-free diet on chronic spontaneous urticaria: a prospective trial Allergy 65:78–83

May CD (1985) Are confusion and controversy about food hypersensitivity really necessary? J Allergy Clin Immunol 75:329–333

Misch K, Black AK, Greaves MW (1983) Almosauri T, Stanworth DR, Passive transfer of cold urticaria to monkeys. Acta Derm Venereol (Stockh) 63:163–164

Morioke S, Takahagi S, Iwamoto K, Shindo H, Mihara S, Kameyoshi Y, Hide M (2010) Pressure challenge test and histopathological inspections for 17 Japanese cases with clinically diagnosed delayed pressure urticaria. Arch Dermatol Res [Epub ahead of print]

10

Murphy GM, Black AK, Greaves MW (1983) Persisting cholinergic erythema – a variant of cholinergic urticaria. Br J Dermatol 109:343–348
Murphy GM, Zollman PE, Greaves MW, Winkelmann RK (1987) Symptomatic dermographism
(factitious urticaria) – passive transfer experiments from human to monkey. Br J Dermatol
116:801–804
Niimi N, Francis DM, Kermani F, Black AK, Barr RM, Grattan CEH, Greaves MW (1996) Dermal
mast cell activation by autoantibodies against the high affinity IgE receptor in chronic urticaria.
J Invest Dermatol 106:1001–1006
O'Donnell BF, Black AK (1995) Urticarial vasculitis. Int Angiol 14:166–174
O'Donell BF, Lawlor F, Simpson J, Morgan M, Greaves MW (1997) The impact of chronic urticaria
on quality of life. Br J Dermatol 136:197–201
O'Donnell BF, Barr RM, Black AK, Francis DM, Greaves MW (1998) Intravenous immunoglobulin
in chronic autoimmune urticaria. Br J Dermatol 138:101–6
O'Donnell BF, O'Neill CM, Francis DM, Niimi N, Barr RM, Barlow RJ, Greaves MW, Welsh K
(1999) Human leucocyte antigen class II associations in chronic idiopathic urticaria. Br J Der-
matol 140:853–858
Ohnishi-Inoue Y, Mitsuya K, Horio T (1998) Aspirin-sensitive urticaria: provocation with a leukotriene receptor antagonist. Br J Dermatol 138:483–485
Ozkaya-Bayazit E, Demir K, Ozgaroglu E, Kaymakoglu S, Ozamagar G (1998) Helicobacter pylori
eradication in patients with chronic urticaria. Arch Dermatol 314:1165–1166
Pachlopnik JM, Horn MP, Fux M, Dahinden M, Mandallaz M, Schneeberger D, Baldi L, Vogel M,
Stadler BM, Miescher SM (2004) Natural anti-FcεRIα autoantibodies may interfere with diagnostic tests for autoimmune urticaria. J Autoimmun 22:43–51
Pachor ML, Lunardi C, Nicolis F, Cortina P, Accordini C, Marchl G, Corrocher R, de Sandre G
(1987) Utilita del propranololo nel trattamento dell'orticaria colinergica. Clin Ter 120:205–210
Pacor ML, Di Lorenzo G, Corrocher R. (2001) Efficacy of leukotriene receptor antagonist in
chronic urticaria. A double-blind, placebo-controlled comparison of treatment with montelukast and cetirizine in patients with chronic urticaria with intolerance to food additive and/or
acetylsalicylic acid. Clin Exp Allergy 31:1607–1614
Pandey V, Mihara S, Fensome-Green A, Bolsover S, Cockcroft S (2004) Monomeric IgE stimulates
NFAT translocation into the nucleus, a rise in cytosol Ca^{2+}, degranulation, and membrane ruf-
fling in the cultured rat basophilic leukemia-2H3 mast cell line. J Immunol 172:4048–4058
Pastorello EA (1995) Evaluating new tests for the diagnosis of food allergy. Allergy 50:289–291
Pirisi A (2000) Antihistamines impair driving as much as alcohol. Lancet 355:905
Ramsay CA (1977) Solar urticaria treatment by inducing tolerance to artificial radiation and natu-
ral light. Arch Dermatol 113:1222–1225
Reimers A, Pichler C, Helbling A, Pichler WJ, Yawalkar N (2002) Zafirlukast has no beneficial ef-
fects in the treatment of chronic urticaria. Clin Exp Allergy 32:1763–1768
Rivera J (2002) Molecular adapters in FcεRI signaling and the allergic response. Curr Opin Immunol 14:688–693
Rorsman H (1961) Basopenia in urticaria. Acta Allergol 16:185–215
Sabroe RA, Francis DM, Barr RM, Black AK, Greaves MW (1998) Anti- FcεRI autoantibodies
and basophil histamine release ability in chronic idiopathic urticaria. J Allergy Clin Immunol
102:651–658
Sabroe RA, Seed PT, Francis DM, Barr RM, Black AK, Greaves MW (1999a) Chronic idiopathic
urticaria: comparison of clinical features of patients with or without anti- FcεRI or anti-IgE
autoantibodies. J Am Acad Dermatol 40:443–450
Sabroe RA, Poon E, Orchard GE, Lane D, Francis DM, Barr RM, Black AK, Greaves MW (1999b)
Cutaneous inflammatory cell infiltrate in chronic idiopathic urticaria: comparison of patients
with and without anti-FcεRIα or anti-IgE autoantibodies. J Allergy Clin Immunol 103:484–493

Sabroe RA, Grattan CEH, Francis DM, Black AK, Barr RM, Greaves MW (1999c) The autologous serum skin test: a screening test for autoantibodies in chronic idiopathic urticaria. Br J Dermatol 140:446–452

Sabroe RA, Fiebiger E, Francis DM, Maurer D, Seed PT, Grattan CE, Black AK, Stingl G, Greaves MW, Barr RM (2002) Classification of anti-FcεRI and anti-IgE autoantibodies in chronic idiopathic urticaria and correlation with disease severity. J Allergy Clin Immunol 110:492–499

Schnyder B, Helbling A, Pichler WJ (1999) Chronic idiopathic urticaria: natural course and association with Helicobacter pylori infection. Int Arch Allergy Immunol 119:60–63

Siebenhaar F, Degener F, Zuberbier T, Martus P, Maurer M (2009) High-dose desloratadine decreases wheal volume and improves cold provocation thresholds compared with standard-dose treatment in patients with acquired cold urticaria: a randomized, placebo-controlled, crossover study J Allergy Clin Immunol.123:672–9

Sibbald RG, Black AK, Eady RAJ, James M, Greaves MW (1981) Aquagenic Urticaria: evidence of a cholinergic and histaminergic basis. Br J Dermatol 105:297–302

Staevska M, Popov TA, Kralimarkova T, Lazarova C, Kraeva S, Popova D, Church DS, Dimitrov V, Church MK (2010) The effectiveness of levocetirizine and desloratadine in up to 4 times conventional doses in difficult-to-treat urticaria J Allergy Clin Immunol.125:676–82

Smith CH, Atkinson B, Morris RW, Hayes N, Foreman JC, Lee TH (1992) Cutaneous responses to vasoactive intestinal polypeptide in chronic idiopathic urticaria. Lancet. 339:91–93

Tam SW, Demissie S, Thomas D, Daeron M (2004) A bispecific antibody against human IgE and human FcγRII that inhibits antigen-induced histamine release by human mast cells and basophils. Allergy 59:772–780

Takahagi S, Tanaka T, Ishii K, Suzuki H, Kameyoshi Y, Shindo H, Hide M (2009) Sweat antigen induces histamine release from basophils of patients with cholinergic urticaria associated with atopic diathesis. Br J Dermatol 160:426–428

Tanaka T, Kameyoshi Y, Hide M (2006) Analysis of the prevalence of subtypes of urticaria and angioedema. Arerugi 55:134–139

Tong LJ, Balakrishnan G, Kochan JP, Kinet J-P, Kaplan AP (1997) Assessment of autoimmunity in chronic urticaria. J Allergy Clin Immunol 99:461–465

Ujiie H, Shimizu T, Natsuga K, Arita K, Tomizawa K, Shimizu H (2006) Severe cholinergic urticaria successfully treated with scopolamine butylbromide in addition to antihistamines. Clin Exp Dermatol 31:588–602

Wedi B, Wagner S, Werfil T, Mann MP, Kapp A (1998) Prevalence of Helicobacter pylori-associated gastritis in chronic urticaria. Int Arch Allergy Immunol 116:288–294

Wolfrom E, Chene G, Boisseau H, Beylot C, Geniaux M, Taleb A (1995) Chronic urticaria and Toxocara canis. Lancet 345:196

Wong E, Eftekhari N, Greaves MW, Milford Ward A (1987) Beneficial effects of danazol on symptoms and laboratory changes in cholinergic urticaria. Br J Dermatol 116:353–356

Ying S, Kikuchi Y, Meng Q, Kay AB, Kaplan AP (2002) TH1/TH2 cytokines and inflammatory cells in skin biopsy specimens from patients with chronic idiopathic urticaria: comparison with the allergen-induced late-phase cutaneous reaction. J Allergy Clin Immunol 109:694–700

Zweiman B, Valenzano M, Atkins PC, Tanus T, Getsy JA (1996) Characteristics of histamine-releasing activity in sera of patients with chronic idiopathic urticaria. J Allergy Clin Immunol 98:89–98

Zuberbier T, Greaves MW, Juhlin L, Kobza-Black A, Maurer D, Stingl G, Henz BM (2001) Definition, classification, and routine diagnosis of urticaria: a consensus report. J Invest Dermatol Symp Proc. 6:123–127

Zuberbier T, Asero R, Bindslev-Jensen C, Canonica W, Church M K, Gimenez-Arnau A, Grattan CEH, Kapp A, Merk HF, Rogala B, Saini S, Sanchez-Borges M, Schmid-Grendelmeier P, Schunemann H, Staubach P, Vena GA, Wedi B, Maurer M (2009) EAACI/GA2LEN/EDF/WAO guideline: definition, classification and diagnosis of urticaria. Allergy 64:1417–26

10

Lichen Planus, Lichenoid Eruptions and Cutaneous Graft-Versus-Host-Reaction

11

Miklós Simon Jr.

Introduction

Lichen planus (LP) is a noncontagious, inflammatory, pruritic, papular mucocutaneous disease of unknown etiology that most commonly affects middle-aged adults. In 1869 Erasmus Wilson described the cutaneous "leichen planus" in 50 case histories and recorded oral lesions in 3 of his patients (Wilson, 1869). Weyl and Wickham noted the surface markings on the papules and pointed out the importance of these marks in establishing the clinical diagnosis of LP (Weyl, 1885; Wickham, 1895). After Neumann, Weyl, Caspary, and Poór, Darier described the histopathology of LP (Darier, 1909), the only important addition has been the demonstration of "colloid bodies" at the dermoepidermal junction by Thyresson and Moberger (1957). The direct immunofluorescence findings in LP have been extensively studied for the first time by Barthelmes and Haustein (1970) and Baart de la Faille Kuyper and Baart de la Faille (1974) as well.

LP has a worldwide distribution. The prevalence of LP in the general population is of the order of 0.9 to 1.2% (Scully & El-Kom, 1985). It appears initially during the fifth or sixth decade and affect women preferentially. LP of childhood is unusual, but familial cases have been observed (Copeman, 1978). A weak association with HLA-A3, B8, B16, B35 and a significantly increased HLA-DR1 (DRB1* 0101) antigen frequency has been reported in patients with idiopathic LP (Simon jr et al., 1984; Powell et al., 1986; La Nasa et al., 1995). In addition, TNF-α, IFN-γ, and IL-18 gene polymorphisms contributing to susceptibility to LP were described, very recently (Carrozzo et al., 2004; Bai et al., 2007).

The cause of LP remained undissolved. Evidence points to the possibility that an alteration of epidermal cell antigens (bacterial/viral infections, contact sensitizers, trauma etc.) induces a cell-mediated immune response similar to that seen in cutaneous graft-versus-host-reaction (cGVHR). Drugs may induce lichenoid eruptions (LDE). LDE (probably by an allergic type IV reaction) produces mucocutaneous lesions that are clinically and histologically indistinguishable from (idiopathic) LP. LDE usually appear as a symmetric eruption on the trunk and extremities and sometimes fail to exhibit classic Wickham striae. Medications commonly associated with the development of LDE are antimalarials, gold, penicillamine, methyldopa, ß-blockers, angiotensin-converting enzyme inhibitors, spironolactone, lithium, cinnarizine, nonsteroidal anti-inflammatory drugs, thiazide, phenothiazine derivatives, allopurinol, tetracycline, and sulfonylurea agents (Ellgehausen et al., 1998).

There have been several reports of patients with LP in association with autoimmune disorders, notably with systemic lupus erythematosus, thymoma, myasthenia gravis, dermatomyositis, ulcerative colitis, primary biliary cirrhosis, chronic active hepatitis, pemphigus vulgaris, dermatitis herpetiformis, bullous pemphigoid, alopecia areata, vitiligo, Sjögren's syndrome, morphea, and systemic sclerosis suggesting there may also be an immunological basis for classical LP (Simon jr, 1985, review).

Immune Pathogenesis

Direct immunofluorescence studies of lesional and uninvolved skin in patients with LP demonstrated an irregular deposition of fibrin and complement along the dermoepidermal junction, especially in the dermal papillary region and around hair follicles, in the active papular lesions. The colloid bodies fluoresced brightly with IgM and with other immunoglobulins and complement components (Barthelmes & Haustein, 1970; Baart de la Faille-Kuyper & Baart de la Faille, 1974; Simon jr et al., 1983). In 1984, Olsen et al. described an LP-specific antigen (LPSA) found by indirect immunofluorescence in the granular or spinous layer of the epidermis of lesional tissue (Olsen et al., 1984). The circulating anti-LPSA antibodies are more likely to be markers of the disease than to be causative.

Touraine et al. (1975) and Saurat et al. (1975) reported a lichenoid eruption that occurred in two men who had received allogenic bone marrow transplants from their sisters. Now, it seems likely that this lichenoid tissue reaction is a later and more chronic manifestation of a GVHR in which the target appears to be the basal cell layer of the epidermis. The clinical picture and the histologic as well as direct immunofluorescence findings were essentially the same as those in idiopathic LP. Recently, immunopathological investigations of lesional skin in GVHR patients revealed intraepidermal a predominance of $CD3^+CD8^+CD11a^+CD16^+CD25^+CDw137^+$T-lymphocytes and a net-like specific positive staining when exposed to HLA-DR, CD54, CD36, CD21, CD16, and CD1 monoclonal antibodies (Simon jr & Hunyadi, 1992; Anasetti, 2004). Cutaneous GVHR occurs most commonly in patients undergoing bone marrow transplantation, following peripheral blood stem cell transfer, after solid organ transplant, but is also seen in fetuses obtaining maternal leukocytes via maternal-fetal transfusion and in blood transfusions transplanting immunocompetent cells into immunodeficient recipients. The precise pathophysiology of GVHR is not known. However, several studies demonstrate that acute GVHR occurring in humans is induced by donor T-lymphocytes reactive against recipient cells expressing different tissue antigens. TNF-α plays a key role in this process. On the other hand, T-cells recognizing host-specific antigens are present in the blood and the skin of patients with chronic GVHR (Aractingi & Chosidow, 1998). Recently, a significant association between polymorphism of the TNF-α, IFN-γ, IL-10, and IL-6 genes and the development of severe GVHR has been demonstrated (Takahashi et al., 2000; Cavet et al., 2001).

The pathologic process in LP is a cell-mediated response localized to the dermoepidermal junction and characterized by degeneration of keratinocytes in the basal layer and disruption of the basement membrane. The basement membrane zone is an interface composed of epidermal basal cell surface glycoproteins, laminin, fibronectin, type IV collagen, and supporting mesenchymal extracellular proteoglycans. These proteins and oligosaccharides may be identified immunohistochemically by monospecific antibodies and high-affinity lectins, respectively. Evidence from oral LP suggests that CD8$^+$ lesional cytotoxic T-lymphocytes recognize a LP-specific antigen associated with MHC class I on lesional keratinocytes. The nature of this antigen is unknown. The antigen may be an autoreactive peptide, defining LP as an autoimmune disease. On the other hand, it may represent an exogenous antigen (viral or other infectious agent, contact allergen, drug), or an unidentified immunogenic target (Sugerman et al., 2000).

The earliest features of LP are changes in, and close to the epidermal basal cell layer, which may occur in the absence of demonstrable changes in the dermis. Studies concerning the evolution of lesions of LP demonstrated, that one of the first observable changes is the appearance of Langerhans cells (Ragaz & Ackerman, 1981). Shortly after the appearance of Langerhans cells, basal keratinocytes undergo flattening and hydropic changes, and their nuclei become injured at an early phase of the mitotic cycle. The changes of basal cells in LP are accompanied by a dense mononuclear inflammatory T-lymphocyte infiltration at the subepidermal area and at the dermoepidermal interface, the location of which makes a relationship most likely to the basal epithelial changes. T-lymphocytes may become activated via antigen-presenting cells or accessory cells (epidermal keratinocytes) in association with members of the MHC II and various cytokines. CD4$^+$ T-lymphocytes may also propagate CD8$^+$ cytotoxic T-lymphocytes (cellular cooperation, release of specific cytokines).

In the course of examining keratinocyte-lymphocyte interactions in vitro, Nickoloff et al. (1988) reported prominent adherence by both allogeneic and autologous T-lymphocytes and monocytes to cultured keratinocytes after pretreatment of keratinocytes with IFN-γ. The binding of these mononuclear cells to IFN-γ-treated keratinocytes involves the lymphocyte function-associated antigen-1 (LFA-1) molecule on T-cells and the intercellular adhesion molecule-1 (ICAM-1) induced by IFN-γ or TNF-α on keratinocytes (Griffiths et al., 1989). Biopsy specimens from lesional skin of LP patients exhibited intraepidermal specific positive stainings when exposed to ICAM-1 (CD54), HLA-DR, NF-kappaB, CXCL9, 10, 11, CD1, and CD120a antibodies (Malmnäs Tjernlund, 1980; Simon jr, 1988; Griffiths et al., 1989; Simon jr & Gruschwitz, 1997; Iijima et al., 2003; Santoro et al., 2003). CD54 and vascular cell adhesion molecule-1 (VCAM-1) expressions in lesional keratinocytes in LP, similar to that in various cutaneous inflammatory conditions (Lange Wantzin et al., 1988; Griffiths et al., 1989), may be important initiators of keratinocyte-lymphocyte interaction, whereas HLA-DR expression in keratinocytes seems to be more important in postadherence antigenic recognition and/or presentation to activated T-lymphocytes (Messadi et al., 1988).

In LP, the cellular infiltrate is predominantly composed of T-lymphocytes and monocytes as detected by hetero- and monoclonal antibodies, nonspecific esterase, lysosyme, and, selectively by peanut agglutinin lectin (Walker, 1976). The role of these T-lymphocytes, probably antigen activated T-cells, is not quite clear, however, autoradiographic investigations revealed a three to four times higher lymphoblast proliferation rate in

LP lesions than in psoriasis or contact dermatitis (Lachapelle & De la Brassine, 1973). Langerhans cells in the epidermis and dermis may also be identified with the use of light microscopy by formalin resistent sulfhydril dependent nucleoside triphosphatase, ultrastructurally by the presence of Birbeck's granules, immunohistochemically by monoclonal antibodies or S-100 calf brain protein. Their participation in LP, and close vicinity to the T-lymphocytes, combined with local and systemic release of various cytokines (e. g. TNF-α, IFN-γ, RANTES, IL-1-α, IL-6, IL-8) both in the skin and in the serum, would seem to provide antigen processing activity and the induction of a hypersensitivity reaction (Giannotti et al., 1983; Soehnchen et al., 1992; Zhang et al., 2008). In addition, soluble mediators of cell damage produced by T-cells may induce keratinocyte apoptosis and formation of colloid bodies.

Examinations of different lymphocyte subpopulations in cutaneous inflammatory infiltrate of active LP revealed the existence of T-lymphocytes of both the CD4+ and the CD8+ phenotypes. In early phases of LP lesions, the lymphocytes observed in close contact with large, non-lymphoid cells, were identified as CD4+T-cells (Bhan et al., 1982). In the late phases of LP lesions, intraepidermal lymphocytes almost constantly exhibited CD8-positivity (Simon jr & Keller, 1984). The dermoepidermal interface, from the pathogenetic point of view probably the most important zone, showed a predominance of HLA-DR+CD25+LFA-1+TNF-R+CCR5+CXCR3+CCL5+CXCL9+CXCL10+CD3+CD8+TCRγδ+T-lymphocytes (Malmnäs Tjernlund, 1980; Simon jr & von den Driesch, 1994; Gadenne et al., 1994; Simon jr & Gruschwitz, 1997; Iijima et al., 2003).

ICAM-1 (CD54) is a ligand for LFA-1 on the surface of lymphocytes, which enhances the interaction of lymphocytes with the antigen presenting cells, and activated, lesional keratinocytes. Laminin-5 as well as collagen types IV and VII are increased in lesional LP, thus allowing enhanced binding of ß1-integrin-positive lymphocytes to the basement membrane. The close interaction between lymphocytes and basement membrane leeds to release of certain metalloproteinases produced by lymphocytes to alter extracellular matrix proteins, and the process eventuates in basement membrane disruption, apoptosis, and subepidermal cleft formation. TNF-α upregulates the expression of matrix metalloproteinase (MMP)-9 in lesional T-lymphocytes, thus further enhancing basement membrane disruption and triggering apoptosis (Ramirez-Amador et al., 1996; Gunduz et al., 2006; Zhou et al., 2009).

The exact mechanisms contributing to apoptosis of keratinocytes in LP are not completely known. Possible mechanisms include T-cell surface CD95L binding CD95 on the keratinocyte, T-cell secreted TNF-α binding to the TNF-αR1 receptor on the keratinocyte surface, and T-cell secreted granzyme B entering the keratinocyte via perforin-induced membrane pores as well, resulting in activation of the keratinocyte caspase cascade, leading to keratinocyte apoptosis (Sugerman et al., 2000; Ammar et al., 2008).

Immunological characterization of different T-lymphocyte subpopulations in peripheral blood of LP patients, by means of the indirect immunofluorescence technique using monoclonal antibodies, clearly documented a reduced percentage of the CD8+T-cell subset, normal pan T-, CD4+T-, and B-lymphocyte values as compared to the controls (Simon jr & Keller, 1984). The phytohemagglutinin response of lymphocytes from LP patients was in the same range as that of healthy controls (Cerni et al., 1976).

A markedly diminished, to the severity of the disease related natural killer cell activity against K562 target cells was revealed in patients with extensive erosive LP of oral mucosa, generalized acute eruptive and moderate cutaneous LP as compared to that of patients with non-erosive LP of oral mucosa and healthy controls. IL-2 failed to restore completely reduced natural killer cell activities in all groups of patients investigated (Simon jr et al., 1989).

The in vitro effect of peripheral blood lymphocytes on syngeneic oral epithelial cells using a modified ^{51}Cr release macro-assay in patients with LP resulted in a substantial lymphocytotoxicity in comparison to the controls. This positive lymphocytotoxicity is probably generated by sensitized effector lymphocytes via specific recognition of foreign antigenic structures on syngeneic oral target cells (Simon jr et al., 1983). Similar results were found using CD8+ T-cell lines and clones cultured from LP lesions against autologous lesional keratinocytes, recently (Sugerman et al., 2000). These findings may be regarded as a functional evidence for the pathogenetic role of CD8$^+$ cytotoxic T-cells in the course of LP.

Clinical features

Lichen planus, lichenoid eruptions

The cutaneous lesions of LP consist of pruritic faintly erythematous to violaceous, flat-topped, polygonal papules, occasionally showing central umbilication. A thin, transparent scale may be discerned atop the lesions. A network of fine white lines or puncta referred to as Wickham striae is present in many well-developed papules (Fig. 1).

LP lesions are usually distributed symmetrically, the disease tends to involve the flexural areas (wrists, arms, legs), preferentially. The thighs, lumbar area, trunk, neck, and the dorsal surfaces of the hands with the nails may also be affected. The face and scalp are usu-

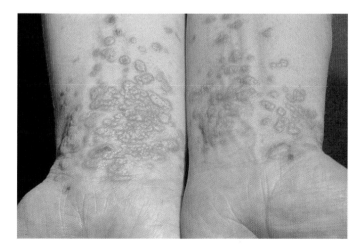

Fig. 1. Typical purple polygonal papules of LP

ally spared in classic LP. Inverse LP affects the axillae, groin, and inframammary regions. Nail changes include longitudinal ridging and splitting of the nail plate, onycholysis, pterygium formation, or complete loss of the nail plate. Mucous membranes are in more than half of the patients additional sites of involvement. Erosive mucosal LP is extremely painful often pursues a chronic course with little tendency to spontaneous resolution. It may predispose to squamous cell carcinoma, but the risk is fairly low. In generalized LP, the eruption often spreads within 1–3 month from onset of the disease. Koebner's isomorphic response (LP develops at the site of exogenous irritation) is common (Fox & Odom, 1985; Boyd & Neldner, 1991).

Clinical variants

Several distinctive variants of LP need to be recognized, since lack of characteristic skin changes in these cases makes the clinical diagnosis difficult. The prototypic papule of LP can be altered / modified in morphology, configuration or anatomic distribution.

Linear LP. Linear group of typical LP papules, are usually located on the extremities. The linear pattern may develop secondary to trauma in zosteriform or segmental arrangement or even in the site of healed herpes zoster.

Annular LP. Annular lesions develop from a ring of typical LP papules that progress peripherally and produce central clearing. Annular lesions are common on the penis and scrotum but may occur on the trunk or extremities.

Bullous LP. Rare variant of LP characterized by the development of bullae on preexisting LP papules. The bullae, which appear mostly on the extremities with mild constitutional symptoms, usually resolve in a few month. Bullae arising from normal skin in LP patients are more characteristic of lichen planus pemphigoides, which is a unique condition with circulating IgG autoantibodies reacting to 180- and / or 200-kDa antigen within the basement membrane zone.

Erosive / ulcerative LP. This is a very rare variant of LP presenting with chronic, painful bullae and ulcerations of the soles of the feet, and sometimes of the mucous membranes associated with cicatricial alopecia of the scalp and permanent loss of the toenails. The lesions on the feet tend not to heal but have a definite risk of development of a squamous cell carcinoma in the chronic ulcerations.

Hypertrophic LP. The extensor sides of the shins and interphalangeal joints are preferentially affected with highly pruritic, lichenified, violaceous, or hyperpigmented plaques (LP verrucous). The lesions are often symmetric, sometimes show accentuated, elevated follicle swellings and chalky hyperkeratoses. Scarring occurs after healing of the lesions. Malignant degeneration is relatively common.

Atrophic LP. In some cases, atrophy of LP papules may produce sharply demarcated, whitish, atrophic maculae. These lesions can coalesce and form larger plaques most commonly on the trunk or lower extremities. This LP variant is rare and needs to be distinguished from lichen sclerosus et atrophicus and guttate morphea.

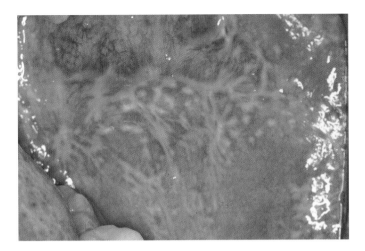

Fig. 2. Reticular LP in buccal mucosa.

Follicular LP. This form of LP may occur alone or simultaneously with other types of mucocutaneous changes of LP. It forms isolated or aggregated, pinhead-sized red papules, which carry a conical acuminated hyperkeratosis (LP acuminatus). Sites of predilection include the trunk, neck, sacral region, and the proximal extremities. Follicular LP of the scalp also occurs in an isolated form and leads to scarred alopecia (LP follicularis decalvans, frontal fibrosing alopecia). This condition affects more women than men. Perifollicular erythema and acuminate keratotic plugs are characteristic features. The symptom combination of follicular LP on the trunk and on the scalp with nail dystrophy has been described as Lassueur-Graham-Little syndrome.

Actinic LP. This variant is more common in the tropics, especially in children and young adults on sun-exposed parts of the body such as the face, the back of the hands, the lower forearms, and the chest. The extremely pruritic papular lesions are hyperpigmented with violaceous-brown color, which frequently show annular configuration. The course is subacute, and the condition tends to heal spontaneously.

Mucosal LP. This form of LP can affect the mucosal sites of mouth, glans penis, vulva, vagina, collum uteri, anus, conjunctiva, nose, larynx, trachea, esophagus, stomach, urethra, bladder, and tympanic membrane.

Oral LP is present in some 60–70% of dermatological patients with LP. As the sole manifestation of the disease, it makes up 15% to 35% of the patient populace. The buccal mucosa (bilateral) and the tongue are most often affected but the gums, floor of the mouth, palate, and lips have also been documented. The mucosal lesions consist of lacy, reticulated white streaks (Fig. 2), white papules and plaques, and erythematous, atrophic or ulcerated patches with painful, burning sensations.

Particular clinical forms are characteristic for certain regions of the oral mucosa. Reticular LP is the most common type. It affects the buccal mucosa predominantly. The margins of the tongue show generally lace-like and / or erosive LP, the dorsal surface exhibits usually round, white plaques or smooth atrophic areas. Most cases of carcinoma appear to arise in patients with longstanding erosive / atrophic LP of the tongue or buccal mucosa. Gingival involvement of LP may potentially lead to the picture of desquamative gingivitis (Scully & El-Kom, 1985).

Lesions of the male genitalia are observed in about 25% of cases. The glans penis is most commonly affected, exhibiting annular lesions frequently. Similar changes can occur on the scrotal skin as well. Occasionally, the glans penis has erosive lesions and is the only site of LP involvement (Alinovi et al., 1983). The female genitalia demonstrate generally patches of leukoplakia or erythroplakia, with variable atrophy. Desquamative vaginitis is most commonly due to LP. The labia minora agglutinate and vaginal adhesions in association with burning pain, may prevent sexual intercourse (Edwards & Friedrich jr, 1988; Soper et al., 1988).

Cutaneous graft-versus-host-reaction (cGVHR)

Mucocutaneous lesions of GVHR develops in 20 to 80% of posttransplant cases after allogeneic bone marrow infusion or haemopoietic stem cell transplantation. Cutaneous eruptions of GVHRs occur after autologous and syngeneic transplantation in up to 10% of patients. There are two forms: i) in the acute form the cutaneous eruption begins between the fifth and fiftieth day; ii) in the chronic form appears two to six months after grafting. Some patients experience both forms of cGVHR, sequentially (Harper, 1987).

11

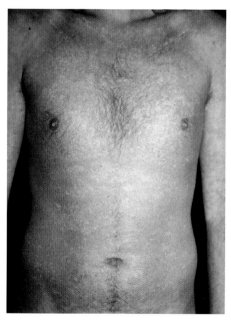

Fig. 3. Disseminated lichenoid GVHR.

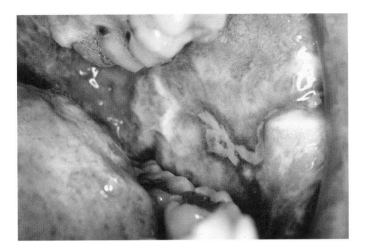

Fig. 4. Erosive buccal lesions in a patient with lichenoid GVHR.

In acute cGVHR the eruption generally begins with tender erythematous macules on the upper trunk, neck, hands, feet, face, and forehead. As a cGVHR evolves, the distribution of erythematous macules increases, becoming confluent over broad body surfaces. At later stages, erythroderma may ensue. Generalized erythroderma with bullae formation and desquamation portend a poor prognosis. The clinical picture of subepidermal bullae with a necrotic roof in these patients greatly resembles toxic epidermal necrolysis. Oral and / or ocular involvement in acute cGVHR may occur but are less common then in chronic cGVHR (Volc-Platzer, 1992; Aractingi & Chosidow, 1998).

The incidence of a chronic cGVHR, divided artificial into lichenoid and sclerodermoid forms, is roughly 25%. This two forms of chronic cGVHR clearly overlap in many patients.

In the lichenoid form, which may also occur soon after transplantation, erythematous to violaceous polygonal papules appear acrally and may be seen on the palms and soles. In addition, lichenoid cGVHR favors the ears, periorbital region, trunk, buttocks, hips, and thighs as well. In some cases lichenoid papules can occur around hair follicles. LP-like cGVHR can also affect the nails, with onychatrophia and pterygium. The disseminated lichenoid eruption in chronic cGVHR is clinically indistinguishable from LP (Fig. 3). Pruritus and postinflammatory hyperpigmentation are also present. Oral involvement is typical, with white lacy patches and / or painful erosions on the tongue and buccal mucosa (Fig. 4).

The sclerodermoid form of a chronic cGVHR greatly resembles scleroderma with variably distributed, hyper- and / or hypopigmented, somewhat atrophic plaques. Some patients develop only few sclerodermoid plaques, other ones develop widespread disease associated with alopecia, chronic cutaneous ischemia with ulceration, joint contractures and debilitating fasciitis. Of note, acrosclerosis and Raynaud phenomenon are uncommon in chronic sclerodermatous GVHR, in contrast to systemic sclerosis. The mucosa of the gums, palate, and lips can become atrophic and occasionally ulcerate. Sicca symptoms often accompany the sclerodermoid form due to diminished salivary and lacrimal output (Volc-Platzer, 1992; Aractingi & Chosidow, 1998).

Despite the apparent simplicity of the traditional classification of GVHR into acute and chronic phases, defined as number of days after transplantation, this separation is not that precise. The lichenoid chronic GVHR may be observed as early as day 30 after transplantation and acute GVHR may appear/persist after day 100 in some cases. Moreover, atypical variants of cGVHR have been described that do not fit into this diagnostic classification either.

Diagnosis

The diagnosis of LP, LDE, cGVHR rests fundamentally on the combination of anamnestic data, clinical, histopathologic, and immunofluorescence/immunohistochemical findings. Special immunophenotypic and T-cell receptor genotypic analyses are sometimes required to define the underlying pathology manifesting as lichenoid dermatitis more precisely.

The clinical differential diagnosis of lichenoid dermatoses, depending on the manifestation of the disease, involves generalized granuloma annulare, psoriasis guttata, papular sarcoid, lichen amyloidosus, scabies, pityriasis rosea, pityriasis rubra pilaris, and papular secondary syphilis. Mucous membrane lesions may be confused with leukoplakia, mucous patches of syphilis, candidiasis, oral hairy leukoplakia, lupus erythematosus, chronic ulcerative stomatitis, paraneoplastic pemphigus, and cicatricial pemphigoid.

Therapy

Lichen planus, lichenoid eruptions

Apart from the very rare instances of possible malignant transformation (ulcerative LP, LP verrucosus, erosive/atrophic mucosal LP), LP is a benign disease with spontaneous remissions and exacerbations. Consequently, any treatment strategy must be safe and unlikely to aggravate the disease. Avoidance of potentially provocative medications (Ellgehausen et al., 1998), unless absolutely required, and minimizing trauma to skin and mucosal tissues are recommended. Patients with actinic LP must be protected by sunscreens. Oral erosive/atrophic LP lesions are painful and are frequently associated with poor oral hygiene. For these patients, good oral hygiene (the use of an antibacterial mouthwash e.g. chlorhexidine) and regular professional dental care need to be encouraged.

Evaluating the efficacy of different forms of treatment in cutaneous LP is difficult since LP tends to regress spontaneously after varying amounts of time. A large variety of topical and systemic therapies are available, and this range of options may be attributed to the chronicity, symptomatology, and variable responsiveness of the disease. In mild cases, treatment should be symptomatic: antihistamines for pruritus and topical glucocorticoids for their antipruritic and anti-inflammatory effects. Severe, acute cases may benefit from a tapered course of systemic glucocorticoids or retinoids for two to eight weeks. Relapses may occur, however, chronic systemic glucocorticoid use should be avoided. Narrowband UVB, ultraviolet A1, PUVA photochemotherapy (or bath PUVA) solely or combined with systemic retinoids may have beneficial effect in such cases. Systemic cyclosporine administration has many side effects, therefore it should be considered as a drug of last resort. Hypertrophic LP may also benefit from intralesional glucocorticoids, or topical glucocorticoids under occlusion, or tar preparations. Peroxisome proliferator-activated receptor gamma agonists seems to be helpful in management of lichen planopilaris of the scalp. Efalizumab and alefacept have been used for generalized or erosive LP. Ulcerative and hypertrophic LP of the palms and soles is frequently disabling and uncomfortable. Use of split-thickness skin grafts to cover these lesions has been proved an effective way to manage such patients (Lendrum, 1974; Simon jr, 1990; Simon jr & Hunyadi, 1990; Simon jr & von den Driesch, 1994; Boyd, 2000; Saricaoglu et al., 2003; Polderman et al., 2004; Fivenson & Mathes, 2006; Mirmirani & Karnik, 2009).

Non-erosive LP of mucous membranes generally does not need any treatment and may resolve spontaneously. Erosive oral and / or genital LP can be exceptionally difficult to control, but may respond to high potency topical glucocorticoids (in Orabase or intralesional), topical retinoic acid (tretinoin or isotretinoin gel), cyclosporine rinses, and topical pimecrolimus or tacrolimus (FK-506) (Hodgson et al., 2003). Recently, 308-nm UVB excimer laser showed encouraging results in these patients (Kollner et al., 2003). Topical anaesthetics also provide symptomatic benefit for patients who have difficulty with eating and chewing. Newer antifungal agents may be useful in mucosal LP with evidence of Candida colonization.

Systemic treatment with oral glucocorticoids and retinoids may be considered for particularly severe erosive mucosal LP lesions, but remissions are short-lived and the risk of serious side-effects is high. Nevertheless, oral glucocorticoids may be of value in the management of acute episodes, when topical or intralesional glucocorticoids alone failed to achieve adequate control. In recalcitrant cases, steroid sparing agents such as azathioprine, mycophenolate mofetil, methotrexate or cyclosporine are generally added. Anecdotal reports have suggested improvement in mucosal erosive LP with a number of systemic agents including griseofulvin, dapsone, hydroxychloroquine, low-molecular-weight heparin, and thalidomide. The administration of low dose cyclophosphamide, the effective inhibitor of denovo protein sysnthesis, for the treatment of severe oral LP, unresponsive to the aforementioned therapies, appears to induce remissions that are sustained. Extracorporeal photochemotherapy has recently been examined for the treatment of erosive LP, mainly involving oral and vulvar tissues. All patients experienced complete remission, and some have showed a durable response. Surgical excision, CO_2 laser, Nd: YAG laser, and cryotherapy have all been used for treatment of recalcitrant mucosal LP. In general, surgery is reserved for removal of dysplastic areas in patients at high risk. Patients under a great deal of stress frequently show improvement when their emotional environment is altered (Boyd, 2000; Setterfield et al., 2000).

Cutaneous graft-versus-host-reaction (cGVHR)

The best way of treating (c)GVHR is to prevent it from occurring by irradiating blood products before transfusion. Patients receiving allogeneic transplants are placed on methotrexate, cyclosporine, or both before marrow infusion. Recent data indicate that FK-506 is more effective than cyclosporine in the prevention of GVHR when each drug is used in combination with methotrexate (Hiraoka et al., 2001).

If acute GVHR has already occurred, initial therapy usually includes systemic glucocorticoids. Anti-thymocyte globulin, azathioprine, mycophenolate mofetil, pentostatin, cyclosporine, FK-506, and monoclonal antibodies, directed against effector cell populations (CDw52, CD25) or cytokines (TNF-α), are used separately or in combination. Narrowband UVB, PUVA or extracorporeal photochemotherapy may be useful in the treatment of patients with acute cGVHR. Keratinocytes treated with UV-A and UV-B are known to produce immunosuppressive cytokines. Depletion and morphologic alterations of dendritic cells also occur (Queen et al., 1989; Aubin et al., 1995; Hale et al., 1996; Richter et al., 1997; Dall'Amico & Zacchello, 1998; Grundmann-Kollmann et al., 2002).

Chronic GVHR is treated similar to acute GVHR. Glucocorticoids, cyclosporine, azathioprine, mycophenolate mofetil, and methotrexate are administered in various combinations, depending on the severity of the disease. Tacrolimus ointment, pimecrolimus cream or PUVA treatment generally control widespread lichenoid GVHR effectively (Volc-Platzer et al., 1990; Choi & Nghiem, 2001). Mucous membrane manifestations may improve with these therapies as well. It is unclear whether PUVA (or bath PUVA) is able to reverse the cutaneous changes in sclerodermatous GVHR (Aubin et al., 1995). Ultraviolet A1 phototherapy may be considered as an appropriate approach for these patients (Calzavara Pinton et al., 2003). Extracorporeal photochemotherapy has also been reported as beneficial (Greinix et al., 2000).

Summary

Lichenoid dermatoses encompass, based on the microscopic pattern of inflammation and skin response, a significant group of dermatologic conditions whose pathophysiologic mechanisms are currently unknown. Lichen planus (LP), the prototype, is an inflammatory disorder with characteristic purple, polygonal, pruritic papules of the skin and may be accompanied by mucosal lesions. There are many similar clinical variants described, ranging from lichenoid drug eruptions (LDE) to association with other diseases such as the cutaneous graft-versus-host-reaction (cGVHR). This chapter delineates some of the recent aspects of the etiopathogenesis, clinical manifestations and treatment modalities of LP, LDE, and cGVHR.

References

Alinovi A, Barella PA, Benoldi D (1983) Erosive lichen planus involving the glans penis alone. Int J Dermatol. 22:37–38

Ammar M, Mokni M, Boubaker S, El Gaied A, Ben Osman A, Louzir H (2008) Involvement of gran-zyme B and granulysin in the cytotoxic response in lichen planus. J Cutan Pathol 35:630–634

Anasetti C (2004) Advances in the prevention of graft-versus-host disease after hematopoietic cell transplantation. Transplantation 77: S79–S83

Aractingi S, Chosidow O (1998) Cutaneous graft-versus-host disease. Arch Dermatol 134:602–612

Aubin F, Brion A, Deconinck E, Plouvier E, Herve P, Humbert P, Cahn JY (1995) Phototherapy in the treatment of cutaneous graft-versus-host disease. Our preliminary experience in resistant patients. Transplantation 59:151–155

Baart de la Faille-Kuyper EH, Baart de la Faille H (1974) An immunofluorescence study of lichen planus. Br J Dermatol. 90:365–371

Bai J, Zhang Y, Lin M, Zeng X, Wang Z, Shen J, Jiang L, Gao F, Chen Q (2007) Interleukin-18 gene polymorphisms and haplotypes in patients with oral lichen planus: a study in an ethnic Chinese cohort. Tissue Antigens 70:390–397

Barthelmes H, Haustein UF (1970) Nachweis von Fibrinablagerungen beim Lichen ruber planus mit Hilfe der Immunfluoreszenzhistologie. Derm Mschr 156:85–96

Bhan AK, Harrist TJ, Murphy GF, Mihm jr MC (1982) T cell subsets and Langerhans cells in lichen planus: In situ characterization using monoclonal antibodies. Br J Dermatol 105:617–622

Boyd AS (2000) New and emerging therapies for lichenoid dermatoses. Dermatol Clin 18:21–29

Boyd AS, Neldner KH (1991) Lichen planus. J Am Acad Dermatol 25:593–619

Calzavara Pinton P, Porta F, Izzi T, Venturini M, Capezzera R, Zane C, Notarangelo LD (2003) Prospects for ultraviolet A1 phototherapy as a treatment for chronic cutaneous graft-versus-host disease. Haematologica 88:1169–1175

Carrozzo M, Uboldi de Capei M, Dametto E, Fasano ME, Arduino P, Broccoletti R, Vezza D, Ren-dine S, Curtoni ES, Gandolfo S (2004) Tumor necrosis factor-alpha and interferon-gamma polymorphisms contribute to susceptibility to oral lichen planus. J Invest Dermatol 122:87–94

Cavet J, Dickinson AM, Norden J, Taylor PR, Jackson GH, Middleton PG (2001) Interferon-gamma and interleukin-6 gene polymorphisms associate with graft-versus-host disease in HLA-matched sibling bone marrow transplantation. Blood 98:1594–1600

Cerni C, Ebner H, Kokoschka E-M (1976) Allgemeiner Immunstatus bei Patienten mit generalisi-ertem Lichen ruber planus. Arch Dermatol Res 256:13–22

Choi CJ, Nghiem P (2001) Tacrolimus ointment in the treatment of chronic cutaneous graft-vs-host disease. A case series of 18 patients. Arch Dermatol 137:1202–1206

Copeman PWM, Tan RSH, Timlin D, Samman PD (1978) Familial lichen planus. Br J Dermatol 98:573–577

Dall'Amico R, Zacchello G (1998) Treatment of graft-versus-host disease with photopheresis. Transplantation 65:1283–1284

Darier J (1909) Précis de Dermatologie. Masson, p 118. Paris

Edwards L, Friedrich jr EG (1988) Desquamative vaginitis: lichen planus in disguise. Obstet Gy-necol. 71:832–836

Ellgehausen P, Elsner P, Burg G (1998) Drug-induced lichen planus. Clin Dermatol 16:325–332

Fivenson DP, Mathes B (2006) Treatment of generalized lichen planus with alefacept. Arch Der-matol 142:151–152

Fox BJ, Odom RB (1985) Papulosquamous diseases: A review. J Am Acad Dermatol 12:597–624

Gadenne AS, Strucke R, Dunn D, Wagner M, Bleicher P, Bigby M (1994) T-cell lines derived from lesional skin of lichen planus patients contain a distinctive population of T-cell receptor γδ-bearing cells. J Invest Dermatol 103:347–351

Giannotti B, De Panfilis G, Manara GC, Allegra F (1983) Macrophage-T-lymphocyte interaction in lichen planus. An electron microscopic and immunocytochemical study. Arch Dermatol Res 275:35–40

Greinix HT, Volc-Platzer B, Knobler RM (2000) Extracorporeal photochemotherapy in the treatment of severe graft-versus-host disease. Leuk Lymphoma 36:425–434

Griffiths CEM, Voorhees JJ, Nickoloff BJ (1989) Characterization of intercellular adhesion molecule-1 and HLA-DR expression in normal and inflamed skin: modulation by recombinant gamma-interferon and tumor necrosis factor. J Am Acad Dermatol 20:617–629

Grundmann-Kollmann M, Martin H, Ludwig R, Klein S, Boehncke WH, Hoelzer D, Kaufmann R, Podda M (2002) Narrowband UV-B phototherapy in the treatment of cutaneous graft versus host disease. Transplantation 74:1631–1634

Gunduz K, Demireli P, Inanir I, Nese N (2006) Expression of matrix metalloproteinases (MMP-2, MMP-3, and MMP-9) and fibronectin in lichen planus. J Cutan Pathol 33:545–550

Hale G, Waldmann H (1996) Recent results using CAMPATH-1 antibodies to control GVHD and graft rejection. Bone Marrow Transplant 17:305–308

Harper JI (1987) Cutaneous graft versus host disease. Br Med J 295:401–402

Hiraoka A, Ohashi Y, Okamoto S, Moriyama Y, Nagao T, Kodera Y, Kanamaru A, Dohy H, Masaoka T; Japanese FK506 BMT (Bone Marrow Transplantation) Study Group (2001) Phase III study comparing tacrolimus (FK506) with cyclosporine for graft-versus-host disease prophylaxis after allogenic bone marrow transplantation. Bone Marrow Transplant 28:181–185

Hodgson TA, Sahni N, Kaliakatsou F, Buchanan JA, Porter SR (2003) Long-term efficacy and safety of topical tacrolimus in the management of ulcerative/erosive oral lichen planus. Eur J Dermatol 13:466–470

Iijima W, Ohtani H, Nakayama T, Sugawara Y, Sato E, Nagura H, Yoshie O, Sasano T (2003) Infiltrating CD8[+] T cells in oral lichen planus predominant express CCR5 and CXCR3 and carry respective chemokine ligands RANTES/CCL5 and IP-10/CXCL10 in their cytolytic granules: a potential self-recruiting mechanism. Am J Pathol 163:261–268

Kollner K, Wimmershoff M, Landthaler M, Hohenleutner U (2003) Treatment of oral lichen planus with the 308 nm UVB excimer laser. Early preliminary results in eight patients. Lasers Surg Med 33:158–160

La Nasa G, Cottoni F, Mulargia M, Carcassi C, Vacca A, Pizzati A, Ledda A, Montesu MA, Cerimele D, Contu L (1995) HLA antigen distribution in different clinical subgroups demonstrates genetic heterogeneity in lichen planus. Br J Dermatol 132:897–900

Lachapelle JM, De la Brassine M (1973) The proliferation of cells in the dermal infiltrate of lichen planus lesions. Br J Dermatol 89:137–141

Lange Wantzin G, Ralfkiaer E, Lisby S, Rothlein R (1988) The role of intercellular adhesion molecules in inflammatory skin reactions. Br J Dermatol 119:141–145

Lendrum J (1974) Surgical treatment of lichen planus of the soles. Br J Plast Surg 27:171–175

Malmnäs Tjernlund U (1980) Ia-like antigens in lichen planus. Acta Derm Venereol (Stockholm) 60:309–314

Messadi DV, Pober JS, Murphy GF (1988) Effects of recombinant gamma-interferon on HLA-DR and DQ expression by skin cells in short-term organ culture. Lab Invest 58:61–67

Mirmirani P, Karnik P (2009) Lichen planopilaris treated with a peroxisome proliferator-activated receptor gamma agonist. Arch Dermatol 145:1363–1366

Nickoloff BJ, Reusch MK, Bensch K, Karasek MA (1988) Preferential binding of monocytes and Leu2[+]T-lymphocytes to interferon-gamma-treated cultured skin endothelial cells and keratinocytes. Arch Dermatol Res 280:235–245

11

Olsen RG, Du Plessis DP, Schulz EJ, Camisa C (1984) Indirect immunofluorescence microscopy of lichen planus. Br J Dermatol 110:9–15

Polderman MCA, Wintzen M, van Leeuwen RL, de Winter S, Pavel S (2004) Ultraviolet A1 in the treatment of generalized lichen planus: A report of 4 cases. J Am Acad Dermatol 50:646–647

Powell FC, Rogers RS, Dickson ER, Breanndan Moore S (1986) An association between HLA-DR1 and lichen planus. Br J Dermatol 114:473–478

Queen C, Schneider WP, Selick HE, Payne PW, Landolfi NF, Duncan JF, Avdalovic NM, Levitt M, Junghans RP, Waldmann TA (1989) A humanized antibody that binds to the interleukin 2 receptor. Proc Natl Acad Sci USA 86:10029–10033

Ragaz A, Ackerman AB (1981) Evaluation, maturation and regression of lesions of lichen planus. Am J Dermatopathol 3:1–4

Ramirez-Amador V, Dekker NP, Lozada-Nur F, Mirowski GW, MacPhail LA, Regezi JA (1996) Altered interface adhesion molecules in oral lichen planus. Oral Dis 2:188–192

Richter HI, Stege H, Ruzicka T, Soehngen D, Heyll A, Krutmann J (1997) Extracorporeal photopheresis in the treatment of acute graft-versus-host disease. J Am Acad Dermatol 36:787–789

Santoro A, Majorana A, Bardellini E, Festa S, Sapelli P, Facchetti F (2003) NF-kappaB expression in oral and cutaneous lichen planus. J Pathol 201:466–472

Saricaoglu H, Karadogan SK, Baskan EB, Tunali S (2003) Narrowband UVB therapy in the treatment of lichen planus. Photodermatol Photoimmunol Photomed 19:265–267

Saurat JH, Didierjean L, Gluckman E, Bussel A (1975) Graft-versus-host-reaction and lichen planus-like eruption in man. Br J Dermatol 92:591–592

Scully C, El-Kom M (1985) Lichen planus: Review and update on pathogenesis. J Oral Pathol 14:431–458

Setterfield JF, Black MM, Challacombe SJ (2000) The management of oral lichen planus. Clin Exp Dermatol 25:176–182

Simon jr M (1985) Lichen ruber planus aus immunologischer Sicht. Zbl Hautkr 150:699–708

Simon jr M (1988) Lesional keratinocytes express OKM5, Leu-8 and Leu-11b antigens in lichen planus. Dermatologica 177:152–158

Simon jr M (1990) Immunopathological aspects of etretinate therapy in lichen planus. J Dermatol (Tokyo) 17:282–286

Simon jr M, Unterpaintner F, Reimer G (1983) Immunphänomene bei Lichen ruber – eine immunfluoreszenzmikroskopische Studie. Z Hautkr 58:121–128

Simon jr M, Reimer G, Schardt M, Hornstein OP (1983) Lymphocytotoxicity for oral mucosa in lichen planus. Dermatologica 167:11–15

Simon jr M, Keller J (1984) Subpopulations of T lymphocytes in peripheral blood and in skin lesions in lichen ruber planus. Dermatologica 169:112–116

Simon jr M, Djawari D, Schönberger A (1984) HLA antigens associated with lichen planus. Clin Exp Dermatol 9:435

Simon jr M, Hunyadi J, Fickentscher H, Hornstein OP (1989) Basic and interleukin-2-augmented natural killer cell activity in lichen planus. Dermatologica 178:141–144

Simon jr M, Hunyadi J (1990) Etretinate suppresses ICAM-1 expression by lesional keratinocytes in healing cutaneous lichen planus. Arch Dermatol Res 282:412–414

Simon jr M, Hunyadi J (1992) Immunopathologische Untersuchungen bei Patienten mit chronischer kutaner Graft-versus-host-Reaktion. Z Hautkr 67:900–903

Simon jr M, Driesch von den P (1994) Expressionsmuster von Adhäsionsmolekülen bei PUVA-behandelten Lichen planus-Patienten. Hautarzt 45:161–165

Simon jr M, Gruschwitz MS (1997) In situ expression and serum levels of tumour necrosis factor alpha receptors in patients with lichen planus. Acta Derm Venereol (Stockholm) 77:191–193

Soehnchen RM, Kaudewitz P, Holler E (1992) Tumour necrosis factor-α is elevated in serum of patients with lichen planus. Arch Dermatol Res 284:27

Soper DE, Patterson JW, Hurt WG, Fantl JA, Blaylock WK (1988) Lichen planus of the vulva. Obstet Gynecol. 72:74–76

Sugerman PB, Satterwhite K, Bigby M (2000) Autocytotoxic T-cell clones in lichen planus. Br J Dermatol 142:449–456

Takahashi H, Furukawa T, Hashimoto S, Suzuki N, Kuroha T, Yamazaki F, Inano K, Takahashi M, Aizawa Y, Koike T (2000) Contribution of TNF-alpha and IL-10 gene polymorphisms to graft-versus-host disease following allo-haematopoietic stem cell transplantation. Bone Marrow Transplant 26:1317–1323

Thyresson N, Moberger G (1957) Cytologic studies in lichen ruber planus. Acta Derm Venereol (Stockholm) 37:191–204

Touraine R, Revuz J, Dreyfus B, Rochant H, Mannoni P (1975) Graft-versus-host-reaction and lichen planus. Br J Dermatol 92:589

Volc-Platzer B (1992) "Graft-versus-host disease" (GvHD). Hautarzt 43:669–677

Volc-Platzer B, Hönigsmann H, Hinterberger W, Wolff K (1990) Photochemotherapy improves chronic cutaneous graft-versus-host disease. J Am Acad Dermatol 23:220–228

Walker DM (1976) Identification of subpopulations of lymphocytes and macrophages in the infiltrate of lichen planus lesions of skin and oral mucosa. Br J Dermatol 94:529–534

Weyl A (1885) Bemerkungen zum Lichen planus. Dtsch Med Wschr 11:624–626

Wickham LF (1895) Sur un signe pathognomonique du lichen de Wilson (lichen plan). Stries et ponctuations grisatres. Annls Derm Syph Paris 6:517–520

Wilson E (1869) On leichen planus. J Cut Med 3:117–132

Zhang Y, Lin M, Zhang S, Wang Z, Jiang L, Shen J, Bai J, Gao F, Zhou M, Chen Q (2008) NF-kappaB-dependent cytokines in saliva and serum from patients with oral lichen planus: a study in an ethnic Chinese population. Cytokine 41:144–149

Zhou L, Yan C, Gieling RG, Kida Y, Garner W, Li W, Han YP (2009) Tumor necrosis factor-alpha induced expression of matrix metalloproteinase-9 through p21-activated kinase-1. BMC Immunol Mar 19; 10:15

11

12

Peter Lamprecht and Wolfgang L. Gross

Introduction

Vasculitis of small blood vessels of the skin, i. e. arterioles, capillaries and venules, is found in cutaneous leukocytoclastic vasculitis (CLA) as well as in systemic vasculitides. CLA is restricted to the skin, whereas ANCA-associated and immune complex-mediated systemic vasculitides – except polyarteritis nodosa – are characterized by an involvement of predominantly small vessels affecting various organs including the skin.

Primary systemic vasculitides, where no underlying disease or agent is known, are distinguished from secondary vasculitides, i. e. secondary from other diseases of either autoimmune or other origin. ANCA-associated and immune complex-mediated vasculitides are the major immunopathogenetic categories which involve small vessels (Table 1) (Gross, 2003).

Pathophysiology

ANCA-associated vasculitides

Substantial evidence from *in vitro* experiments and animal models supports the view, that anti-neutrophil cytoplasmic antibodies (ANCA) have a role in the immunopathogenesis of *Wegener`s granulomatosis (WG)* and *microscopic polyangiitis (MPA)*, giving rise to the "ANCA-cytokine sequence theory" (Fig. 1.) (Gross et al., 1991, Gross, 2003). The main target autoantigens proteinase 3 (PR3) in WG and myeloperoxidase (MPO) in MPA are constituents of neutrophil azurophilic granula. ANCA (usually with MPO specificity) are less frequently detected in Churg-Strauss syndrome (CSS). High constitutive membrane PR3 (mPR3) expression is associated with an increased risk of relapse and increased relapse rate in WG (Rarok et al., 2002). Following cytokine priming, PR3 and MPO are translocated from intracellular azurophilic granules to the membrane of neutrophils. Binding of

Table 1. Small vessel vasculitides affecting the skin

Primary systemic vasculitis	**ANCA-associated vasculitis**
	1. Wegener's granulomatosis (WG)
	2. Microscopic polyangiitis (MPA)
	3. Churg-Strauss syndrome
	Immune complex-mediated primary systemic vasculitis
	1. Cutaneous leukocytoklastic angiitis (CLA)
	2. Henoch-Schönlein purpura (HSP)
	3. Essential cryoglobulinemic vasculitis (ECV)
Secondary systemic vasculitis	**Immune complex-mediated secondary systemic vasculitis**
	1. Rheumatoid vasculitis (RV)
	2. HCV-associated CV
	3. Secondary vasculitis or CV in SLE, Sjögren's syndrome and other connective tissue diseases
	4. Secondary vasculitis or CV in infectious diseases, e.g. bacterial endocarditis
	5. Paraneoplastic vasculitis

Abbreviations: ANCA = anti-neutrophil cytoplasmic antibody; HCV = hepatitis C virus; SLE = systemic lupus erythematosus

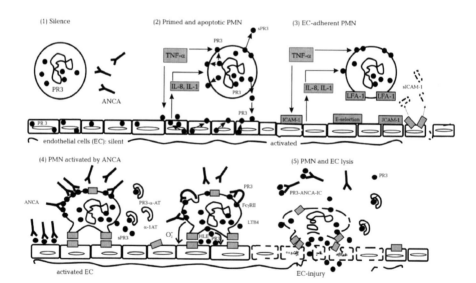

Fig. 1. ANCA-cytokine sequence theory: Cytokine primed polymorphonuclear leukocytes (PMN) translocate and express intracytoplasmic proteinase 3 (PR3) or myeloperoxidase (MPO) on their cell surface. PR3 or MPO become accessible to anti-neutrophil cytoplasmic antibodies (ANCA). ANCA bind via Fc and Fab proportions to PMN. Activated PMN adhere to endothelial cells via adhesion molecule interaction and release oxygen radicals (ROS) and other substances. As a consequence endothelial damage is found (Gross et al., 1991, Gross, 2003)

the ANCA to both mPR3 or mMPO and the Fc-γ(R)eceptor is necessary for the full activation of the neutrophils (Falk et al., 1988, Jenne et al., 1990, Falk et al., 1990, Csernok et al., 1990, Porges et al., 1994, Kocher et al., 1998). Moreover, neutrophil extracellular traps (NETs) containing the target-autoantigens PR3 and MPO are released from ANCA-stimulated neutrophils, thereby perpetuating the autoimmune response against neutrophil components and triggering vasculitis (Kessenbrock et al., 2009).

ANCA-activated neutrophil granulocytes up-regulate gene expression of inflammatory mediators and release cytokines such as IL-8 and leukotrienes (Grimminger et al., 1996, Yang et al., 2002). Production of IL-8 by ANCA stimulated neutrophils and monocytes within the intravascular department and/or endothelial cells may frustrate transendothelial leukocyte migration and favor premature degranulation with subsequent endothelial damage (Cockwell et al., 1999). ANCA also favor firm adhesion of rolling neutrophil granulocytes and promote their migration *in vitro* (Radford et al., 2001). Pauci-immune, necrotizing vasculitis is seen as a result of the complex interaction of ANCA, neutrophil granulocytes and endothelial cells. An *in vivo* animal model has provided further support of the pivotal role of ANCA and neutrophil granulocytes for the induction of vasculitis (Xiao et al., 2002).

Granulomatous lesions in WG and CSS

The inciting agent(s) triggering the pathophysiological cascade in ANCA-associated vasculitides are still unknown. One of the most striking features of WG and CSS is their inherent propensity for granulomatous inflammation of the upper and/or lower respiratory tract. The earliest symptoms of WG and CSS are usually confined to the upper and/or lower airways and herald generalisation with systemic vasculitis in both diseases. Moreover, so-called "grumbling disease" related to persistent granulomatous disease activity within the ENT tract and/or lower respiratory tract is seen in many WG- and CSS-patients, who are defined as being otherwise in clinical remission, and precedes relapses. Thus, granulomatous inflammation plays a role both in local tissue destruction (e.g. saddle nose deformity) and in triggering systemic vasculitis (Lamprecht & Gross, 2008, Lamprecht et al., 2009). Interestingly, about 10% of the WG-patients remain in the localized stage (i.e. WG-restricted to the respiratory tract). Localized and generalized WG as well as ANCA-positive and -negative CSS are characterized by differences in predisposing genetic risk factors (Wieczorek et al., 2008, Wieczorek et al., 2010).

Barrier dysfunction with abnormal microbial mucosa-invasiveness and -composition triggering inflammation plays a crucial role in many chronic inflammatory diseases such as Crohn's disease. More recently, impaired respiratory ciliar function, which could predispose to chronic granulomatous inflammation, has been demonstrated in WG (Ullrich et al., 2009). Intriguingly, neoformation of ectopic lymphoid structures within chronic inflamed tissue and T-cell alterations are found in WG as well as in other autoimmune diseases such as rheumatoid arthritis and Sjögren's syndrome (Voswinkel et al., 2006, Müller et al., 2008, Capraru et al., 2008). In animal models infectious agents trigger chronic inflammation with ectopic lymphoid structure neoformation, subsequent break of tolerance and induction of autoimmune disease (Lang et al., 2005).

Immune complex-mediated vasculitides

Deposition or in situ formation of immune complexes in the vessel wall may result in the subsequent evolution of vasculitis. Additional factors such as the size of the complexes, composition, charge, complement activation, hydrostatic pressure on the wall and efficiency or ineffectivity of reparative mechanisms determine, whether the initial lesion will eventually progress to a necrotizing vasculitis (Gross, 2003). Immune complexes formed in antigen excess circulate until the aforementioned factors contribute to their deposition in blood vessel walls. Activation of neutrophils, up-regulation of endothelial adhesion molecules and cytokine release facilitate further leukocyte recruitment. The membrane attack complex of complement plays a significant role in altering the endothelial cell membrane integrity. Activated neutrophils release proteolytic enzymes, especially collagenases

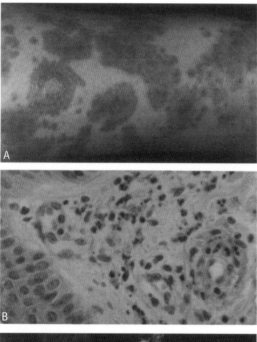

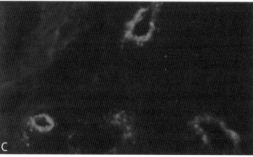

Fig. 2. Immune complex vasculitis. **A**. Clinical presentation with petechial purpura of the lower legs. **B**. Histopathology with diapedesis of erythrocytes and fragmentation of neutrophil granulocytes. **C**. Depositis of immune complexes around dermal blood vessels detected by direct immunofluorescence microscopy

and elastases, along with free oxygen radicals that further damage the vessel wall (Claudy, 1998).

Cryoglobulinemic vasculitis (CV) is an immune complex-mediated vasculitis predominately affecting small vessels. Cryoglobulins are cold-precipitable monoclonal or polyclonal immunoglobulins. Cryoglobulins can induce cold-dependent activation of complement and hypocomplementemia, followed by leukocyte attraction and vessel damage (Wei et al., 1997). The skin is frequently involved. CV is usually found in the presence of type II cryoglobulinemia, i. e. mixed monoclonal IgMκ and polyclonal IgG cryoglobulinemia. The monoclonal IgM component often (> 75%) has rheumatoid factor activity (Ferri & Mascia, 2006). The non-enveloped HCV core protein is a constitutive component of type II cryoglobulins and might contribute to cryoprecipitation in hepatitis C virus (HCV)-associated CV. Binding of HCV core protein to the globular domain of the C1q receptor on the surface of both leukocytes and endothelial cells may favor the interaction of HCV core protein-containing type II cryoglobulin and endothelial cells (Sansonno et al., 2003).

Clinical classification and manifestations

Classification

ANCA-associated, pauci-immune vasculitides (WG, MPA, CSS) and immune complex-mediated vasculitides (CLA, Henoch-Schönlein purpura / HSP, essential CV / ECV) comprise the group of primary systemic vasculitides affecting predominantly small vessels according to the definition of the Chapel Hill Consensus (CHC) conference. Further, large vessel vasculitides (giant cell arteritis and Takayasu arteritis) and vasculitides of medium-sized vessels (polyarteritis nodosa and Kawasaki disease) are discerned (Jennette et al., 1994).

Skin manifestations

The typical aspect of CLA and skin involvement in systemic small vessel vasculitides is the *palpable purpura* (Csernok and Gross, 2000). Purpura is a manifestation mainly of the postvenule capillary vasculitis. The lower limbs are most frequently affected by the palpable purpura due to the higher hydrostatic pressure in these vessels (Hautmann et al., 1999). Hydrostatic pressure may also account for the accentuation of the purpura during the day seen in some patients. *Petechiae* may occur secondary to widespread capillary damage. *Urticaria vasculitis* results from a progression of small vessel vasculitis to fibrinoid necrosis in postcapillary venules, i. e. necrotizing vasculitis. Urticaria typically persists for more than 24 hours in these cases (Schur, 1993).

Small hemorrhages with slightly nodular character at the tips of the fingers (*Osler's nodes*) and on the palms, especially on the thenar eminences (*Janeway lesions*) are seen in secondary immune complex-mediated small vessel vasculitides in infectious endocarditis. These lesions indicate an important differential diagnosis with regard to the etiology of vasculitis (Schur et al., 1993). *Pyoderma gangrenosum* or *dermatitis ulcerosa* may be encountered in several systemic diseases, e. g. inflammatory bowel diseases, and in small vessel vasculitides (Powell et al., 1985)

Nailfold splinter hemorrhages and infarcts are vasculitic manifestations mainly of the arterioles and small arteries. The vasculitis may progress and include small arteries causing cutaneous ulcers and acral necrosis. Pathologic examination often reveals fibrinoid necrosis and thrombosis with little inflammatory infiltration. Vasospasm of dermal ascending arterioles with hyperperfusion of unaffected vessels gives rise to livedo reticularis. Progression to *livedo vasculitis* may result in purpura, cutaneous nodules and ulceration predominantly of the lower extremities (Schur, 1993).

Systemic vasculitis

Constitutional signs such as malaise, weight loss, fever, arthralgia and myalgia may proceed other symptoms of systemic vasculitis. Multi-organ involvement may be found in every systemic small vessel vasculitis. However, mono- or oligosymptomatic courses may be encountered at times. Vasculitides differ with respect to the preferential involvement of distinct vascular areas (Table 2): Pulmonary-renal syndrome is more likely in WG and MPA, whereas other diseases such as systemic lupus erythemtosus (SLE) less often cause this syndrome. Purpura and renal involvement are common in CV, pulmonary infiltrates in WG and CSS, polyneuropathy and gastrointestinal vasculitis in CV and CSS, and cardiac involvement in CSS. Proceeding nasal obstruction, crusting, epistaxis and/or otitis media and mastoiditis is often found in WG. Episcleritis is seen in WG and MPA. Asthma bronchiale, eosinophilia and pulmonary infiltrations together with cardiac involvement and/or polyneuropathy are typically seen in CSS. Severe renal disease is less frequent in CSS compared to WG and MPA. Neuropathy and cardiac disease are frequently encountered in severe CSS. Coronary arteritis and myocarditis are the principle causes of morbidity and mortality in CSS (Jennette and Falk, 1997; Sablé-Fourtassou et al., 2005). CSS may evolve over a period of time starting with allergic rhinitis, asthma bronchiale. Thereafter, a hypereosinophilic syndrome with infiltrative eosinophilic disease, e. g. eosinophilc pneumonia and gastroenteritis will ensue, and finally small vessel vasculitis with granulomatous lesions is seen in CSS (Lanham et al., 1984). The triad of arthralgia, purpura and weakness (so-called Meltzer's triad) is frequently seen in essential CV (ECV) and in HCV-associated CV. CV frequently involves the kidneys and peripheral nerves (Ferri & Mascia, 2006). Purpura, cutaneous ulcers and polyneuropathy in a patient with long-standing rheumatoid arthritis (RA) is suggestive of rheumatoid vasculitis (RV). Purpura, arthritis, and abdominal pain in a child with a nephritic sediment is found in Henoch-Schönlein purpura (HSP). HSP has a peak incidence at the age of five years. The disease often begins after an upper respiratory tract infection (Jennette and Falk, 1997).

Small vessel vasculitides may affect different structures within the same organ or body region giving rise to a variety of symptoms: Affection of the ear in WG may include sensoneurinal deafness due to vasculitis of the inner ear and/or cochlear nerve, otitis media, and mastoiditis. CSS and CV may cause abdominal pain due to gastro-intestinal vasculi-

Table 2. Typical aspects of ANCA-associated vasculitides (WG, MPA, CSS) and immune complex-mediated vasculitides (CLA, CV, sec. SVV in SLE, RV)

Vasculitis	Clinical findings	Laboratory findings	Histology
WG	Starts in the upper respiratory tract, pulm.-renal syndr.	Compl. ↔ or ↑, C-ANCA, PR3-ANCA	Granulomatous lesions, pauci-imm. vasc.
MPA	Pulm-renal syndr.	Compl. ↔ or ↑, P-ANCA, MPO-ANCA	Pauci-imm. vasc.
CSS	Asthma, pulmonary infiltration, PNP, cardiac involvement	Eosinophilia, compl. ↔ or ↑, less often: ANCA	Pauci-imm. vasc., eosinophil infiltration
CLA	Purpura	Compl. ↔ or ↓	Leukocyt. vasculitis
ECV, HCV-ass. CV	Purpura, arthralgia, weakness, PNP, GN	Compl. ↓, RF, cryoglobulin, HCV-ab., HCV-RNA	Imm. compl. vasc.
Sec. vasculitis in SLE	Purpura, PNP, GN, cerebral vasculitis	Compl. ↓, ANA, ds-DNA ab., anti-Sm ab.	Imm. compl. vasc.
RV	Purpura, ulcers, PNP	Compl. ↓, RF	Imm. compl. vasc.
HSP	Purpura, arthralgia, GN, abdominal pain	Compl. ↓, IgA ↑	Imm. compl. vasc. with IgA

Abbreviations: ANCA = anti-neutrophil cytoplasmic antibody (Immunofluorescence patterns: C-ANCA = cytoplasmic pattern ANCA, P-ANCA = perinuclear pattern ANCA; ELISA: PR3-ANCA = proteinase 3 ANCA, MPO = myeloperoxidase ANCA), WG = Wegener's granulomatosis, MPA = microscopic polyangiitis, CSS = Churg Strauss syndrome, CLA = cutaneous leukocytoclastic angiitis, CV = cryoglobulinemic vasculitis (ECV = essential CV, HCV-ass. CV = hepatitis C virus associated CV), sec. = secondary, GN = glomerulonephritis, PNP = polyneuropathy, RA = rheumatoid arthritis, SVV = small vessel vasculitis, SLE = sytemic lupus erythematosus, RV = rheumatoid vasculitis, ab. = antibody, Imm. compl. vasc. = immune complex-mediated vasculitis, Compl. = complement, ANA = antinuclear ab., ds-DNA ab. = double strand DNA ab, Leukocyt. vasc. = leukocytoclastic vasculitis, Immune compl.–med. vasc. = immune complex-mediated vascultis

tis or vasculitis of the gall bladder. Renal involvement in immune complex-mediated vasculitis may result in mesangioproliferative and other forms of glomerulonephritis, whereas focal and segment necrotizing glomerulonephritis is more common in ANCA-associated vasculitis (Jennette and Falk, 1997). Renal vasculitis of small and medium sized renal arteries is seen at least in one third of the patients with cryoglobulinemic glomerulonephritis (D'Amico, 1998, Ferri & Mascia, 2006). Pulmonary small vessel vasculitis may result in dyspnoea, cough, hemoptysis due to either bronchial ulcerations or frank hemorrhagic alveolitis. Full-blown pulmonary-renal syndrome will cause renal and respiratory failure. Central nervous involvement may cause cranial nerve palsies, seizures, stroke and other symptoms. Cardiac involvement may be indicated by arrhythmias due to coronariitis or myocarditis, pericardial effusion, and angina pectoris (Jennette and Falk, 1997).

Secondary vasculitides in SLE and other connective tissue diseases or rheumatoid arthritis are usually preceded by typical symptoms of their underlying autoimmune disease. Thus, rheumatoid vasculitis is usually encountered after previous long-lasting rheumatoid arthritis. In case of unusual symptom constellations paraneoplastic vasculitis, secondary vasculitis in infectious diseases such as bacterial endocarditis, and drug-induced vasculitides should be excluded. It has to be kept in mind, that small vessel vasculitides are also seen in primary immunodeficiencies, e. g. bare lymphocyte syndrome (TAP-deficiency and others), CVID, hyperimmunoglobulinemia D and periodic fever syndrome (HIDS), and tumor necrosis factor receptor-associated periodic syndrome (TRAPS) (Moins-Teisserenc et al., 1999, Sais et al., 1996, Lamprecht et al., 2004)

Diagnosis

Clinical parameters

A detailed patient history, physical examination and focused laboratory investigation are vital in diagnosing vasculitic disorders. The goals of the work-up include identification of a cause of the disease and / or the underlying immunopathogenetic mechanism, classification of the disease, and determination of the disease activity and extent. A detailed patient history and physical examination should give rise to a preliminary diagnosis. CLA requires a detailed drug history as drugs cause ca. 10% of vasculitic skin lesions. Drugs that have been implicated are penicillins, aminopenicillins, sulfonamides, allopurinol, thiazides, hydantoins and propylthiouracil (Jennette and Falk, 1997).

Laboratory tests

Laboratory tests are used to ascertain the type of vasculitis. Erythrocyte sedimentation rate (ESR) and C-reactive protein (CRP) indicate inflammation. Low complement levels are seen in immune complex-mediated vasculitides including CV, whereas normal or elevated complement levels are found in ANCA-associated vasculitides. Furthermore, low complement levels may indicate hereditary complement deficiencies, which may cause SLE-like diseases with secondary vasculitides. C-ANCA are strongly associated with "classic" WG. The principle target antigen for C-ANCA in WG is PR3. Only few WG patients (< 5%) have a P-ANCA with MPO specificity. Despite their high sensitivity and specificity for WG, C-ANCA and PR3-ANCA may be found in other diseases than WG, e. g. subacute bacterial endocarditis or severe CV (Choi et al., 2000). Rheumatoid factor (RF) may be found in various conditions such as RV, CV and endocarditis. Autoantibodies, e. g. ANA, ds-DNA antibodies, anti Sm, anti SSA, anti-SSB etc., will be seen in secondary vasculitides in SLE, Sjögren's syndrome and other connective tissue diseases. Low level autoantibodies such as ANA and RF may also be found in CV. ANA may be seen in RV and a variety of other diseases. Serum levels of IgA are elevated in half of the patients with HSP. As infections may cause secondary vasculitis, HBV, HCV, HIV, and bacterial infections should be excluded.

Serial blood cultures may be necessary. ALT and AST may not necessarily be elevated in HCV-associated CV. Procalcitonin may help to differentiate between autoimmune diseases and bacterial infections and sepsis (Lamprecht et al., 2009b).

Additional diagnostics

Echocardiography should rule out vegetations on the heart valves. Primary immunodeficiencies also have to be considered. Quantitative assessment of immunoglobulin classes including IgD, lymphocyte subpopulations, standardized cutaneous tests for various T-cell specific antigens, complement levels, MHC-class I and II expression, tests for the assessment of the functional status of various neutrophils, lymphocytes etc., and moleculargenetic analysis of mutations of the MEFV-gene (Familial Mediterranean fever), MVK-gene (HIDS), or TNFRSF1A-gene (TRAPS) may be necessary in selected patients (Lamprecht et al., 2009b).

Arteriogramms are helpful in identifying vasculitis of medium-sized arteries, e.g. renal, coronar or intestinal vessels, or even larger arteries. These vascular areas may sometimes be involved in addition to the small vessel vasculitis. The definite diagnosis of vasculitis is dependent on the demonstration of vascular involvement by biopsy. Biopsy specimen should be obtained from clinically involved tissue. Applying immunohistochemistry is helpful in distinguishing immune complex mediated from pauci-immune (ANCA-associated) vasculitides (Lamprecht et al., 2009b)

Therapy

Cutaneous leukocytoclastic vasculitis (CLA)

CLA is usually limited to a single episode that resolves spontaneously within weeks or a few months. Approximately 10% will have recurrent disease at intervals of months to years. Drugs that could cause the disease should be stopped. Oral corticosteroid therapy is indicated in severe cutaneous disease. Progressive, steroid resistant CLA is rarely encountered and may necessitate additional immunosuppressive therapy such as azathioprine. Critical reevaluation of the diagnosis should also take place in such cases (Jennette and Falk, 1997).

ANCA-associated vasculitides (WG, MPA, CSS)

Induction of remission is achieved with combined oral corticosteroids and oral cyclophosphamide in life threatening conditions and severe, progressive vasculitis in WG, MPA and CSS. Oral cyclophosphamide at 2 mg/kg/day is preferentially used in severe conditions ("Fauci's scheme" or "NIH standard"), whereas cyclophosphamide i.v. (15 mg/kg every 3 weeks) may be an alternative in patients with less severe disease (Reinhold-Keller et al.,

1994, Jayne et al., 2003). Reduction of the corticosteroid dose should be started carefully as cyclophosphamide therapy becomes effective after 7–10 days. Tapering of corticosteroids is aimed at reaching the lowest effective dose after having achieved a stable remission for more than three months. Doses should at least range below the so-called "Cushing" level at this time in order to prevent adverse effects (Jayne et al., 2003, Lamprecht et al., 2009b). Rituximab is effective in refractory cases (Jones et al., 2009).

Corticosteroids and cyclophosphamide predispose patients to serious adverse effects. Cyclophosphamide causes premalignant hemorrhagic cystitis, ovarian and testicular failure and myelodysplastic syndrome (Hoffman et al., 1992; Reinhold-Keller et al., 2000). Mesna is beneficial in avoiding hemorrhagic cystitis (Reinhold-Keller et al., 2000). Less toxic treatment is highly desirable. WG- and MPA-patients without life threatening disease manifestations can be treated with methotrexate (0.3 mg / kg / week i. v.) and corticosteroids for the induction of remission (De Groot, 2005). Azathioprine is given for the maintenance of remission after induction of remission with cyclophosphamide (Jayne et al., 2003). Alternatives for the maintenance of remission in WG and MPA are methotrexate and leflunomide (Metzler et al., 2007). Nasal *S. aureus* carriage is associated with activity of WG in the upper respiratory tract. A prophylaxis with trimethoprim / sulfamethoxazole results in a significant reduction in the relapse rate (Stegeman et al., 1996).

CSS is often controlled with high-dose corticosteroid treatment. Refractory and relapsing disease may require addition of a cytotoxic drug similar to the treatment of WG and MPA (Jennette and Falk, 1997). Interferon-α (IFN-α) therapy has been reported to induce remission in CSS and substantial reduction of the prednisolone requirement in patients who had attained incomplete remission with cyclophosphamide or methotrexate. The mechanism of action of IFN-α in CSS has not been clearly established, but switch in the cytokine profile as well as down-regulation of IgE receptors on eosinophils and lymphocytes may be relevant (Tatsis et al., 1998; Metzler et al., 2008). The Th2-type cytokine IL-5 may be a another target for therapy in CSS. Treatment with mepolizumab, a monoclonal anti-IL-5-antibody, was efficiently steroid-sparing in the hypereosinophilic syndrome (not associated with FIP-PDGFR mutation) and in prednisolone-dependent asthma with sputum eosinophilia. Mepolizumab is currently tested in CSS in an open-study (Nair et al., 2009).

Cryoglobulinemic vasculitis

Essential CV, i. e. non-infection or other disease related CV, is treated similar to the treatment protocol for WG and MPA. Plasmapheresis has been recommended in life-threatening conditions, progressive glomerulonephritis and polyneuropathy. Rituximab and PEG-IFN-α plus ribavirin induce remission in severe and refractory HCV-associated cryoglobulinemic vasculitis. Based on the currently available evidence, combined treatment with rituximab and PEG-IFN-α plus ribavirin should be considered as first line treatment in patients with active disease resistant to anti-viral treatment and patients with severe manifestations and activity of cryoglobulinemic vasculitis (e. g. rapidly deteriorating renal function, gastro-intestinal vasculitis, central nervous system (CNS) involvement, hyper-viscosity syndrome). PEG-IFN-α plus ribavirin without preceding rituximab may be efficient in less severe cases. In HCV-negative "idiopathic" cryoglobulinemic vasculitis rituximab represents a new treatment option in cases resistant to conventional immunosuppressive therapy, too. Moreover, IFN-α has been reported to induce remission in 2 cases of severe HCV-negative cryoglobulinemic vasculitis, presumably based on its anti-proliferative effect (Ferri & Mascia, 2006, Saadoun et al., 2008).

Henoch-Schönlein Purpura

HSP has a good prognosis in general. Pulmonary disease, rapidly progressive renal failure and peripheral polyneuropathy are uncommon (Jennette and Falk, 1997). Adult onset HSP is rare. Corticosteroids and azathioprine may be beneficial in patients with progressive renal insufficiency (Bergstein et al., 1998).

Miscellaneous secondary vasculitides

RV shows histopathological similarities to polyarteritis nodosa and requires equally aggressive therapy. Intermittent intravenous pulse cyclophosphamide plus methylprednisolone for the induction of remission has been demonstrated to improve healing of vasculitic lesions including leg ulcers and neuropathy. Pulse therapy results in a lower incidence of relapse and a lower mortality compared to other treatments. Comparatively high doses of cyclophosphamide (15–20 mg / kg per pulse) and short treatment intervals (14 and 21 days) are necessary to control the often aggressive course of the disease (Scott & Bacon, 1984). Although there are no controlled studies for the maintenance of remission in RV, practical considerations suggest to treat the patient with DMARDS used in RA, preferably methotrexate.

Secondary vasculitis in SLE is treated with intermittent intravenous pulse cyclophosphamide and corticosteroids according to the Austin's scheme. The original Austin's scheme included monthly intermittent intravenous bolus cyclophosphamide (0.5–1.0 g / m² body surface area) plus low-dose oral prednisolone (starting with up to 0.5 mg / kg per day) (Austin et al., 1986; Boumpas et al., 1991). Secondary vasculitides in other connective tissue diseases are treated analogous to the Austin's scheme in SLE.

Secondary vasculitis in bacterial endocarditis is treated with antibiotics. Paraneoplastic vasculitis may require treatment similar to the treatment protocol for WG and MPA for the vasculitic manifestations, e. g. cutaneous ulcers, acral necrosis, or polyneuropathy. Therapy of the underlying neoplasm is essential for the control of the vasculitis. Rheumatic symptoms and vasculitis secondary to primary immunodeficiencies may improve upon intravenous immunoglobulin administration in some disease conditions, e. g. CVID (Sais et al., 1996) and in TAP deficiency (Gadola et al., 2000).

Summary

Small vessel vasculitides affecting the skin are seen in primary systemic vasculitides, i. e. the ANCA-associated vasculitides (WG, MPA, CSS) and the immune complex-mediated vasculitides (ECV, HSP, CLA). Secondary immune complex-mediated vasculitides, e. g. in SLE and other connective tissue diseases, paraneoplastic conditions, and in infectious diseases, also frequently involve small vessels of the skin. Diagnosis is made upon a detailed patient history, physical examination, focused laboratory investigation, and demonstration of vasculitis by biopsy. Stage-adopted therapy aims at inducing and maintaining remission of the respective vasculitis. Treatment of underlying diseases may be necessary in secondary vasculitides.

References

Austin HA 3d, Klippel JH, Balow JE, le Riche NG, Steinberg AD, Plotz PH, Decker JL (1986) Therapy of lupus nephritis. Controlled trial of prednisone and cytotoxic drugs. N Engl J Med 314:614–619

Bergstein J, Leiser J, Andreoli SP (1998) Response of crescentic Henoch-Schoenlein purpura nephritis to corticosteroid and azathioprine therapy. Clin Nephrol 49:9–14

Boumpas DT, Yamada H, Patronas NJ, Scott D, Klippel JH, Balow JE (1991) Pulse cyclophosphamide for severe neuropsychiatric lupus. Q J Med 81:975–984

Capraru D, Müller A, Csernok E, Gross WL, Holl-Ulrich K, Northfield J, Klenerman P, Herlyn K, Holle J, Gottschlich S, Voswinkel J, Spies T, Fagin U, Jabs WJ, Lamprecht P (2008) Expansion of circulating NKG2D+ effector memory T-cells and expression of NKG2D-ligand MIC in granulomaous lesions in Wegener's granulomatosis. Clin Immunol 127:144–150

Choi HK, Lamprecht P, Niles JL, Gross WL, Merkel PA (2000) Subacute bacterial endocarditis with positive C-ANCA and antiproteinase 3 antibodies. Arthritis Rheum 43:226–231

Claudy A (1998) Pathogenesis of leukocytoclastic vasculitis. Eur J Dermatol 8:75–79

Cockwell P, Brooks CJ, Adu D, Savage COS (1999) Interleukin-8: pathogenetic role in antineutrophil cytoplasmic autoantibody-associated glomerulonephritis. Kidney Int 55:852–863

Csernok E, Gross WL (2000) Primary vasculitides and vasculitis confined to the skin: clinical features and new pathogenic aspects. Arch Dermatol Res 292:427–436

De Groot K, Rasmussen N, Bacon PA, Tervaert JW, Feighery C, Gregorini G, Gross WL, Luqmani R, Jayne DR (2005) Randomized trial of cyclophosphamide versus methotrexate for induction of remission in early systemic antineutrophil cytoplasmic antibody-associated vasculitis. Arthritis Rheum 52:2461–2469

Falk RJ, Jennette JC (1988) Anti-neutrophil cytoplasmic autoantibodies with specificity for myeloperoxidase in patients with systemic vasculitis and idiopathic necrotizing and crescentic glomerulonephritis. N Engl J Med 318:1651–1657

Falk RJ, Terrell RS, Charles LA, Jennette JC (1990) Anti-neutrophil cytoplasmic autoantibodies induce neutrophils to degranulate and produce oxygen radicals in vitro. Proc Natl Acad Sci USA 87:4115–4119

Ferri C, Mascia MT (2006) Cryoglobulinemic vasculitis. Curr Opin Rheumatol 18:54–63

Gadola SD, Moins-Teisserenc HT, Trowsdale J, Gross WL, Cerundolo V (2000) TAP deficiency syndrome. Clin Exp Immunol 121:173–178

Grimminger F, Hattar K, Papavassilis C, Temmesfeld B, Csernok E, Gross WL, Seeger W, Sibelius U (1996) Neutrophil activation by anti-proteinase 3 antibodies in Wegener's granulomatosis: role of exogenous arachidonic acid and leukotrien B4 generation. J Exp Med 184:1567–1572

Gross WL, Csernok E, Schmitt WH (1991) Antineutrophil cytoplasmic autoantibodies: immunobiolgical aspects. Klin Wochenschr 69:558–566

Gross WL (2003) Immunopathogenesis of vasculitis. In: Klippel JH, Dieppe PA (eds) Rheumatology. 3rd ed. Mosby, London, chapter 7.19, p. 1–8

Hautmann G, Campanile G, Lotti TM (1999) The many faces of cutaneous vasculitis. *Clin Dermatol* 17:515–531

Hoffman GS, Kerr GS, Leavitt RY, Hallahan CW, Lebovics RS, Travis WD, Rottem M, Fauci AS (1992) Wegener granulomatosis: an analysis of 158 patients. Ann Intern Med 116:488–498

Jayne D, Rasmussen N, Andrassy K, Bacon PA, Cohen Tervaert JW, Dadoniene J, Ekstrand A, Gaskin G, Gregorini G, deGroot K, Gross WL, Hagen EC, Mirapeix E, Pettersson E, Siegert C, Sinico A, Tesar V, Westman K, Pusey C, for the European Vasculitis Study Group (2003) A randomized trial of maintenance therapy for vasculitis associated with antineutrophil autoantibodies. N Engl J Med 349:36–44

Jennette JC, Falk RJ, Andrassy K, Bacon PA, Churg J, Gross WL, Hagen EC, Hoffman GS, Hunder GG, Kallenberg CG, McCluskey RT, Sinico A, Rees AJ, van Es LA, Waldherr R, Wiik A (1994) Nomenclature of systemic vasculitides. Proposal of an international consensus conference. Arthritis Rheum 37:187–192

Jennette JC, Falk R. (1997) Small-vessel vasculitis. N Engl J Med 337:1512–1523

Jones RB, Ferraro AJ, Chaudhry AN, Brogan P, Salama AD, Smith KG, Savage CO, Jayne DR (2009) A multicenter survey of rituximab therapy for refractory antineutrophil cytoplasmic antibody-associated vasculitis. Arthritis Rheum 60:2156–2168

Kessenbrock K, Krumbholz M, Schönermarck U, Back W, Gross WL, Werb Z, Gröne HJ, Brinkmann VJ, Jenne DE (2009) Netting neutrophils in autoimmune small-vessel vasculitis. Nat Med 15:623–625

Kocher M, Edberg JC, Fleit HB, Kimberly RP (1998) Antineutrophil cytoplasm antibodies preferentially engage Fc gammaRIIIb on human neutrophils. J Immunol 161:6909–6914

Lamprecht P, Moosig F, Adam-Klages S, Mrowietz U, Csernok E, Kirrstetter M, Ahmadi-Simab K, Schröder JO, Gross WL (2004) Small vessel vasculitis and relapsing panniculitis in tumor necrosis factor receptor-associated periodic syndrome (TRAPS). Ann Rheum Dis 63:1518–1520

Lamprecht P, Gross WL (2008) Antineutrophil cytoplasmic antibody-associated vasculitis: autoinflammation, autodestruction and autoimmunity – key to new therapies. Trends Immunol 29:587–588

Lamprecht P, Wieczorek S, Epplen JT, Ambrosch P, Kallenberg CG (2009a) Granuloma formation in ANCA-associated vasculitides. APMIS Suppl. 127:32–6

Lamprecht P, Holle J, Gross WL (2009b) Update on clinical, pathophysiological and therapeutic aspects in ANCA-associated vasculitides. Curr Drug Discov Technol 6:241–251

Lang KS, Recher M, Junt T, Navarini AA, Harris NL, Freigang S, Odermatt B, Conrad C, Ittner LM, Bauer S, Luther SA, Uematsu S, Akira S, Hengartner H, Zinkernagel RM (2005) Toll-like receptor engagement converts T-cell autoreactivity into overt autoimmune disease. Nat Med 11:138–145

Lanham JG, Elkon KB, Pusey CD, Hughes GR (1984) Systemic vasculitis with asthma and eosinophilia: a clinical approach to the Churg-Strauss syndrome. Medicine (Baltimore) 63:65–81

Metzler C, Miehle N, Manger K, Iking-Konert C, de Groot K, Hellmich B, Gross WL, Reinhold-Keller E; German Network of Rheumatic Diseases (2007) Elevated relapse rate under oral methotrexate versus leflunomide for maintenance of remission in Wegener's granulomatosis. Rheumatology (Oxford) 46:1087–1091

Metzler C, Schnabel A, Gross WL, Hellmich B (2008) A phase II study of interferon-alpha for the treatment of refractory Churg-Strauss syndrome. Clin Exp Rheumatol 26(3 Suppl 49): S35–40

Moins-Teisserenc HT, Gadola SD, Cella M, Dunbar PR, Exley A, Blake N, Baycal C, Lambert J, Bigliardi P, Willemsen M, Jones M, Buechner S, Colonna M, Gross WL, Cerundolo V (1999) Association of a syndrome resembling Wegener's granulomatosis with low surface expression of HLA class-I molecules. Lancet 354:1598–1603

Müller A, Holl-Ulrich K, Lamprecht P, Gross WL (2008) Germinal centre-like structures in Wegener's granuloma: the morphological basis for autoimmunity. Rheumatology (Oxford) 47:1111–1113

Nair P, Pizzichini MM, Kjarsgaard M, Inman MD, Efthimiadis A, Pizzichini E, Hargreave FE, O'Byrne PM (2009) Mepolizumab for prednisone-dependent asthma with sputum eosinophilia. N Engl J Med 360:985–993

Porges AJ, Redecha PB, Kimberly WT, Csernok E, Gross WL, Kimberly RP (1994) Anti-neutrophil cytoplasmic antibodies engage and activate human neutrophils via Fc gamma RIIa. J Immunol 153:1271–1280

Powell FC, Schroeter AL, Su WPD, Perry HO (1985) Pyoderma gangrenosum: A review of 86 patients. Q J Med 55:173–82

Radford DJ, Luu NT, Hewins P, Nash GB, Savage CO (2000) Antineutrophil cytoplasmic antibodies stabilize adhesion and promote migration of flowing neutrophils on endothelial cells. Arthritis Rheum 44:2851–2861

Rarok AA, Stegeman CA, Limburg PC, Kallenberg CG (2002) Neutrophil membrane expression of proteinase 3 (PR3) is related to relapse in PR3-ANCA-associated vasculitis. J Am Soc Nephrol 13:2232–2238

Reinhold-Keller E, Kekow J, Schnabel A, Schmitt WH, Heller M, Beigel A, Duncker G, Gross WL (1994) Influence of disease manifestation and antineutrophil cytoplasmic antibody titer on the response to pulse cyclophosphamide therapy in patients with Wegener's granulomatosis. Arthritis Rheum 37:919–924

Reinhold-Keller E, Beuge N, Latza U, de Groot K, Rudert H, Nolle B, Heller M, Gross WL (2000) An interdisciplinary approach to the care of patients with Wegener's granulomatosis: long-term outcome in 155 patients. Arthritis Rheum 43:1021–1032

Saadoun D, Delluc A, Piette JC, Cacoub P (2008) Treatment of hepatitis C-associated mixed cryoglobulinemia vasculitis. Curr Opin Rheumatol 20:23–28

Sablé-Fourtassou R, Cohen P, Mahr A, Pagnoux C, Mouthon L, Jayne D, Blockmans D, Cordier JF, Delaval P, Puechal X, Lauque D, Viallard JF, Zoulim A, Guillevin L; French Vasculitis Study Group (2005) Antineutrophil cytoplasmic antibodies and the Churg-Strauss syndrome. Ann Intern Med 143:632–638

Sais G, Vidaller A, Servitje O, Jucgla A, Peyri J (1996) Leukocytoclastic vasculitis and common variable immunodeficiency: successful treatment with intravenous immune globulin. J Allergy Clin Immunol 98:232–233

Sansonno D, Lauletta G, Nisi L, Gatti P, Pesola F, Pansini N, Dammacco F (2003) Non-enveloped HCV core protein as constitutive antigen of cold-precipitable immune complex in type II mixed cryoglobulinemia. Clin Exp Immunol 133:275–282

Schur PH (1993) Clinical features of SLE. In: Kelley WN, Harris ED Jr, Ruddy S, Sledge CB (eds) Textbook of Rheumatology, Volume 2. WB Saunders Company, Philadelphia London Toronto Montreal Sydney Tokyo, pp 1017–1042

Scott DG, Bacon PA (1984) Intravenous cyclophosphamide plus methylprednisolone in treatment of systemic rheumatoid vasculitis. Am J Med 76:377–384

Stegeman CA, Cohen Tervaert JW, de Jong PE, Kallenberg CGM (1996) Trimethoprim-sulfmethoxazole (Co-trimoxazole) for the prevention of relapses in Wegener's granulomatosis. N Engl J Med 335:16–20

Tatsis E, Schnabel A, Gross WL (1998) Interferon-alpha treatment of four patients with the Churg-Strauss syndrome. Ann Intern Med 129:370–374

Ullrich S, Gustke H, Lamprecht P, Gross WL, Schumacher U, Ambrosch P, Laudien M (2009) Severe impaired respiratory ciliary function in Wegener granulomatosis. Ann Rheum Dis 68:1067–1071

Voswinkel J, Mueller A, Kraemer JA, Lamprecht P, Herlyn K, Holl-Ulrich K, Feller AC, Pitann S, Gause A, Gross WL (2006) B lymphocyte maturation in Wegener's granulomatosis: a comparative analysis of VH genes from endonasal lesions Ann Rheum Dis 65:859–864

12

Wei G, Yano S, Kuroiwa T, Hiromura K, Maezawa A (1997) Hepatitis C virus (HCV)-induced IgG-IgM rheumatoid factor (RF) complex may be the main causal factor for cold-dependent activation of complement in patients with rheumatic disease. *Clin Exp Immunol* 107:83–88

Wieczorek S, Hellmich B, Arning L, Moosig F, Lamprecht P, Gross WL, Epplen JT (2008) Functionally relevant variations of the interleukin-10 gene associated with antineutrophil cytoplasmic antibody-negative Churg-Strauss syndrome, but not with Wegener's granulomatosis. Arthritis Rheum 58:1839–1848

Wieczorek S, Holle JU, Müller S, Fricke H, Gross WL, Epplen JT (2010). A functionally relevant IRF5 haplotype is associated with reduced risk to Wegener's granulomatosis. J Mol Med 88:413–421

Xiao H, Heeringa P, Hu P, Liu Z, Zhao M, Aratani Y, Maeda N, Falk RJ, Jennette JC (2002) Antineutrophil cytoplasmic autoantibodies specific for myeloperoxidase cause glomerulonephritis and vasculitis in mice. J Clin Invest 110:955–963

Yang JJ, Preston GA, Alcorta DA, Waga I, Munger WE, Hogan SL, Sekura SB, Phillips BD, Thomas RP, Jennette JC, Falk RJ (2002) Expression profile of leukocyte genes activated by anti-neutrophil cytoplasmic autoantibodies (ANCA). Kidney Int 62:1638–1649

Skin Manifestations of Rheumatic Diseases

13

Camille Francès and Nicolas Kluger

Introduction

This chapter focuses on cutaneous manifestations observed in autoimmune rheumatic diseases, particularly the main systemic vasculitides, rheumatoid arthritis and relapsing polychondritis. Clinical correlation between these manifestations and internal organ involvement is highlighted.

Skin Manifestations in Systemic Vasculitis

Even though a certain number of syndromes have been described, a patient may present with symptoms that overlap with another clinical diagnosis making a diagnosis "at first sight" impossible. Skin manifestations are frequently observed in almost all-systemic vasculitis (Carlson et al., 2006, Kluger et al., 2008, Crowson et al., 2003, Fiorentino, 2003). Some of them correspond to a skin localization of the systemic vasculitis while others result from a different pathologic process. As biopsy of dermatological lesions is easy to obtain, it has a great interest in confirming the diagnosis. However, its contribution to determine the type of vasculitis is not guaranteed. In fact, neither clinical nor pathologic features of the skin are specific of a given type. Furthermore, skin and systemic vasculitis may be coincident, as when skin involvement is drug-induced or follows a transient viral infection.

Skin Manifestations

Skin manifestations of vasculitis

Clinical features

Skin vasculitis presents as a spectrum of clinical lesions including erythema, purpura, papules, pustules, nodules, livedo, necrosis, ulcerations and bullae. These various lesions come often altogether giving a pleomorphic appearance of the eruption.

Palpable purpura is unquestionably the most frequent manifestation. Lesions usually begin as tiny red macules that later become papules and plaques ranging from several millimetres to several centimetres. Larger lesions are ecchymotic. Color range may change from red to purple to brownish yellow, as extravasated blood is progressively broken. Palpable purpura is most common on the legs, ankles and feet but other areas of the body can be affected (Fig. 1).

Urticarial vasculitis is characterized by the presence of wheals that persist two to three days unlike ordinary urticaria expected to clear within 24 hours. Pruritus is less intense. Lesions may become purpuric. They are mainly located on the trunk and the limbs (Fig. 2). Elsewhere, other papules, neither purpuric nor urticarial, may also correspond to skin vasculitis, especially when found on the outer aspects of the limbs. Some papules appear red

13

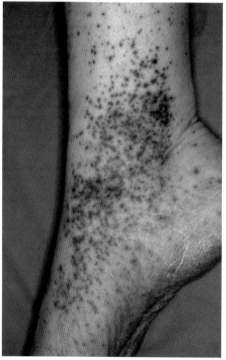

Fig. 1. Infiltrated purpura of the ankles

to purple, then become brown to yellow and follow a chronic evolution as in erythema elevatum diutinum.

Pustular vasculitis is usually non-follicular, underlined by erythema. Other frequently observed pustules may result from secondary infection of necrotic lesions.

Nodules of vasculitis are typically inflammatory, tender, red and small-sized (Fig. 3). They are mainly located on the lower limbs (legs, soles), where they can be surrounded by livedo reticularis, but are also observed on other sites such as the dorsal aspect of upper limbs or rarely the trunk. Nodules may also gather in groups along the course of superficial arteries.

Livedo reticularis is a reddish blue mottling of the skin in a "fishnet" reticular pattern. It is typically irregular with broken meshes (Fig. 4). Some infiltrated areas are found on careful examination. When associated with vasculitis, livedo persists indefinitely with some fluctuations in intensity and extensiveness as temperature varies.

Necrosis results from the obstruction of dermal vessels (Fig. 5). Its extension and depth are highly variable depending on extension and depth of involved vessels. Localized necrotic lesions may turn into vesicles. Pustules may appear due to secondary infection. When necrosis is extensive, painful purpura is followed by a black necrotic plaque with active purpuric border and bullous lesions. After removal of necrotic tissue, ulcerations of various sizes take place.

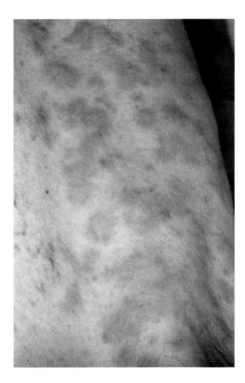

Fig. 2. Urticarial vasculitis on the limbs

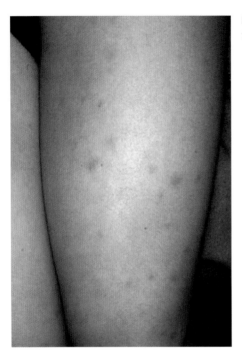

Fig. 3. Nodules on the lower limbs in a patient with cutaneous periarteritis nodosa

13

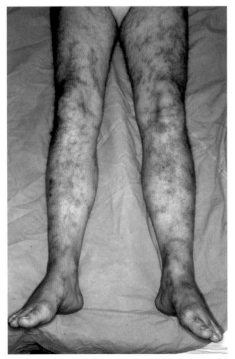

Fig. 4. Infiltrated, irregular livedo reticularis of vasculitis (livedo racemosa)

Fig. 5. Necrotic lesions secondary to a vasculitis involving both the superficial and deep dermal vessels.

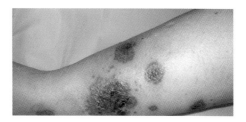

Histopathology and clinical-pathological correlation (Crowson et al., 2003)

The hallmark pathologic pattern of purpuric lesions is leukocytoclastic vasculitis of the small dermal vessels. Post-capillary venules are preferentially involved. Leukocytoclastic vasculitis is characterized by vascular alterations and dermal cellular infiltrates.

Vascular alterations consist of endothelial cell swelling, activation of nuclei, wrinkling of nuclear membranes, necrosis with deposition of fibrinoid material and sometimes thrombosis. The fibrinoid material is predominantly made of fibrin but also contains necrotic endothelial cells and deposits of immuno-reactants (immunoglobulins and / or complement proteins).

Dermal infiltrates vary in intensity. They are usually peri-vascular but at times widely dispersed. Neutrophils with nucleus fragmentation (karyorrhexis or leukocytoclasia) are the main cells. In other cases or at a later stage, lymphocytes and monocytes may predominate.

In some patients, especially those with immune complex-mediated vasculitis and extensive complement activation, dermal small-vessel vasculitis generates focal oedema with subsequent urticaria.

Nodular vasculitis results from inflammation of vessel walls at the dermo-hypodermal junction or in subcutaneous fat. When arterioles are involved, pathologic features become similar to those observed in cutaneous polyarteritis nodosa. Endothelial swelling and fibrinoid necrosis of the media are often severe with inconstant thrombosis. Invasion of the vessel wall with neutrophils is usual in the acute phase although leukocytoclasis is less frequently observed. In other cases, the infiltrate can be initially granulomatous. In the healing phase, the vessel wall is invaded by granulation tissue and replaced by a fibrous scar. Continuous proliferation of capillaries occurs.

In summary, palpable purpura and papular lesions such as urticaria correspond to a leukocytoclastic or lymphocytic vasculitis of the small vessels of the dermis. Nodules correspond to a vasculitis of arterioles or vessels at the dermo-hypodermal junction or in the subcutaneous fat. Necrosis and livedo occur when either small and / or larger vessels are involved.

Other skin manifestations associated with systemic vasculitis.

Extravascular necrotizing granuloma

Initially described by Churg and Strauss in 1951 as a manifestation of allergic angiitis (Churg-Strauss syndrome), the extravascular granuloma has been further reported in a large variety of other systemic vasculitis and connective tissue diseases (Guillevin et al., 1999, Davis et al., 1997, Obermoser et al., 2002). Papular or nodular lesions vary in size, from 2 mm to 2 cm or more, and colour, from red to purple. Central crusting and / or ulceration are frequent. Rarely, other aspects are reported like vesicles, pustules, arciform plaques or firm mass. Sites of involvement are the extensor aspects of the elbows, the fingers where they are usually multiple, often symmetrical, and less frequently the buttocks, the scalp, the knees, the hands, the dorsum of feet, the neck, the forehead, the ears…

Histological features include endothelial necrosis and oedema, fibrinoid necrosis of the collagen and granulomas containing eosinophils, histiocytes and lymphocytes. The centre of the granuloma consists of basophilic fibrillar necrosis in which bands (sometimes linear) of destroyed tissue are interspersed with poly-morpho-nuclear leukocytes and leukocytoclastic debris. This necrotic area is surrounded by a granulomatous mass of histiocytes, often in a palisade array. Decrease or absence of elastic fibres is observed in foci of degenerated collagen. No relationship is noted between the clinical appearance of lesions, the histological features, and the associated systemic disease. However, tissue eosinophilia is more frequently reported in patients with Churg-Strauss syndrome. The profound alteration of the T-cell response including Th1 and Th17 responses, anomalously NK-receptor-expressing 'NK-like' T cells, and dysfunctional regulatory T cells could facilitate and sustain granuloma formation and autoimmunity (Lamprecht et al., 2009).

Panniculitis

Cutaneous eruption consists of recurrent crops of erythematous, oedematous and tender subcutaneous nodules. The nodule size is around 1 or 2 cm but could be much larger. In lobular panniculitis, lesions are usually of symmetrical distribution on the thighs and the lower legs. They usually regress spontaneously with hypopigmented and atrophic scar due to fat necrosis. Occasionally, they may suppurate. In septal panniculitis, nodular lesions are primarily located over the extensor aspects of the lower limbs. They regress spontaneously without atrophic scar.

A lobular infiltrate of lymphocytes, plasma cells, and histiocytes with fat necrosis is common in lobular panniculitis while in septal panniculitis the infiltrate surrounds vessels of the septa.

Pyoderma gangrenosum

Pyoderma gangrenosum lesions usually begin as deep-seated, painful nodules or as superficial hemorrhagic pustules, either de novo or after minimal trauma. They further break down and ulcerate discharging purulent and haemorrhagic exudates. Ulcers spread reaching 10 cm or more, partially regress or remain indolent for a long period. The irregular edges are raised, red or purplish, undermined, soggy and often perforated. The most commonly affected sites are the lower extremities, the buttocks and the abdomen but other areas of the body may be involved. Lesions are usually solitary but may arise in clusters,

13

which then coalesce to form polycyclic irregular ulcerations. When healing occurs, an atrophic and often cribriform scar is left.

The histological features consist of a large, sterile abscess in which thrombosis of small- and medium-sized vessels, haemorrhage and necrosis are present. Neutrophils are numerous but epithelioid, giant, and mononuclear cells are also seen especially in forms that are more chronic. Leukocytoclastic or lymphocytic vasculitis may be observed, particularly in the active border of the lesion. These changes are not pathognomonic and the diagnosis is essentially based on the clinical aspects.

Granuloma

Granulomatous lesions with neither vasculitis nor central necrosis may be observed in systemic vasculitis, especially Wegener's granulomatosis. Clinical aspect is highly variable ranging from papules, nodules, subcutaneous infiltration, and pseudo-tumour to chronic ulcers. Any site of the body may be involved: breasts, scrotum, face, gums... Other granulomatous diseases have to be considered in the differential diagnosis like sarcoidosis, metastatic Crohn's disease, mycobacterium infections, and foreign bodies granulomas.

Superficial thrombophlebitis

Thrombophlebitis of a superficial vein is sometimes clinically evident due to the presence of painful induration of the vein with redness and increased heat. In other cases, the clinical aspect is a non-specific red nodule and diagnosis is only confirmed by histological examination of a deep skin biopsy. Such lesions are essentially observed in thromboangiitis obliterans, Behçet's disease, Crohn's disease and relapsing polychondritis.

Gangrene

Gangrene resulting from arterial occlusion may be observed in all vasculitis involving medium or large-sized arteries. It is initially characterized by a sharply demarcated blue-black colour of the extremities. The main differential diagnoses are thrombosis, without inflammation of the vessel walls, and emboli. Angiography visualizes occlusion or stenosis of arteries and does not help distinguishing these different pathologic processes.

Raynaud's phenomenon

Bilateral Raynaud's phenomenon may occur in 5 to 30% of randomly questioned population. It is classically associated with all types of vasculitis. However, its prevalence is unknown in many vasculitis and its diagnostic value is very low. In contrast, unilateral Raynaud's phenomenon suggests an obstructive arterial disease and is mainly observed in Takayasu's arteritis.

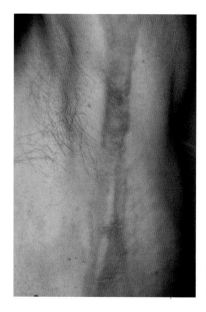

Fig. 6. Palpable cord on the lateral aspects of the trunk (the rope sign) of interstititial granulomatous dermatitis.

Interstitial granulomatous dermatitis (IGD)

IGD is a histological term describing the association of a characteristic inflammatory infiltrate and other clinical findings including linear cord-like lesions (Fig. 6). It is an uncommon disorder. Skin manifestations include typical erythematous, asymptomatic, palpable cords on the lateral aspects of the trunk (the rope sign) or slight burning and multiple, bilateral, somewhat symmetrical, erythematous plaques, mainly involving the lateral chest wall, abdomen and medial thighs (Crowson et al., 2009).

Histopathologically, IGD is quite distinct and characterized by a dense, diffuse dermal inflammatory infiltrate composed primarily of histiocytes distributed interstitially and in palisaded array. In the deep reticular dermis, small foci of degenerated collagen are enveloped by large numbers of neutrophils and/or eosinophils.

IGD may be associated with various auto-immune vascular diseases, including rheumatoid arthritis, SLE, Still's disease, Churg-Strauss syndrome, microscopic polyangiitis, thyroiditis and vitiligo. Although its cause remains unknown, its association with autoimmune diseases makes an immune complex-mediated pathogenesis likely.

Dermatological Findings in the main systemic vasculitides (Table 1)

Henoch-Schönlein purpura

The association of purpuric lesions with arthritis, gastrointestinal symptoms, and IgA nephritis is considered as a distinctive entity among the group of angiitis and called Henoch-

Table 1. Dermatologic manifestations in systemic vasculities

Systemic vasculitis	Most frequent dermatologic lesions	Most typical dermatologic lesions
Henoch-Schönlein purpura	Purpura, Urticaria	Purpura, Urticaria
Essential cryoglobulinemic vasculitis	Purpura	Pigmented purpura
Polyarteritis nodosa	Purpura	Nodules, Livedo
Microscopic polyangiitis	Purpura, Nodules	Purpura
Churg and Strauss syndrome	Purpura	Extravascular necrotizing granuloma
Wegener's granulomatosis	Purpura	Oral ulcers Gingival hyperplasia

Schonlein purpura. Synonyms for this illness are Henoch-Schonlein syndrome, anaphylactoid purpura, allergic purpura and haemorrhagic capillary toxicosis. This type of vasculitis predominantly occurs in children although all ages can be affected. There is no seasonal pattern but higher incidence in winter and lower incidence in summer have been recorded. In adults over 41 years of age, a malignancy, especially solid tumours, may be associated with this vasculitis. There were no distinctive features of HSP associated with malignancy. Although the frequency of this association has not been evaluated extensively, adult patients without indentifiable triggers of HSP should be evaluated for underlying malignancy (Mitsui et al., 2009, Solans-Laqué et al., 2008).

Skin lesions begin as a crop of red macules, some of which resolve in the early stage while others become papular, urticarial or purpuric. In some cases, the characteristic urticarial component of the rash is missing and purpura is the only sign. When inflammation and exudation are severe with involvement of all superficial vessels, haemorrhagic vesicles, bulla, necrosis, and ulcers develop. The sites of predilection are the extensor aspects of the limbs, the buttocks, the back, and occasionally the face. Rarely, oral mucosa is involved. Lesions occur in successive waves then resolve spontaneously. On histology, early changes are essentially those of leukocytoclastic vasculitis with extravasation of erythrocytes. In the later stages, mononuclear cells may predominate. The superficial dermal vessels are quite exclusively involved. The frequency of dermal IgA vessel deposits varies depending on series. These IgA deposits are sometimes included in the diagnostic criteria of dermatology series and thus are present in 100% of cases. Inversely, these deposits are present in only 50% of patients of nephrology series where IgA nephropathy is present in 100% of cases. These dermal IgA deposits are not specific of Henoch-Schonlein purpura; they may be encountered in a large variety of cutaneous vasculitis (Tancrede-Bohin et al., 1997).

Cryoglobulinemic vasculitis

Cryoglobulins are immunoglobulins that persist in the serum, precipitate with cold temperature, and resolubilize when rewarmed. Three types have been described. Mixed type II and III cryoglobulins induce mainly vasculitis by immune-complex deposition while monoclonal Type I cryoglobulin induces more vessels occlusions than an inflammatory vasculitis. Main causes of mixed cryoglobulinemia include mainly hepatitis C chronic infection, B-cell lymphoproliferative disorders and autoimmune diseases (systemic lupus and Sjögren's syndrome). Nowadays, "essential" mixed cryoglobulinemia represents barely between 10 to 30% of all cases (Ferri, 2008)

Skin manifestations occur in 60% to100% of patients with symptomatic cryoglobulinemia (Cohen et al., 1991). They are a frequent presenting complaint and often come along with arthralgia and weakness. The disease has a tendency to wax and wane. Women outnumber men with a sex ratio W / M of 1.3 / 1. The average age of onset is 50 years. The interval between the first skin manifestation and diagnosis of cryoglobulinemia varies from 0 to 10 years. Palpable purpura of the lower extremities is the main manifestation, present from 30 to 100% of the patients. The lesions may extend progressively to the abdomen. Purpura often displays seasonal triggering (winter time, cold exposure) or related to prolonged standing, physical exertion, or trauma. Purpuric lesions can first start by a preceding burning sensation and leave a brown residual pigmentation (dermite ocre) within 10 days. Post-inflammatory pigmentation is noted in 40% of patients and can retrospectively evoke the diagnosis. Infarction, haemorrhagic crusts and ulcers are present in 10 to 25% of patients. Widespread necrotic areas, head and mucosal involvement, livedoid vasculitis, Raynaud's phenomenon and cold induced acrocyanosis are relatively more common in type I cryoglobulinemia.

On histology, purpura corresponds to a leukocytoclastic vasculitis of the small dermal vessels. DIF studies have shown IgM, IgG, and C3 deposits in some patients with acute vasculitis. In type I cryoglobulinemia, thrombosis is the main histological feature, sometimes associated with vasculitis.

As HCV infection is the main identified etiology of essential mixed cryoglobulinemia (especially type II), the influence of this infection on clinical presentation has been studied. Globally, the clinical and histological aspects of purpura are not different wether HCV infection is present or not (Dupin et al., 1995).

Polyarteritis nodosa (PAN)

According to the names and definitions of vasculitis adopted by the Chapel Hill consensus conference on the nomenclature of systemic vasculitides, classic polyarteritis nodosa (PAN) is characterized by a necrotizing inflammation of medium-sized or small arteries without glomerulonephritis or vasculitis in arterioles, capillaries or venules (Jennette et al., 1994).

Systemic PAN is actually very rare; its evolution is acute with skin manifestations different from those observed in chronic cutaneous PAN.

The skin hallmarks of **cutaneous PAN** are nodules. These cutaneous or subcutaneous nodules are the first sign of the disease and appear in groups along the course of superficial arteries. They measure between 5 and 25 mm in diameter and are mainly located on the lower legs, especially around the knees and on the feet. Arms, trunk, head, and buttocks also can be involved. The number of nodules is highly variable, according to each flare. Each nodule displays a course ranging from a few days to more than 2 months. Nodules may leave a violaceous livedoid color or pigmentation that persists for months to years. Livedo reticularis may precede, come along, or follow the onset of nodules. In PAN, livedo reticularis is typically located on the lower limbs, the dorsal aspects of upper limbs and rarely the trunk. The fishnet reticular pattern is irregular with broken meshes. On careful examination, infiltrated areas of the fishnet pattern are palpable. Painful ulcerations are frequently associated with tender and firm plaques resulting from coalescent nodules (Fig. 7). Some patients may present atrophic, ivory-colored, stellate-shaped scars (atrophie blanche) (Mimouni et al., 2003). These clinical features are characteristic of cutaneous PAN which, by definition, only affects small arteries of the skin. A full-thickness excison of an active inflammatory nodule will show a necrotizing arteritis with variable amounts of fibrinoid necrosis and leukocytoclasia, edema, and inflammatory cells. DIF may show non specific immunoglobulins IgM and complement deposits (Diaz-Pérez et al., 2007).

These chronic, benign limited cutaneous forms of periarteritis nodosa are in fact frequently associated with arthralgia and pure sensitive neuropathy. Systemic acute disease rarely occurs in the course of cutaneous PAN.

Cutaneous manifestations, occurring during systemic PAN, have been reported from 28% to 60% , 44% in our experience (Kluger et al., 2008). They were one of the presenting manifestations in 33% of cases. The most frequent skin lesions were palpable purpura (19%), livedo (17%) and nodules (15%). Other manifestations may be observed such as urticaria, transient erythema, superficial phlebitis, Raynaud's phenomenon, splinter haemorrhages, digital necrosis. Localized oedema is usually associated with underlying muscular involvement. Although this systemic disease mainly affects the medium-sized arteries of the kidney, liver, heart and gastrointestinal tract, the most common cutaneous finding was small vessel leukocytoclastic vasculitis.

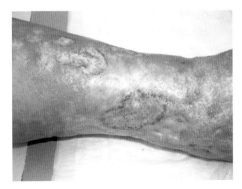

Fig. 7. Fibrous ulcerations and livedoid vasculitis during the course of cutaneous PAN. Erythematous periphery of the ulcers indicates the beginning of ulcer healing under immunosuppressive therapy

Microscopic polyangiitis (MPA)

The microscopic form of PAN, now called microscopic polyangiitis (MPA), is defined as a systemic vasculitis of small-sized vessels (i. e. capillaries, venules or arterioles) without ex-travacular granuloma. MPA is associated with segmental necrotizing glomerulonephritis and anti-neutrophil cytoplasm antibodies (ANCA) of the myeloperoxidase type.

Dermatologic manifestations occur in 25 to 60% of patients (Kluger et al., 2008, Guillevin et al., 1999). Purpuric lesions of the lower limbs are the most frequent. Other lesions have been reported such as erythematous macules, vesicles, bullae, splinter haemorrhages, annular purpura, nodules, palmar erythema, erythema elevatum diutinum, oral ulcers, facial oedema and pyoderma gangrenosum-like lesion. All these skin lesions rapidly disappear with treatment.

Leukocytoclastic vasculitis of the small vessels of dermis is usually observed. Sometimes, arterioles or smaller vessels of the deep dermis and subcutaneous fat are also involved, explaining the nodular appearance of skin lesions. DIF is usually negative but the presence of vascular deposits of immunoglobulins and complement does not exclude the diagnosis. Of note, neither the cutaneous manifestations, nor the skin histological studies contribute to the distinction between PAN and MPA (Kluger et al., 2008).

Churg and Strauss syndrome

In 1951, Churg and Strauss defined allergic granulomatosis as a distinct entity occurring in asthmatic adults and associated with fever, eosinophilia, systemic vasculitis and extra-vascular granulomas.

Skin lesions have been observed in 40 to 75% of cases depending on series. They are rarely (6%) the presenting symptom (Davis et al., 1997, Guillevin et al., 1999). Palpable purpura, petechia, ecchymoses, hemorrhagic bullae on lower extremities are the most frequent cutaneous manifestation (50%). Cutaneous nodules (30%) or papules are also very frequent, sometimes with an urticarial appearance, located on the lower limbs or on the extensor side of the elbows, fingers, scalp and / or breast. Lesions of the fingers are usually multiple, often symmetrical, and most commonly localized at both lateral sides of the distal inter-phalangeal joint. These nodules or papules of the upper limbs have frequently central crusting or ulceration. Their consistence is usually firm. A pustular or vesicular component is rarely noted. Various other dermatologic lesions have been reported: maculo-papules resembling erythema multiforme, ulcerations, livedo reticularis, patchy and migratory urticarial rash, nail fold infarction with splinter haemorrhages, and facial oedema (Davis et al., 1997).

Histologically, three distinct patterns – that can be associated on a biopsy – are noted during CSS: i) a small vessel eosinophil rich neutrophilic vasculitis of the superficial and mid dermis, ii), dermal eosinophilia and iii) palisading neutrophilic and granulomatous inflammation with degenerated collagen bundles (so called "red" granulomas). Nodules correspond to granulomatous vasculitis, or necrotizing vasculitis of arterioles of the deep dermis or hypodermis (similar to those observed in PAN) or to extra-vascular granuloma. Conversely extra-vascular granuloma correlates, in the majority of patients, with papules and nodules on the extensor aspects of the elbows. Finally, histological findings of skin lesions can be disappointing, typical granuloma and eosinophilia not being detected in more than half of patients. Skin lesions rapidly respond to systemic corticosteroids and eosinophilia may be absent. DIF is usually negative.

Wegener's granulomatosis

Wegener's granulomatosis (WG) is a systemic vasculitis characterized by granulomatous necrotizing inflammatory lesions of the upper and lower respiratory tractus, usually accompanied by rapidly progressing glomerulonephritis. Any other organ system may be affected. Detection of ANCA is an essential clue to the diagnosis. In this systemic vasculitis, ANCA have typically a diffuse cytoplasmic immunfluorescence pattern (C-ANCA) and anti-proteinase 3 specificity (Guillevin et al., 1997).

Dermatologic lesions are frequently encountered and occasionally may be the initial manifestations (8–13%). Their prevalences during the course of the disease, varies according to the series (Guillevin et al., 1997, Hoffman et al., 1992) from 12 to 67% of cases.

Palpable purpura of the lower extremities is undoubtedly the most frequent clinical manifestation. It is usually secondary to leukocytoclastic vasculitis affecting mainly the small vessel (post-capillary venules) of the upper dermis but also larger vessels, especially in case of associated necrosis (Francès et al., 1994).

Oral ulcers are present in 10% to 50% of cases depending on series. Unlike aphthae, they are persistent and not recurrent (Fig. 8). Their number and localization are highly variable. They were observed on cheeks, tongue, floor of the mouth, lips, palate, gingivae,

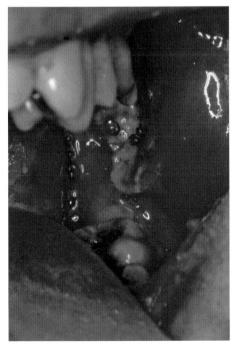

Fig. 8. Cheek ulceration in a patient with Wegener Granulomatosis

tonsils, posterior palate. Genital ulcers are uncommon although penile necrosis has previously been described. Histopathologic findings of oral ulcers in WG tend to be nonspecific, showing only acute and chronic inflammation (Patten et al., 1993). In a few cases, an extravascular granuloma has been reported (Francès et al., 1994).

Papulo-necrotic lesions are ulcerated papules that are present on the extensor surfaces of the limbs closed to elbows, knees, hands and feet. They can occur as well on the face and scalp. Occasionally, they can resemble erythema elevatum diutinum and may be associated with IgA paraproteinemia. Found in 10% of WG, patients these lesions may be mistaken for rheumatoid nodules. Unlike rheumatoid nodules, they tend to ulcerate and are mobile within the dermis (Fiorentino, 2003). They correspond to leukocytoclastic or granulomatous vasculitis involving small vessels or to extra-vascular granuloma.

Nodules are quite frequent, mainly localized on the limbs. They are related to a necrotizing vasculitis involving medium-sized arterioles of the deep dermis or hypodermis, which may be suggestive of periarteritis nodosa for the pathologist. In other cases, these nodules are related to granulomatous vasculitis of medium-sized arterioles, to extra-vascular granuloma or non specific septal panniculitis.

Extensive and painful cutaneous ulcerations may precede in weeks to years other systemic manifestations. These ulcers are sometimes described as "pyoderma gangrenosum-like lesions", especially when they follow a localized traumatism or the breakdown of painful nodules or pustules. However, they usually lack the typical raised, tender, undermined border of pyoderma gangrenosum. Sometimes numerous, they are located on the limbs, the trunk, the face (pre-auricular area), the breasts (mimicking adeno-carcinoma with possible nipple retraction and galactorrhea) and the perineum. The histopathologic pattern of pyoderma-like ulcerations differs from that observed in pyoderma gangrenosum as it is characterized by foci of palisaded neutrophilic and granulomatous dermatitis, prominent granulomatous and neutrophilic necrotizing vasculitis and basophilic collagen degeneration.

Digital gangrene is occasionally reported. An unusual and distinctive gingivitis considered pathognomonic of WG in early stages occurs in some patients (Manchanda et al., 2003). This gingivitis is characterized by an exophytic hyperplasia with petechial flecks and a red, friable, granular appearance that begins focally in the interdental papillae and quickly spreads to produce a segmental or panoral gingivitis (Fig. 9). It may be associated with alveolar bone loss and tooth mobility. Pain and bleeding are common. Biopsy specimens generally show chronic inflammation with histiocytes and eosinophils, in some instance forming microabscesses. Giant cells are often present.

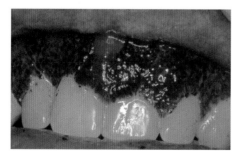

Fig. 9. Gingival hyperplasia in a patient with Wegener Granulomatosis

Florid xanthelasma is usually associated with longstanding granulomatous orbital and periorbital infiltration.

Although WG is considered a pauci-immune systemic vasculitis based on the absence of immune deposits in renal biopsies of patients with active disease, a susbstantial number of skin biopsies showed immune deposits (24–71%). C3 deposition in and around dermal vessels is the most frequent finding. IgM, IgG and/or IgA deposits may also be detected without similar immune deposits in the kidney biopsies (Brons et al., 2001, Daoud et al., 1994).

Dermatologic lesions of WG may correlate with the activity, distribution and course of the disease, thus serving as prognostic indicators (Barksdale et al., 1995). They were found to be associated with a higher frequency of articular and renal involvement (Francès et al., 1994). According to the Mayo clinic series (Daoud et al., 1994), patients with cutaneous lesions had an 80% chance of kidney involvement developing during the course of the disease whereas the overall risk was 33.4% in this study group.

A correlation was also demonstrated between the histopathologic subgroups and different clinical courses of WG. Patients with leukocytoclastic vasculitis had more rapidly progressive and widespread WG than patients with granulomatous skin lesions or patients without skin lesions. A marked excess of joint and musculoskeletal symptoms and renal disease was seen in patients with leukocytoclastic vasculitis. Patients with granulomatous inflammation had less systemic involvement and progressed at a slower rate than that of the patients with leukocyctoclastic vasculitis (Barksdale et al., 1995).

Localized WG may be localized in lungs, sinus or skin. When present only on skin, ulcerations and nodules are proeminent on the face and not on the limbs as in systemic disease (Kuchel et al., 2003). Cutaneous lesions may also be associated with sole sinus involvement. This bipolar WG has usually a subacute or chronic course without life-threatening localization. Generally, patients suffer from chronic sinusitis and nodules of the limbs. These localized subtypes of WG are characterized histologically by the presence of granuloma or granulomatous vasculitis. PBMCs from localized WG exhibited higher spontaneous IFN-gamma and IL10 production (Muller et al., 2000). A larger fraction of in situ CD4(+)CD28(-) T-cells displayed CCR5 expression compared to generalized WG (Lamprecht et al., 2003). This immune blood and tissue response may explain the best prognosis of these localized subtypes. However severe multi-organ system involvement may develop several years later requiring a long-term follow up.

Takayasu arteritis (TA)
(Perniciaro et al., 1987, Francès et al., 1990, Skaria et al., 2000, Pascual-Lopez et al. 204)

TA is a rare chronic inflammatory arteriopathy of unknown origin that predominantly affects the aorta and its main branches. Two, eventually overlapping, stages of this disease have been distinguished: a first systemic nonspecific inflammatory stage followed by an occlusive stage characterized by inflammation of the media and adventitial layers of the large vessels wall resulting in vascular stenosis and/or aneurysm formation.

Skin manifestations have been reported in 2.8 to 28% of patients. Some are directly related to large vessels occlusion such as unilateral Raynaud's phenomenon, digital gangrene or unilateral digital clubbing. Other skin manifestations were frequently thought to be related to this vasculitis i. e. ulcerated or non ulcerated nodules of the lower limbs, pyoderma gangrenosum, livedo reticularis, papular or papulo-necrotic lesions, superficial phlebitis, Sweet lesions. Other manifestations are occasionally related without evident relationship with TA: urticaria, angioedema, erythema multiforme, erythematous eruptions and "dermatitis". The prevalence of these different skin lesions greatly varies from Asian to European countries. In northern America and Europe, acute or sub-acute inflammatory nodules are the most commonly observed skin lesions. Erythema induratum corresponds to ulcerated sub-acute nodular lesions. The histological features of these nodules are variable. They may correspond to granulomatous or necrotizing vasculitis of small-sized or medium-sized arterioles of the dermis or hypodermis, extra-vascular granuloma, septal or lobular panniculitis. Usually, there is no correlation between the localization of the nodules and alterations of large vessels revealed by angiography. Furthermore, these nodules can occur at any stage of the disease. Tuberculoid infiltration has been reported in biopsies from papular or papulo-necrotic lesions raising the problem of an infectious origin of the disease. These lesions mainly occur at the occlusive stage of the disease. In Japan, pyoderma gangrenosum-like lesions are frequent, especially at the occlusive stage; this type of lesions has also been reported in patients from Northern Africa. The relationship between skin manifestations and TA is based on the absence of other aetiology and on the parallel course of skin lesions and vasculitis. Whatever is the stage of the disease, recurrence of skin lesions is strongly suggestive of arteritis reactivation.

Giant cell arteritis (GCA)

GCA is a systemic vasculitis with a predilection for small- to medium-sized cranial arteries in elderly patients. It represents less than 1% of all cutaneous vasculitis. Skin manifestations are often observed in the late stages of the disease (Currey, 1997). Therefore, they are actually rare due to an early diagnosis. According to a French retrospective study of 260 patients, cutaneous symptoms represent only 2% of the inaugural symptoms and they don't develop solely (Becourt-Verlomme et al., 2001).

Classically, scalp and temples are tender and red. Tender cordlike nodules are palpable over the course of temporal, occipital or facial arteries. Pulsations in these arteries are diminished or absent. Exceptionally, multiple scalp aneurysms have been reported..

The majority of other skin lesions are the consequence of ischemia related to cranial arteries occlusion and localized on the tongue and the scalp. Glossitis occurs in 10% of patients, and may sometimes be revealing. The tongue has a red, raw-beef colour and may become blistered, scaling or gangrenous. Necrosis usually occurs in the anterior two-thirds (Monteiro et al., 2002, Matsushima et al., 2003, Campbell et al., 2003). Lesions may start as crusts of the scalp that misdiagnosed for herpes zoster lesions. Bullae, ulcers or massive necrosis may then affect the scalp. Patients with scalp necrosis represent a subgroup of severe GCA with older age of onset and frequent serious complications such as visual loss, gangrene of the tongue or nasal septum necrosis. The mean interval between onset of symptoms of GCA and scalp necrosis is 3.0 months. Under treatment, scalp healing is complete or satisfactory in 75% of cases. In other cases, skin grafts are possible. Less severe chronic ischemia of the scalp leads to thinning or loss of hair. Ischemic skin lesions of the neck or the cheeks are occasionally reported. Rarely, vessels of the lower limbs are involved leading to ischemic ulcerations or distal gangrene. Skin biopsy of the border of ulceration or necrotic tissue is rarely contributive since granulomatous vasculitis has been shown in only 2 of 24 biopsies from patients with scalp necrosis. Other skin manifestations have been published as case-reports: nodules of the lower limbs with granulomatous vasculitis in the hypodermis or septal panniculitis, butterfly rash with transient oedema. Senile purpura is frequent on sun-exposed skin areas in elderly patients, especially when treated with corticosteroids. However, palpable purpura of the lower limbs due to vasculitis is exceptional.

Skin Manifestations in Rheumatoid Arthritis (Ra)

Extra-articular complications including dermatologic manifestations occur in more aggressive and long-standing forms of RA (Sayah et al., 2005, Yamamoto, 2009). Three main distinctive pathological patterns are recognized , namely extravascular palisading inflammation, active vasculopathy encompassing lymphocyte-dominant, neutrophil rich and granulomatous vasculitis, and interstitial and/or subcuticular neutrophilia. In most cases an overlap of the three reaction patterns is seen (Magro et al., 2003).

Palisading Granulomas

Rheumatoid nodules

Classic rheumatoid nodules are present in about 25% of patients and are the most common extra-articular manifestation of RA (Fig. 10). About 90 percent of patients with rheumatoid nodules are rheumatoid factor positive. They generally develop as a later manifestation of active arthritic disease though some nodules can form prior to joint disease. Involved most often are areas prone to mild, repetitive irritation such as extensor surfaces of

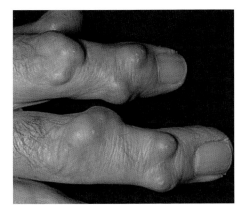

Fig. 10. Rheumatoid nodules

the forearms, the elbows, the hands – especially the fingers joints –, sacral prominences, the Achilles' tendon and less often the ears and the head. Rarely, rheumatoid nodules may be located in tendons, synovium, bones, sclera, dura, even vocal cords and internal organs, particularly the lungs and the heart. The size of these mostly indolent, hard, flesh-coloured, dome-shaped nodules varies from 5 to 15 mm; they may be visible above the skin level or palpable only subcutaneously or even in the soft parts. The characteristic histological features of rheumatoid nodules are dense deposits of fibrin surrounded by palisades of histiocytes, lymphocytes, plasma cells, and occasionally neutrophils and neutrophilic dust. The majority of patients with rheumatoid nodules suffers from severe forms of sero-positive RA, which subsequently lead to a clinically poorer outcome. Only rare complications of nodules are noted such as ulcerations, infections, sepsis, and fistula formation require surgical intervention. Accelerated growth of rheumatoid nodules (*rheumatoid nodulosis*) can be observed in RA patients under treatment with methotrexate.

Other cutaneous granulomas in rheumatoid arthritis

Pseudorheumatoid nodules are mostly seen in children but also in some adults of whom not all have rheumatic disease. They mainly occur on scalp and lower legs and are considered a deep, or juxta-articular form of granuloma annulare.

Palisaded neutrophilic granumomatous dermatitis (PNGD) is a rare dermatologic condition which shows various clinical and histopathological features. In our opinion, this entity is similar to interstitial granumatous dermatis (IGD). Initial lesions can be urticarial and later evolve to skin-coloured nodules. On the elbows, they may clinically resemble rheumatoid nodules. In other patients, cutaneous plaques, or linear cords are seen, especially on the lateral aspects of the trunk. The histologic appearance of PNGD vary from diffuse interstitial inflammation composed of lymphocytes, histiocytes and eosinophils and little neutrophils to dense neutrophilic infiltrates with degenerated collagen, leukocytoclastic debris and palisading granuloma with fibrosis and scant neutrophilic debris. *Cutaneous mucinous nodules* described mostly in Japanese patients with rheumatoid arthritis may represent another variant of PNGD clinically and pathologically characterized by extensive subcutaneous mucin deposition.

Rheumatoid Vasculitis (RV)

RV is a rare inflammatory condition of the small- and medium-sized vessels that affects a subset of approximately 1 to 5% of the patients with established RA (Genta et al., 2006). It is defined as an exclusion diagnosis after having ruled out all other causes of vasculitis during RA (infection, drug hypersensitivity, malignancy, or other vasculitides :WG, cryoglobulinemia, PAN…). Skin is the most commonly affected in 90% of the cases with focal digital infarcts with nailfold involvement appearing as dark perinungual macules (Bywaters lesions), maculopapular erythema, palpable purpura, haemorrhagic blisters, ulcers, and gangrene. Petechiae and purpura occur mostly in the lower extremities and has no specific characteristics. Ulcers are usually deep, painful, with a punched-out aspect and tend to be found in the lower extremities in unusual locations, such as the dorsum of the foot or the tibia. Moreover, subcutaneous nodules, livedo reticularis, atrophie blanche, pyoderma gangrenosum and erythema elevatum diutinum have been also reported. Chen *et al.* described three different pathological pattern upon histology of cutaneous lesions of RV : i) dermal necrotizing venulitis with predominance of neutrophilic infiltrates (leucocytoclastic vasculitis) related to purpura, haemorrhagic bullae, maculopapular erythema and erythema elevatum diutinum; ii) acute or healed arteritis at the junction of dermis and subcutis, histologically resembling cutaneous polyarteritis nodosa, in nodules, livedo reticularis and ulcerations and iii) coexistence of arteritis and dermal venulitis in subcutaneous nodules, atrophie blanche and purpura. DIF disclosed dermal small vessel wall depositions of immunoglobulin (IgM) and / or C3 (Chen et al., 2002). Cutaneous RV overlaps both the characteristics of cutaneous necrotizing venulitis and cutaneous polyarteritis nodosa. Leucocytoclastic vasculitis in RA patients does not necessarily indicate a favourable prognosis (Chen et al., 2002).

Neutrophilic Dermatoses

Pyoderma gangrenosum (PG)

PG is the most severe of this heterogeneous group of inflammatory neutrophilic skin diseases; it may occur in about 10% of patients with RA, more often in women, but is also seen in association with other chronic inflammatory and autoimmune disorders such as Crohn´s disease or with lymphoproliferative malignancies or presents as an idiopathic disorder without apparent underlying disease.

PG start with single or multiple small bullous lesions or pustules, mostly on the legs, in the abdominal or genital-anal area; however, PG can occur elsewhere including on mucous membranes. The initial lesions may coalesce and rapidly progress to mature into ulcerative superficial granulomas and large necrotic and painful ulcers with a purulent base and characteristic reddish-blue undermined borders that extend centrifugally (Fig. 11). Single lesions can show a size of 20 cm in diameters and more, multiple lesions tend to

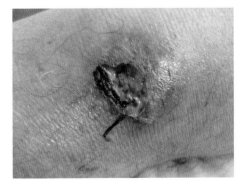

Fig. 11. Pyoderma gangrenosum of the arm in a patient with Rheumatoid arthritis

be smaller The PG ulcers can take years to heal and often requires high-dose corticosteroids and/or immuno-suppressant treatment leaving behind atrophic often hyperpigmented scars.

Rheumatoid neutrophilic dermatitis (RND)

RND is a rare cutaneous finding in patients with severe RA. Clinically, the eruption is characterized by symmetric erythematous papules or plaques. Sometimes, vesicles are seen on the extensor surfaces of the arms and hands.

On histological examination, a dense interstitial dermal neutrophilic infiltrate without signs of leukocytoclastic vasculitis is seen. In most cases, topical treatment with potent corticosteroids is sufficient.

Acute febrile neutrophilic dermatosis (Sweet´s syndrome) may closely resemble RND on histology. Clinically, this prototype of neutrophilic dermatosis has a more acute onset with fever and develops with markedly inflamed and edematous coin- or dome-shaped tender infiltrates and plaques, often in the shoulder areas and on the face.

Cutaneous Side Effects of RA Treatment

It is estimated that up to 40% of RA patients develop cutaneous drug toxicity in the course of their treatment. These reactions are mild in most cases, occur within the first few weeks of treatment, and manifest as vasculitis, urticaria or skin rash. Rash may be maculo-papular, vesiculous, bullous or pustular , often affecting the whole integument and the mucosal surfaces; the most severe of these allergic drug reaction to anti-rheumatic drugs are the Stevens-Johnson syndromes (SJS) and the toxic epidermal necrolysis (TEN, Lyell syndrome) which bears a mortality of more than 40 percent especially in the elderly.

Non-steroidal anti-inflammatory drugs (NSAID)

Skin reactions to *aspirin* are rare (< 1%) in the general population but much more common among patients with asthma or chronic urticaria. These reactions are mostly of a non-immunological nature but related to pharmacologic intolerance and linked to arachidonic acid metabolism and leukotriene release. On the other side, NSAID´s such as the many *pyrazol* and *pyrazolon derivates* including oxicam belong together with antibiotics, anti-HIV- medications, anti-epileptic drug thiazide-type diuretics, and allopurinol to those drugs with a high risk for allergic skin reactions, ranging from transient rash resembling viral exanthema to toxic epidermal necrolysis (TEN). However, the absolute risks of Stevens Johnson syndrome (SJS) and TEN associated with NSAID treatment are low; oxicams have higher risks of SJS and TEN than the other NSAID and patients who recently began treatment should be carefully monitored (Ward et al., 2010). Selective cyclo-oxygenase-2 inhibitors have been less frequently reported to be associated with serious drug reactions; in fact, it seems that they are well tolerated by most of the NSAID-sensitive and aspirin-intolerant patients.

13

Disease-modifying antirheumatic drugs

Sulfasalazine or its major metabolites *5-aminosalicylic acid* and *sulfapyridine* can cause an itchy rash that usually resolves once the drugs are stopped. Sulfasalazine causes a peculiar orange-tinged discoloration of sweat. Rare adverse muco-cutaneous side effects include oral ulcerations, hypersensitivity syndrome (lichenoid skin eruption, leukocytopenia, thrombocytopenia, fever) and SJS or TEN.

Chloroquine and hydroxychloroquine are known to induce pruritus, increased photosensitivity, premature greying of hair and characteristic greyish-blue hyperpigmentation of glaborous skin and mucosal surfaces. Since antimalarials were claimed to exacerbate psoriasis and psoriatic arthritis, they are not usually prescribed in these conditions.

Muco-cutaneous side effects to *gold compounds* (oral or intramuscular) are not infrequent and are estimated to occur in about 10 to 20 percent of treated patients. Within weeks or after a delay of several months, generalized skin rash closely resembling lichen planus, pityriasis rosea or eczema may be seen; urticarial, hyperpigmented (*Chrysiasis*) or vasculitic lesions are less frequent; SJS and TEN are extremely rare. The gold dermatitis often responds to topical treatment with mid-potent corticosteroids and continuation of treatment in lower dosage may be tried.

Cutaneous toxicity from *d-penicillamine* can be a major problem requiring definite discontinuation of the drug; besides eczematous or lichenoid skin rashes as seen with other antirheumatic medications, d-penicillamine can uniquely induce or exacerbate autoimmune diseases such as SLE, dermatomyositis, myasthenia gravis and – most notably – pemphigus vulgaris or foliaceus. D-penicillamine contains sulfhydril groups that are speculated to interact with the pemphigus autoantigens desmoglein 1 and 3.

Biologics

The introduction of biological therapies that target specific proinflammatory cytokines have gained great impact as new treatment options for patients with RA.

Adverse reactions to the IL-1 blocker anakinra and to the TNF-α inhibitors infliximab, etanercept and adalimumab have been estimated to occur in about 25% of RA patients treated with biologics (Scheinfeld, 2004, Lee et al., 2007).

These cutaneous reactions are of special interests to dermatologists, since most of the biologics are also used for inflammatory skin disorders such as psoriasis.

Local reactions

Inflammatory reactions at injection sites are common, up to 60%, in RA patients undergoing treatment with *anakinra*. Reaction occurs within the first month as well-defined erythema and oedema involving the injection sites (Vila et al., 2005). More severe reaction such as a case of wells' cellulitis of the thigh has been reported at the site of injection (Livory et al., 2008). Similar erythematous or edematous lesions occur mostly within 12 to 24 hours following subcutaneous injection of *etanercept* and usually disappear within 3 to 5 days without topical treatment.

A matter of concern are generalized cutaneous reactions seen either immediately or with a delay of several days in 10 to 20% of RA patients after intravenous administration of *infliximab*; these reactions present with a disseminated erythematous flush or with acute urticaria and pruritus; when these skin reactions recur with the following injections or are accompanied by systemic symptoms such as fever, dizziness or hypotension, withdrawal of infliximab treatment may become necessary. However, anaphylactic reaction to infliximab requiring intensive care intervention is very rare.

Skin infections

About one third of skin changes related to treatment with biologics are infections, such as pityriasis versicolor; herpes simplex or bacterial infections are less frequent.

Inflammatory skin eruptions

Generalized or localized inflammatory skin reactions resembling atopic dermatitis, eczema, or psoriasis are the most frequent cutaneous adverse effects related to treatment with biologics. Psoriasiform eruptions seem to be a class effect common to infliximab, etanercept or adalimumab; the eruption may already appear after the first injection or several months after, and tend to become pustular often resembling palmoplantar pustular psoriasis, especially in RA patients treated with infliximab; but psoriasis vulgaris may also occur. The mechanisms involved remain elusive. In some patients, the switch to another TNF alpha-blocker results in clearing of the skin; in others discontinuation of biologics altogether and instalment of an anti-psoriatic treatment is necessary.

Sarcoid-like granulomatosis is rare but not exceptional in patients treated with TNF blockers (Fig. 12). It does not seem to be related to gender, rheumatic disease or the type of anti-TNF drug used. Clinical manifestations are mainly pulmonary and cutaneous. Discontinuation of anti-TNF usually leads to recovery. When anti-TNF is required to control the underlying rheumatic disease, a switch from a soluble receptor format to mono-

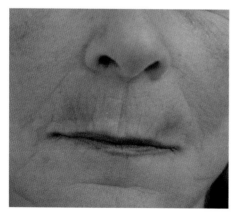

Fig. 12. Sarcoid like lesions in a patient with rheumatoid arthritis treated with adalimumab.

clonal antibodies and the converse may be recommended as recurrence is not usual (Da-ïen et al., 2009).

Of note, anecdotal case of psoriasis (Gonzales-Lopez et al., 2008) and interstitial granulomatous reaction (Regula et al., 2008) have been reported with *anakinra*.

Drug-induced lupus erythematosus

Antinuclear antibodies (ANA) are a frequent serologic finding in RA patients treated with TNF alpha inhibitors. Lupus-like skin manifestations resembling subacute or discoid cutaneous lupus erythematosus, or lupus erythematosus tumidus are, however, very rare and are estimated to occur in less than 0.5 percent of RA patients treated with TNF alpha inhibitors. About two third of these patients have typical systemic manifestations characterized by arthritis, polyserositis, myositis, vasculitis and other complications including renal disease; serologically, antibodies to double-stranded DNA and hypocomplementemia are often present. TNF alpha-induced SLE differs markedly from drug-induced SLE due to other medications (Vedove et al., 2009). Other patients develop discoid lupus erythematosus with erythemato-squamous lesions in UV-exposed skin, alopecia, chilblain-like lesions, and vasculitis or overlap syndromes such as mixed connective tissue disease. In many patients, the lupus reaction resolves after withdrawal of the TNF alpha-blocker treatment.

Besides LE or lupus-like syndromes other autoimmune diseases may develop under therapy with biologics; these include hypocomplementemic systemic vasculitis and IgA-nephritis.

Cutaneous Manifestations In Subsets Of Rheumatoid Arthritis

Cutaneous manifestations of *Felty syndrome* are rheumatoid nodules, hyperpigmentation and leg ulcers. The incidence of rheumatoid nodules in Felty syndrome is about 70 percent and thus much higher than in RA. The leg ulcers may be secondary to pyoderma gangrenosum or medium-sized vessel vasculitis with ulcerations. They are frequently refractory with a risk of secondary infection, due to underlying immune defects present in some patients with Felty syndrome.

Juvenile onset Still's disease is in up to 90 percent characterized by a typical transient, pink macular rash over the trunk, axillae face and extremities that is non-pruritic and coincides with acute febrile episodes of the disease. The patient's skin is hypersensitive often demonstrating urticarial dermographism. Other cutaneous features include persistent linear plaques and periorbital edema and erythema. Rheumatoid nodules are rare but may appear in the course of treatment with methotrexate.

The transient, asymptomatic skin rash of *adult-onset Still's disease* also accompanies fever spikes and shows a characteristic salmon-pink colour. The rash is most often macular or slightly urticarial and appears over pressure points. Persistent red-brownish papules and plaques may be also seen in adult patients with Still's disease.

The differential diagnosis of the rash in Still's disease includes various viral exanthemas, drug eruptions, and erythema marginatum rheumaticum seen in *acute rheumatic fe-*

ver. This rapidly spreading annular erythema occurs mostly on the trunk and is -in contrast to Still's disease- not associated with fever spikes. The presence of neutrophilic infiltrates in the dermis was frequently observed in adult-onset Still's disease eruption (Kieffer et al., 2009).

Dermatologic Manifestations of Relapsing Polychondritis (Francès et al., 2001)

Relapsing polychondritis (RP) is a rare disease which is characterized by attacks of chondritis, occurring in a relapsing-remitting pattern. More than 30 percent of patients have an associated disease, mainly of autoimmune origin (table II).

Inflammatory episodes generally last a few days or weeks and may subside spontaneously or upon treatment; recurrences after weeks or months occur and result subsequently in cartilage destruction. Auricular chondritis is the most frequent (85%), causing pain, redness, and swelling of the cartilaginous portion of the pinna, sparing the non cartilaginous lobe (Fig. 13). Biopsy of the auricular cartilage is no more necessary for diagnosis. The histology shows perichondrial inflammation and the loss of the normal cartilaginous basophilia. After several attacks, the pinna may become soft and sloppy with a cauliflower

Table 2. Main conditions associated with relapsing polychondritis and / or with smiliar manifestations

Autoimmune diseases	Vasculitides
Rheumatoid arthritis	Leukocytoclastic
Systemic lupus erythematosus	Wegener's granulomatosis
Sjögren syndrome	Polyarteritis nodosa
Mixed connective tissue disease	Microscopic polyangitis
Thyroid autoimmune disease	Churg-Strauss syndrome
Diabetes mellitus	Behçet's disease
Hematologic disorders	Takayasu arteritis
Myelodysplastic syndromes	**Intestinal diseases**
IgA myeloma	Crohn's disease
Others	Ulcerative colitis
Skin diseases	**Others**
Vitiligo	Reiter's syndrome
Psoriasis	Ankylosing spondylitis
Alopecia areata	
Lichen planus	

13

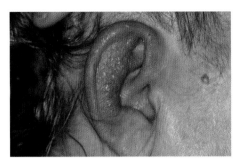

Fig. 13. Auricular chondritis sparing the earlobe

aspect (Fig. 14); sometimes it is stiff due to calcifications. Nasal chondritis (65%) is less inflammatory, presenting with nasal pain, stuffiness, rhinorrhea and sometimes epistaxis. The characteristic saddle-nose deformity may appear secondly or without previous inflammatory episodes. Respiratory tract chondritis, though uncommon at presentation, occurs in up to 50% of patients, and may be lethal. Costochondritis (35%) induce parietal pains which may also compromise respiration.

Dermatologic manifestations are sometimes the presenting feature of RP (12%), noticed subsequently in more than 1/3 of patients of a large series (Francès et al., 2001). They are non specific including nodules on the limbs, purpura, oral or complex aphthosis, papules, sterile pustules, superficial phlebitis, livedo reticularis, ulcerations on the limbs, distal necrosis. They appeared concomitantly or not with attacks of chondritis. Pathological features included inflammatory or thrombotic vascular lesions, neutrophil infiltrates as in neutrophilic dermatosis, inflammation of the dermis or subcutis. Patients with and without dermatologic manifestations have similar clinical manifestations of RP. However, the frequency of dermatologic manifestations (>90%), age at first chondritis and male/female ratio seems higher when RP is associated with myelodysplasia; so, their presence in an old man warrants repeated blood cell counts to detect a smouldering myelodysplasia.

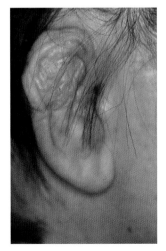

Fig. 14. Soft and sloppy pinna with a cauliflower aspect.

The frequency of aphthosis lead Firestein et al. in 1985 (Firestein et al., 1985) to create the term "MAGIC syndrome" (Mouth And Genital ulcers with Inflamed Cartilage). All other skin lesions observed in RP such as leukocytolastic vasculitis, septal panniculitis, superficial phlebitis, or neutrophilic dermatosis, also may be observed in Behçet's disease as well as in Crohn's disease. So the distinction between associated disease or other conditions sharing clinical manifestations is sometimes difficult.

Summary

Dermatologic manifestations are currently observed in autoimmune rheumatic diseases, particularly in the main systemic vasculitides, rheumatoid arthritis and relapsing polychondritis. In systemic vasculitides, some skin lesions correspond to a skin localization of the systemic vasculitis while others result from a different pathologic process. As biopsies of dermatological lesions are easy to obtain, they have a great impact on confirming the diagnosis. However, its contribution to determine the type of vasculitis is not guaranteed. In fact, neither clinical nor pathologic features of the skin are specific of a given type. The result of the biopsy has to be correlated to direct immunofluorescence data, medical history, physical examination, laboratory and radiological findings leading to the correct diagnosis and effective treatment.

Rheumatoid nodules and vasculitis are the most frequent extra-articular manifestation of rheumatoid arthritis, often indicative of advanced disease and poor prognosis. Cutaneous side effects of antirheumatic drugs range from transient skin rashes to life-threatening toxic epidermal necrolysis. Biological therapies induce local reactions, skin infections and inflammatory lesions such as psoriasiform eruptions which seem to be a class effect. Sarcoid-like granulomatosis is rare but not exceptional. Antinuclear antibodies are a frequent serologic finding in rheumatoid arthritis patients treated with TNF alpha inhibitors while lupus-like skin manifestations are rare. The most frequent dermatologic manifestations in relapsing chondritis are aphthosis with sometimes complex aphthosis, nodular or purpuric lesions, and superficial phlebitis. Histologically these dermatological lesions correspond to non specific inflammatory infiltrates, vasculitis or thrombosis. Similar dermatological manifestations are observed in Behçet's syndrome and in inflammatory bowel diseases. Old men with relapsing polychondritis and dermatologic manifestations have usually a myelodysplasia.

References

Barksdale SK, Hallahan CW, Kerr GS, Fauci AS, Stern JB, Travis WD (1995) Cutaneous pathology in Wegener's granulomatosis. A clinicopathologic study of 75 biopsies in 46 patients. Am J Surg Pathol 19:161–72

Becourt-Verlomme C, Barouky R, Alexandre C, Gonthier R, Laurent H, Vital Durand D, Rousset H (2001) Inaugural symptoms of Horton's disease in a series of 260 patients. Rev Med Interne. 22:631–637

Brons RH, de Jong MC, de Boer NK, Stegeman CA, Kallenberg CG, Tervaert JW (2001) Detection of immune deposits in skin lesions of patients with Wegener's granulomatosis. Ann Rheum Dis 60:1097–1102

Campbell FA, Clark C, Holmes S (2003) Scalp necrosis in temporal arteritis. Clin Exp Dermatol 28:488–490

Carlson JA, Cavaliere LF, Grant-Kels JM (2006) Cutaneous vasculitis: diagnosis and management. Clin Dermatol 24 :414–429

Chen KR, Toyohara A, Suzuki A, Miyakawa S (2002) Clinical and histopathological spectrum of cutaneous vasculitis in rheumatoid arthritis. Br J Dermatol 147:905–913

Cohen SJ, Pittelkow MR, Su WP (1991) Cutaneous manifestations of cryoglobulinemia: clinical and histopathologic study of seventy-two patients. J Am Acad Dermatol 25:21–27

Crowson AN, Mihm MC Jr, Magro CM (2003) Cutaneous vasculitis: a review. J Cutan Pathol 30:161–173

Crowson AN, Magro C (2004) Interstitial granulomatous dermatitis with arthritis. Hum Pathol.35:779–780

Currey J (1997) Scalp necrosis in giant cell arteritis and review of the literature. Br J Rheumatol. 36:814–816

Daïen CI, Monnier A, Claudepierre P, Constantin A, Eschard JP, Houvenagel E, Samimi M, Pavy S, Pertuiset E, Toussirot E, Combe B, Morel J (2009) Club Rhumatismes et Inflammation (CRI). Sarcoid-like granulomatosis in patients treated with tumor necrosis factor blockers:10 cases. Rheumatology (Oxford). 48:883–886

Daoud MS, Gibson LE, De Remee RA, Specks U, El-Azhary RA, Su WPD (1994) Cutaneous Wegener's granulomatosus: clinical, histopathologic and immunopathologic features of thirty patients. J Am Acad Dermatol 31:605–612

Davis MD, Daoud MS, McEvoy MT, Su WP (1997) Cutaneous manifestations of Churg-Strauss syndrome: a clinicopathologic correlation. J Am Acad Dermatol 37:199–203

Díaz-Pérez JL, De Lagrán ZM, Díaz-Ramón JL, Winkelmann RK (2007) Cutaneous polyarteritis nodosa. Semin Cutan Med Surg 26:77–86

Dupin N, Chosidow O, Lunel F, Cacoub P, Musset L, Cresta P, Frangeul L, Piette JC, Godeau P, Opolon P (1995) Essential mixed cryoglobulinemia. A comparative study of dermatologic manifestations in patients infected or noninfected with hepatitis C virus. Arch Dermatol 131:1124–1127

Ferri C (2008) Mixed cryoglobulinemia. Orphanet J Rare Dis 16:3:25

Fiorentino DF (2003) Cutaneous vasculitis. J Am Acad Dermatol 48:311–40

Firestein GS, Gruber HE, Weisman MH, Zvaifler NJ, Barber J, O'Duffy JD (1985) Mouth and genital ulcers with inflamed cartilage: MAGIC syndrome. Five patients with features of relapsing polychondritis and Behçet's disease. Am J Med 79:65–72

Francès C, Boisnic S, Blétry O, Dallot A, Thomas D, Kieffer E, Godeau P (1990) Cutaneous manifestations of Takayasu arteritis. A retrospective study of 80 cases. Dermatologica. 181:266–272

Francès C, Lê Thi Huong D, Piette JC, Saada V, Boisnic S, Wechsler B, Blétry O, Godeau P (1994) Wegener's granulomatosis. Dermatological manifestations in 75 cases with clinicopathologic correlation. Arch Dermatol 130:861–867

Francès C, El Rassi R, Laporte JL, Rybojad M, Papo T, Piette JC (2001) Dermatologic manifestations of relapsing polychondritis. A study of 200 cases at a single center. Medicine (Baltimore) 80:173–179

Genta MS, Genta RM, Gabay C (2006) Systemic rheumatoid vasculitis: a review. Semin Arthritis Rheum 36:88–98

González-López MA, Martínez-Taboada VM, González-Vela MC, Fernández-Llaca H, Val-Bernal JF (2008) New-onset psoriasis following treatment with the interleukin-1 receptor antagonist anakinra. Br J Dermatol 158:1146–1148.

Guillevin L, Cordier JF, Lhote F, Cohen P, Jarrousse B, Royer I, et al. (1997) A prospective, multicenter, randomized trial comparing steroids and pulse cyclophosphamide versus steroids and oral cyclophosphamide in the treatment of generalized Wegener's granulomatosis. Arthritis Rheum 40, 2187–2198

Guillevin L, Cohen P, Gayraud M, Lhote F, Jarrousse B, Casassus P (1999) Churg-Strauss syndrome. Clinical study and long-term follow-up of 96 patients. Medicine (Baltimore) 78:26–37

Guillevin L, Durand-Gasselin B, Cevallos R, Gayraud M, Lhote F, Callard P, Amouroux J, Casassus P, Jarrousse B (1999) Microscopic polyangiitis: clinical and laboratory findings in eighty-five patients. Arthritis Rheum 42:421–430

Hoffman GS, Kerr GS, Leavitt RY, Hallahan CW, Lebovics RS, Travis WD, Rottem M, Fauci AS (1992) Wegener granulomatosis: an analysis of 158 patients. Ann Intern Med 116:488–498

Jennette JC, Falk RJ, Andrassy K, Bacon PA, Churg J, Gross WL, Hagen EC, Hoffman GS, Hunder GG, Kallenberg CG, et al. (1994) Nomenclature of systemic vasculitides. Proposal of an international consensus conference. Arthritis Rheum 37:187–192

Kieffer C, Cribier B, Lipsker D (2009) Neutrophilic urticarial dermatosis: a variant of neutrophilic urticaria strongly associated with systemic disease. Report of 9 new cases and review of the literature. Medicine (Baltimore) 88:23–31

Kluger N, Pagnoux C, Guillevin L, Francès C; French Vasculitis Study Group (2008) Comparison of cutaneous manifestations in systemic polyarteritis nodosa and microscopic polyangiitis. Br J Dermatol 159:615–20

Kuchel J, Lee S (2003) Cutaneous Wegener's granulomatosis: a variant or atypical localized form. Aust J Dermatol 44:129–135

Lamprecht P, Bruhl H, Erdmann A, Holl-Ulrich K, Csernok E, Seitzer U, Mack M, Feller AC, Reinhold-Keller E, Gross WL, Muller A (2003) Differences in CCR5 expression on peripheral blood CD4+CD28- T-cells and in granulomatous lesions between localized and generalized Wegener's granulomatosis. Clin Immunol.108:1–7

Lamprecht P, Wieczorek S, Epplen JT, Ambrosch P, Kallenberg CG (2009) Granuloma formation in ANCA-associated vasculitides. APMIS Suppl .127:32–36

Lee HH, Song IH, Friedrich M, Gauliard A, Detert J, Röwert J, Audring H, Kary S, Burmester GR, Sterry W, Worm M (2007) Cutaneous side-effects in patients with rheumatic diseases during application of tumour necrosis factor-alpha antagonists. Br J Dermatol. 156:486–91

Livory M, Wechsler J, Revuz J, Bagot M, Chevalier X, Poszepczynska-Guigné E (2008) Wells' cellulitis and bacterial necrotizing cellulitis induced by anakinra. Ann Dermatol Venereol 135:839–842

Magro CM, Crowson AN (2003) The spectrum of cutaneous lesions in rheumatoid arthritis : a clinical and pathological study of 43 patients.J Cutan Pathol 30 :1–10

Manchanda Y, Tejasvi T, Handa R, Ramam M (2003) Strawberry gingiva: a distinctive sign in Wegener's granulomatosis. J Am Acad Dermatol 49:335–7

Matsushima M, Yamanaka K, Mori H, Murakami T, Hakamada A, Isoda K, Mizutani H (2003) Bilateral scalp necrosis with giant cell arteritis. J Dermatol. 30:210–215

Mimouni D, Ng PP, Rencic A, Nikolskaia OV, Bernstein BD, Nousari HC (2003) Cutaneous polyarteritis nodosa in patients presenting with atrophie blanche. Br J Dermatol 148:789–794

Mitsui H, Shibagaki N, Kawamura T, Matsue H, Shimada S (2009) A clinical study of Henoch-Schönlein Purpura associated with malignancy. J Eur Acad Dermatol Venereol.23:394–401

Monteiro C, Fernandes B, Reis I, Tellechea O, Freitas J, Figueiredo A (2002) Temporal arteritis presenting with scalp ulceration. J Eur Acad Dermatol Venereol. 16:615–617

Müller A, Trabandt A, Gloeckner-Hofmann K, Seitzer U, Csernok E, Schönermarck U, Feller AC, Gross WL (2000) Localized Wegener's granulomatosis: predominance of CD26 and IFN-gamma expression. J Pathol. 192:113–120

Obermoser G, Zelger B, Zangerle R, Sepp N (2002) Extravascular necrotizing palisaded granulomas as the presenting skin sign of systemic lupus erythematosus. Br J Dermatol 147:371–374

Pascual-López M, Hernández-Núñez A, Aragüés-Montañés M, Daudén E, Fraga J, García-Díez A (2004) Takayasu's disease with cutaneous involvement. Dermatology 208:10–15

Patten SF, Tomecki KJ (1993) Wegener's granulomatosis: cutaneous and oral mucosal disease. J Am Acad Dermatol 28:710–718

Perniciaro CV, Winkelmann RK, Hunder GG (1987) Cutaneous manifestations of Takayasu's arteritis. A clinicopathologic correlation. J Am Acad Dermatol 17:998–1005

Regula CG, Hennessy J, Clarke LE, Adams DR, Ioffreda MD, Graber EM, Helm KF (2008) Interstitial granulomatous drug reaction to anakinra. J Am Acad Dermatol. 59(2 Suppl 1):S25–S27

Sayah A, English J (2005) Rheumatoid arthritis: A review of the cutaneous manifestations. J Am Acad Dermatol 53:191–209

Scheinfeld N (2004) A comprehensive review and evaluation of the side effects of the tumor necrosis factor alpha blockers etanercept, infliximab and adalimumab. J Dermatol Treat 15, 280–294

Skaria AM, Ruffieux P, Piletta P, Chavaz P, Saurat JH, Borradori L (2000) Takayasu arteritis and cutaneous necrotizing vasculitis. Dermatology 200:139–143

Solans-Laqué R, Bosch-Gil JA, Pérez-Bocanegra C, Selva-O'Callaghan A, Simeón-Aznar CP, Vilardell-Tarres M (2008) Paraneoplastic vasculitis in patients with solid tumors: report of 15 cases. J Rheumatol 35:294–304

Tancrede-Bohin E, Ochonisky S, Vignon-Pennamen MD, Flageul B, Morel P, Rybojad M (1997) Schönlein-Henoch purpura in adult patients. Predictive factors for IgA glomerulonephritis in a retrospective study of 57 cases. Arch Dermatol 133:438–442

Vedove CD, Del Giglio M, Schena D, Girolomoni G (2009) Drug-induced lupus erythematosus. Arch Dermatol Res 301:99–105

Vila AT, Puig L, Fernández-Figueras MT, Laiz AM, Vidal D, Alomar A (2005) Adverse cutaneous reactions to anakinra in patients with rheumatoid arthritis: clinicopathological study of five patients. Br J Dermatol 153:417–423

Ward KE, Archambault R, Mersfelder TL (2010) Severe adverse skin reactions to nonsteroidal anti-inflammatory drugs: A review of the literature. Am J Health Syst Pharm.67:206–213

Yamamoto T (2009) Cutaneous manifestations associated with rheumatoid arthritis. Rheumatol Int 29:979–988

Vitiligo

14

Karin U. Schallreuter

Introduction

Vitiligo (from vitula (latin) = calf, vitium (latin) = mistake) is an acquired idiopathic epidermal pigment loss which can occur anywhere on the body. The onset of the disease can be at any time in life. Besides rare spontaneous repigmentation in most cases vitiligo is an unpredictable progressive disorder.

The incidence of vitiligo in Europe is around 0.5%. A recent analysis of the published data shows that the worldwide incidence is ranging from 0.04–2.16% in adults and from 0.06–1.2% in children (Fig. 1), but only 28% of the patients are actually very concerned about this disease and actually seek medical help (Johnson and Roberts, 1978, Krüger et al. submitted). However, those concerned patients or the parents of affected children are confronting Dermatologists worldwide. Despite major efforts the cause of this ancient disease is yet unknown. Most publications describe decreased numbers of functioning melanocytes or the complete absence of these cells in the depigmented epidermis (Ortonne and Bose, 1993, LePoole et al., 1993a, LePoole et al., 1993b, Xie et al., 1999, Schallreuter et al., 2008a). A study by Tobin et al. proved that melanocytes are still present, even in long standing vitiligo (Tobin et al., 2000). In addition there are many reports invoking participation of keratinocytes and Langerhans cells in the pathogenesis of this disease (for review Schallreuter et al., 2008a). Several hypotheses have been put forward in effort to elucidate the sudden depigmentation process but none of them can explain conclusively the plethora of clinical and basic scientific data (LePoole et al., 1993a, Gauthier et al., 2003, Dell'Anna and Picardo, 2006, Schallreuter et al., 2008a). The most popular hypothesis is still selective autoimmunity to melanocytes.

Considering the substantial *in vivo* and *in vitro* evidence for generation / accumulation of ROS and recently reactive nitrogen species (RNS) in the epidermis and consequently in the system of patients with vitiligo (for review Schallreuter et al., 2008a, Salem et al., 2009), it is the aim of this contribution to dissect and translate the possible effect of ROS / RNS on pro and contras of various hypotheses including autoimmunity in vitiligo.

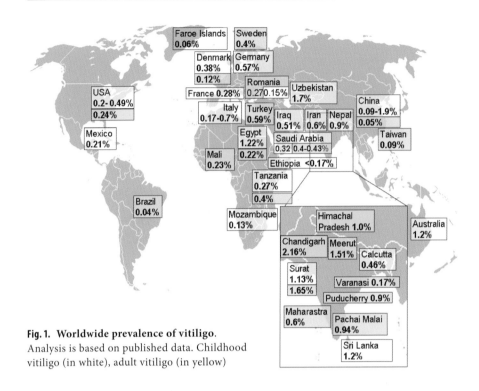

Fig. 1. Worldwide prevalence of vitiligo.
Analysis is based on published data. Childhood
vitiligo (in white), adult vitiligo (in yellow)

Clinical picture and classification

14

The classical skin lesion of vitiligo shows chalk white patches in different sizes and location
sometimes associated with early greying of the hair or bundles of white hair (poliosis). The
disease is usually diagnosed by eye but a distinct fluorescence of the depigmented epidermis upon Wood's light examination (UVA 351 nm) exposure due to the presence of oxidised pterins proves the diagnosis (Schallreuter et al., 1994a). A comparison of vitiligo and
laser induced leucoderma is shown in Fig. 2A/B. Notably, the same fluorescence is present
in Piebald lesions pointing to the involvement of redox imbalance in this disorder besides
the well established genetic defect (Vafaee et al., 2009). Acute vitiligo is often characterised by multiple pinpoint needle sized white lesions or by a mottled expression of the skin
colour mimicking trichrome / quadrichrome vitiligo or fungal infection (Fig. 2C). Vitiligo
can be associated with pruritus in the progressive depigmenting skin (Schallreuter et al.,
2008a) and Koebnerisation is present in more than 40% of the patients (Ortonne and Bose,
1993, Schallreuter et al., 2008b).

The view on, whether vitiligo is truly associated with other autoimmune diseases is controversial. In our clinic association of classical autoimmune disorders together with vitiligo
is a rather rare event. The majority of patients presents only vitiligo (unpublished data on
>6000 patients, KUS). These data are in agreement with an earlier clinical study involving
320 German patients with vitiligo which failed to support a strong association with classical autoimmunity disorders (Schallreuter et al., 1994d).

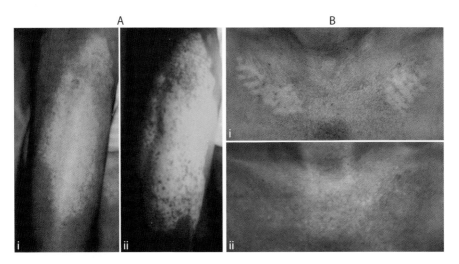

Fig. 2. Differential diagnosis of clinical leucoderma upon WOOD's light (351 nm) examination
A **Vitiligo vulgaris**
  i. Clinical picture
  ii. N.B. Presence of bluish fluorescence is characteristic for vitiligo.
B **Laser induced leucoderma**
  i. Clinical picture
  ii. N.B. Absence of any fluorescence under WOOD's light

Vitiligo shows several characteristic clinical patterns which can involve the entire skin surface including mucosa, palms and soles. The clinical location of the white spots has formed the basis for classification of subtypes.

- Focal vitiligo appears in one or more isolated macules anywhere on the body.
- Segmental vitiligo is characterised by unilateral appearance in dermatomal or near dermatomal distribution. This form can be mixed with generalised vitiligo (Schallreuter et al., 2008b) (Fig. 3A).
- In Blaschkolinear vitiligo the depigmentation pattern follows Blaschko lines. It can occur isolated or in association with vitiligo vulgaris (Schallreuter et al., 2007a).
- Generalised vitiligo (vitiligo vulgaris) is often characterised by symmetrical distribution of white areas anywhere on the integument.
- Acrofacial vitiligo involves distal digits and acrofacial as well as genito-anal areas.
- Universal vitiligo describes depigmentation in > 80% of the entire integument.
- Inflammatory vitiligo is characterised by a red, often slightly scaly border around the depigmented lesion.

Here it should be mentioned that a new classification has been put forward by the European task force group (Taïeb and Picardo, 2007). Classification in segmental vitiligo (SV) and nonsegmental vitiligo (NSV) do not account for mixed forms and those occur and are not extremely rare.

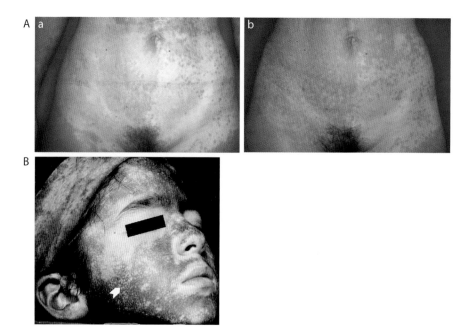

Fig. 3.
A Segmental vitiligo mixed with generalised vitiligo (vulgaris)
   a. Before treatment
   b. After treatment with low dose narrowband UVB activated pseudocatalase (PC-KUS)
   NB. The repigmentation of segmental vitiligo is considerably slower!
B Acute facial vitiligo
N.B. Pinpoint sized depigmentation which is characterised with high H_2O_2 levels evidenced by *in vivo* FT-Raman spectroscopy

14

Frequently vitiligo can be associated with Halo Nevi. Whether this entity is part of vitiligo or whether it presents an own disorder has been subject of several controversies. Recently it was shown that Halo Nevi are an independent entity which can occur together with vitiligo but these lesions seem to have their own distinct pathogenesis and clinical outcome (Schallreuter et al., 2003b).

Pathomechanisms in vitiligo – What do we know?

I. ROS and RNS induced stress in vitiligo

Although most studies have concentrated on the fate of pigment forming cell in the pathogogenesis of vitiligo, there are several lines of evidence that vitiligo is a disease affecting the entire epidermis including keratinocytes and Langerhans cells (Nordlund and Ortonne, 1992, Prignano et al., 2009, Schallreuter et al., 1999a, Schallreuter, 1999b, Schallreuter et al., 2008a, Salem et al., 2009, Tobin et al., 2000). Various degrees of vacuolation and deposition of debris in all epidermal cells including dilation of the rough endoplasmic reticulum and mitochondrial alteration have been documented (Moellmann et al., 1982, Bhawan and Bhutani, 1983, Boissy et al., 1991, Tobin et al., 2000, Prignano et al., 2009). In 2000 these data were reconciled on the basis of H_2O_2-mediated stress (Tobin et al., 2000). Signs for oxidative stress were even observed in melanocytes and keratinocytes under *in vitro* conditions unless these cells were not protected by anti-oxidant enzymes, for instance catalase (Medrano and Nordlund, 1990, Tobin et al., 2000). Low epidermal catalase levels in epidermal suction blister tissue extracts from patients with vitiligo supported the involvement of a perturbed redox imbalance in this disease (Schallreuter et al., 1991). These early data were confirmed *in vitro* showing that melanocytes established from the non-lesional skin of these patients contained lower than normal catalase activities (Yohn et al., 1991, Maresca et al., 1997). Here it is notable that the expression of catalase mRNA remains unaltered (Schallreuter et al., 2004). The proof of H_2O_2-mediated oxidative stress in vitiligo has been accomplished *in vivo*® by depigmented epidermis using non-invasive Fourier Transform (FT) Raman spectroscopy (Schallreuter et al., 1999a). Importantly, epidermal H_2O_2 can be reduced by a synthetic catalyst that oxidises H_2O_2 to O_2 and H_2O, thus mimicking the reaction catalysed by natural catalase. The active catalyst is a low dose NB-UVB-activated bis Mn^{III} (EDTA)$_2$ (HCO^{3-})$_2$ complex and has been named pseudocatalase PC-KUS (Schallreuter et al., 1995b, Schallreuter et al., 2008a, Schallreuter et al., 2008b). This pseudocatalase can arrest the progress of the disease after topical application in 95% of all patients and it initiates repigmentation in those patients, who hold a normal L-phenylalanine metabolism, regardless of the duration and expansion of the disease (Schallreuter et al., 1995b, Schallreuter et al., 1999a, Schallreuter et al., 2008b).

The biochemical basis for the accumulation of H_2O_2 and the recent identification of reactive nitric oxide species (RNS) based on the presence of 3-nitro tyrosine residues in patient's skin has been target of much research (for review Schallreuter et al., 2008a, Salem et al., 2009). In the skin of patients with vitiligo several sources have been identified and documented.

1. Increased NADPH-oxidases activities from neutrophils and macrophages of the perilesional infiltrate (Darr and Fridowich, 1994, Marks et al., 1996).
2. Increased epidermal monoamine oxidase A activities (Schallreuter et al., 1996a).
3. Increased epidermal TNFα levels (Moretti et al., 2002, Schallreuter et al., 2008a).
4. Photo-oxidation of epidermal 6-biopterin and sepiapterin (Rokos et al., 2002).
5. Increased estrogen / progesterone mediated H_2O_2-generation (Anderson et al., 2003).
6. Perturbed phenylalanine hydroxylase activity via 7BH$_4$ due to deactivation of 6BH$_4$ recycling (Schallreuter et al., 1994a, Schallreuter et al., 2005, Pey et al., 2006).
7. Epidermal xanthine oxidase activity contributes to H_2O_2 oxidising its product uric acid to allantoin (Shalbaf et al., 2008).
8. Increased epidermal inducible nitric oxide synthase (Schallreuter et al., 2005, Salem et al., 2009).
9. Increased peroxynitrite formation (ONOO$^-$) (Salem et al., 2009).

Taken together, to date there is ample evidence that epidermal H_2O_2 / ONOO$^-$ accumulation in vitiligo is a fact.

What are possible consequences of mM H_2O_2-concentrations in the epidermis of these patients?

Most important for the contribution presented herein is the question, whether we can link these findings to the autoimmune response in this disease.

H_2O_2-mediated oxidation affects the epidermal anti-oxidant defence machinery and its repair mechanisms

- H_2O_2 concentrations in the mM range deactivate catalase due to oxidation of the porphyrin ring as well as methionine and tryptophan residues in the structure of the enzyme active and the cofactor NADPH-binding site (Aronoff, 1965, Maresca et al., 2006, Wood and Schallreuter, 2006, Gibbons et al., 2006, Wood et al., 2008). The net result is a decrease in protein expression and activities (Schallreuter et al., 1991, Schallreuter et al., 2008a, Salem et al., 2009).
- The same mode of action has been recognised for thioredoxin reductase due to oxidation of the enzyme active and the NADPH cofactor binding site (Gibbons et al., 2006). Low enzyme activities and low protein expression have indeed been shown in vitiligo (Schallreuter et al., 1986, Schallreuter et al., 1987, Schallreuter et al., 2008a). Moreover, low glutathione peroxidase serum levels have been documented (Beazley et al., 1999).
- Oxidation of methionine sulfoxide reductase A leads to compromised protein repair after oxidation of methionine residues to methionine sulfoxide. Low epidermal enzyme levels and activities were demonstrated in vitiligo (Schallreuter, 2006a, Schallreuter et al., 2008d).

In summary, in vitiligo H_2O_2 alters its entire degradation machinery due to oxidation of methionine, tryptophan and cysteine/selenocysteine residues in the structure of antioxidant enzymes. In addition, in the presence of $ONOO^-$, nitration of tyrosine and cysteine residues needs to be taken into account as effective contributors to alter protein structure and folding.

H_2O_2 affects the essential cofactor (6R)-L-erythro 5,6,7,8 tetrahydrobiopterin (6BH$_4$) and consequently cofactor dependent mechanisms

In 1994 it was proven that the fluorescent compounds present in vitiliginous skin are oxidised pterins (Schallreuter et al., 1994a, Schallreuter et al., 1994b). Accumulation of epidermal oxidised pterins revealed the presence of a defective de novo synthesis/recycling/regulation of the essential cofactor (6R)-L-erythro 5,6,7,8 tetrahydrobiopterin (6BH$_4$) in vitiligo (Schallreuter et al., 1994a, Schallreuter et al., 1994b). It is the defective recycling of 6BH$_4$ causing formation and accumulation of its isomer 7BH$_4$ which in turn inhibits phenylalanine hydroxylase (PAH), thus preventing the turnover from L-phenylalanine to L-tyrosine (Davis et al., 1992, Pey et al., 2006). L-phenylalanine build up was documented in vivo by FT-Raman spectroscopy (Schallreuter et al., 1998). Moreover, H_2O_2-mediated oxi-

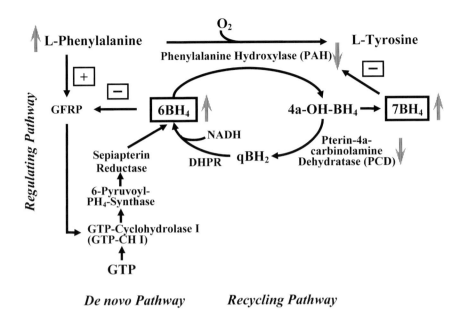

De novo Pathway   **Recycling Pathway**

Fig. 4. Defective 6BH4 synthesis leading to 7BH4 production in vitiligo. Both epidermal melanocytes and keratinocytes have the full capacity for *de novo* synthesis / recycling of 6BH$_4$ (Schallreuter et al., 1994a, Schallreuter et al., 1994b). The rate limiting step for the *de novo* synthesis of 6BH$_4$ is GTP-cyclohydrolase I (GTP-CH-I) which is regulated by H$_2$O$_2$ (Shimizu et al., 2003). This enzyme is also controlled by L-phenylalanine (positive feedback) via the GTP-CH-I feedback regulatory protein (GFRP), as well as several cytokines (TNFα, IL-2, IFNγ, MGF). 6BH$_4$ down regulates GTP-CH-I via GFRP. Furthermore, 6BH$_4$ is the essential cofactor (a) for phenylalanine hydroxylase to metabolise L-phenylalanine to L-tyrosine in melanocytes and keratinocytes, and (b) for tyrosine hydroxylase to convert L-tyrosine to L-dopa in catecholamine biosynthesis in epidermal keratinocytes and melanocytes. It is also a regulator of tyrosinase activity in melanocytes, inhibiting the enzyme by an allosteric mechanism. The recycling of 6BH$_4$ is catalysed by the rate-limiting pterin-4a-carbinolamine dehydratase (PCD) via quinonoid dihydropterin (qBH$_2$) and its reduction by dihydropteridine reductase (DHPR) in the presence of NADH. If 6BH$_4$ is overproduced, as in vitiligo, then 4a-hydroxy-BH$_4$ is non-enzymatically converted to high levels of 7BH$_4$, which in turn inhibits phenylalanine hydroxylase, yielding a compromised L-tyrosine supply.

dation leads to deactivation of the rate limiting recycling enzyme 4a-carbinolamine dehydratase (PCD) (Schallreuter et al., 2001) (Fig. 4). H$_2$O$_2$ rapidly oxidises 6BH$_4$ to L-biopterin and this oxidation product is cytotoxic to melanocytes with an LC$_{50}$ 1×10^{-7} M (Schallreuter et al., 1994c). Further investigation revealed the presence of pterin 6-carboxylic acid as the final oxidation product of L-biopterin and other pterins. This photo-oxidation coincides with the generation of H$_2$O$_2$ (Rokos et al., 2002). Hence, defective pterin synthesis coupled to oxidative stress can directly influence melanocyte populations and integrity in vitiligo primarily due to the cytotoxicity of L-biopterin and other oxidised pterins.

H_2O_2 compromises the epidermal cholinergic signal

Iyengar was the first to report high epidermal acetylcholine levels in patients with vitiligo (Iyengar, 1989). Later this result was confirmed and the mechanism behind could be explained by H_2O_2-mediated deactivation of the enzyme active site of both acetylcholinesterase and butyrylcholinesterase (Schallreuter et al., 2004, Schallreuter et al., 2006b, Schallreuter et al., 2007b). In addition, it was shown that the tetramerisation domain as well as the EF-hand calcium binding domain are affected in the latter enzyme (Schallreuter et al., 2007c, Grando et al., 2006). The presence of high epidermal acetylcholine levels have been implicated in pruritus in the case of acute vitiligo (Schallreuter et al., 2008a). Moreover, elevated acetylcholine levels are in agreement with impaired sweating in these patients (Elwary et al., 1997).

H_2O_2 affects POMC cleavage and POMC-derived peptides

Decreased epidermal α-MSH levels have been reported in vitiligo (Thody et al., 1993, Spencer et al., 2007). These results were reconciled in the context of H_2O_2-mediated oxidation affecting POMC cleavage as well as the structure and function of POMC-derived peptides including ACTH, α-MSH and β-endorphin whereas β-MSH is not affected (Spencer et al., 2007; Spencer et al., 2008, Spencer and Schallreuter, 2009).

H_2O_2 affects epidermal calcium homeostasis in vitiligo

The influence of oxidative stress on calcium uptake / efflux has been known for a long time (Marks et al., 1996). Studies on the transport of radio-labelled [45]calcium within keratinocytes and melanocytes established from the depigmented epidermis of patients with vitiligo revealed a significant decrease in the rates for calcium uptake in these cells (Schallreuter et al., 1988, Schallreuter et al., 1996b). Since extracellular calcium concentration controls the kinetics for its uptake and efflux, this was a fundamental observation. In this context it is of interest that dendritic outgrowth of melanocytes requires calcium (Hara et al., 1994). In vitiligo several calcium dependent mechanisms have been identified as target for H_2O_2-mediated oxidation, including POMC-cleavage via the prohormone convertases and furin (Spencer et al., 2008), albumin (Rokos et al., 2004), butyrylcholinesterase (Schallreuter et al., 2006b) and calmodulin (Schallreutert et al., 2007d). Calcium is also directly involved in L-phenylalanine transport via the sodium / calcium ATP-ase antiporter system and the uptake can be severely hampered in vitiligo (Schallreuter et al., 1999c, Schallreuter et al., 2005). Since the majority of eumelanin is synthesised in melanocytes from autocrine conversion of L-phenylalanine to L-tyrosine via PAH, then the perturbation of calcium homeostasis in these cells could contribute significantly to impaired melanogenesis in vitiliginous melanocytes (Schallreuter et al., 1996b, Schallreuter et al., 1999c, Schallreuter et al., 2008c). This assumption is in agreement with low epidermal PAH and high epidermal phenylalanine levels in patients compared to controls (Schallreuter et al., 2005).

14

In vitiligo epidermal H_2O_2 is transferred to the vascular system

After reduction of epidermal H_2O_2 with a topical applied pseudocatalase PC-KUS epidermal and systemic enzyme levels recover (Schallreuter et al., 2008a, Salem et al., 2009). In this context it was shown that systemic H_2O_2 levels influence the cholinergic pathway via acetylcholine esterase (Schallreuter et al., 2004) and dihydropteridine reductase (DHPR), the last step in $6BH_4$ recycling (Hasse et al., 2004). Based on these results it was concluded that the systemic redox-status is under control of epidermal H_2O_2 and that this ROS is transferred from the epidermal compartment to the vascular system in patients with vitiligo.

Increased DNA damage does not induce skin cancer in patients with vitiligo despite the presence of high H_2O_2- and $ONOO^-$ levels

Considering that oxidative stress in vitiligo is massive, the question arises, how do these patients combat with this constant threat?

Clearly under these oxidative conditions DNA damage would be an expected must. Here it is noteworthy that these patients have persistent elevated levels of functioning wild type p53 protein in their entire skin (Schallreuter et al., 2003, Salem et al., 2009). Given that the p53 tumour suppressor protein is constitutively expressed and its nuclear presence is important in response to any genotoxic stress (Jiminez et al., 1999), this avenue was recently re-explored (Salem et al., 2009).

It was recognised that elevated epidermal p53 levels in the cytosol and in the nucleus are associated with significantly increased DNA damage as evidenced by significantly increased 8-oxo guanine (8-oxoG) levels in patient's skin and plasma. The presence of this oxidised DNA base is linked to up-regulated epidermal hOgg1, APE1 and DNA polymerase β levels, pointing to enhanced short patch base excision repair (BER). Moreover, functionality of the up-regulated p53 in vitiligo including phosphorylation of p53 via ATM and acetylation via PCAF was proven by the presence of phosphorylated ser 9 & ser 15 and acetylated lys 373 & lys 382 residues of increased p53 protein in association with induction of Gadd45, p21 and PCNA. The presence of significantly up-regulated epidermal Bcl2 protein expression in association with decreased cytochrome c, capase 3 and acetylcholinesterase levels argues against the presence of increased apoptosis in vitiligo (Boissy and Nordlund, 1997, van den Wijngaard et al., 2000, Tobin et al., 2000, Kemp et al., 2001, Schallreuter et al., 2003a, Salem et al., 2009). Induction of epidermal p76MDM^2 levels in association with normal p90MDM^2 expression could provide a conclusive rationale for the constant up-regulated p53 in this disease. Besides accumulation of epidermal H_2O_2 there are significantly elevated epidermal 3-nitro tyrosine levels present in vitiligo which in turn point to the presence of $ONOO^-$, thus adding this radical to the list of oxidative stress inducers in vitiligo (Salem et al., 2009).

Why show these patients no increased photo-damage / premature aging and high numbers of solar induced non-melanoma skin cancer despite the presence of abnormal high H_2O_2 and $ONOO^-$ levels and the absence of pigment in the affected skin (Calanchini-Postizzi and Frenk, 1987, Westerhof and Schallreuter, 1997, Schallreuter et al., 2002, Salem et al., 2009)?

p53 has many functions including induction of DNA repair via base patch excision. In addition this protein has a DNA binding domain which can directly act as DNA repair. In this context it was shown that the binding capacity of human wild-type p53 is significantly enhanced in the presence of 10^{-3} M H_2O_2 and ONOO‾ concentrations (Salem et al., 2009). Hence, up-regulated p53 in vitiligo could act in two ways to support DNA repair which could in turn explain the normal prevalence of solar induced skin cancer and the absence of premature skin aging despite massive oxidative stress and partial absence of pigment (Calanchini-Postizzi and Frenk, 1987, Schallreuter et al., 2002, Salem et al., 2009). Consequently it is tempting to invoke p53 as a possible master conductor in the scenario of vitiligo.

II. The neural hypothesis

For a long time it was believed that neurochemical mediators, released from nerve endings, can cause destruction of melanocytes in vitiligo. It was proposed that some intermediates or endproducts of catecholamines destroy the pigment (reviewed in Nordlund et al., 1988). Moreover, it was suggested that abnormal release of catecholamines from autonomic nerve endings contributes to an etiological role in the onset of vitiligo via toxic catecholamine generated radicals (Picardo et al., 1993). Taking into consideration that the human skin holds the capacity for autocrine catecholamine synthesis and degradation, contribution of these *in loco* produced neurotransmitters are becoming even more valid in the pathogenesis of vitiligo (Schallreuter et al., 1992). Both keratinocytes and melanocytes express tyrosine hydroxylase (TH) isoform I, the rate limiting step for catecholamine synthesis (Schallreuter et al., 1995a, Marles et al., 2003). Moreover, the presence of autocrine synthesis/regulation of the essential cofactor for the aromatic hydroxylases (6R)-5,6,7,8-tetra hydrobiopterin in epidermal cells has been extensively documented (Schallreuter et al., 1994a; Schallreuter et al., 1994b). Without this cofactor neither L-phenylalanine nor L-tyrosine and L-tryptophan could be metabolised via the aromatic hydroxylases. Moreover, this cofactor is also required by the nitric oxide synthases (NOS) (Thöny et al., 2000).

In the above context it has been reported that patients with active vitiligo have elevated noradrenaline levels in skin and plasma, as well as high levels of catecholamine metabolites in their urine which even correlate with early phase disease activity (Schallreuter et al., 1994b, Morrone et al., 1992, Cucci et al., 2003). Increased noradrenaline synthesis in the epidermis of these patients causes the induction of the two catecholamine degrading enzymes monoamine oxidase A (MAO-A) and catecholamine-O-methyl-transferase (COMT) (LePoole et al., 1994, Schallreuter et al., 1996a). Here it should be noted that adrenaline can stimulate melanogenesis via the β_2-adrenoceptor induced cAMP signal (Gillbro et al., 2004, Sivamani et al., 2009). Since melanocytes are noradrenergic cells due to the lack of phenylethanolamine-N-methyltransferase (PNMT) activity, these cells rely on keratinocyte produced adrenalin. But keratinocytes established from patients with vitiligo have significantly lower PNMT activities (Schallreuter et al., 1994b). Therefore the net results are low adrenalin- and high noradrenalin levels in the epidermal compartment of these patients. Given that β_2-adrenoceptors downregulate immature Langerhans cell function leading to down regulation of antigen presentation there is good evidence that catecholamines are major players in the immune response (Seiffert et al., 2002). Besides elevation of noradrenalin levels, epidermal dopamine levels are also elevated in vitiligo (Park et al., 2007). This metabolite is cytotoxic to melanocytes. Since dopamine induces ROS production and quinone toxicity, it could be an additional contributor to the loss of functioning melanocytes in affected individuals (Park et al., 2007). In this context it should also be noted that a significantly higher sensitivity to quinones has been documented in peripheral blood lymphocytes from patients with vitiligo (Schallreuter et al., 2006c).

Considering that melanocytes synthesise both catecholamines and melanin by the oxidation of L-tyrosine via L-dopa to L-dopaquinone and the latter metabolite generates indoles and ROS, both catecholamine- and melanin precursors have the potential for contribution to the depigmentation process in vitiligo (Boissy and Manga, 2004, Kroll et al., 2005, Picardo et al., 1993, Dell'Anna and Picardo, 2006, Park et al., 2007).

III. Virus and vitiligo

Virus has been implicated in the pathogenesis of vitiligo (Grimes et al., 1996, Grimes et al., 1999). Using PCR techniques, cytomegalovirus (CMV) and Epstein Barr virus (EBV) were detected in the epidermis of patients with this disorder. A later study on the same subject involving 72 German patients with vitiligo compared to healthy controls ($n = 70$) could not confirm those results (Würfel et al., 2000). Despite of these controversial findings, a viral involved 'hit / run' mechanism cannot be excluded. In fact, it has been shown in animal models that virus infection can trigger an autoimmune response due to molecular mimicry of viral peptide sequences activating in turn subsets of T-cells. In these models the virus, causing autoimmunity, escaped detection after the onset of the disease (Herrath and Oldstone, 1996, Morse et al., 1999). Taken together, viral induced T-cells could act against melanocytes. However, it would also be possible that virus can attract leukocytes and macrophages leading in turn to the 'oxygen burst' via NADPH-oxidase concomitant with the production of ROS, such as superoxide anion radical (O_2^-) and H_2O_2, thus feeding back to the ROS pool in vitiligo.

IV. Genetic factors in vitiligo

The use of FT-Raman spectroscopy for *in vivo* analysis of the depigmented epidermis proved the presence of high levels of H_2O_2 by following the peak at $875\,cm^{-1}$ (Schallreuter et al., 1999a). In addition, all patients tested have higher phenylalanine levels in their depigmented skin documented *in vivo* by the same method paralleled by low epidermal PAH activities (Schallreuter et al., 1994a, Schallreuter et al., 1998, Schallreuter et al., 2005). Moreover, an impaired phenylalanine metabolism has also been recognised in the systemic turnover of L-phenylalanine in this patient group ($n > 1000$) after receiving an oral loading with this essential amino acid (Schallreuter et al., 1998). Interestingly, 40% of the patients tested, revealed pathological L-phe / L-tyr ratios, similar to phenylketonurea heterozygotes, some patients present a mild hyperphenylalaninaemia and others have an impaired L-phenylalanine up-take (Schallreuter et al., 1998, Schallreuter et al., 2005, Schallreuter unpublished results). Despite major effort, so far there is no evidence for any mutation on the PAH gene nor in the transporter gene (Schallreuter et al., 2005). The defective recycling of 6BH$_4$ via pterin 4a-carbinolamine dehydratase (PCD) suggested another possibility of a polymorphism in this gene (Schallreuter et al., 1994a, Schallreuter et al., 1994b), but it was shown that PCD is directly deactivated by H$_2$O$_2$-mediated oxidation (Schallreuter et al., 2001). Examination of the PCD gene revealed only wild type enzyme (Schallreuter et al., 2001). Another report suggested that vitiligo might be caused by a mutation in GTP-cyclo-hydrolase I (GTP-CH-I), the rate limiting enzyme for 6BH$_4$ synthesis (De la Fuente-Fernandez, 1997), but this result could also not be substantiated (Schallreuter and Blau, 1997, Blau et al., 1996). An attempt to search for a possible mutation in the regulatory protein GFRP revealed again only wild type sequence for the 6BH$_4$ binding domain.

However, there is some evidence for polymorphism in the catalase gene of affected individuals which could account for vitiligo susceptibility (Casp et al., 2002, Wood et al., 2008). The involvement of the catalase gene in vitiligo would certainly correlate with ROS induction and its consequences discussed above. Although computer simulation of those documented SNPs strongly supports that the enzyme structure is substantially altered by H$_2$O$_2$-mediated oxidation, these data need confirmation by functional studies with catalase containing the documented SNPs (Wood et al., 2008). Other genetic studies support 'autoimmune' vitiligo strongly linked with autoimmune disease associated genes including *AIS1*, *AIS2,* and *SLEV1* while *AIS3* has been put forward for vitiligo without any association of other autoimmune diseases (Spritz et al., 2004). Moreover, a possible contribution of innate immune response via NALP1 SNPs has been postulated (Jin et al., 2007).

V. Autoimmunity and vitiligo – bringing the facts together

Question number 1

Could formation of neoantigens through ROS / RNS mediated oxidation and failing degradation / turnover foster production of autoantibodies in vitiligo?

Various antibodies are present in the circulating periphery of patients with vitiligo (Naughton et al., 1983a, Naughton et al., 1983b, Naughton et al.1986a, Naughton et al., 1986b, Galbraith et al., 1988, Farrokhi S et al., 2005). There is some debate how these antibodies arise but there is not yet a common consensus (Kemp et al., 2007). A correlation has been described between the frequency and the level of melanocyte antibodies and disease activity (Harning et al., 1991). Antibodies are directed against antigens of different sizes (Cui et al., 1992, Cui et al., 1993, Cui et al., 1995). Several autoantigens were identified including tyrosinase, TRP1, TRP2, melanosomal matrix protein gp100 (Pmel17), the melanocyte transcription factor SOX 10 and melanocyte concentrating hormone receptor (MCHR1) (Kemp et al., 2007). Whether melanocyte autoantibodies are indeed able to cause vitiligo is still under dicussion. There is some evidence that these antibodies destroy melanocytes under *in vitro* conditions via complement mediated cytotoxicity or *per se* in an antibody dependent cellular manner (Norris et al., 1998).

Over the past much research has focused on the detection of antibodies against tyrosinase and tyrosinase related proteins 1 and 2 (TRP-1 and TRP-2) (Song et al., 1994, Baharav et al., 1996, Kemp et al., 1997a, Kemp et al., 1997b, Kemp et al., 1998 and Okamato et al., 1998). Since tyrosinase is a glycoprotein which is extremely stable to proteolytic digestion, it appeared to be a good candidate for the elicitation of an immune response (Laskin and Piccinini, 1996). In addition to tyrosinase, TRP-1 and TRP-2 are other key proteins in control of pigmentation. TRP-1 is a melanosomal membrane associated protein which has 43% sequence homology with tyrosinase and it controls both the activity and stability of this key enzyme (Halaban and Moellmann, 1990, Orlow et al., 1993). Halaban and Moellmann were the first to demonstrate that TRP-1 has catalase / peroxidase activities and these authors suggested that it functions by protecting tyrosinase from oxidative degradation (Halaban and Moellmann, 1990). In this context, it has been established that H_2O_2 exercises a concentration dependent dual action ranging from activation to inactivation. H_2O_2 in higher concentrations is a potent competitive inhibitor of human tyrosinase. Moreover, superoxide anion radical is a better activator of the enzyme compared to molecular oxygen (Wood and Schallreuter, 1991). Thus, melanogenesis including the end product melanin has been considered as effective anti-oxidant defence mechanism protecting the melanocyte against oxidative stress (Wood et al., 1999). Jimbow et al. reported that melanocytes established from perilesional skin of patients with vitiligo expressed a TRP-1 containing 11 additional amino acids at the C-terminal end of its sequence. This sequence was identical to murine TRP-1 (Jimbow et al., 2001). The initial transcript for human and murine TRP-1 shows 93% sequence homology (Boissy et al., 1998). However, post-translational processing via an unidentified protease occurs in the human system producing a protein lacking 11 residues from the C-terminal. It was proposed that this protease appears to be lost, inhibited or inactivated in vitiligo (Jimbow et al., 2001). Interestingly, in vitiliginous melanocytes the murine form of TRP-1 is expressed and this protein loses its function for protecting melanosome integrity due to defective interactions with both tyrosinase as well as the melanosome chaperone calnexin (Jimbow et al., 2001, Manga et al., 2000). Animal models lacking active TRP-1 develop an adaptive autoimmune response to melanocytes, thus providing a good example in support of a potential role triggering an immune response (Rutault et al., 1999, Austin and Boissy, 1995).

To date the results obtained on tyrosinase antibodies in vitiligo are controversial. Xie et al. could not confirm the presence of antibodies to tyrosinase in 54 patients' sera (Xie et al., 1999). These authors reported a non-specific protein co-migrating with tyrosinase at 62 kD (Xie et al., 1999). Therefore, it was concluded that this protein most likely gave false positive results as reported by Song et al. (Xie et al., 1999, Song et al., 1994). Kemp et al. have re-examined these antibodies and this group delineated epitope regions on tyrosinase reacting with the antibodies utilised (Kemp et al., 1999). Accordingly, three epitope regions were found in the centre of the tyrosinase molecule (i. e. amino acids 240–255, 289–294 and 295–300) and two others towards the C-terminal end (i. e. amino acids 435–447 and 461–479). The centrally located epitopes had sequence homology with regions of TRP-1 and TRP-2, which consequently could explain the cross reactivity observed for these closely related proteins (Kwon, 1993, Yokoyama et al., 1994). Two of the five patients examined cross-reacted with both TRP-1 and TRP-2 and one patient reacted only with the 289–294 and 295–300 regions of tyrosinase (Kemp et al., 1999). Two patients reacted only with tyrosinase 435–447 and 461–479 and did not recognise TRP-1 or TRP-2 (Kemp et al., 1999). Based on these results, it can be concluded that multiple autoantibodies to tyrosinase could occur. Similar low frequencies for TRP-1 and TRP-2 were found in vitiligo patients (i.e. 5 out of 53) (Kemp et al., 1997a, Kemp et al., 1997b, Kemp et al., 1998). It should be mentioned that during the period from 1994 to 1999 autoantibodies to tyrosinase in vitiligo have lost their scientific significance from 61% down to 0–5% (Xie et al., 1999, Song et al., 1994, Kemp et al., 1999). Recently haptenation of tyrosinase due to oxidation of cysteine residues in the sequence of the enzyme via catechols has been put forward to explain the presence of tyrosinase antibodies in vitiligo (Westerhof and d'Ischia, 2007). Given that H_2O_2-mediated oxidation of methionine 374 in the active site of tyrosinase completely abrogates enzyme activity and that methionine sulfoxide cannot be repaired under these conditions as MSRA and MSRB are also subject to deactivation by H_2O_2-mediated oxidation, both altered proteins could offer ground for the formation of *neo*antigens, if complete degradation is not in place (Schallreuter et al., 2008d, Wood et al., 2009). Here, it is tempting to add the formation of thyroid peroxidase and other tissue antibodies as the result of protein alteration due to ROS/RNS induced changes and incomplete clearing of the affected proteins or protein fragments. This concept could be certainly valid in the case of Hashimoto-thyreoditis.

Question number 2

ROS / RNS and induction of T-cell response – the possible link to auto immunity in vitiligo?

Given the *in vivo* and *in vitro* evidence for ROS/RNS in vitiligo, it is tempting to analyse their possible role in the cellular immune response. ROS are instrumental in regulating cellular functions (Sahaf et al., 2003; Cross and Templeton, 2006). As discussed above in the case of vitiligo production of ROS/RNS is associated with oxidative stress, which in turn is characterized by a major shift in the cellular redox-balance and by ROS-mediated damage (Valko et al., 2007; Salem et al., 2009). However, ROS can also induce changes in the redox-balance to regulate cellular activity (Saran, 2003). Redox regulation involves subtle oxidations that might involve modifications in proteins by, for example, modifying methionine residues and cysteine cross-linking to name a few, in turn altering protein function (Hogg, 2003; Sahaf et al., 2005; Laragione et al., 2003; DeYulia et al., 2005). Importantly, T-cells have been shown to be targets for redox regulation (Gmunder et al., 1990; Angelini et al., 2002) and it is documented that exposure of T-cells to ROS down regulates T-cell activity (Gelderman et al., 2006; Gringhuis et al., 2000; Forman and Torres, 2001). Hence, T-cells require a reducing milieu for optimal proliferation and activation. In addition to the extracellular redox level, intracellular redox levels also influence T-cells, where a decrease in the intracellular redox-balance impairs T-cell function. Apart from the observation that ROS influence activation of T-cells, it has been shown that the type of T-cell response is also influenced by ROS. Some more support to this scenario could stem from the cellular infiltrate in the perilesional skin of patients (Prignano et al., 2009). The presence of this infiltrate indicates the likelihood of a biological 'oxygen burst' leading to the generation of superoxide anion radical (O_2^-) from O_2 via NADPH-oxidase (Darr and Fridovich, 1994, Marks et al., 1996, Stark, 1998). In inflammatory reactions O_2^- concentrations can increase up to 20-fold. After disproportionation this concentration would produce a 10-fold increase in H_2O_2 (Darr and Fridovich, 1994). However, the numbers of infiltrating neutrophils and macrophages as well as T-cells are usually very low or even absent in long lasting disease. Therefore, it is very difficult to assess the H_2O_2 contribution deriving from this infiltrate. In this context it is important to remember that cells in the perilesional epidermis in vitiligo show the same degree of vacuolation (i. e. lipid peroxidation) as cells in lesional and non-lesional skin (Tobin et al., 2000, Schallreuter et al., 1999a). Given that H_2O_2 can also activate peripheral blood dendritic cells by up-regulating surface markers known to be involved in T-cell interactions (Rutault et al., 1999) and this H_2O_2 driven process can promote interaction with MHC class II molecules (DQ and DR) as well as costimulatory molecules CD 40 and CD 86 (Rutault et al., 1999), it is also possible that a direct immune response can be stimulated via ROS. More support stems from an observation that dendritic cells promote T-cell proliferation after exposure to H_2O_2 (Rutault et al., 1999). The effect of H_2O_2 can be blocked *in vitro* upon the addition of the anti-oxidant N-acetyl cysteine (Rutault et al., 1999). In the same context, it has been shown that solar simulated irradiation up-regulates epidermal Langerhans cell B7.1 and B7.2 costimulatory molecules (Laihia and Jansen, 1997). Again H_2O_2 is generated by UVB (311 nm) and UVA 340nm (Schallreuter et al., 1999a). Therefore it is tempting to conclude that H_2O_2 modulates also the response of epidermal Langerhans cells and other dendritic cells in vitiligo (Tobin et al., 2000, Schallreuter et al., 1999a, Laihia and Jansen, 1997). These data could directly link oxidative stress from H_2O_2 to the onset of an adaptive immune response (Laihia and Jansen, 1997).

To date there is a plethora of evidence for the involvement of cytotoxic T-cells in the skin and in peripheral blood of these patients. T-cells are more prevalent in vitiligo perilesional skin than in lesional and non lesional skin. The infiltrate consists mainly of CD8 with lesser CD4 cells (Le Poole et al., 1996). It is currently believed that granzyme / perforin in T-cells mediates melanocyte cytotoxicity. In this context it has been proposed that in the absence of regulatory T-cells, cytotoxic T-cells enter the skin followed by targeting melanocytes causing in turn cellular damage and finally depigmentation (Oyarbide-Valencia et al., 2006).

Along this line there are reports that vitiligo occurred in patients after bone marrow transplantation where donor-derived alloreactive cytotoxic T-lymphocytes have been implied in the onset of the pigment loss (Cathcart and Morrell, 2007). In some cases the donor had vitiligo and the host developed the disease. Consequently adoptive transfer of the disease after allogeneic peripheral stem cell transplant has been put forward (Neumeister et al., 2000). Moreover, vitiligo occurred also in immune suppressed HIV positive individuals. Here the question arises, could the virus be the trigger factor as discussed above? Clearly these data strongly support immunological triggered vitiligo. However, one could also argue that these individuals might have been potential carriers for vitiligo susceptibility and that the onset of the disease was triggered by a severely perturbed cellular homeostasis including dramatic changes in the redox-balance and ROS related stress response. Considering the numbers of immune suppressed patients, the incidence of vitiligo would be expected to be significantly higher in these special patients if immunosuppression would be a strong contributor in the onset of vitiligo.

Newer treatment concepts

Based on the evidence provided herein, to date there is no doubt that epidermal generation/accumulation of H_2O_2 and $ONOO^-$ plays a central role in vitiligo.

This concept is in agreement with the clinical observation, that patients with this disorder, regardless of the time of onset and duration of the disease, age, gender and skin phototype respond to a topically applied pseudocatalase (PC-KUS) with a reduction of epidermal and systemic H_2O_2 accumulation concomitant with repigmentation (Schallreuter et al., 2008a, Schallreuter et al., 2008b, Salem et al., 2009) (Fig. 5B).

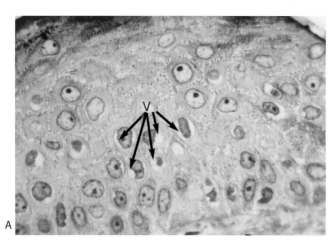

A

14

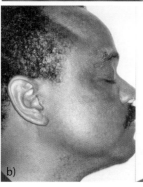

B a)

Fig. 5.
A Epidermal oxidative stress in acute vitiligo
   Toluidine blue staining
   NB. The extensive vacuolation (V) is based on lipid
   peroxidative damage due to H_2O_2 (Tobin et al., 2000).
B Extensive facial vitiligo in skin phototype VI
   (Fitzpatrick Classification)
   a Before treatment
   b After treatment with low dose narrowband UVB
     activated pseudocatalase (PC-KUS)

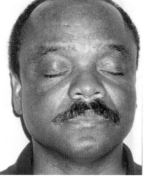
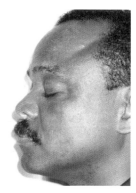

b)

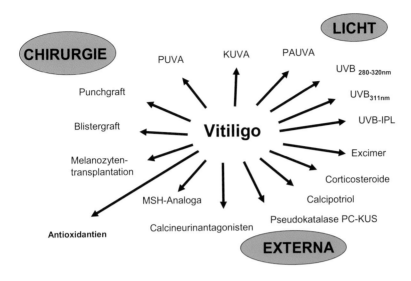

Fig. 6. Current treatment modalities for vitiligo

Despite substantial evidence for autoimmunity in vitiligo, the use of topical or systemic immuno suppressive drugs in the treatment is disappointing. Topical application of tacrolimus and pimecrolimus as local treatment modalities are effective in the repigmentation of facial vitiligo but fail the management of other body areas. Apart from pseudocatalase (PC-KUS) the most promising treatment at the present time seems to be the use of NB-UVB (311nm) with increasing doses twice or 3 times per week at least over 1 year. The precise mechanism of action remains to be established (Westerhof et al., 1999, Hamzavi et al., 2004). Oral supplementation of an antioxidant pool containing vitamin C and E, polyunsaturated fatty acid and α-lipoic acid significantly improved the clinical effectiveness of NB-UVB (Dell'Anna et al., 2007) supporting a role for ROS mediated stress in vitiligo. The many different approaches of the current treatment modalities are summarised in Fig. 6 underlining the dilemma in the search of an effective management for the affected patient.

Summary and conclusion

What is the overall take home message?

Vitiligo affects the entire epidermal compartment and not only melanocytes. These patients have no increased risk to develop skin cancer despite the absence of pigment and massive oxidative stress via H_2O_2 and $ONOO^-$. The disease is associated with DNA damage which is effectively repaired by a functioning persistent up-regulated wild type functioning p53 coupled to induction of both short patch and long patch base excision repair as well as

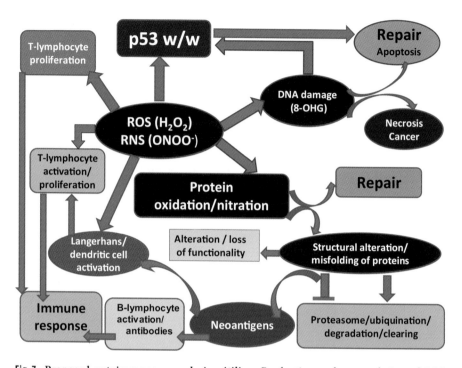

Fig. 7. Proposed autoimmune cascade in vitiligo. Production and accumulation of ROS (H_2O_2) / RNS ($ONOO^-$) leads to DNA-damage associated with increased 8-OHG levels in skin and in plasma (Salem et al., 2009). Both DNA damage and ROS / RNS induce and activate wild type p53 which in turn induces short patch and long patch excision repair (Schallreuter et al., 2003, Salem et al., 2009). H_2O_2 leads to oxidation of many protein structures including the entire antioxidant enzyme machinery leading to deactivation or loss of full functionality (for review Schallreuter et al., 2008a). Methionine sulfoxide is reduced to methionine by MSRA and MSRB, but the enzymes are subject to H_2O_2-mediated oxidation (Schallreuter et al., 2008d, Gibbons et al., 2006). The net results are altered proteins (for review Schallreuter et al., 2008a). Normally these are eliminated from the system via proteasome / ubiquitin degradation. However, in the case of leaky clearing protein fragments or complete oxidised / nitrated proteins neoantigens can be formed after B-cell activation providing ground for antibody production. ROS-activated dendritic cells and Langerhans cells initiate a cellular immune response (Rutault et al., 1999, Kemp et al., 2007). Furthermore ROS / RNS can stimulate and activate T-lymphocytes leading to immune response including cytokine release (TNFα, γIFN, Il 1β, Il 6 etc) (Oyarbide-Valencia K 2006). Both ROS / RNS can stimulate NFkB affecting a number of cellular processes including inflammation, cellular proliferation, transformation and tumorigenesis. Epidermal generation of H_2O_2 and its accumulation is supported by low catalase levels and a leaky catalase due to various SNP's in the gene (Schallreuter et al., 1991, Casp et al., 2002, Wood et al., 2008). Enhanced autoimmune reactivity could be paired with the respective autoimmune genes recently identified (Spritz et al., 2004, Jin et al., 2007). However, there is evidence for direct cellular melanocyte toxicity due to quinones, phenols and oxidised pterins to name a few (Schallreuter et al., 2007, Boissy et al., 2004, Schallreuter et al., 1994c). Moreover, cellular homeostasis can be affected by impaired calcium-uptake, perturbed L-phenylalanine up-take, cAMP-signalling and many more. Taken together, there is substantial evidence for different pathways leading to vitiligo.

enhanced DNA-binding capacity in the presence of H_2O_2 and $ONOO^-$. Degradation of p53 is prevented by p76 MDM^2. There is no evidence for increased skin cancer / photodamage and epidermal apoptosis in this disease (Schallreuter et al., 2003a, Salem et al., 2009).

Evidence to date supports ROS mediated T-cell activation and T-cell response as well as the possibility of *neo*antigen formation due to H_2O_2 / $ONOO^-$-mediated oxidation / nitration of proteins. Considering that normally oxidised proteins and oxidatively-modified biomolecules are cleared by the proteasome / ubiquination system or lysosomes, it could be possible that H_2O_2-mediated oxidation and the presence of $ONOO^-$ and its protonated peroxinitrious acid (ONOOH) leads to dysfunction or even deactivation of this important machinery (Grune et al., 1997, Halliwemm, 2002, Ullrich and Hofrichter, 2007). Preliminary data from our lab support a dysfunctional degradation axis (Schallreuter, unpublished results). At this point it is tempting to propose incomplete proteasomal degradation / ubiquination for ineffective clearing of altered proteins leading in turn to the formation of antibodies against melanocytes and other tissues which then can elicitate a cellular immune response in this disease. The proposed cascade is summarised in Fig. 7.

Whether other autoimmune disorders are a conditio sine qua non in the pathomechanism of vitiligo remains to be shown. In the light of epidermal and systemic H_2O_2 accumulation, it is tempting to speculate that environmental (exogenous) or systemic (endogenous) trigger factors could be the mechanisms for the 'hit' that increases H_2O_2 production via NADPH-oxidase in the microenvironment. This could tip the balance and cause the initial loss of constitutive pigment due to the generation of hydroxyl radicals (OH$^{\cdot}$) from H_2O_2 via the UV-catalysed Haber-Weiss reaction in susceptible individuals. However, in the subsequent process of the disease, the origin of H_2O_2 derives from various sources, which could well foster the 'run' mechanism, where H_2O_2 activates T-cell proliferation with consequent activation of T-cell clones (Rutault et al., 1999, LePoole et al., 2004). The abundance of $ONOO^-$ in the epidermis of patients opens new avenues. Our knowledge on the effect of $ONOO^-$ in vitiligo is just at the tip of an ice berg.

In conclusion, there is strong evidence that autoantigens / autoantibodies and T-cell response play a major role in the pathogenesis of vitiligo.

However, it is tempting to propose that the clinical picture of vitiligo might be rather a clinical symptom for different vitiligo / depigmentation entities. Some support for this hypothesis stems from vitiligo-like depigmentation in association with melanoma, or syndromes including Vogt-Koyanagi-Harada syndrome, Schmidt's syndrome and the autoimmune polyglandular-syndromes.

Very recently significant associations between generalized vitiligo and SNPs at several loci previously associated with other autoimmune diseases were detected. These included genes encoding major-histocompatibility-complex class I molecules and class II molecules PTPN22, LPP, IL2RA UBASH3A and C1QTNF6. Moreover, associations SNPs in two additional immune-related loci, RERE and GZMB and in a locus containing TYR (P=$1.60\times10-18$), encoding tyrosinase were documented.

References

Anderson D, Schmid TE, Baumgartner A, Cemeli-Carratala E, Brinkworth MH, Wood JM (2003) Oestrogenic compounds and oxidative stress (in human sperm and lymphocytes in the Comet assay). Mutat Res 544(2-3):173–180

Angelini G, Gardella S, Ardy M, Ciriolo MR, Filomeni G, Di Trapani G, Clarke F, Sitia R, Rubartelli A (2002) Antigen-presenting dendritic cells provide the reducing extracellular microenvironment required for T lymphocyte activation. Proc Natl Acad. Sci USA 99:1491–1496

Aronoff S (1965) Catalase: kinetics of photo-oxidation. Science 150:72–73

Austin LM, Boissy RE (1995) Mammalian tyrosinase related protein-1 is recognised by autoantibodies from vitiliginous Smyth chickens. Am J Pathol 146:1529–1541

Baharav E, Merimski O, Shoenfeld Y, Zigelman R, Gilbrud B, Yecheskel G, Youinou P, Fishman P (1996) Tyrosinase as an autoantigen in patients with vitiligo. Clin Exp Immunol 105:84–88

Beazley WD, Gaze DC, Panske A, Panzig E, Schallreuter KU (1999) Serum selenium levels and glutathione peroxidase activities in vitiligo. Br J Dermatol 141:301–303

Bhawan J, Bhutani LK (1983) Keratinocyte damage in vitiligo. J Cutaneous Path 10:207–212

Blau N, Barnes I, Dhondt JL (1996) International database of tetrahydrobiopterin deficiences. J Inherit Metab Dis 19:8–14

Boissy R, Liu YY, Medrano EE, Nordlund JJ (1991) Structural aberration of the rough endoplasmic reticulum and melanosome compartmentalisation in long term cultures of melanocytes from vitiligo patients. J Invest Dermatol 97:395–404

Boissy, RE, Nordlund, J. J. (1997) Molecular basis of congenital hypopigmentary disorders in humans: a review. Pigment Cell Res. 10:12–24

Boissy RE, Sakai C, Zhao H, Kobayashi T, Hearing VJ (1998) Human tyrosinase related protein-1 (TRP-1). Exp Dermatol 7:198–204

Boissy RE, Manga P (2004) On the etiology of contact/occupational vitiligo. Pigment Cell Res 17:208–14

Calanchini-Postizzi E, Frenk E (1987) Long-term actinic damage in sun-exposed vitiligo and normally pigmented skin. Dermatologica 174:266–71

Casp CB, She JX, McCormack WT (2002) Genetic association of the catalase gene (CAT) with vitiligo susceptibility. Pigment Cell Res 15:62–66

Cathcart S, Morrell D (2007) Vitiligo as a post-bone marrow transplantation complication. J Pediatr Hematol Oncol 29(7):485–7

Cross JV, Templeton DJ (2006) Regulation of signal transduction through protein cysteine oxidation. Antioxid Redox Signal 8:1819–1827

Cucci ML, Frattini P, Santagostino G, Preda S, Orrecchia G (2003) catecholamines increase in the urine of non-segmental vitiligo especially during its active phase Pigment Cell Res 16(2):111–116

Cui J, Harning R, Henn M, Bystryn J-C (1992) Identification of pigment cells antigens defined by vitiligo antibodies. J Invest Dermatol 98:162–165

Cui J, Arita Y, Bystryn J-C (1993) Cytolytic antibodies to melanocytes in vitiligo. J Invest Dermatol 100:812–815

Cui J, Chen D, Misfeldt ML, Swinfard RW, Bystryn J-C (1995) Antimelanoma antibodies in swine with spontaneously regressing melanoma. Pigment Cell Res 8:60–63

Darr D, Fridovich I (1994) Free radicals in cutaneous biology. J Invest Dermatol 102:671–675

Davis MD, Ribeiro P, Tipper J, Kaufman S (1992) 7-Tetrahydrobiopterin, a naturally occurring analogue of tetrahydrobiopterin, is a cofactor for and a potential inhibitor of the aromatic amino acid hydrolases. Proc Natl Acad Sci USA 89:10108–10113

De la Fuente-Fernandez R (1997) Mutations in GTP-cyclohydrolase I gene and vitiligo. Lancet 350:640

Dell'Anna ML, Picardo M (2006) A review and a new hypothesis for non-immunological pathogenetic mechanisms in vitiligo. Pigment Cell Res 19:406–411

Dell'Anna ML, Mastrofrancesco A, Sala R, Venturini M, Ottaviani M, Vidolin AP, Leone G, Calzavara PG, Westerhof W, Picardo M (2007) Antioxidents and narrowband-UVB in the treatment of vitiligo: a double-blind placebo controlled trial. Clin Exp Dermatol 32:631–636

DeYulia GJ Jr., Carcamo JM, Borquez-Ojeda O, Shelton CC, Golde DW (2005) Hydrogen peroxide generated extracellularly by receptor-ligand interaction facilitates cell signaling. Proc Natl Acad Sci USA. 102:5044–5049

Elwary SM, Headley K, Schallreuter KU (1997) Calcium homeostasis influences epidermal sweating in patients with vitiligo. Br J Dermatol. 137(1):81–85

Farrokhi S, Hojjat-Farsangi M, Noohpisheh MK, Tahmasbi R, Rezaei N (2005) Assessment of the immune system in 55 Iranian patients with vitiligo. J Eur Acad Dermatol Venereol 19(6):706–11

Forman HJ, Torres M (2001) Signaling by the respiratory burst in macrophages. IUBMB Life. 51:365–371

Galbraith GM, Miller D, Emerson DL (1988) Western blot analysis of serum antibody reactivity with human melanoma cell antigens in alopecia areata and vitiligo. Clin Immunol Immunopathol 48:317–324

Gauthier Y, Cario-Andre M, Taieb A (2003) A critical appraisal of vitiligo etiologic theories. Is melanocyte loss a melanocytorrhagy? Pigment Cell Res 16:322–332

Gelderman KA, Hultqvist M, Holmberg J, Olofsson P, Holmdahl R (2006) T cell surface redox levels determine T cell reactivity and arthritis susceptibility. Proc Natl Acad Sci USA 103:12831–12836

Gibbons NC, Wood JM, Rokos H, Schallreuter KU (2006) Computer simulation of native epidermal enzyme structures in the presence and absence of hydrogen peroxide (H_2O_2): potential and pitfalls. J Invest Dermatol. 126(12):2576–82

Gillbro JM, Marles LK, Hibberts NA, Schallreuter KU (2004) Autocrine catecholamine biosynthesis and the beta-adrenoceptor signal promote pigmentation in human epidermal melanocytes. J Invest Dermatol 123(2):346–53

Gmunder H, Eck HP, Benninghoff B, Roth S, Droge W (1990) Macrophages regulate intracellular glutathione levels of lymphocytes. Evidence for an immunoregulatory role of cysteine. Cell Immunol 129:32–46

Grando SA, Pittelkow MR, Schallreuter KU (2006) Adrenergic and cholinergic control in the biology of epidermis: physiological and clinical significance. J Invest Dermatol. 126(9):1948–65

Grimes PE, Sevall JS, Vojdani A (1996) Cytomegalovirus DNA identified in skin biopsy specimens of patients with vitiligo. J Am Acad Dermatol 35:21–26

Grimes PE, Elkadi T, Sanders, J (1999) Epstein-Barr virus infection in patients with vitiligo (abstr). J Invest Dermatol 112:604

Gringhuis SI, Leow A, Papendrecht-Van Der Voort EA, Remans PH, Breedveld FC, Verweij CL (2000) Displacement of linker for activation of T cells from the plasma membrane due to redox balance alterations results in hyporesponsiveness of synovial fluid T lymphocytes in rheumatoid arthritis. J. Immunol 164:2170–2179

Grune T, Reinheckel T, Davies KJ (1997) Degradation of oxidized proteins in mammalian cells. FASEB J 11:526–534

Hara I, Yaar M, Tang A, Eller MS, Reenstra W, Gilchrist BA (1994) Role of integrins in melanocyte attachment and dendricity. J Cell Sci107:2739–2748

Halaban R, Moellmann GE (1990) Murine and human b-locus pigmentation genes encode a glycoprotein (gp75) with catalase activity. Proc Nat Acad Sci USA 87:4809–4813

Halliwell B (2002) Proteosomal dysfunction. Ann N Y Acad Sci 962:182–195

Hamzavi I, Jain H, Mclean D, Shapiro J, Zeng H, Lui H (2004) Parametric modelling of narrowband UVB phototherapy for vitiligo using a novel quantitative tool: the Vitiligo Area Scoring Index. Arch Dermatol 140:677–83

Harning R, Cui J, Bystryn J-C (1991) Relation between the incidence and level of pigment cell antibodies and disease activity in vitiligo. J Invest Dermatol 97:1078–1080

Hasse S, Gibbons NC, Rokos H, Marles LK, Schallreuter KU (2004) Perturbed 6-tetrahydrobiopterin recycling via decreased dihydropteridine reductase in vitiligo: more evidence for H_2O_2 stress. J Invest Dermatol 122:307–313

Herrath MG, Oldstone MB (1996) Virus induced autoimmune disease. Curr Opin Immunol 8:878–885

Hogg PJ (2003) Disulfide bonds as switches for protein function. Trends Biochem. Sci. 28:210–214

Iyengar B (1989) Modulation of melanocytic activity by acetylcholine. Acta Anat (Basel) 36:139–141

Jimbow K, Chen H, Park JS, Thomas P (2001) Increased sensitivity of melanocytes to oxidative stress and abnormal expression of tyrosinase related protein in vitiligo. Br J Dermatol 144:55–65

Jimenez GS, Khan SH, Stommel JM, Wahl GM (1999) p53 regulation by post-translational modification and nuclear retention in response to diverse stresses. Oncogene 18:7656–7665

Jin Y, Mailloux CM, Gowan K, Riccardi SL, LaBerge G, Bennett DC, Fain PR, Spritz RA (2007) NALP1 in vitiligo-associated multiple autoimmune disease. N Engl J Med 356(12):1216–25

Johnson MT, Roberts J (1978) Skin conditions and related need for medical care among persons 1–74 years. United States 1971–1974. Vital Health Stat 11:212 I-V 1–72

Kemp EH, Gawkrodger DJ, MacNeil S, Watson PF, Weetman AP (1997a) Detection of tyrosinase autoantibodies in vitiligo patients using ^{35}S-labelled recombinant human tyrosinase in a radioimmunoassay. J Invest Dermatol 109:69–73

Kemp EH, Gawkrodger DJ, Watson PF, Weetman AP (1997b) Immunoprecipitation of melanogenic enzyme autoantigens with vitiligo sera: evidence for cross-reactive autoantibodies to tyrosinase and tyrosinase-related protein-2 (TRP-2). Clin Exp Immunol 109:495–500

Kemp EH, Waterman, Gawkrodger DJ, Watson PF, Weetman AP (1998) Autoantibodies to tyrosinase-related protein-1 (TRP-1) detected in the sera of vitiligo patients using a quantitative radiobinding assay. Br J Dermatol 139:798–805

Kemp EH, Waterman EA, Gawkrodger DJ, Watson PF, Weetman AP (1999) Identification of epitopes on tyrosinase which are recognised by autoantibodies from patients with vitiligo. J Invest Dermatol 113:267–271

Kemp, EH, Waterman, EA, Weetman, AP (2001) Autoimmune aspects of vitiligo. Autoimmunity 34:65–77

Kemp EH, Gavalas NG, Gawkrodger DJ, Weetman AP (2007) Autoantibody responses to melanocytes in the depigmenting skin disease vitiligo. Autoimmun Rev 6(3):138–42

Kroll TM, Bommiasamy H, Boissy RE, Hernandez C, Nickoloff BJ, Mestril R, Lepoole IC (2005) 4-tertiarybutyl phenol exposure sensitizes human melanocytes to dendritic cell mediated killing: relevance in vitiligo J Invest Dermatol 124:798–806

Krüger C, Smythe JW, Spencer JD, Hasse S, Panske A, Chiuchiarelli G, Schallreuter KU (2010) Combined climatotherapy at the Dead Sea significantly improves quality of life and supports coping with the disease in patients with vitiligo. Acta Derm Venereol (submitted)

Kwon BS (1993) Pigmentation genes: the tyrosinase gene family and the pmel17 gene family. J Invest Dermatol 100:134S–140S

Laihia JK, Jansen CT (1997) Upregulation of human epidermal Langerhans cell B7-1 and B7-2 costimulatory molecules in vivo by solar stimulating irradiation. Eur J Immunol 27:984–989

Laragione T, Bonetto V, Casoni F, Massignan T, Bianchi G, Gianazza E Ghezzi P (2003) Redox regulation of surface protein thiols: identification of integrin alpha-4 as a molecular target by using redox proteomics. Proc Natl Acad. Sci USA 100:14737–14741

Laskin JD, Piccinini LA (1986) Tyrosinase isozyme heterogeneity in differentiating B16/C3 melanoma. J Biol Chem 261:16626–16635

LePoole IC, Das PK, van den Wijngaard RM, Bos JD, Westerhof W (1993a) Review of the etiopathomechanism of vitiligo: A convergence theory. Exp Dermatol 2:146–153

14

LePoole IC, van den Wijngaard RM, Westerhof W, Dutrieux RP, Das PK (1993b) Presence or absence of melanocytes in vitiligo lesions: an immunohistochemical investigation. J Invest Dermatol 100:816–82

LePoole C, Wijngaard van den, Smit NPM, Oosting J, Westerhof W, Pavel S (1994) Catechol-O-methyl transferase in vitiligo. Arch Dermatol Res 286:81–86

Le Poole IC, van den Wijngaard RM, Westerhof W, Das PK (1996) Presence of T cells and macrophages in inflammatory vitiligo skin parallels melanocyte disappearance. Am J Pathol 148(4):1219–28

Le Poole IC, Wankowicz-Kalinska A, van den Wijngaard RMJGJ, Nickoloff BJ, Das PK (2004) Autoimmune aspects of depigmentation in vitiligo. J Invest Dermatol Symp Proc 9:68–72

Manga P, Sato K, Ye L, Beerman F, Lamoreux ML, Orlow SJ (2000) Mutational analysis of the modulation of tyrosinase by tyrosinase related proteins 1 and 2 in vitro. J Pigment Cell Res 13:364–374

Maresca V, Roccella M, Roccella F, Camera E, Del Porto G, Passi S, Grammatico P, Picardo M (1997) Increased sensitivity to peroxidative agents as a possible pathogenic factor of melanocyte damage in vitiligo. J Invest Dermatol 109:310–313

Maresca V, Flori E, Briganti S, Camera E, Cario-André M, Taïeb A, Picardo M (2006) UVA-induced modification of catalase charge properties in the epidermis is correlated with the skin phototype. J Invest Dermatol 126(1):182–90

Marks DB, Marks AD, Smith CM (1996) Oxygen metabolism and oxygen toxicity. In: Basic Medical Biochemistry: A Clinical Approach. Baltimore: Williams and Wilkins 327–340

Marles LK, Peters EM, Tobin DJ, Hibberts NA, Schallreuter KU (2003) Tyrosine hydroxylase isoenzyme I is present in human melanosomes: a possible novel function in pigmentation. Exp Dermatol 12:61–70

Medrano EE and Nordlund JJ (1990) Successful culture of adult human melanocytes obtained from normal and vitiligo donors. J Invest Dermatol 95:441–445

Moellmann G, Klein-Angerer S, Scollay DA, Nordlund JJ, Lerner AB (1982) Extracellular granular material and degeneration of keratinocytes in the normally pigmented epidermis of patients with vitiligo. J Invest Dermatol 79:321–330

Moretti S, Spallanzani A, Amato L et al. (2002) New insights into the pathogenesis of vitiligo: imbalance of epidermal cytokines at sites of lesions. Pigment Cell Res 15:87–92

Morrone A, Picardo M, De Luca C, Terminali O, Passi S, Ippolito F (1992) Catecholamines and vitiligo. Pigment Cell Res 5:58–62

Morse SS, Sakaguchi N, Sakaguchi S (1999) Virus and autoimmunity: induction of autoimmune disease in mice by mouse T-lymphotropic virus (MTLV) destroying CD4 and T cells. J Immunol 162:5309–5316

Naughton GK, Eisinger M, Bystryn J-C (1983a) Antibodies to normal human melanocytes in vitiligo. J Exp Med 158:246–251

Naughton GK, Eisinger M, Bystryn J-C (1983b) Detection of antibodies to melanocytes in vitiligo by specific immunoprecipitation. J Invest Dermatol 81:540–542

Naughton GK, Reggiardo MD, Bystryn J-C (1986a) Correlation between vitiligo antibodies and extent of depigmentation in vitiligo. J Am Acad Dermatol 15:978–981

Naughton GK, Mahaffey M, Bystryn J-C (1986b) Antibodies to surface antigens of pigment cells in animals with vitiligo. Proc Soc Exp Biol Med 181:423–426

Neumeister P, Strunk D, Apfelbeck U, Sill H, Linkesch W (2000) Adoptive transfer of vitiligo after allogeneic bone marrow transplantation for non-Hodgkin's lymphoma. Lancet 355(9212):1334–50

Nordlund JJ, Ortonne JP (1992) Vitiligo and depigmentation. Curr Prob Dermatol 4:3–30

Nordlund JJ, Boissy RE, Hearing VJ, King RA, Ortonne JP (eds) (1998) The pigmentary system. Physiology and Pathophysiology. Oxford University Press, Oxford

Norris DA, Kissinger RM, Naughton GK, Bystryn J-C (1998) Evidence for immunologic mechanisms in human vitiligo: patients' sera induce damage to human melanocytes in vitro by complement-mediated damage and antibody-dependent cellular toxicity. J Invest Dermatol 90:783–789

Okamoto T, Irie RF, Fujii S, Huang SKS, Nizze AJ, Morton DL, Hoon DSB (1998) Anti-tyrosinase related protein-2 immune response in vitiligo patients and melanoma patients receiving active-specific immunotherapy. J Invest Dermatol 111:1034–1039

Orlow SJ, Boissy RE, Moran D, Pifka-Hinst S (1993) Subcellular distribution of tyrosinase and tyrosinase related protein 1: Implications for melanosomal biogenesis. J Invest Dermatol 100:55–64

Ortonne JP, Bose SK (1993) Vitiligo: Where do we stand? Pigment Cell Res 8:61–72

Oyarbide-Valencia K, van den Boorn JG, Denman CJ, Li M, Carlson JM, Hernandez C, Nishimura MI, Das PK, Luiten RM, Le Poole IC (2006) Therapeutic implications of autoimmune vitiligo T cells. Autoimmun Rev 5(7):486–92

Park ES, Kim SY, Na JI, Ryu HS, Youn SW, Kim DS, Yun HY, Park KC (2007) Glutathione prevented dopamine-induced apoptosis of melanocytes and its signaling. J Dermatol Sci 47(2):141–49

Pey AL, Martinez A, Charubala R, Maitland DJ, Teigen K, Calvo A, Pfleiderer W, Wood JM, Schallreuter KU (2006) Specific interaction of the diastereomers 7(R)- and 7(S)-tetrahydrobiopterin with phenylalanine hydroxylase: implications for understanding primapterinuria and vitiligo. FASEB J 20:2130–2132

Picardo M, Passi S, Morrone, A, Grandinetti M, Di Carlo A, Ippolito F (1993) Antioxidant Status in the blood of patients with active vitiligo. Pigment Cell Res 7(2):110–115

Prignano F, Pescitelli L, Becatti M, Di Gennaro P, Fiorillo C, Taddei N, Lotti T (2009) Ultrastructural and functional alterations of mitochondria in perilesional vitiligo skin. J Dermatol Sci 54(3):157–67

Rokos H, Beazley WD, Schallreuter KU (2002) Oxidative stress in vitiligo: photo-oxidation of pterins produces H_2O_2 and pterin-6-carboxylic acid. Biochem Biophys Res Commun 292:805–11

Rokos H, Moore J, Hasse S, Gillbro JM, Wood JM, Schallreuter KU (2004) In vivo Fluorescence Excitation Spectroscopy and in vivo FT-Raman Spectroscopy in human skin: Evidence of H_2O_2 oxidation of epidermal albumin in patients with vitiligo. J Raman Spectrosc 35:125–130

Rutault K, Alderman C, Chain BM, Katz DR (1999) Reactive oxygen species activate human peripheral blood dendritic cells. Free Radic Biol Med 26:232–238

Sahaf B, Heydari K, Herzenberg LA, Herzenberg LA (2003). Lymphocyte surface thiol levels. Proc Natl Acad Sci USA 100:4001–4005

Sahaf B, Heydari K, Herzenberg LA, Herzenberg LA (2005) The extracellular microenvironment plays a key role in regulating the redox status of cell surface proteins in HIV-infected subjects. Arch Biochem Biophys 434:26–32

Salem MM, Shalbaf M, Gibbons NC, Chavan B, Thornton JM, Schallreuter KU (2009) Enhanced DNA binding capacity on up-regulated epidermal wild-type p53 in vitiligo by H_2O_2-mediated oxidation: a possible repair mechanism for DNA damage. FASEB J 23(11):3790–807

Saran M (2003) To what end does nature produce superoxide? NADPH oxidase as an autocrine modifier of membrane phospholipids generating paracrine lipid messengers. Free Radic Res 37:1045–1059

Schallreuter KU, Pittelkow MR, Wood JM (1986) Free radical reduction by thioredoxin reductase at the surface of normal and vitiliginous human keratinocytes. J Invest Dermatol 87:728–732

Schallreuter KU, Hordinsky, Wood JM (1986) Thioredoxin reductase – Role in free radical reduction in different hypopigmentaion disorders. Arch Dermatol 123:615–619

Schallreuter KU, Pittelkow MR (1988) Defective calcium uptake in keratinocyte cell cultures from vitiliginous skin. Arch Dermatol Res 280:137–139

Schallreuter KU, Wood JM, Berger J (1991) Low catalase levels in the epidermis of patients with vitiligo. J Invest Dermatol 97:1081–1085

Schallreuter KU, Wood JM, Lemke R, Le Poole C, Das P, Westerhof W, Pittelkow, MR, Thody AJ (1992) Production of catecholamines in the human epidermis. Biochem Biophys Res Communs 189:72–78

Schallreuter KU, Wood JM, Pittelkow MR, Gütlich M, Lemke KR, Rödl W, Swanson NN, Hitzemann K, Ziegler I (1994a) Regulation of melanin biosynthesis in the human epidermis by tetrahydrobiopterin. Science 263:1444–1446

14

Schallreuter KU, Wood JM, Ziegler I, Lemke KR, Pittelkow MR, Lindsey NJ, Gütlich M (1994b) Defective tetrahydrobiopterin and catecholamine biosynthesis in the depigmentation disorder vitiligo. Biochim Biophys Acta 1226:181–192

Schallreuter KU, Büttner G, Pittelkow MR, Wood JM, Swanson NN, Körner C (1994c) Cytotoxicity of 6-biopterin to human melanocytes. Biochem Biophys Res Communs 204:43–48

Schallreuter KU, Lemke R, Brandt O, Schwartz R, Westhofen M, Montz R, Berger J (1994d) Vitiligo and other diseases: coexistence or true association? Hamburg study on 321 patients. Dermatology 188(4):269–275

Schallreuter KU, Lemke KR, Pittelkow MR, Wood JM, Körner C, Malik R (1995a) Catecholamines and keratinocyte differentiation. J Invest Dermatol 104:953–957

Schallreuter KU, Wood JM, Lemke KR, Levenig C (1995b) Treatment of vitiligo with a topical application of pseudocatalase and calcium in combination with short-term UVB exposure: a case study on 33 patients. Dermatol 190:223–229

Schallreuter KU, Wood JM, Pittelkow MR, Büttner G, Swanson NN, Körner C, Ehrke C (1996a) Increased monoamine oxidase A activity in the epidermis of patients with vitiligo. Arch Dermatol Res 288:14–18

Schallreuter KU, Pittelkow MR, Swanson NN (1996b) Defective calcium transport in vitiliginous melanocytes. Arch Dermatol Res 288:11–13

Schallreuter KU, Blau N (1997) GTP-cyclohydrolase and vitiligo. Lancet 350:1254

Schallreuter KU, Zschiesche M, Moore J, Panske A, Hibberts NA, Herrmann FH, Metelmann HR, Sawatzki J (1998) *In vivo* evidence for compromised phenylalanine metabolism in vitiligo. Biochem Biophys Res Commun 243:395–399

Schallreuter KU, Moore J, Wood JM, Beazley WD, Gaze DC, Tobin DJ, Marshall HS, Panske A, Panzig E, Hibberts NA (1999a) *In vivo* and *in vitro* evidence for hydrogen peroxide (H_2O_2) accumulation in the epidermis of patients with vitiligo and its successful removal by a UVB-activated pseudocatalase. J Invest Dermatol Symp Proc 4:91–96

Schallreuter KU (1999b) Successful treatment of oxidative stress in vitiligo. Skin Pharmacol Appl Skin Physiol 12:132–138

Schallreuter KU, Wood JM (1999c) The importance of L-phenylalanine transport and its autocrine turnover to L-tyrosine for melanogenesis in human epidermal melanocytes. Biochem Biophys Res Communs 262:423–428

Schallreuter KU, Moore J, Wood JM, Beazley WD, Peters EMJ, Marles LK, Behrens-Williams SC, Dummer R, Blau N, Thöny B (2001) Epidermal H_2O_2 accumulation alters tetrahydrobiopterin ($6BH_4$) recycling in vitiligo: Identification of a general mechanism in regulation of all $6BH_4$ dependent processes? J Invest Dermatol 116:167–74

Schallreuter KU, Tobin DJ, Panske A (2002) Decreased photodamage and low incidence of non-melanoma skin cancer in 136 sun-exposed caucasian patients with vitiligo. Dermatology 204:194–201

Schallreuter KU, Behrens-Williams S, Khaliq TP et al. (2003a) Increased epidermal functioning wild-type p53 expression in vitiligo. Exp Dermatol 12:268–277

Schallreuter KU, Kothari S, Elwary S, Rokos H, Hasse S, Panske A (2003b) Molecular evidence that halo in Sutton's naevus is not vitiligo Arch Derm Res 295:223–228

Schallreuter KU, Elwary SM, Gibbons NC, Rokos H, Wood JM (2004) Activation / deactivation of acetylcholinesterase by H_2O_2: more evidence for oxidative stress in vitiligo. Biochem Biophys Res Commun 315:502–508

Schallreuter KU, Chavan B, Rokos H, Hibberts N, Panske A, Wood JM (2005) Decreased phenylalanine uptake and turnover in patients with vitiligo. Mol Genet Metab 86 Suppl 1: S27–33

Schallreuter KU (2006a) Functioning methionine-S-sulfoxide reductases A and B are present in human skin. J Invest Dermatol 126(5):947–949

Schallreuter KU, Gibbons NC, Zothner C, Elwary SM, Rokos H, Wood JM (2006b) Butyrylcholinesterase is present in the human epidermis and is regulated by H_2O_2: more evidence for oxidative stress in vitiligo. Biochem Biophys Res Commun 349(3):931–938

Schallreuter KU, Chiuchiarelli G, Cemeli E, Elwary SM, GillbroJM, Spencer JD, Rokos H, Panske A, Chavan B, Wood JM, Anderson D (2006c) Estrogens can contribute to hydrogen peroxide generation and quinone-mediated DNA damage in peripheral blood lymphocytes from patients with vitiligo J Invest Dermatol 126:1036–1042

Schallreuter KU, Krüger C, Rokos H, Hasse S, Zothner C, Panske A (2007a) Basic research confirms coexistence of acquired Blaschkolinear Vitiligo and acrofacial Vitiligo. Arch Dermatol Res 299(5-6):225–230

Schallreuter KU, Elwary S (2007b) Hydrogen peroxide regulates the cholinergic signal in a concentration dependent manner. Life Sci 80(24-25):2221–2226

Schallreuter KU, Gibbons NC, Elwary SM, Parkin SM, Wood JM (2007c) Calcium-activated butyrylcholinesterase in human skin protects acetylcholinesterase against suicide inhibition by neurotoxic organophosphates. Biochem Biophys Res Commun 355(4):1069–1074

Schallreuter KU, Gibbons NCJ, Zothner C, Abou Ellouf MM, Wood JM (2007d) Hydrogen peroxide –mediated oxidative stress disrupts calcium binding on calmodulin: More evidence for oxidative stress in vitiligo. Biochem Biophys Res Commun 360:70–75

Schallreuter KU, Bahadoran P, Picardo M et al. (2008a) Vitiligo pathogenesis: autoimmune disease, genetic defect, excessive reactive oxygen species, calcium imbalance, or what else? Exp Dermatol 17(2):139–160

Schallreuter KU, Krüger C, Würfel BA, Panske A, Wood JM (2008b) From basic research to the bedside: efficacy of topical treatment with pseudocatalase PC-KUS in 71 children with vitiligo. Int J Dermatol 47(7):743–53

Schallreuter KU, Kothari S, Chavan B, Spencer JD (2008c) Regulation of melanogenesis – controversies and new concepts. Exp Dermatol 17(5):395–404

Schallreuter KU, Rübsam K, Gibbons NC, Maitland DJ, Chavan B, Zothner C, Rokos H, Wood JM (2008d) Methionine sulfoxide reductases A and B are deactivated by hydrogen peroxide (H_2O_2) in the epidermis of patients with vitiligo. J Invest Dermatol 128(4):808–815

Seiffert K, Hosoi J, Torii H ..(2002) Catecholamines inhibit the antigen-presenting capabilityof epidermal Langerjans cell. J Immunol 168:6128–6135

Shalbaf M, Gibbons NC, Wood JM, Maitland DJ, Rokos H, Elwary SM, Marles LK, Schallreuter KU (2008) Presence of epidermal allantoin further supports oxidative stress in vitiligo. Exp Dermatol 17(9):761–770

Sivamani RK, Porter SM, Isseroff RR (2009) An epinephrine-dependent mechanism for the control of UV-induced pigmentation. J Invest Dermatol 129(3):784–787

Song Y, Connor E, Li Y, Zorovich B, Balducci P, Maclaren N (1994) The role of tyrosinase in autoimmune vitiligo. Lancet 344:1049–1052

Spencer JD, Gibbons NC, Rokos H, Peters EM, Wood JM, Schallreuter KU (2007) Oxidative stress via hydrogen peroxide affects proopiomelanocortin peptides directly in the epidermis of patients with vitiligo. J Invest Dermatol 127(2):411–20

Spencer JD, Gibbons NC, Böhm M, Schallreuter KU (2008) The Ca^{2+}-binding capacity of epidermal furin is disrupted by H_2O_2-mediated oxidation in vitiligo. Endocrinology 149(4):1638–45

Spencer JD, Schallreuter KU (2009) Regulation of pigmentation in human epidermal melanocytes by functional high-affinity beta-melanocyte-stimulating hormone / melanocortin-4 receptor signalling. Endocrinology 150(3):1250–1258

Spritz RA, Gowan K, Bennett DC, Fain PR (2004) Novel vitiligo susceptibility loci on chromosomes 7 (AIS2) and 8 (AIS3), confirmation of SLEV1 on chromosome 17, and their roles in an autoimmune diathesis. Am J Hum Genet 74:188–91

Stark JM (1998) Immunological adjuvance of metabolic origin: oxidative stress, postulated impaired function of thiol proteases and immunogenicity. Scand J Immunol 48:475–479

Taïeb A, Picardo M (2007) The definition and assessment of vitiligo: a consensus report of the Vitiligo European Task Force. Pigment Cell Res 20(1):27–35

Thody AJ, Hunt G, Donatien PD, Todd C (1993) Human Melanocytes Express Functional Melanocyte-Stimulating Hormone Receptors. Annals of the New York Academy of Sciences 680, Issue The Melanotropic Peptides, 381–390.

14

Thöny B, Auerbach G, Blau N (2000) Tetrahydrobiopterin biosynthesis, regeneration and functions. Biochem J 347 Pt 1:1–16

Tobin DJ, Swanson NN, Pittelkow MR, Peters EMJ, Schallreuter KU (2000) Melanocytes are not absent in lesional skin of long duration vitiligo. J Pathol 191:407–416

Ullrich R, Hofrichter M (2007) Enzymatic hydroxylation of aromatic compounds. Cell Mol Life Sci 64:271–293

Vafaee T, Rokos H, Salem MM, Schallreuter KU (2010) In *vivo* and in *vitro* evidence for epidermal HO-mediated oxidative stress in piebaldism. Exp Dermatol [Epub ahead of print]

Valko M, Leibfritz D, Moncol J, Cronin MT, Mazur M, Telser J (2007) Free radicals and antioxidants in normal physiological functions and human disease. *Int J Biochem Cell Biol* 39:44–84

van den Wijngaard RM, Aten J, Scheepmaker A, Le Poole IC, Tigges AJ, Westerhof W, Das PK (2000) Expression and modulation of apoptosis regulatory molecules in human melanocytes: significance in vitiligo. Br J Dermatol 143(3):573–581

Westerhof, W, Schallreuter, KU (1997) PUVA for vitiligo and skin cancer. Clin Exp Dermatol 22:54

Westerhof W, Nieuweboer-Krobotova L, Mulder PG, Glazenburg EJ (1999) Left-right comparison study of the combination of fluticasone propionate and UVA vs either fluticasone propionate or UVA alone for the long term treatment of vitiligo. Arch Dermatol 135:1061–1066

Westerhof W, d'Ischia M (2007) Vitiligo puzzle: the pieces fall in place. Pigment Cell Res 20(5):345–59

Wood JM, Schallreuter KU (1991) Studies on the reactions between human tryosinase, superoxide anion, hydrogen peroxide and thiols. Biochim Biophys Acta 1074:378–385

Wood JM, Jimbow K, Boissy RE, Slominski A, Plonka PM, Slawinski J, Wortsman J, Tosk J (1999) What's the use of generating melanin? Exp Dermatol 8:133–164

Wood JM, Schallreuter KU (2006) UVA-irradiated pheomelanin alters the structure of catalase and decreases its activity in human skin. J Invest Dermatol. 126(1):13–14

Wood JM, Gibbons NC, Chavan B, Schallreuter KU (2008) Computer simulation of heterogeneous single nucleotide polymorphisms in the catalase gene indicates structural changes in the enzyme active site, NADPH-binding and tetramerization domains: a genetic predisposition for an altered catalase in patients with vitiligo? Exp Dermatol 17(4):366–371

Wood JM, Decker H, Hartmann H, Chavan B, Rokos H, Spencer JD, Hasse S, Thornton MJ, Shalbaf M, Paus R, Schallreuter KU (2009) Senile hair graying: H_2O_2-mediated oxidative stress affects human hair color by blunting methionine sulfoxide repair. FASEB J 23(7):2065–75

Würfel F, Panske A, Schallreuter KU (2000) Are viral infections a possible cause for the manifestation of vitiligo? Pigment Cell Res 13:404

Xie Z, Chen D, Jiao D, Bystryn J-C (1999) Vitiligo antibodies are not directed to tyrosinase. Arch Dermatol 135:417–422

Ying Jin, Stanca A. Birlea, Pamela R. Fain, Katherine Gowan, Sheri L. Riccardi, Paulene J. Holland, Christina M. Mailloux, Alexandra J.D. Sufit, Saunie M. Hutton, Anita Amadi-Myers, Dorothy C. Bennett, Margaret R. Wallace, Wayne T. McCormack, E. Helen Kemp, David J. Gawkrodger, Anthony P. Weetman, Mauro Picardo, Giovanni Leone, Alain Taïeb, Thomas Jouary, Khaled Ezzedine, Nanny van Geel, Jo Lambert, Andreas Overbeck, and Richard A. Spritz,. (2010) Variant of TYR and Autoimmunity Susceptibility Loci in Generalized Vitiligo N Engl J Med; 362:1686–1697

Yohn JJ, Norris DA, Yrastorza G, Buno IJ, Leff JA, Hake SS, Repine JE (1991) Disparate antioxidant enzyme activities in cultured human cutaneous fibroblasts, keratinocytes and melanocytes. J Invest Dermatol 97:405–409

Yokoyama K, Suzuki H, Yasumoto K, Tomita Y, Shibahara S (1994) Molecular cloning and functional analysis of a cDNA coding for human DOPAchrome tautomerase/tyrosinase-related protein-2. Biochim Biophys Acta 1217:317–321

Alopecia Areata

15

Pia Freyschmidt-Paul, Kevin McElwee, and Rolf Hoffmann

Classification / Clinical appearance

Alopecia areata (AA) is the symptomless loss of hair in either small circumscribed patches (Fig. 1), which may remain discrete or may expand into total loss of all scalp (Fig. 2) and even body hair. AA is a common human disease with a lifetime risk of 1.7% in the general population (Safavi et al., 1995). It is characterized by a reversible patchy hair loss most commonly involving the scalp although other regions of the head, including eyelashes and beard, may also be affected. The typical patient with AA notes the sudden appearance of a circular patch of hair loss. Areas of activity in the lesion may be indicated by the presence of "exclamation mark" hairs (Fig. 3) which are usually 2–4 mm long and may have a dark expanded tip and a depigmented root. The disease may sometimes lead to complete scalp baldness (Alopecia areata totalis) or even total body hair loss (Alopecia areata universalis). AA band-like hair loss in parieto-temporo-occipital area is described as Alopecia areata ophiasis (Alkhalifah et al., 2010). AA may be observed at any age and has no clear sex pre-

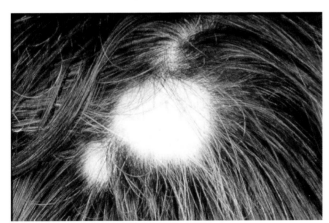

Fig. 1. Patchy alopecia areata: Two small round bald patches in a child.

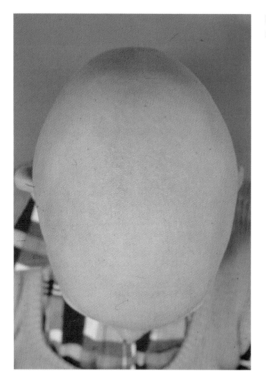

Fig. 2. Alopecia areata totalis: Involvement of the entire scalp.

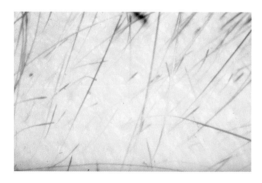

Fig. 3. Exclamation point hairs at advancing edge of patch of alopecia areata.

dominance. However, AA is more likely to first occur in adolescents suggesting a potential relationship to hormonal activity. AA is not life-threatening but it is psychologically and socially disturbing.

The course of AA is unpredictable and typically characterized by phases of acute hair loss followed by spontaneous hair regrowth and waxing and waning of the lesions. However, in severe forms hair loss can persist for many years. Very often AA shows a mild clinical course with only a few small bald patches and hair regrowth after some weeks or months. However, the severe forms are usually chronic. The prognosis for AA is defined

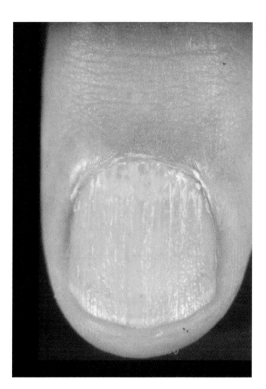

Fig. 4. Mild nail dystrophy in alopecia areata with pitting and ridging.

by the age at disease onset, duration, nail signs, the extent of hair loss and the presence of atopic dermatitis. This means that a patient with AA universalis for many years, with a first episode of AA during childhood, associated nail changes and atopic dermatitis, has only a small chance to experience hair regrowth.

No other organs are affected by AA except for the nails, which may show typical signs of AA such as small pits, red spotted lunulae or verticular ridging (Fig. 4). Nail involvement tends to be associated with more wide spread AA (Kasumagic-Halilovic and Prohic, 2009). Sometimes small nail pits are the first signs of developing AA and hair loss may occur later. Only exceptionally nails may fall off (Onychomadesis) due to a severe nail AA and sometimes all nails are affected.

There are some publications which describe the association of AA with other autoimmune diseases, such as vitiligo or an increased association with type 1 diabetes mellitus in relatives of patients (Muller and Winkelmann, 1963; Wang et al., 1994). However, there is considerable debate about the practical value of these observations and whether there is a truly significant relationship. In our view, only Hashimotos thyroiditis tends to be more common in AA affected individuals (Kurtev and Iliev, 2005).

Just as hair loss is sudden, hair regrowth occurs without any indicators. The initial hair regrowth after an episode of AA is often white due to a delay in repigmentation of hairs. Interestingly, the last hairs to be affected by AA are white hairs, explaining how scalp hair can appear to become white overnight (Helm and Milgrom, 1970).

Diagnosis

The clinical history of abrupt onset of patchy hair loss, the lack of infection, black dots, ex-clamation mark hairs, are all suggestive of the diagnosis of AA and in most cases the di-agnosis of AA can be made clinically. There is no blood test to confirm or to rule out the diagnosis. In rare cases differential diagnosis such as chronic discoid lupus erythemato-sus, lichen planopilaris, syphilis, traction alopecia, metastasis to the scalp, mycosis fungoi-des or alopecia mucinosa must be taken into consideration. Especially in AA of the diffuse type it might be difficult to make the diagnosis. Then a scalp biopsy is indicated (Alkhali-fah et al., 2010).

Histopathology

Histopathological features of AA include peri- and intrafollicular lymphocytic infiltrates involving only anagen hair follicles with subsequent miniaturization of these follicles (Whiting, 2003). The lymphocytic infiltrate is located around the hair bulb with some lym-phocytes invading the hair follicle (Fig. 5). As a consequence, edema, microvesiculation, pigment incontinence, keratinocyte cell apoptosis, and vacuolar damage may be seen in and around the affected hair follicles (Tobin, 1997). Destruction of hair follicles or scarring usually does not occur in AA and therefore hair regrowth is possible at any time point of the disease, either spontaneously or due to a successful treatment. The process usually in-volves terminal hairs but can affect vellus hairs as well.

Molecular genetics – the present knowledge

AA has been proposed to be an autoimmune disease based on several indirect observa-tions in humans and animal models of the disease (McElwee et al., 1999c). Genetic influ-ence has been clearly demonstrated in most other autoimmune diseases and one would ex-pect that AA is no exception. AA is a complex disease which does not segregate according to the rules of Mendelian inheritance (Van der Steen et al., 1992a; Shellow et al., 1992; Co-lombe et al., 1995; Sharma et al., 1996a). As with other autoimmune diseases, AA is most likely a polygenic disorder where susceptibility is dictated by several major genes and the phenotype may be modified by numerous minor genes.

Rodent models

Isolated examples of AA have been identified in several species. However, the limited characterization or availability of these examples restricts their usefulness in any genetic research for AA (McElwee et al., 1998b). Two rodent models have been developed and characterized for use in AA research, the Dundee experimental bald rat (DEBR) and the C3H/HeJ mouse (Michie et al., 1991; Sundberg et al., 1994). Both models are inbred strains. Despite their inbred nature, rodents may have a wide variety of hair loss presenta-

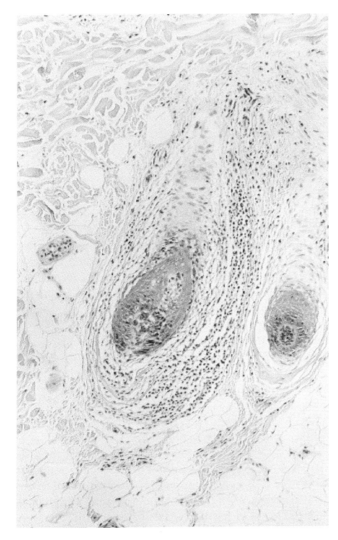

Fig. 5. Histopathology of alopecia areata. Lymphocytes are clustered around the hair bulb and extend into the dermal papilla (LM × 100).

tions from isolated patches, or diffuse AA, to near universal hair loss. AA in both rodent models has been shown to be an autosomal polygenic trait with partial phenotype penetrance by analysis of breeding programs.

The DEBR, originally a hybrid between BDIX and Wistar rats, has been intercrossed for over 35 generations. Two separate inbred DEBR sub-strains exist, one black hooded and the other brown, but with similar AA phenotype properties. Hair loss is associated with a primarily CD4+ and CD8+ lymphocytic cell infiltrate of anagen stage hair follicles and production of hair follicle specific antibodies (Zhang and Oliver, 1994; McElwee et al., 1996). Spontaneous expression of AA develops in 42% of individuals with onset from 7 months of age in both males and females. Hair loss typically first develops in symmetrical bald patches on the flanks. Multiple patches may develop to affect the head, dorsal and ventral skin with approximately 15% of affected individuals reaching a near universal hair loss state. DEBR have been cross bred with PVG/OlaHsd rats yielding 21% affected F1 offspring (Oliver, personal communication) suggesting PVG/OlaHsd rats contain few AA susceptibility genes. PVG/OlaHsd rats may be one of several strains suitable for use in an intercross or backcross breeding strategy to identify AA susceptibility and severity modifying genes by linkage disequilibrium.

C3H/HeJ mice have existed as a unique inbred strain at the Jackson Laboratory since 1947, but onset of the AA phenotype was first observed in several individuals of a C3H/HeJ mouse colony in 1993. The mouse breeding pattern permitted tracing the genetic history of the affected mice to a single breeding pair at generation F198 (Sundberg et al., 1994), suggesting a genetic modification of the strain in one parent. The frequency of spontaneous AA expression in aged mice, up to 18 months old, increased to approximately 20% in 3–4 generations for over 300 mice evaluated (Sundberg et al., 1994). Both males and females are affected with initially ventral hair loss typically developing in females from 6 months and in males from 10 months of age. Hair loss may progress to the dorsal surface and reach near universal loss in 10% of affected individuals. Histopathology shows all affected anagen stage hair follicles to be affected by non-scaring focal inflammation of primarily CD4$^+$ and CD8$^+$ lymphocytes and hair follicle specific autoantibodies are present at a high titer (Tobin et al., 1997; Freyschmidt-Paul et al., 1999).

Recent studies have demonstrated that all adult C3H/HeJ mice are susceptible to AA. Grafting skin from spontaneous AA affected mice to normal haired C3H/HeJ mice consistently promotes onset of AA 8–10 weeks after grafting (McElwee et al., 1998a). Skin grafts from AA affected mice to the histocompatible C3H/OuJ and C3HeB/FeJ inbred strains promotes AA onset with a similar phenotype and pathology, but in only 40% of graft recipients (McElwee et al., 1998a). Crosses between C3H/HeJ mice with AA and mice from the closely related strain with no history of age associated alopecia, yielded F1 and subsequent generation mice with an AA expression frequency of 10–12% (Sundberg et al., 1994). The AA induction technique suggests that while inbred C3H/HeJ mice may all be genetically susceptible, the AA phenotype must be activated. It is possible that the environment provides a trigger for initial disease onset. The apparent reduced susceptibility of the C3H/OuJ and C3HeB/FeJ strains to AA suggest that these strains carry fewer AA susceptibility genes as compared to the C3H/HeJ strain. The segregation pattern of phenotypes suggests that AA in laboratory mice is under the control of one or more dominant gene alleles.

C3H/HeJ mice cross bred with C57/BL6J mice yield 7% of affected F1 generation mice (10% affected females, 2% affected males). Intercross studies are in progress with up to 13 candidate gene loci under investigation supporting the hypothesis that AA is a polygenic disease (Sundberg et al., 2003, 2004).

Human epidemiology

There is a higher incidence of AA in genetically related individuals. This suggests that at least some people are genetically predisposed to develop AA. The triggers for the onset of AA may be environmental, but the resistance of the AA lesion to treatment, its persistence and regression, and its extent over the body may be influenced by the presence and interaction of multiple genes. Several studies suggest that AA has a genetic basis (Van der Steen et al., 1992a; Colombe et al., 1995). AA with similar times of onset or similar hair loss patterns has been reported in monozygotic twins (Hendren, 1949; Weidman et al., 1956; Bonjean et al., 1968; Stankler, 1979; Cole and Herzlinger, 1984; Scerri and Pace, 1992; Al-saleh et al., 1995). Families with several generations of AA affected individuals also suggest AA may be a genetically determined disease (Shelton and Hollander, 1942; Goldstein and Chipizhenko, 1978; Hordinsky et al., 1984; Valsecchi et al., 1985; Van der Steen et al., 1992a; Sharma et al., 1996a; Sharma et al., 1996b).

Epidemiological studies provide basic evidence for AA susceptibility genes. Numerous studies suggest AA may be more frequently expressed in genetically related individuals. Typically, 10 to 20% of patients with AA indicate at least one other affected family member (Table 1). In contrast, the lifetime risk of AA expression in the general population has been suggested to be 1.7% (Safavi et al., 1995). Familial incidence may be significantly higher than reported in epidemiological studies as the marked psycho-social consequences of hair loss inhibit some individuals from seeking diagnosis. In addition, some may not be aware of their hair loss if it is limited or develops in an area not immediately visible to the individual.

A strong association has been observed between AA and trisomy 21 (Down's syndrome). From 1000 patients and 1000 control subjects, Du Vivier and Munro observed 60 cases of trisomy 21 individuals with AA versus 1 control (Du Vivier and Munro, 1975). Carter and Jegasothy identified 19 cases of AA in 214 trisomy 21 affected patients and the statistical relationship is further supported in other studies (Wunderlich and Braun-Falco, 1965; Carter and Jegasothy, 1976). The genetic mutation for autoimmune polyendocrinopathy syndrome type 1 (AIRE, autoimmune regulator gene) (Finnish-German APECED Consortium 1997) is also associated with a 29 to 37% prevalence of AA (Betterle et al., 1998). These studies suggest that candidate gene loci for AA susceptibility may be present on human chromosome 21.

Associations of AA with other autoimmune diseases have also been reported. Between 7% and 27% of AA affected patients may also have a thyroid disease, including goiter presence, myxedema and Hashimoto's thyroiditis (Cunliffe et al., 1969; Milgraum et al., 1987; Shellow et al., 1992; Puavilai et al., 1994). Co-expression of vitiligo and AA has also been reported at between 4% and 9% (Muller and Winkelmann, 1963; Main et al., 1975). However, the statistical significance of these disease associations when compared to appropriate control populations has been disputed elsewhere (Salamon et al., 1971; Gollinck and Orfanos, 1990; Schallreuter et al., 1994). Numerous case reports detail concordant presence of AA with other autoimmune diseases, such as diabetes and myasthenia gravis, although the statistical significance is unknown (McElwee et al., 1998b).

HLA genes

Human leukocyte antigen (HLA) genes on human chromosome 6 code for the major histocompatibility complex (MHC) proteins that are important in presentation of antigens

Table 1. Incidence of alopecia areata in reported epidemiological studies

Percentage with family history	Geographic location	Source
3%	UK	Barber 1921
20%	UK	Brown 1929
20%	France	Sabouraud 1929
19%	UK	Anderson 1950
10%	USA	Muller and Winkelmann 1963
3.4%	Italy	Olivetti and Bubola 1965
6.3%	Portugal	Bastos Araujo and Poiares Baptista 1967
25%	UK	Cunliffe et al., 1969
17%	Sweden	Gip et al., 1969
27%	USA	Sauder et al., 1980
24%	UK	Friedmann 1981
11%	Belgium	De Weert et al., 1984
6.6%	Germany	Lutz and Bauer 1988
18%	Netherlands	De Waard 1989
11.4%	Germany	Gollinck and Orfanos 1990
16%	Germany	Van der Steen et al., 1992
42%	USA	Shellow et al., 1992
11.5%	Korea	Ro Bi 1995
9%	India	Sharma et al., 1996a
12.4%*	India	Sharma et al., 1996b

*children aged 16 or younger

15

and self recognition by immune cells. MHC class I antigens comprise the HLA-B, HLA-C and HLA-A loci in this order. MHC class II is coded by genes in the HLA-D region that is subdivided into gene clusters HLA-DP, HLA-DQ, and HLA-DR (Vogel and Motulsky, 1997). MHC class I antigens are expressed on almost all nucleated cells. $CD8^+$ lymphocytes have the capacity to recognize cellular antigens presented in association with MHC class I via their T cell receptors. In contrast, MHC class II antigens are normally expressed on antigen presenting cells (APCs), such as macrophages and Langerhans' cells, and expression may be induced on other nucleated cells during inflammatory processes such as AA (Messenger and Bleehen, 1985; Bröcker et al., 1987). $CD4^+$ lymphocytes may recognize antigen plus MHC class II complexes on APCs. Different MHC proteins may have superior presenting properties for particular antigens compared to other MHC complexes and consequently some antigen-MHC complexes will be more effective in their activation of lymphocytes than others. In part, this may determine the ability of lymphocytes to respond to the hair follicle antigen(s) targeted in AA and may define how potent an immune response against a particular antigen will be.

Genetic research in other autoimmune diseases has shown HLA encoding alleles to segregate with specific disease phenotypes. However, inconsistent results have been found with analysis of HLA class I haplotypes of the A and B series and AA. Some studies report statistically significant associations, but other studies found no HLA class I association (Kuntz et al., 1977; Zlotogorski et al., 1990). HLA-A2, B40 and Aw32, B18 have each been reported as associated with AA (Hordinsky et al., 1984; Valsecchi et al., 1985). Associations between HLA-B12 in Finnish patients, HLA-B18 in Israelis, B13 and B27 in Russians have also been suggested (Kianto et al., 1977; Hacham-Zadeh et al., 1981; Averbakh and Pospelov, 1986).

Genetic analysis studies in AA have primarily focused on the HLA-D genes (MHC class II encoding) as the most likely region for genes that regulate susceptibility, severity of, or resistance to disease (Duvic et al., 1991). Consistent associations have been observed between class II haplotypes and AA including DR4 (Friedman, 1985; Frentz et al., 1986; Orecchia et al., 1987; Duvic et al., 1991; de Andrade et al., 1999), DR5 (Friedman, 1985; Frentz et al., 1986; Orecchia et al., 1987), DR6 (de Andrade et al., 1999), DR7 (Averbakh and Pospelov, 1986) and broad antigen DQ3 (Welsh et al., 1994; Colombe et al., 1995; Colombe et al., 1999). More recent research has shown allele DRB1*1104 (DR11) to be present with significant increased expression in patients with AA (Colombe et al., 1995; Colombe et al., 1999) and this was confirmed in other studies (Morling et al., 1991; Welsh et al., 1994; Duvic et al., 1995). Allele DRB1*0401 (DR4) was strongly associated with AA totalis or universalis sub-groups (Colombe et al., 1999). DQB1*0301 (DQ7 by serology) was also significantly expressed only in association with AA totalis and universalis (Colombe et al., 1995; Duvic et al., 1995; Colombe et al., 1999). Other studies implicate other DQB1 alleles, DQB1*0302, DQB1*0601, and DQB1*0603, in AA (de Andrade et al., 1999). The current consensus is that AA in humans has a genetic basis, but is not always in a familial aggregation (Van der Steen et al., 1992; Colombe et al., 1995).

It has been suggested that the HLA gene products, the MHC antigens, could be important for the presentation of an unknown AA antigen. Aberrant expression of MHC proteins within AA affected hair follicles is frequently found, but the question of its true significance remains (Messenger and Bleehen, 1985; Bröcker et al., 1987). There are many more alleles that code for other factors within, and outside of, the immune system that may be vital in the development of AA.

Non HLA genes

The HLA gene region is likely to be only one of several gene loci involved in AA, but limited research has been conducted in other areas of the genome. One investigation has shown an association between AA and allele 2 of a 5 allele polymorphism for the IL-1rn gene on human chromosome 2 that codes for the IL-1 receptor antagonist (Tarlow et al., 1994). Results indicated allele 2 was present in 41% of controls versus 44% in individuals with patchy AA, 66% of those with alopecia totalis and 77% of alopecia universalis affected individuals (Tarlow et al., 1994). Allele 2 is known to influence IL-1ß production. Galbraith et al. identified the IL-1ß-1,2 genotype as significantly increased in frequency for individuals with extensive, but not patchy, AA further suggesting that the severe form of disease may be associated with increased IL-1ß production (Galbraith et al., 1999).

Genes for immunoglobulin heavy (Gm) and light (Km) chain genotypes on human chromosome 14 have also been implicated in AA susceptibility (Galbraith et al., 1984; Galbraith and Pandey, 1989) with the suggestion that IL-1ß (IL-1ß-1,2) and light chain (KM-1,3) genotypes may interact to increase AA susceptibility (Galbraith et al., 1999). TNFα gene polymorphisms, or adjacent genes in the HLA region may also influence AA susceptibility (Galbraith and Pandey, 1995; Cork et al., 1996). Involvement of all these gene loci, as susceptibility or severity modifying genes, is consistent with an autoimmune pathogenesis of AA.

More recently, investigation of AA genetics has progressed to genome wide association studies. Data is still preliminary, but at least one investigation of 804 unrelated AA affected individuals and 2229 controls suggested potential linkage to seven distinct loci (Petukhova et al., 2010).

Conclusions

Rodent model research has shown that AA is an immune mediated disease and strongly suggests that the mechanism is autoimmune in nature (McElwee et al., 1999c). It is probable that AA susceptibility and severity modifying genes will primarily be involved in the immune system, but other susceptibility genes may control hair follicle function. From observation in humans and animal models, AA can be described as a polygenic disease with a variable spectrum of severity. While previous research studies have understandably focused on the HLA region and identification of marker genes segregating with the AA phenotype, there is a clear need for genome wide association studies to define further candidate susceptibility, severity modifying, and possibly resistance gene loci. Human population analysis suggests potential gene loci may be located on Chromosomes 2, 6, 14, and 21 (Du Vivier and Mundo, 1975; Colombe et al., 1995; Duvic et al., 1995; Galbraith et al., 1999). Careful categorization of DNA samples based on phenotypic presentation of hair loss in the individual will be important for defining sub-categories of AA. It might be possible to define specific alleles with association to particular AA phenotypes such as patchy AA, AA totalis, or AA universalis.

Pathogenesis

Circumstantial evidence for AA as an autoimmune disease

The complete pathogenesis picture for AA has yet to be determined. However, recent research has made much progress in our understanding of the disease mechanism. There is numerous circumstantial evidence in support of the notion that AA is fundamentally an inflammation driven disease and may be autoimmune in nature. Observation of a peri- and intra-follicular inflammation of the target anagen hair follicle primarily by T lymphocytes in both humans and animal models is the most compelling morphological evidence (Perret et al., 1984; Ranki et al., 1984; Zhang et al., 1994; Sundberg et al., 1994). In addition to a lymphocytic infiltrate there is increased presence of antigen presenting cells such as macrophages and particularly Langerhans cells around, and sometimes within, dystrophic hair follicles (Wiesner-Menzel and Happle, 1984; Zhang et al., 1994). Furthermore, inflammatory markers include up regulation of ICAM and ELAM expression on the endothelium of blood vessels closely associated with affected hair follicles (Nickloff and Griffiths, 1991; McDonagh et al., 1993; Zhang et al., 1994). Changes in cytokine levels, particularly activating cytokines such as IL-2 and IFN-γ, have been noted during AA inflammation with corresponding alteration of cytokine concentrations after successful topical counter irritant therapy (Hoffmann et al., 1994). MHC class I and II expression on hair follicle epithelial structures normally devoid of MHC expression is associated with hair follicle inflammation and AA (Bröcker et al., 1987; McDonagh et al., 1993). Certain MHC class II haplotypes seem to be associated with predisposal of the individual towards AA, a common observation in autoimmune diseases (Duvic et al., 1991; Colombe et al., 1999). Hair follicle specific IgG autoantibodies have been found in increased concentrations in the peripheral blood of AA affected individuals compared to normal, non-affected humans (Tobin et al., 1994a, Tobin et al., 1994b). AA may respond to a range of immunomodulatory treatments (Hoffmann and Happle, 1999). All these and other circumstantial evidence (McElwee et al., 1999c; McElwee et al., 2002b) are of some assistance in understanding the pathogenesis of AA. However, detailed characterization and functional studies are required to demonstrate the significance of these circumstantial observations and to elucidate disease mechanisms. Primarily due to ethical limitations, functional studies cannot readily be conducted in humans. Consequently, animal models of human AA are required.

Immune system targets

AA is generally believed to have an autoimmune pathogenesis (Paus et al., 1993; McDonagh and Messenger, 1996). While the evidence in support of this idea is compelling, the primary requirement to prove the autoimmune nature of AA, to identify a self antigen as the primary target that can initiate the disease mechanism and lead to development of the phenotype, has yet to be proven. Without this evidence, AA can only be described as a putative autoimmune disease. Using a SCID-human model of AA, Gilhar et al. claimed melanogenesis related antigens to be inciting agents for the activation of pathogenic cells involved in AA (Gilhar et al., 2001). Circumstantially, there are several claimed cases of selective pigmented hair loss and white hair survival in AA affected individuals (Plinck et al., 1993; Messenger and Simpson, 1997; Camacho, 1997). Much has been made of this observed phenomenon in defining potential targets of inflammation in AA. However, there are many more unreported examples of AA affected individuals losing both pigmented and non-pigmented hair and in a mouse model of AA white hair can be successfully targeted by inflammatory cells (McElwee et al., 2001a).

While it is quite possible for melanocyte derived antigens to be involved in AA, they need not be the primary agents in precipitating disease onset. Downstream of the disease activation event it is likely that the phenomena of epitope spreading (Chan et al., 1998) results in the targeting of numerous antigenic epitopes from diverse sources within the hair follicles. Logically, one would expect the primary target for follicular inflammation to be a key component in hair fiber production, the targeting of which would lead to growth cessation. While follicular dermal papilla cells may be a candidate source of the primary antigenic target for inflammatory cells (Nutbrown et al., 1996), the most likely source of the primary inciting agent are follicular keratinocytes. Circumstantial evidence in support of this view includes the identification of hair follicle specific autoantibodies which target keratinocyte derived epitopes and that intra-follicular penetrating inflammatory cells in humans and animal models primarily take up residence in keratinocyte comprised root sheath and matrix locations (McElwee et al., 2003b). However, beyond these speculations, little is known about the nature of the antigenic targets on which inflammatory cells focus in AA. It is quite possible that different clinical AA presentations may be associated with different antigenic epitope targeting patterns.

The humoral immune system in AA

Autoantibodies against hair follicle antigen have been identified in both humans and animal models of AA with significantly increased frequency compared to the general population. Tobin et al. demonstrated production of antibodies with heterogeneous targeting of hair follicle structures and similar heterogeneity of morphological targeting has been found in mouse and rat models of AA (McElwee et al., 1996a; Tobin et al., 1997). Trichohyalin and specific keratins have been defined as targets for some of the antibodies (Tobin et al., 2003). The diversity of autoantibody production with no consistent structure targeting observed in serum samples from different patients, suggests autoantibodies are not the dominant factor in AA development. Other evidence also supports this view with time line evaluation studies on a mouse model for AA indicating cellular targeting for the follicle occurs prior to an upregulation in genes associated with antibody production (Carroll et al., 2002). Transfer of serum from AA patients to skin in a SCID-human model also failed to regenerate the disease phenotype (Gilhar et al., 1992). However, this does not invalidate antibody investigation. Autoantibodies in serum from AA patients may hold important clues to the targets for cellular inflammation in AA. Autoantibodies may yet be shown to play a secondary role in the disease pathogenesis. One small study involving the transfer of equine AA-derived antibodies to normal haired mice promoted an increase in telogen state hair follicles, although no apparent development of cellular inflammation was induced and systemic AA did not develop (Tobin et al., 1998). Autoantibodies then may play a secondary role accentuating the chronic disease state but it seems unlikely they are the primary mediators of AA.

15

The cellular immune system in AA

In many autoimmune diseases and animal models of autoimmune disease lymphocytes are identified as the primary disease mediator. Most commonly, CD4$^+$ lymphocytes have been identified as the primary pathogenic cell subset retaining the ability to transfer many autoimmune diseases, but other subsets including CD8$^+$ cells have also been identified as important in disease pathogenesis (eg. Ablamunits et al., 1999; Huseby et al., 2001). The predominantly CD4$^+$ and CD8$^+$ lymphocyte inflammation of hair follicles suggests these cells to be the primary instigators of the disease phenotype in AA. Depleting the inflammatory cell number with immunosuppressive therapies reinforces the general view that these cells hold the key to hair growth inhibition in AA (Freyschmidt-Paul et al., 2001). In rodent models this has been taken a step further with the selective removal of CD4$^+$ or CD8$^+$ cells by injections of monoclonal antibodies. Depletion of one or other lymphocyte population permits hair regrowth, but with replacement of the depleted cell population the AA phenotype redevelops (McElwee et al., 1996b; McElwee et al., 1999b; Carroll et al., 2002).

Recent cell subset transfer studies have further characterized the importance of CD4$^+$ and CD8$^+$ lymphocytes in AA. Human AA-affected, skin-derived cells have been shown to reinduce inflammatory hair loss in xenografts of previously AA affected skin grafted to *scid/scid* mice (Gilhar et al., 1998). Separation of CD4$^+$ and CD8$^+$ cell subsets and their transfer to this model suggested each cell type alone was not capable of reinducing hair loss, but in combination hair loss redeveloped (Gilhar et al., 2002). In C3H/HeJ mice subcutaneous injection of CD8$^+$ cells led to the rapid development of localized hair loss at the site of injection but no further development of hair loss. In contrast, injection of CD4$^+$/CD25$^-$ cells resulted in little localized hair loss but successful transfer of the disease systemically with the development of multiple alopecia patches (McElwee et al., 2005). Thus, it is the CD4$^+$/CD25$^-$ cell population in the C3H/HeJ mouse model that retains the capacity to transfer the systemic AA phenotype to naïve hosts and most likely promotes AA via promotion of APC activity and subsequent stimulation of hair follicle autoreactive CD8$^+$ cells. This pathogenic activity defines the CD4$^+$/CD25$^-$ cell population as a key component of AA and a prime target for the development of therapeutic strategies. CD8$^+$ cells, although apparently the primary effectors of the actual hair loss phenotype, are largely under the control of CD4$^+$/CD25$^-$ cells.

Mechanisms of cellular action on the hair follicle

It seems then that the cellular immune system is the principal promoter of AA. The question remains how might leukocytes act on hair follicles to promote hair loss. Studies so far implicate a combination of mechanisms. Cytotoxicity may be mediated through Fas – Fas ligand (FasL) interaction. The binding of Fas expressed on target cells by FasL on activated lymphocytes leads to apoptosis of the Fas expressing cell. This mechanism of tissue destruction is not MHC restricted and has the potential to damage innocent bystander cells not directly targeted by the pathogenic lymphocyte clones. Fas – FasL signaling is also believed to promote antigen presentation (Siegel et al., 2000). In the C3H/HeJ mouse model for AA, Fas and FasL are significantly differentially expressed in skin infiltrating lymphocytes and Fas is highly expressed on human and mouse dystrophic hair follicle keratinocytes (Bodemer et al., 2000; McElwee et al., 2002a; Freyschmidt-Paul et al., 2003). Histocompatible mice deficient in Fas or FasL are comparatively resistant to the induction of AA. This resistance was in part localized to the skin as Fas and FasL deficient skin transplanted to AA affected mice resisted immune activity and continued to grow hair (Freyschmidt-Paul et al., 2003). The possibility of an autocrine and paracrine action of Fas and FasL within and between hair follicle keratinocytes may add to the action of the inflammatory infiltrate and may explain why FasL deficient hair follicles were also relatively resistant to AA.

Perforin, produced by cytotoxic T cells, is a potent mediator of cell lysis (Russell and Ley, 2002). For perforin induced lysis of target cells to occur, the T cell receptor of an autoreactive cell must ligand with the relevant antigenic peptide presented in conjunction with MHC on the target cell. Whether perforin mediated cell destruction occurs in AA is unknown, but the presence of highly activated CD8+ cells within dystrophic hair follicles and the high expression of MHC molecules on hair follicle keratinocytes circumstantially suggests MHC restricted, perforin mediated, tissue damage could occur. Granzymes, that may gain access to target cells via perforin or induce apoptosis independent of perforin through binding cell surface receptors (Motyka et al., 2000), have been identified as highly expressed in human AA (Bodemer et al., 2000; Carroll et al., 2002). Inducible nitric oxide synthase expression is apparent during mouse AA development which may suggest a role for nitric oxide in disease pathogenesis (McElwee, personal observations).

Lymphocytes need not have close contact with hair follicle keratinocytes to exert an effect. Cytokines such as TNFα may have a negative impact on the survival of hair follicle keratinocytes in AA (Janssen et al., 2003). IFNγ may inhibit cell proliferation and promote keratinocyte expression of MHC molecules that will aid other inflammatory mechanisms (Schroder et al., 2004). Other cytokines may negatively regulate keratinocyte cell proliferation and encourage hair follicles to truncate their growth cycle and enter a telogen resting state (Randall, 2001). Overall, cytokines may be significant modulators of hair follicle disruption.

Disease modulating factors

While the fundamental mechanism of AA is essentially self contained it is likely there are exterior factors that influence the disease course. Thus far various, candidate genetic influences have been identified in human and rodent model AA (described elsewhere). In addition, environmental factors are also probably involved in determining an individual's susceptibility to AA. Influencing factors may be both susceptibility and severity modifiers of AA and act in two ways: They may modify an individual's general susceptibility to a disease activation event. Alternatively, they may be involved in determining the future prognoses for hair loss in terms of extent, hair loss pattern, duration or chronicity of disease, and/or resistance to treatment, once onset of overt hair loss has been initiated.

Recently, using the C3H/HeJ mouse model, IFNγ has been identified as a key player in precipitating onset of hair loss (Freyschmidt-Paul et al., 2006). Injecting IFNγ into mice known to be genetically susceptible to AA brings forward the time at which AA onset develops and increases the frequency of mice expressing the AA while transgenic knockout mice genetically deficient in IFNγ are incapable of developing AA. In the real world, IFNγ expression is increased in response to a variety of insults, particularly infectious agents (Schroder et al., 2004). It is generally accepted that an infectious agent might promote autoimmune disease onset through mimicry of antigenic epitopes (Wucherpfennig, 2001). If an infectious agent expresses antigens that are similar to self antigens found naturally in hair follicles then exposure to the pathogen may elicit a cross reactivity to the hair follicle located antigens. However, the knowledge that IFNγ is involved in disease development suggests that there need not be a specific relationship between pathogen-expressed antigens and hair follicle antigens. Rather, responses to the general "viral load" might play a key role in AA for some (Stewart and Smoller, 1993; Kissler et al., 2001). It is conceivable then that an individual genetically susceptible to AA might experience onset of hair loss subsequent to infectious agent exposure or exposure to any other factor that promotes in an increase in IFNγ. Chronic exposure or cumulative exposure to multiple pathogens may increase the level of susceptibility to disease onset.

Increased levels of IFNγ alone are unlikely to induce AA onset in any one individual. If this were true, AA would be expressed with a much higher frequency within the population than is the case. It is likely that multiple genetic and environmental factors must interact correctly for actual disease onset to occur. Rodent model research has shown that hormones can influence the degree of susceptibility to AA induction. Ovariectomized mice had a relatively reduced rate of AA development compared to estradiol supplemented mice. In contrast mice supplemented with testosterone were fully resistant to AA development compared to gonadectomized mice (McElwee et al., 2001b). Hormonal influence in humans is suggested by old case reports asserting temporary hair growth in AA affected women during the late stages of pregnancy or improvement with onset of menopause (Sabouraud, 1913; Lévy-Franckel, 1925; Walker, 1950). Model research has also shown that increased dietary soy oil content can reduce AA susceptibility (McElwee et al., 2003a). While this is of little practical value in understanding human AA, it demonstrates the potential influence of environmental factors on AA susceptibility.

To protect against inappropriate immune system activation and to calm down activated immune cells after a pathogenic challenge has been cleared, immune regulatory mechanisms are exploited. CD4$^+$/CD25$^+$ cells have been identified as one of probably several lymphocyte regulatory cell subsets that can restrain pathogenic cell activity. CD4$^+$/CD25$^+$ cells are essential for maintaining homeostasis, are able to suppress the induction of autoimmune disease, suppress CD4$^+$/CD25$^-$ cells, and can inhibit the effector function of autoreactive CD8$^+$ cells (Suri-Payer et al., 1998; Gao et al., 1999; Annacker et al., 2001). Little is currently known about immune regulatory mechanisms in human AA. Studies in the skin graft induced AA mouse model have revealed that CD4$^+$/CD25$^+$ cell levels drop significantly on activation of AA and prior to the onset of overt hair loss (Zöller et al., 2002). In contrast, sham grafted mice are able to maintain CD4$^+$/CD25$^+$ cell numbers and quickly recover normal inflammatory cell numbers after injury. This apparent active depression of regulatory cells in AA challenged mice may be a key factor in AA susceptibility. CD4$^+$/CD25$^-$ cells or CD8$^+$ cells from AA affected mice transferred to unaffected mice can induce some form of AA, but if CD4$^+$/CD25$^+$ cells are added to the mixture the disease onset is partially inhibited (McElwee et al., 2005). This indicates the potential importance of regulatory cell failure in AA development. Why regulatory cells fail appropriately and restrain onset of AA is not known but further examination of CD4$^+$/CD25$^+$ cells and other regulatory cells may reveal significant insights into AA susceptibility and development.

There are likely other factors that modulate AA. Stress has been suggested as a potential instigator of autoimmune diseases possibly through glucocorticoid modulation of inflammatory cytokine expression (Elenkov and Chrousos, 2002). Stress has also been postulated as a potential influence on AA development although the evidence is largely circumstantial (Mehlman and Griesemer, 1968; Colon et al., 1991; Liakopoulou et al., 1997; Kavak et al., 2002). Recent studies with the AA mouse model suggest that AA onset is associated with significant changes in the hypothalamic-pituitary-adrenal (HPA) tone and activity centrally and peripherally in the skin and lymph nodes. Exposing AA affected mice to stress further exacerbated changes in AA mouse HPA activity and the mice had a deficit in habituation to repeated restraint stress (McElwee et al., 2009).

AA frequency and severity is apparently associated with a greater frequency of allergies as compared to the general population (Muller and Winkelmann, 1963; Ikeda, 1965; Penders, 1968; De Waard-van der Spek et al., 1989; Weise et al., 1996). Whether there is a direct relationship whereby an allergic response is capable of increasing immune system sensitivity and instability such that AA susceptibility increases, or whether the increased frequency of allergies in AA patients is merely a reflection of genetically determined immune system sensitivity remains to be determined. Other promoters of the immune system in autoimmune diseases may include drugs and toxins (Bigazzi, 1994; Elkayam et al., 1999; Holsapple, 2002). In principle, one or more of these factors may modulate the immune system in AA, but in practice little is known about the effects of environmental stimuli on AA in rodent models or humans.

With time and changes in factors that may influence AA, so the degree of susceptibility to AA will fluctuate. While an individual may have a genetic susceptibility to AA that may be regarded as an unmovable baseline, additional factors may increase or depress overall AA susceptibility. Only if an individual receives multiple signals that cumulatively increase the susceptibility to disease above a threshold level for expression will an episode of AA actually develop. This may also help explain why the presentation of the AA phenotype is so varied. Individuals with chronic extensive AA, versus those with an isolated AA patch, may have a dominant genetic susceptibility to disease and relatively minor environmental modification of this genetic susceptibility. In others who whose AA waxes and wanes, or who present with multiple episodes of AA expression and remission may be more greatly impacted by environmental factors and their changing influence with time.

Disease initiation

We still do not know the disease phenotype precipitating event, but one hypothesis is that AA develops in susceptible individuals due to a failure in hair follicle immunoprotection. Anagen stage hair follicles are regarded as immune privileged sites (Westgate et al., 1991; Paus et al., 1999), but follicle immunoprotection is likely only transient due to the nature of the hair follicle cycle. Research suggests the onset of catagen is associated with an infiltration of immune cells, candidate antigen presenting cells (Parakkal, 1969; Westgate et al.,

1991; Paus, 1996; Eichmüller et al., 1998). Regression of the hair follicle in catagen involves high levels of apoptosis and significant remodeling of the lower transient portion of the hair follicle (Weedon and Strutton, 1981; Lindner et al., 1997). It is possible then that the immune system is constantly exposed to low levels of hair follicle derived antigens as hair follicles cycle through catagen and given the ability of dendritic cells to present apoptosis derived antigens. Autoimmune disease is not regarded as an all or nothing event. Rather, there are degrees of autoreactivity and a threshold level above which overt autoimmune disease is induced (McElwee et al., 2001b; Ludewig et al., 2001). A reflection of this may be the low level of hair follicle specific antibodies found in some humans and rodents in the absence of overt AA (Tobin et al., 1994a; Tobin et al., 1994b; Tobin et al., 1997). If however, catagen regression became disordered and the immune cell infiltrate associated with catagen inappropriately presented antigenic peptides in association with expression of costimulatory molecules, antigen presentation to the immune system might breach the threshold for stimulation of autoreactive cells. In a genetically susceptible individual, resident in a permissible environment, AA might follow.

Summary

Overall, we still cannot claim AA is an autoimmune disease with complete confidence, but all the evidence produced so far points in that direction and provides compelling supporting evidence. Circumstantial evidence from observing the state of humans with AA has been supplemented with indirect, functional evidence from a variety of animal models. In the near future, animal model and human genome screening will likely define loci involved in AA susceptibility and resistance. With further research, the contribution of specific genes to the disease onset may provide much information on the disease pathogenesis.

Therapy

Various methods to treat AA have been described, but for many of them only anecdotal reports exist and the alleged treatment success might be attributed to spontaneous remission. Because of the high rate of spontaneous hair regrowth in AA, the only treatments that can be regarded as evidence-based are those proven to be effective either after exclusion of spontaneous remission by treating every patient on one half of the scalp only or in a double-blind, placebo controlled study including a very large number of patients. Furthermore, studies evaluating a treatment for AA should preferably include patients with AA totalis, AA universalis and extensive patchy AA (> 25% scalp hair loss) persisting longer than 3 months, because these patients have a worse prognosis than patients with limited patchy AA. These patients are also the ones who are most in need of an effective treatment. Any treatment has to be suitable for long-term therapy, because AA is a disease that can persist for many years or even life. Hence, all therapeutic approaches showing severe side-effects are inappropriate for AA in the long run.

Immunosuppressive Treatment

Corticosteroids

Topical, intralesional, and systemic corticosteroids have been used for the treatment of AA with different rates of success and side effects.

Topical corticosteroids

Corticosteroid creams, ointments or lotions are frequently used for the treatment of AA. However, only two placebo-controlled studies fulfilling the criteria of evidence-based medicine reported a treatment response, both using clobetasol propionate 0.05% (Tosti et al., 2003; Tosti et al., 2006). In 9% of patients with patchy AA treated with a clobetasol propionate 0.05% foam hair regrowth > 75% was observed, 20% of patients experienced hair regrowth > 50% (Tosti et al., 2006). However, patients with AA totalis or AA universalis did not respond to treatment with the clobetasol foam. A more effective treatment for patients with AA totalis or AA universalis is the application of clobetasol propionate 0.05% ointment under occlusion. Tosti reported a treatment success of 17.8% in patients with AA totalis and AA universalis when clobetasol propionate 0.05% ointment was applied under occlusion 6 nights a week for 6 months (Tosti et al., 2006). Therefore, topical corticosteroids can only be recommended when clobetasol propionate 0.05% is used and even then it will only be effective in a subgroup of patients with severe AA when occlusive application is used or exclusively in patients with patchy AA, when clobetasol-foam is applied.

15

Intralesional corticosteroids

Intralesional injections of corticosteroid crystal suspensions, primarily triamcinolone acetonide, have been used for the treatment of AA for more than 40 years (Kalkoff and Macher, 1958). Several studies reported hair regrowth at the site of injection in the majority of cases (Kalkoff and Macher, 1958; Orentreich et al., 1960; Porter and Burton, 1971; Fülöp and Vajda, 1971; Abell and Munro, 1973; Frentz, 1977). Most of these studies tried to exclude spontaneous hair regrowth by comparing the injected sites of the scalp with uninjected areas, especially in alopecia totalis. However, in practice it is impossible to treat the whole scalp by intralesional injections of corticosteroids and so this treatment is only indicated in patchy AA with longstanding bald areas. Apart from the sometimes painful procedure of injection, permanent skin atrophy can occur after injection. Taken together, intralesional injection of corticosteroids is a reasonable treatment in selected cases of longstanding small patches of AA, but has potentially significant side effects.

Systemic corticosteroids

Since 1975 several authors have performed pulsed administration of corticosteroids in single doses, given once monthly in order to reduce the side effects of corticosteroids to an acceptable level. Major side effects have not been observed in pulsed administration of corticosteroids to AA patients, side effects that occurred were striae, nausea, flushing, headache, polymenorrhea, fatigue, palpitations, dyspnea, and giddiness. The way pulse therapy was performed varied between the studies; some authors applied the corticosteroids intravenously, using either 500 mg methylprednisolone i.v. for 3 days or 8 mg methylprednisolone / kg body weight on 3 consecutive days at 4-week intervals for at least 3 courses. Other groups applied the corticosteroids orally with a median dose of 5 mg prednisolone / kg body weight once monthly for 3–9 months or 80 mg predonine for 3 consecutive days once every 3 months (reviewed in Freyschmidt-Paul et al., 2001, 2003; Kurosawa et al., 2006; Luggen and Hunziker, 2008; Seiter et al., 2001). Some authors observed cosmetically acceptable hair regrowth in patients treated by pulsed administration of corticosteroids, but their studies were not controlled and the majority of patients responding to treatment had patchy AA, which usually shows a high rate of spontaneous remission. Hence, the observed hair regrowth after treatment may as well be due to spontaneous remission. Moreover, other studies reported a treatment failure after corticosteroid pulse therapy, especially in patients suffering from AA totalis and universalis (reviewed in Freyschmidt-Paul et al., 2001, 2003; Kälin and Hunziker, 2008; Luggen and Hunziker, 2008; Seiter et al., 2001). Therefore, controlled studies are urgently required to prove the efficacy and long-term value of this treatment. In particular, the efficacy in interrupting acute phases of rapid hair loss by pulsed administration of oral corticosteroids should be investigated.

Photochemotherapy (PUVA)

Several studies have been performed on the treatment of AA with PUVA using either oral application of 8-methoxypsoralen (8-MOP) with ultraviolet A radiation (UVA) of the scalp or the whole body, or topical application of 8-MOP and UVA radiation on the scalp, including one study with topical application of psoralen via the PUVA-turban (Larkö and Swanbeck, 1983; Claudy and Gagnaire, 1983; Lassus et al., 1984; Mitchell and Douglass, 1985; Healy and Rogers, 1993; Taylor and Hawk, 1995; Behrens-Williams et al., 2001). Some investigations seemed to show good results (Claudy and Gagnaire, 1983; Lassus et al., 1984; Healy and Rogers, 1993; Taylor and Hawk, 1995; Behrens-Williams et al., 2001, Whitmont and Cooper, 2003), but there were no controls in any of the studies. Moreover, there were a high number of AA recurrences in most of the studies (between 30% and 50% of successfully treated patients) after initial hair regrowth that strongly decreases the efficacy of PUVA treatment for AA (Claudy and Gagnaire, 1983; Lassus et al., 1984; Healy and Rogers, 1993; Taylor and Hawk, 1995). This high number of relapses is most likely due to the fact that regrown hair inhibits the UVA light from reaching the skin. Technical improvements, such as a comb emitting UVA light, have been tried, but so far no results have been reported. Unfortunately, a continuous hair regrowth after the initial response has to be actively maintained for several years in most cases of AA, bearing an increased risk of skin malignancies after long-term PUVA therapy.

308 nm-excimer laser

Using the immunosuppressive properties of the 308 nm-excimer laser, four within-patient controlled studies have been performed recently, that demonstrated a successful treatment of patchy AA in children and adults. Treatment was performed for about 3 months in 24–27 sessions using $0.2–7.6 J/cm^2$ resulting in a cumulative dose varying between 3.9 and $52.6 J/cm^2$. However, the 308 nm-excimer laser was not able to treat AA totalis or AA universalis in these studies (Zakaria et al., 2004; Gundogan et al., 2004; Al-Mutiri, 2007, 2009). Within an observation period of 6 months after treatment about 50% of the successfully treated patients showed a recurrence of hair loss. Therefore, the 308 nm Excimer laser might be a therapeutic option for patchy AA, but further studies are needed to assess the safety and the long-term results of this treatment.

Immunomodulatory treatments

Diphenylcyclopropenone and squaric acid dibutylester

AA has been treated with contact sensitizers for more than 25 years. Dinitrochlorobenzene (DNCB) was the first sensitizer that was used for the treatment of AA (Happle and Echternacht, 1977), but because it has been shown to be mutagenic in the Ames test, it can no longer be used (Happle, 1979, 1985). Today diphenylcyclopropenone (DCP) or squaric acid dibutylester (SADBE), that are not mutagenic in the Ames test, are widely used in European states and in Canada.

15

Treatment protocol

Treatment with contact sensitizers is preceded by sensitization of the patient with 2% DCP solution on a small area of the scalp. Two weeks later, treatment is initiated by application of a 0.001% DCP solution, followed by weekly application of increasing concentrations of DCP until a mild eczematous reaction is obtained. In this way, an appropriate eliciting concentration of DCP for each patient is identified. This concentration has to be applied once a week to induce a mild eczematous reaction that is characterized by itching and erythema, without blistering or oozing. SADBE is used in those patients who become tolerant to DCP. It is applied in the same way and shows a similar rate of response.

Initial hair regrowth is usually visible after 8–12 weeks. Treatment has to be continued once weekly until complete hair regrowth is obtained. Treatment intervals are then decreased and eventually treatment may be discontinued. However, if a relapse occurs after discontinuation of therapy, treatment can be restarted immediately to stop further progression of AA and induce renewed hair growth. Treatment should initially always be applied

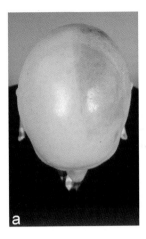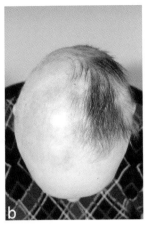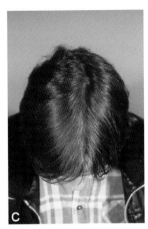

Fig. 6. Treatment of alopecia areata with a contact sensitizer. Unilateral contact dermatitis after application of a contact sensitizer on the left side of the scalp (a); unilateral hair growth on the treated side (b); complete hair growth after treatment of boths sides (c).

on one half of the scalp and the other side left untreated to exclude a spontaneous hair regrowth coincidental to treatment initiation. Treatment is continued on both sides only after the treated side has shown a response in the form of better hair growth on the treated side (Fig. 6).

Side effects

A mild eczematous reaction and enlargement of retroauricular lymph nodes are desired reactions and inherent to treatment. They are usually well tolerated if the patients are informed that these reactions are desirable for the therapeutic effect. Undesired side effects are noted in 2–5% of patients (Hoffmann and Happle, 1996). Vesicular or bullous reactions sometimes occur at the beginning of treatment before the individual appropriate concentration has been determined. Dissemination of allergic contact dermatitis, urticarial or erythema multiforme-like reactions may occur (Perret et al., 1990) but can be successfully treated with topical corticosteroids. Pigmentary disturbances such as postinflammatory hyperpigmentation with spotty hypopigmentation ("dyschromia in confetti") have been observed, especially in patients with dark skin, but resolved within 1 year after discontinuation of treatment in most cases (Hoffmann and Happle, 1996; van der Steen and Happle, 1992). Apart from these acute and subacute side effects, no long-term side effects have been reported after 20 years of DCP (23 years of SADBE) treatment worldwide of about 10,000 patients, including children. However, it should be borne in mind that DCP and SADBE are not approved therapeutic substances.

Clinical trials

More than 25 studies have been performed to test the efficacy of AA treatment with a contact sensitizer. The most significant controlled studies are listed in Table 2. In contrast to corticosteroid and PUVA treatment studies, the majority of contact sensitizer treatment studies were controlled, most of them using the untreated side of the scalp as a control. When comparing the rates of response obtained in various therapeutic modalities, one should bear in mind that spontaneous regrowth is excluded in these controlled, within-patient studies, but not in the uncontrolled ones. The response rate of treatment with a contact sensitizer varies between 29% and 78% (see Table 2). The differences may be explained in part by the different extent and duration of AA prior to treatment in the patients of each study, and in part by differences in the method of treatment. However, the median response rate of all studies is 49%, rendering contact sensitizers an effective therapeutic tool for AA.

Mode of action

The mode of action of the treatment with contact sensitizers is so far poorly understood. It has been shown that treatment with a contact sensitizer changes the composition and localization of the perifollicular infiltrate in humans and in the C3H / HeJ mouse-model for AA (Happle et al., 1986; Freyschmidt-Paul et al., 1999). In both, mice and men, the localization of the inflammatory infiltrate shows a shift from peribulbar before treatment to the upper dermis after therapy. However, in human AA the CD4:CD8 ratio changes from 4:1 before to 1:1 after therapy, while in mice successful treatment with a contact sensitizer is associated with an increase in the number of $CD4^+$ cells and a decrease in the number of $CD8^+$ cells. Hoffmann et al. demonstrated that after treatment with a contact sensitizer the mRNA-expression of IFN-γ is reduced while the expression of IL-10 is increased (Hoffmann et al., 1994). Whether this is due to a Th1-Th2 shift or whether it is caused by the introduction of regulatory T-cells with a type 2 cytokine profile is the object of current investigations. Immunohistochemical studies furthermore have shown in humans and in the C3H / HeJ mouse-model of AA, that treatment with a contact sensitizer reduces the aberrant expression of MHC-I and MHC-II molecules on the lower hair follicle epithelium (Bröcker et al., 1987; Freyschmidt-Paul et al., 1999). From these data it can be concluded that treatment with a contact sensitizer restores the immune priviledge of the lower hair follicle epithelium.

Other treatments

Irritant contact dermatitis – anthralin

While treatment of AA with an allergic contact dermatitis has been proven to be effective, treatment of AA with an irritant contact dermatitis has never been shown to be successful in a controlled study. In a half-side controlled study, using 0.1% anthralin that resulted in a mild irritant contact dermatitis, no difference between treated and untreated side was

Table 2. Treatment of alopecia areata with contact sensitizers, controlled studies including patients with severe, longstanding disease

Reference	Contact Sensitizer	Clinical form of AA (number of patients)			Controlled study	Number of patients	Cosmetically acceptable hair regrowth
		Patchy AA	AA totalis	AA universalis			
Happle et al., 1983	DCP	5	22	0	Yes (ULT)	27	68%
Happle et al., 1984	DCP	8	37	0	Yes (ULT)	45	58%
Ochsendorf et al., 1988	DCP	18	8	1	Yes (ULT)	27	37%
Macdonald Hull and Norris, 1988	DCP	8	20	0	Yes (ULT)	28	29%
Monk, 1989	DCP	0		14	Yes (ULT)	14	43%
Steen van der et al., 1991	DCP	78	32	29	Yes (ULT)	139	50.4%
Macdonald Hull et al., 1991	DCP	4	8	0	Yes (ULT)	12 children	33%
Macdonald Hull et al., 1991	DCP	33	45	0	Yes (ULT)	78	55%
Hoting and Boehm, 1992	DCP	11	20	14	Yes (ULT)	45	51%
Gordon et al., 1996	DCP	12	36	0	Yes (ULT)	48	38%
Schuttelaar et al., 1996	DCP	10	16	0	Yes (ULT)	26 children	32%
Weise et al., 1996	DCP	43	22	40	Yes (ULT)	105	48%
Cotellessa et al., 2001	DCP	14	42	0	Yes (ULT)	56	48%
Wiseman et al., 2001	DCP	113	35	0	Yes (ULT)	148	77.9%
Avgerinou et al., 2007	DCP	48	6		Yes (ULT)	54	39%
Happle et al., 1980	SADBE	26	27	0	Yes (ULT)	53	70%
Case et al., 1984	SADBE	11		10	Yes (ULT)	21	52%
Caserio 1987	SADBE	2	5	7	Yes (ULT)	14	29%
Micali et al., 1996	SADBE	129	8	0	Yes (ULT)	137	64%

ULT, unilateral treatment, untreated side serves as control

observed (Nelson and Spielvogel, 1985). Therefore, anthralin cannot be recommended for the treatment of AA.

Minoxidil

Because the antihypertensive agent minoxidil causes hypertrichosis as a side-effect, Weiss et al. attempted to use it as a treatment for various forms of hair loss, including alopecia areata (Weiss et al., 1984). But all studies that claim successful treatment of AA with minoxidil did not fulfill the criteria of evidence based treatment of AA (Weiss et al., 1984; Fiedler-Weiss et al., 1986; Price, 1987a, b; Ranchoff et al., 1989). Six other placebo-controlled studies performed by various groups did not show a statistically significant difference between the hair growth of patients treated with the placebo or with minoxidil (Frentz, 1984; Maitland et al., 1984; Vanderveen et al., 1984; White and Friedmann, 1985; Vestey and Savin, 1986; Fransway and Muller, 1988). In three of these studies cosmetically acceptable hair regrowth was not even observed in any patient (Vanderveen et al., 1984; White and Friedmann, 1985; Fransway and Muller, 1988). In summary, minoxidil is not useful in the treatment of AA.

Biologics

Based on the knowledge that AA is a T-cell mediated autoimmune disease, various biologicals which have been proven to be effective in psoriasis-therapy also have been tried to treat AA. However, neither TNF-α inhibitors like etanercept or infliximab nor the LFA-3 inhibitor alefacept were shown to be effective in treating AA (Price et al., 2006; Strober et al., 2009). It seems that TNF-α inhibitors may actually worsen the course of the disease (Eggefagh et al., 2004; Hernandez et al., 2009).

15

Summary

Alopecia areata is regarded as a T-cell mediated autoimmune disease that is directed against a so far unknown autoantigen of the hair follicle. There is a genetic predisposition to develop AA, whereas environmental triggers have so far not been identified. The diagnosis can be established by characteristic clinical features of AA including its severe forms AA totalis and AA universalis. Nail changes may help confirm the diagnosis. In some cases a histopathological examination may be necessary, whereas other laboratory investigations are unnecessary. Because of the high rate of spontaneous remission, the efficacy of a rational treatment for AA has to be proven in controlled studies. An ideal treatment should be highly effective but associated with only minor side effects. According to the rules of evidence-based medicine, treatment with a contact sensitizer is at present the most effective treatment of AA showing only mild side effects. However, it is a time-consuming and in some cases ineffective therapeutic approach, which is why it is necessary to develop new, more specific forms of treatment.

References

Abell E, Munro DD (1973) Intralesional treatment of alopecia areata with triamcinolone acetonide by jet injector. Br J Dermatol 88:55–9

Ablamunits V, Elias D, Cohen IR (1999) The pathogenicity of islet-infiltrating lymphocytes in the non-obese diabetic (NOD) mouse. Clin Exp Immunol 115:260–7

Alkhalifah A, Alsantali A, Wang E, McElwee KJ, Shapiro J (2010) Alopecia areata update: part I. Clinical picture, histopathology, and pathogenesis. J Am Acad Dermatol 62:177–88

Al-Mutiri N (2007) 308-nm excimer laser for the treatment of alopecia areata. Dermatologic surgery 33:1483–86

Al-Mutiri N (2009) 308-nm excimer laser for the treatment of alopecia areata in children. Pediatric Dermatol 26:547–550

Alsaleh QA, Nanda A, al-Hasawi F, el-Kashlan M (1995) Concurrent appearance of alopecia areata in siblings. Pediatr Dermatol 12:285–6

Anderson I (1950) Alopecia areata: A clinical study. Br Med J 2:1250–2

Andrade M de, Jackow CM, Dahm N, Hordinsky M, Reveille JD, Duvic M (1999) Alopecia areata in families: Association with the HLA locus. J Invest Dermatol Symp Proc 4:220–3

Annacker O, Pimenta-Araujo R, Burlen-Defranoux O, Barbosa TC, Cumano A, Bandeira A (2001) CD25+ CD4+ T cells regulate the expansion of peripheral CD4 T cells through the production of IL-10. J Immunol 166:3008–18

Averbakh EV, Pospelov LE (1986) HLA antigens in patients with alopecia areata. *Vestn* Dermatol Venerol 1:24–6

Avgerinou G, Gregoriou S, Rigopoulos D, Stratigos A, Kalogeromitros D, Katsambas A (2008) Alopecia areata: topical immunotherapy treatment with diphencyprone. JEADV 22:320–323

Barber HW (1921) Alopecia areata. Br J Dermatol and Syph 33:1–14

Bastos Araujo A, Poiares Baptista A (1967) Algunas consideracions sobre 300 casos de pelada. Trabalhos da Sociedad Portugesa de Dermatologia e Venereologia 25:135–41

Behrens-Williams S, Leiter U, Schiener R, Weidmann M, Peter RU, Kerscher M (2001) The PUVA-turban as a new option of applying a dilute psoralen solution selectively to the scalp of patients with alopecia areata. J Am Acad Dermatol 44:248–252

Betterle C, Greggio NA, Volpato M (1998) Clinical review 93 Autoimmune polyglandular syndrome type 1. J Clin Endocrinol Metab 83:1049–55

Bigazzi PE (1994) Autoimmunity and heavy metals. Lupus 3:449–53

Bodemer C, Peuchmaur M, Fraitaig S, Chatenoud L, Brousse N, De Prost Y (2000) Role of cytotoxic T cells in chronic alopecia areata. J Invest Dermatol 114:112–6

Bonjean M, Prime A, Avon P. Pelade chez deux jumeges homozygotes (sic) (1968) Lyon Med 219:1852–3

Bröcker EB, Echternacht-Happle K, Hamm H, Happle R (1987) Abnormal expression of class I and class II major histocompatibility antigens in alopecia areata: Modulation by topical immunotherapy. J Invest Dermatol 88:564–8

Brown WH (1929) The aetiology of alopecia areata and its relationship to vitiligo and possibly scleroderma. Br J Dermatol and Syph 41:299–323

Burton JL, Shuster S (1975) Large doses of glucocorticoid in the treatment of alopecia areata. Acta Derm Venereol (Stockh) 55:493–6

Camacho F Anagenic and telogenic effluvia (1997) In: Trichology: Diseases of the pilosebaceous follicle, Camacho F, Montagna W, eds.; Aula Medica Group: Madrid pp. 387–96

Carroll JM, McElwee KJ, E King L, Byrne MC, Sundberg JP (2002) Gene array profiling and immunomodulation studies define a cell-mediated immune response underlying the pathogenesis of alopecia areata in a mouse model and humans. J Invest Dermatol 119:392–402

Carter DM, Jegasothy BV (1976) Alopecia areata and Down syndrome. Arch Dermatol 112:1397–9

Caserio RJ (1987) Treatment of alopecia areata with squaric acid dibutylester. Arch Dermatol 123:1036–41

Chan LS, Vanderlugt CJ, Hashimoto T, Nishikawa T, Zone JJ, Black MM, Wojnarowska F, Stevens SR, Chen M, Fairley JA, Woodley DT, Miller SD, Gordon KB (1998) Epitope spreading: lessons from autoimmune skin diseases. J Invest Dermatol 110:103–9

Claudy AL, Gagnaire D (1983) PUVA treatment of alopecia areata. Arch Dermatol 119:975–8

Cole GW, Herzlinger D (1984) Alopecia universalis in identical twins. Int J Dermatol 23:283

Colombe BW, Price VH, Khoury EL, Garovoy MR, Lou CD (1995) HLA class II antigen associations help define two types of alopecia areata. J Am Acad Dermatol 33:757–64

Colombe BW, Lou CD, Price VH (1999) The genetic basis of alopecia areata: HLA associations with patchy alopecia areata versus alopecia totalis and alopecia universalis. J Invest Dermatol Symp Proc 4:216–9

Colon EA, Popkin MK, Callies AL, Dessert NJ, Hordinsky MK (1991) Lifetime prevalence of psychiatric disorders in patients with alopecia areata. Compr Psychiatry 32:245–51

Cork MJ, Crane AM, Duff GW (1996) Genetic control of cytokines: Cytokine gene polymorphisms in alopecia areata. Dermatol Clin 14:671–8

Cotellessa C, Peris K, Caracciolo E, Mordenti C, Chimenti S (2001) The use of topical diphenylcyclopropenone for the treatment of extensive alopecia areata. J Am Acad Dermatol 44:73–6

Cunliffe WJ, Hall R, Stevenson CJ, Weightman D (1969) Alopecia areata, thyroid disease and autoimmunity. Br J Dermatol 81:877–81

De Waard-van der Spek FB, Oranje AP, De Raeymaecker DM, Peereboom-Wynia JD (1989) Juvenile versus maturity-onset al.opecia areata – a comparative retrospective clinical study. Clin Exp Dermatol 14:429–33

De Weert J, Temmerman L, Kint A (1984) Alopecia areata: A clinical study. Dermatologica 168:224–9

Dillaha CJ, Rothman S (1952) Therapeutic experiments in alopecia areata with orally administered cortisone. J Am Med Ass 150:546–50

Du Vivier A, Munro DD (1975) Alopecia areata, autoimmunity, and Down's syndrome. Br Med J I:191–2

Duvic M, Hordinsky MK, Fiedler VC, O'Brien WR, Young R, Reveille JD (1991) HLA-D locus associations in alopecia areata. Arch Dermatol 127:64–8

Duvic M, Welsh EA, Jackow C, Papadopoulos E, Reveille JD, Amos C (1995) Analysis of HLA-D locus alleles in alopecia areata patients and families. J Invest Dermatol 104(suppl):5S–6S

Eggefagh L, Neorost S, Mirmirani P (2004) Alopecia areata in a patient using infliximab: new insights into the role of tumor necrosis factor on human hair follicle. Arch Dermatol 140:1012

Eichmüller S, van der Veen C, Moll I, Hermes B, Hofmann U, Muller-Rover S, Paus R (1998) Clusters of perifollicular macrophages in normal murine skin: physiological degeneration of selected hair follicles by programmed organ deletion. J Histochem Cytochem 46:361–70

Elenkov IJ, Chrousos GP (2002) Stress hormones, proinflammatory and antiinflammatory cytokines, and autoimmunity. Ann N Y Acad Sci 966:290–303

Elkayam O, Yaron M, Caspi D (1999) Minocycline-induced autoimmune syndromes: an overview. Semin Arthritis Rheum 28:392–7

Fiedler-Weiss VC, West DP, Buys CM, Rumsfield JA (1986) Topical minoxidil dose-response effect in alopecia areata. Arch Dermatol 122:180–82

Finnish-German APECED Consortium (1997) An autoimmune disease, APECED, caused by mutations in a novel gene featuring two PHD-type zinc-finger domains. Nature Genet 17:399–403

Fransway AF, Muller SA (1988) 3 percent topical minoxidil compared with placebo for the treatment of chronic severe alopecia areata. Cutis 41:431–435

Frentz G (1977) Topical treatment of extended alopecia. Dermatologica 155:147–154

15

Frentz G (1985) Topical minoxidil for extended areate alopecia. Acta Derm Venereol 65:172–175
Frentz G, Thomsen K, Jakobsen BK, Svejgaard A (1986) HLA-DR4 in alopecia areata. J Am Acad Dermatol 14:129–30
Freyschmidt-Paul P, Sundberg JP, Happle R, McElwee KJ, Metz S, Boggess D, Hoffmann R (1999) Successful treatment of alopecia areata-like hair loss with the contact sensitizer squaric acid dibutylester (SADBE) in C3H/HeJ mice. J Invest Dermatol 113:61–8
Freyschmidt-Paul P, Hoffmann R, Levine E, Sundberg JP, Happle R, McElwee KJ (2001) Current and potential agents for the treatment of alopecia areata. Curr Pharm Des 7:213–30
Freyschmidt-Paul P, Happle R, McElwee KJ, Hoffmann R (2003) Alopecia areata: treatment today and potential treatments of tomorrow. J Invest Dermatol Symp Proc 8:12–17
Freyschmidt-Paul P, McElwee KJ, Botchkarev V, Kissling S, Wenzel E, Sundberg JP, Happle R, Hoffmann R (2003) Fas-deficient C3.MRL-Tnfrsf6(lpr) mice and Fas ligand-deficient C3H/HeJ-Tnfsf6(gld) mice are relatively resistant to the induction of alopecia areata by grafting of alopecia areata-affected skin from C3H/HeJ mice. J Investig Dermatol Symp Proc 8:104–8
Freyschmidt-Paul P, McElwee KJ, Hoffmann R, Sundberg JP, Vitacolonna M, Kissling S, Zöller M (2006) Interferon-gamma-deficient mice are resistant to the development of alopecia areata. Br J Dermatol 155:515–21
Friedli A, Labarthe MP, Engelhardt E, Feldman R, Salomon D, Saurat JH (1998) Pulse methyprednisolone therapy for severe alopecia areata: an open prospective study of 45 patients. J Am Acad Deramtol 39:597–602
Friedmann PS (1981) Alopecia areata and autoimmunity. Br J Dermatol 105:153–157
Friedman PS (1985) Clinical and immunologic association of alopecia areata. Semin Dermatol 4:9–15
Fülöp E, Vajda Z (1971) Experimentelle Untersuchungen über die therapeutische und schädigende Wirkung der intrafokalen Steroidbehandlung. Dermatol Monatsschr 157:269–77
Galbraith GM, Thiers BH, Pandey JP (1984) Gm allotype associated resistance and susceptibility to alopecia areata. Clin Exp Immunol 56:149–52
Galbraith GM, Pandey JP (1989) Km1 allotype association with one subgroup of alopecia areata. Am J Hum Genet 44:426–8
Galbraith GM, Palesch Y, Gore EA, Pandey JP (1999) Contribution of interleukin 1beta and KM loci to alopecia areata. Hum Hered 49:85–9
Galbraith GM, Pandey JP (1995) Tumor necrosis factor alpha (TNF-alpha) gene polymorphism in alopecia areata. Hum Genet 96:433–6
Gao Q, Rouse TM, Kazmerzak K, Field EH (1999) CD4+CD25+ cells regulate CD8 cell anergy in neonatal tolerant mice. Transplant 68:1891–7
Gilhar A, Pillar T, Assay B, David M (1992) Failure of passive transfer of serum from patients with alopecia areata and alopecia universalis to inhibit hair growth in transplants of human scalp skin grafted on to nude mice. Br J Dermatol 126:166–71
Gilhar A, Ullmann Y, Berkutzki T, Assy B, Kalish RS (1998) Autoimmune hair loss (alopecia areata) transferred by T lymphocytes to human scalp explants on SCID mice. J Clin Invest 101:62–7
Gilhar A, Landau M, Assy B, Shalaginov R, Serafimovich S, Kalish RS (2001) Melanocyte-associated T cell epitopes can function as autoantigens for transfer of alopecia areata to human scalp explants on Prkdc(scid) mice. J Invest Dermatol 117:1357–62
Gilhar A, Landau M, Assy B, Shalaginov R, Serafimovich S, Kalish RS (2002) Mediation of alopecia areata by cooperation between CD4+ and CD8+ T lymphocytes: transfer to human scalp explants on Prkdc(scid) mice. Arch Dermatol 138:916–22
Gip L, Lodin A, Molin L (1969) Alopecia areata: A follow-up investigation of outpatient material. Acta Derm Venereol 49:180–8
Goldshtein LM, Chipizhenko VA (1978) Familial alopecia areata. Vestn Dermatol Venerol 10:36–8

Gollinck H, Orfanos CE (1990) Alopecia areata: pathogenesis and clinical picture. In: Orfanos CE, Happle R, eds. Hair and Hair Diseases. Berlin: Springer-Verlag, 529–69

Gordon PM, Aldridge RD, McVittie E, Hunter JAA (1996) Topical diphencyprone for alopecia areata: evaluation of 48 cases after 30 months' follow up. Br J Dermatol 134:869–71

Gundogan C, Greve B, Raulin C (2004) Treatment of alopecia areata with the 308-nm xenon chloride excimer laser: case report of two successful treatments with the excimer laser. Lasers Surg Med 34:86–90

Hacham-Zadeh S, Brautbar C, Cohen C, Cohen T (1981) HLA and alopecia areata in Jerusalem. Tissue Antigens 18:71–4

Happle R, Echternacht K (1977) Induction of hair growth in alopecia areata with D.N.C.B. Lancet 2:1002–3

Happle R (1979) Hinweis zur DNCB-Therapie bei Alopecia areata. Hautarzt 30:556

Happle R, Kalveram KJ, Büchner U, Echternacht-Happle K, Göggelmann W, Summer KH (1980) Contact allergy as a therapeutic tool for alopecia areata: application of squaric acid dibutylester. Dermatologica 161:289–97

Happle R, Hausen BM, Wiesner-Menzel L (1983) Diphencyprone in the treatment of alopecia areata. Acta Derm Venereol (Stockh) 63:49–52

Happle R, Perret C, Wiesner-Menzel L (1984) Treatment of alopecia areata with diphencyprone induces hair regrowth and affects the composition of peribulbar infiltrates. In Immunodermatology MacDonald, DM Ed.; Butterworth: London pp. 279–86

Happle R (1985) The potential hazards of dinitrochlorobenzene. Arch Dermatol 121:330–331

Happle R, Klein HM, Macher E (1986) Topical immunotherapy changes the composition of the peribulbar infiltrate in alopecia areata. Arch Dermatol Res 278:214–8

Healy E, Rogers S (1993) PUVA treatment for alopecia areata: does it work? A retrospective review of 102 cases. Br J Dermatol 129:42–4

Helm F, Milgrom H (1970) Can scalp hair suddenly turn white? A case of canities subita. Arch Dermatol 102:102–3

Hendren S (1949) Identical alopecia areata in identical twins. Arch Dermatol 60:793–5

Hernandez MV, Nogues S, Ruiz-Esquide V, Alsina M, Canetti JD, Sanmarti R (2009) Development of alopecia areata after biological therapy with TNF-α blockers: description of a case and review of the literature. Clin Exp Rheumatol 27:892–3

Hoffmann R, Happle R (1999) Alopecia areata. 1: Clinical aspects, etiology, pathogenesis. Hautarzt 50: W222–31

Hoffmann R, Wenzel E, Huth A, van der Steen P, Schäufele M, Henninger HP, Happle R (1994) Cytokine mRNA levels in Alopecia areata before and after treatment with the contact allergen diphenylcyclopropenone. J Invest Dermatol 103:530–3

Hoffmann R, Happle R (1996) Topical immunotherapy in alopecai areata: what; how; and why? Dermatol Clin 14:739–44

Holsapple MP (2002) Autoimmunity by pesticides: a critical review of the state of the science. Toxicol Lett 127:101–9

Hordinsky MK, Hallgren H, Nelson D, Filipovich AH (1984) Familial alopecia areata. HLA antigens and autoantibody formation in an American family. Arch Dermatol 120:464–8

Hoting E, Boehm A (1992) Therapy of alopecia areata with diphencyprone. Br J Dermatol 127:625–9

Huseby ES, Liggitt D, Brabb T, Schnabel B, Ohlen C, Goverman J (2001) A pathogenic role for myelin-specific CD8(+) T cells in a model for multiple sclerosis. J Exp Med 194:669–76

Ikeda T (1965) A new classification of alopecia areata. Dermatologica 131:421–45

Jansen BJ, van Ruissen F, Cerneus S, Cloin W, Bergers M, van Erp PE, Schalkwijk J (2003) Tumor necrosis factor related apoptosis inducing ligand triggers apoptosis in dividing but not in differentiating human epidermal keratinocytes. J Invest Dermatol 121:1433–9

Kälin U, Hunziker T (2008) Letter to the editor. JDDG 6:895

15

Kalkoff KW, Macher E (1958) Über das Nachwachsen der Haare bei der Alopecia areata und maligna nach intracutaner Hydrocortisoninjektion. Hautarzt 9:441–51

Kasumagic-Halilovic E, Prohic A (2009) Nail changes in alopecia areata: frequency and clinical presentation. J Eur Acad Dermatol Venereol 23:240–1

Kavak A, Yesildal N, Parlak AH (2002) Effect of two consecutive earthquakes on outbreaks of alopecia areata. J Dermatol 29:414–8

Kianto U, Reunala T, Karvonen J, Lassus A, Tiilikainen A (1977) HLA-B12 in alopecia areata. Arch Dermatol 113:1716

Kissler S, Anderton SM, Wraith DC (2001) Antigen-presenting cell activation: a link between infection and autoimmunity? J Autoimmun 16:303–8

Kuntz BM, Selzle D, Braun-Falco O (1977) HLA antigens in alopecia areata. Arch Dermatol 113:1717

Kurosawa M, Nakagawa S, Mizuashi M, Sasaki Y, Kawamura M, Saito M, Aiba S (2006) A comparison of the efficacy, relapse rate and side effects among three modalities of systemic corticosteroid therapy for alopecia areata. Dermatology 212:361–5

Kurtev A, Iliev E (2005) Thyroid autoimmunity in children and adolescents with alopecia areata. Int J Dermatol 44:457–61

Larkö O, Swanbeck G (1983) PUVA treatment for alopecia totalis. Acta Derm Venereol (Stockh) 63:546–9

Larsson M, Fonteneau JF, Bhardwaj N (2001) Dendritic cells resurrect antigens from dead cells. Trends Immunol 22:141–8

Lassus A, Eskelinen A, Johansson E (1984) Treatment of alopecia areata with three different PUVA modalities. Photodermatology 1:141–4

Lévy-Franckel A, Juster E La pelade (1925) J de Medecine de Paris 44:631–5

Liakopoulou M, Alifieraki T, Katideniou A, Kakourou T, Tselalidou E, Tsiantis J, Stratigos J (1997) Children with alopecia areata: psychiatric symptomatology and life events. J Am Acad Child Adolesc Psychiatry 36:678–84

Lindner G, Botchkarev VA, Botchkareva NV, Ling G, van der Veen C, Paus R (1997) Analysis of apoptosis during hair follicle regression (catagen). Am J Pathol 151:1601–17

Ludewig B, Junt T, Hengartner H, Zinkernagel RM (2001) Dendritic cells in autoimmune diseases. Curr Opin Immunol 13:657–62

Luggen P, Hunziker T (2008) High-dose intravenous corticosteroid pulse therapy in alopecia areata: Own experience compared with the literature. JDDG 6:375–8

Lutz G, Bauer R (1988) Autoimmunity in alopecia areata: An assessment in 100 patients. Hautarzt 39:5–11

Macdonald Hull S, Cunliffe WJ (1991) Successful treatment of alopecia areata using the contact allergen diphencyprone. Br J Dermatol 124:212–3

Macdonald Hull S, Norris JF (1988) Diphencyprone in the treatment of long-standing alopecia areata. Br J Dermatol 119:367–74

Macdonald Hull S, Pepall L, Cunliffe WJ (1991) Alopecia areata in children: response to treatment with diphencyprone. Br J Dermatol 125:164–8

Main RA, Robbie RB, Gray ES, Donald D, Horne CH (1975) Smooth muscle antibodies and alopecia areata. Br J Dermatol 92:389–93

Maitland JM, Alridge RD, Main RA, White MI, Ormerod AD (1984) Topical minoxidil in the treatment of alopecia areata. Br Med J 288:794

McDonagh AJ, Messenger AG (1996) The pathogenesis of alopecia areata. Dermatol Clin 14:661–70

McElwee KJ, Pickett P, Oliver RF (1996a) The DEBR rat, alopecia areata and autoantibodies to the hair follicle. Br J Dermatol 134:55–63

McElwee KJ, Spiers EM, Oliver RF (1996b) In vivo depletion of CD8+ T cells restores hair growth in the DEBR model for alopecia areata. Br J Dermatol 135:211–7

McElwee KJ, Boggess D, King LE Jr, Sundberg JP (1998a) Experimental induction of alopecia areata-like hair loss in C3H/HeJ mice using full-thickness skin grafts. J Invest Dermatol 111:797–803

McElwee KJ, Boggess D, Olivry T, Oliver RF, Whiting D, Tobin DJ, Bystryn JC, King LE Jr, Sundberg JP (1998b) Comparison of alopecia areata in human and nonhuman mammalian species. Pathobiology 66:90–107

McElwee KJ, Spiers EM, Oliver RF (1999b) Partial restoration of hair growth in the DEBR model for Alopecia areata after in vivo depletion of CD4+ T cells. Br J Dermatol 140:432–7

McElwee KJ, Tobin DJ, Bystryn JC, King LE Jr, Sundberg JP (1999c) Alopecia areata: An autoimmune disease? Exp Dermatol 8:371–9

McElwee K, Freyschmidt-Paul P, Ziegler A, Happle R, Hoffmann R (2001a) Genetic susceptibility and severity of alopecia areata in human and animal models. Eur J Dermatol 11:11–6

McElwee KJ, Silva K, Beamer WG, King LE Jr, Sundberg JP (2001b) Melanocyte and gonad activity as potential severity modifying factors in C3H/HeJ mouse alopecia areata. Exp Dermatol 10:420–429

McElwee KJ, Hoffmann R (2002a) Alopecia areata – animal models. Clin Exp Dermatol 27:414–21

McElwee KJ, Hoffmann R, Freyschmidt-Paul P, Wenzel E, Kissling S, Sundberg JP, Zöller M (2002b) Resistance to alopecia areata in C3H/HeJ mice is associated with increased expression of regulatory cytokines and a failure to recruit CD4⁺ and CD8⁺ cells. J Invest Dermatol 119:1426–33

McElwee KJ, Niiyama S, Freyschmidt-Paul P, Wenzel E, Kissling S, Sundberg JP, Hoffmann R (2003a) Dietary soy oil content and soy-derived phytoestrogen genistein increase resistance to alopecia areata onset in C3H/HeJ mice. Exp Dermatol 12:30–6

McElwee KJ, Silva K, Boggess D, Bechtold L, King LE Jr, Sundberg JP (2003b) Alopecia areata in C3H/HeJ mice involves leukocyte-mediated root sheath disruption in advance of overt hair loss. Vet Pathol 40:643–50

McElwee KJ, Freyschmidt-Paul P, Hoffmann R, Kissling S, Hummel S, Vitacolonna M, Zöller M (2005) Transfer of CD8+ cells induce localized hair loss while CD4+/CD25- cells promote systemic alopecia areata and CD4+/CD25+ cells blockade disease onset in the C3H/HeJ mouse model. J Invest Dermatol 124:947–57

Mehlman RD, Griesemer RD (1968) Alopecia areata in the very young. Am J Psychiatry 125:605–14

Messenger AG, Bleehen SS (1985) Expression of HLA-DR by anagen hair follicles in alopecia areata. J Invest Dermatol 85:569–72

Messenger AG, Simpson NB (1997) Alopecia areata. In: Diseases of the hair and scalp. Dawber R, ed.; Blackwell Science Oxford pp. 338–69

Micali G, Cicero RL, Nasca MR, Sapuppo A (1996) Treatment of alopecia areata with squaric acid dibutylester. Int J Dermatol 35:52–6

Michie HJ, Jahoda CA, Oliver RF, Johnson BE (1991) The DEBR rat: An animal model of human alopecia areata. Br J Dermatol 125:94–100

Milgraum SS, Mitchell AJ, Bacon GE, Rasmussen JE (1987) Alopecia areata, endocrine function, and autoantibodies in patients 16 years of age or younger. J Am Acad Dermatol 17:57–61

Mitchell AJ, Douglass MC (1985) Topical photochemotherapy for alopecia areata. J Am Acad Dermatol 12:644–9

Monk B (1989) Induction of hair growth in alopecia totalis with diphencyprone sensitization: Clin Exp Dermtol 14:154–7

Morling N, Frentz G, Fugger L, Georgsen J, Jakobsen B, Odum N, Svejgaard A (1991) DNA polymorphism of HLA class II genes in alopecia areata. Dis Markers 9:35–42

Motyka B, Korbutt G, Pinkoski MJ, Heibein JA, Caputo A, Hobman M, Barry M, Shostak I, Sawchuk T, Holmes CF, Gauldie J, Bleackley RC (2000) Mannose 6-phosphate/insulin-like growth factor II receptor is a death receptor for granzyme B during cytotoxic T cell-induced apoptosis. Cell 103:491–500

15

Muller SA, Winkelmann RK (1963) Alopecia areata: An evaluation of 736 patients. Arch Dermatol 88:290–7

Nelson DA, Spielvogel RL (1985) Anthralin therapy fo alopecia areata. Int J Dermatol 24:606–7

Nutbrown M, MacDonald Hull SP, Baker TG, Cunliffe WJ, Randall VA (1996) Ultrastructural abnormalities in the dermal papillae of both lesional and clinically normal follicles from alopecia areata scalps. Br J Dermatol 135:204–10

Ochsendorf FR, Mitrou G, Milbradt R (1988) Therapie der Alopecia Areata mit Diphenylcyclopropenone. Z Hautkr 63:94–100

Olivetti L, Bubola D (1965) Clinical observations on 160 cases of "area celsi". / G It Dermatol Minerva Dermatol 106:367–72

Orecchia G, Belvedere MC, Martinetti M, Capelli E, Rabbiosi G (1987) Human leukocyte antigen region involvement in the genetic predisposition to alopecia areata. Dermatologica 175:10–14

Orentreich N, Sturm HM, Weidman AI, Pelzig A (1960) Local Injection of steroids and hair regrowth in alopecias. Arch Dermatol 82:894–902

Parakkal PF (1969) Role of macrophages in collagen resorption during hair growth cycle. J Ultrastruct Res 29:210–7

Paus R (1996) Control of the hair cycle and hair diseases as cycling disorders. Curr Opin Dermatol 3:248–58

Paus R, Christoph T, Muller-Rover S (1999) Immunology of the hair follicle: a short journey into terra incognita. J Investig Dermatol Symp Proc 4:226–34

Paus R, Slominski A, Czarnetzki BM (1993) Is alopecia areata an autoimmune-response against melanogenesis-related proteins, exposed by abnormal MHC class I expression in the anagen hair bulb? Yale J Biol Med 66:541–54

Penders AJ (1968) Alopecia areata and atopy. Dermatologica 136:395–9

Perret C, Wiesner-Menzel L, Happle R (1984) Immunohistochemical analysis of T-cell subsets in the peribulbar and intrabulbar infiltrates of alopecia areata. Acta Derm Venereol 64:26–30

Perret CM, Steijlen PM, Happle R (1990) Erythema multiforme-like eruptions: a rare side effect of topical immunotherapy with diphenylcyclopropenone. Dermatologica 180:5–7

Perriard-Wolfensberger J, Pasche-Koo F, Mainetti C, Labarthe MP, Salomon D, Saurat J (1993) Pulse of methylprednisolone in alopecia areata. Dermatology 187:282–5

Petukhova L, Duvic M, Hordinsky M, Norris D, Price V, Shimomura Y, et al. (2010) Genome-wide association study in alopecia areata implicates both innate and adaptive immunity. Nature 466:113-7

Plinck E P, Peereboom-Wynia J D, Vuzevski V D, Westerhof W, Stolz E (1993) Turning white overnight, is it possible? Ned Tijdschr Geneeskd 137:207–10

Porter D, Burton JL (1971) A comparison of intra-lesional triamcinolone hexacetonide and triamcinolone acetonide in alopecia areata. Br J Dermatol 85:272

Price VH (1987) Double-blind, placebo-controlled evaluation of topical minoxidil in extensive alopecia areata. J Am Acad Dermatol 16:730–36

Price VH (1987) Topical minoxidil (3%) in extensive alopecia areata, including long-term efficacy. J Am Acad Dermatol 16:737–44

Price V, Hordinsky M, Leonardi C, Roberts J, Olsen E, Rafal E, Korman N, Leung H, Garovoy M, Caro I, Whiting D (2006) Safety and efficacy results of a clinical study of efalizumab in patients with alopecia areata. J Invest Dermatol 126:105

Puavilai S, Puavilai G, Charuwichitratana S, Sakuntabhai A, Sriprachya-Anunt S. (1994) Prevalence of thyroid diseases in patients with alopecia areata. Int J Dermatol 33:632–3

Ranchoff RE, Bergfeld WF, Steck WD, Subichin SJ (1989) Extensive alopecia areata. Results of treatment with 3% topical minoxidil. Cleve Clin J Med 56:149–154

Randall VA (2001) Is alopecia areata an autoimmune disease? Lancet 358:1922–24

Ranki A, Kianto U, Kanerva L, Tolvanen E, Johansson E (1984) Immunohistochemical and electron microscopic characterization of the cellular infiltrate in alopecia (areata, totalis, and universalis). J Invest Dermatol 83:7–11

Ro BI (1995) Alopecia areata in Korea (1982–1994) J Dermatol 22:858–64

Russell JH, Ley TJ (2002) Lymphocyte-mediated cytotoxicity. Annu Rev Immunol 20:323–70

Sabouraud R (1913) Nouvelles recherches sur l'étiologie de la pelade (pelade et ménopause). Annales de Dermatologie et de syphiligraphie 5:88–97

Sabouraud R (1896) Sur les origines de la pelade. Annales de Dermatologie et syphiligraphie 3:253–77

Sabouraud R (1929) Sur l'étiologie de la pelade Arch Dermato-Syphiligr Clin Hop St Louis 1:31–49

Safavi KH, Muller SA, Suman VJ, Moshell AN, Melton LJ 3rd (1995) Incidence of alopecia areata in Olmsted County, Minnesota, 1975 through 1989. Mayo Clin Proc 70:628–33

Salamon T, Musafija A, Milicevic M (1971) Alopecia areata and diseases of the thyroid gland. Dermatologica 142:62–3

Sauder DN, Bergfeld WF, Krakauer RS (1980) Alopecia areata: An inherited autoimmune disease. In: Hair, trace elements and human disease. Brown AC, Crounse AG eds. New York: Praeger, 343

Scerri L, Pace JL (1992) Identical twins with identical alopecia areata. J Am Acad Dermatol 27:766–7

Schallreuter KU, Lemke R, Brandt O, Schwartz R, Westhofen M, Montz R, Berger J (1994) Vitiligo and other diseases: coexistence or true association? Hamburg study on 321 patients. Dermatology 188:269–75

Schroder K, Hertzog PJ, Ravasi T, Hume DA (2004) Interferon-gamma: an overview of signals, mechanisms and functions. J Leukoc Biol 75:163–89

Schulz A, Hamm H, Weiglein U, Axt M, Bröcker EB (1996) Dexamethasone pulse therapy in severe long-standing alopecia areata: a treatment failure. Eur J Dermatol 6:26–9

Schuttelaar M-LA, Hamstra JJ, Plinck EP, Peereboom-Wynia JDR, Vuzevski VD, Mulder PGH, Oranje AP (1996) Alopecia areata in children: treatment with diphencyprone. Br J Dermatol 135:581–5

Seiter S, Ugurel S, Tilgen W, Reinhold U (2001) High-Dose pulse corticosteroid therapy in the treatment of severe alopecia areata. Dermatology 202:230–234

Sharma VK (1996a) Pulsed administration of corticosteroids in the treatment of alopecia areata. Int J Dermatol 35:133–136

Sharma VK, Dawn G, Kumar B (1996b) Profile of alopecia areata in Northern India. Int J Dermatol 35:22–7

Sharma VK, Kumar B, Dawn G (1996c) A clinical study of childhood alopecia areata in Chandigarh, India. Pediatr Dermatol 13:372–7

Sharma VK, Muralidhar S (1998) Treatment of widespread alopecia areata in young patients with monthly oral corticosteroid pulse. Pediatr Dermatol 15:313–7

Shellow WV, Edwards JE, Koo JY (1992) Profile of alopecia areata: A questionnaire analysis of patient and family. Int J Dermatol 31:186–9

Shelton JM, Hollander L (1942) Alopecia totalis in father and daughter. Arch Dermatol Syph 46:137–8

Siegel RM, Chan FK, Chun HJ, Lenardo MJ (2000) The multifaceted role of Fas signaling in immune cell homeostasis and autoimmunity. Nat Immunol 1:469–74

Stankler L (1979) Synchronous alopecia areata in two siblings: a possible viral aetiology. Lancet 1:1303–4

Stewart MI, Smoller BR (1993) Alopecia universalis in an HIV-positive patient: possible insight into pathogenesis. J Cutan Pathol 20:180–3

Strober BE, Menon K, McMichael A, Hordinsky M, Krueger G, Panko J, Siu K, Lustgarten JL, Ross E, Shapiro J. Alefacept for severe alopecia areata. Arch Dermatol 145:1262–1266

Sundberg JP, Boggess D, Silva KA, McElwee KJ, King LE, Li R, Churchill G, Cox GA (2003) Major locus on mouse chromosome 17 and minor locus on mouse chromosome 9 are linked with alopecia areata in C3H/HeJ mice. J Invest Dermatol. 120:771–5

15

Sundberg JP, Silva KA, Li R, Cox GA, King LE (2004) Adult-onset Alopecia areata is a complex polygenic trait in the C3H/HeJ mouse model. J Invest Dermatol 123:294–7

Sundberg JP, Cordy WR, King LE Jr. (1994) Alopecia areata in aging C3H/HeJ mice. J Invest Dermatol 102:847–56

Suri-Payer E, Amar AZ, Thornton AM, Shevach EM (1998) CD4+CD25+ T cells inhibit both the induction and effector function of autoreactive T cells and represent a unique lineage of immunoregulatory cells. J Immunol 160:1212–8

Tarlow JK, Clay FE, Cork MJ, Blakemore AI, McDonagh AJ, Messenger AG, Duff GW. (1994) Severity of alopecia areata is associated with a polymorphism in the interleukin-1 receptor antagonist gene. J Invest Dermatol 103:387–90

Taylor CR, Hawk JLM (1995) PUVA treatment of alopecia areata partialis, totalis and universalis: audit of 10 years' experience at St John's Institute of Dermatology. Br J Dermatol 133:914–8

Tobin DJ, Orentreich N, Bystryn JC (1994a) Autoantibodies to hair follicles in normal individuals. Arch Dermatol 130:395–6

Tobin DJ, Orentreich N, Fenton DA, Bystryn JC (1994b) Antibodies to hair follicles in alopecia areata. J Invest Dermatol 102:721–4

Tobin DJ, Sundberg JP, King LE Jr, Boggess D, Bystryn JC (1997) Autoantibodies to hair follicles in C3H/HeJ mice with alopecia areata-like hair loss. J Invest Dermatol 109:329–33

Tobin DJ (1997) Morphological analysis of hair follicles in alopecia areata. Microsc Res Tech 38:443–451

Tobin DJ, Alhaidari Z, Olivry T (1998) Equine alopecia areata autoantibodies target multiple hair follicle antigens and may alter hair growth. A preliminary study. Exp Dermatol 7:289–97

Tobin DJ (2003) Characterization of hair follicle antigens targeted by the anti-hair follicle immune response. J Investig Dermatol Symp Proc 8:176–81

Tosti A, Piraccini B, Pazzaglia M, Vincenzi C (2003) Clobetasol propionate 0.05% under occlusion in the treatment of alopecia totalis/universalis. J Am Acad Dermatol 49:96–98

Tosti A, Iorizzo M, Botta GL, Milani M (2006) Efficacy and safety of a new clobetasol propionate 0.05% foam in alopecia areata: a randomized, double-blind placebo-controlled trial. JEADV 20:1243–7

Valsecchi R, Vicari O, Frigeni A, Foiadelli L, Naldi L, Cainelli T (1985) Familial alopecia areata – genetic susceptibility or coincidence? Acta Derm Venereol 65:175–7

Van der Steen PH, Baar van JMJ, Perret C, Happle R (1991) Treatment of alopecia areata with diphenylcyclopropenone. J Am Acad Dermatol 24:253–7

Van der Steen P, Traupe H, Happle R, Boezeman J, Strater R, Hamm H (1992a) The genetic risk for alopecia areata in first degree relatives of severely affected patients. Acta Derm Venereol (Stockh) 72:373–5

Van der Steen PH, Happle R (1992b) Dyschromia in confetti as a side effect of topical immunotherapy with diphenylcyclopropenone. Arch Dermatol 128:518–20

Van der Veen EE, Ellis CN, Kang S, Case P, Headington JT, Voorhees JJ, Swanson NA (1984) Topical minoxidil for hair regrowth. J Am Acad Dermatol 11:416–421

Vestey JP, Savin JA (1986) A trial of 1% minoxidil used topically for severe alopecia areata. Acta Derm Venereol (Stockh) 66:179–80

Vogel F, Motulsky AG (1997) Human Genetics: Problems and Approaches. 3rd ed. Berlin: Springer-Verlag, 223–6

Walker SA, Rothman S (1950) Alopecia areata. A statistical study and consideration of endocrine influences. J Invest Dermatol 14:403–413

Wang SJ, Shohat T, Vadheim C, Shellow W, Edwards J, Rotter JI (1994) Increased risk for type I (insulin-dependent) diabetes in relatives of patients with alopecia areata (AA). Am J Med Genet 51:234–9

Weedon D, Strutton G (1981) Apoptosis as the mechanism of the involution of hair follicles in catagen transformation. Acta Derm Venereol 61:335–9

Weidman AI, Zion LS, Mamelok AE (1956) Alopecia areata occurring simultaneously in identical twins. Arch Dermatol 74:424–6

Weise K, Kretzschmar L, John SM, Hamm H (1996) Topical immunotherapy in alopecia areata: anamnestic and clinical criteria of prognostic significance. Dermatology 192:129–133

Weiss VC, West DP, Fu TS, Robinson LA, Cook B, Cohen RL, Chambers DA (1984) Alopecia areata treated with topical minoxidil. Arch Dermatol 120:457–63

Welsh EA, Clark HH, Epstein SZ, Reveille JD, Duvic M (1994) Human leukocyte antigen-DQB1*03 alleles are associated with alopecia areata. J Invest Dermatol 103:758–63

Westgate GE, Craggs RI, Gibson WT (1991) Immune privilege in hair growth. J Invest Dermatol 97:417–420

White SI, Friedmann PS (1985) Topical minoxidil lacks efficacy in alopecia areata. Arch Dermatol 121:591

Whiting DA (2003) Histopathologic features of alopecia areata: a new look. Arch Dermatol 139:1555–9

Whitmont K, Cooper A (2003) PUVA treatment of alopecia areata totalis and universalis: a retrospective study. Australas J Dermatol 44:106–109

Wiseman MC, Shapiro J, MacDonald N, Lui H (2001) Predictive model for immunotherapy of alopecia areata with diphencyprone. Arch Dermatol 137:1063–1068

Wucherpfennig KW (2001) Mechanisms for the induction of autoimmunity by infectious agents. J Clin Invest 108:1097–104

Wunderlich C, Braun-Falco O (1965) Mongolismus und Alopecia areata. Med Welt 10:477–81

Zakaria W, Passeron T, Ostovari N, Lacour JP, Ortonne JP (2004) 308-nm excimer laser therapy in alopecia areata. J Am Acad Dermatol 51:837–8

Zandman-Goddard G, Shoenfeld Y (2002) HIV and autoimmunity. Autoimmun Rev 1:329–37

Zhang JG, Oliver RF (1994) Immunohistological study of the development of the cellular infiltrate in the pelage follicles of the DEBR model for alopecia areata. Br J Dermatol 130:405–14

Zhang X, Yu M, Yu W, Weinberg J, Shapiro J, McElwee KJ (2009) Development of alopecia areata is associated with higher central and peripheral hypothalamic-pituitary-adrenal tone in the skin graft induced C3H/HeJ mouse model. J Invest Dermatol 129:1527–38

Zlotogorski A, Weinrauch L, Brautbar C (1990) Familial alopecia areata: No linkage with HLA. Tissue Antigens 36:40–1

Zöller M, McElwee KJ, Engel P, Hoffmann R (2002) Transient CD44 variant isoform expression and reduction in CD4(+)/CD25(+) regulatory T cells in C3H/HeJ mice with alopecia areata. J Invest Dermatol 118:983–92

15

Autoimmune Phenomena in Atopic Dermatitis 16

Caroline Bussmann and Natalija Novak

Introduction

Atopic dermatitis (AD) is a chronic inflammatory skin disease, which is characterised by relapsing eczema and intense pruritus. It affects about 15–20% of children and 1–3% of adults in the industrialized countries.

The atopic career starts frequently after the 2nd month of life with AD. AD is often associated with food allergy in about 30% of children (Sampson, 2004). Most common are sensitizations against hen's egg and cow's milk. Additionally, allergic asthma may occur together with sensitizations against indoor allergens such as house dust mites. Later on, concomitant allergic rhinitis and sensitizations against pollen, mainly birch and grass-pollen, may appear in adolescence until adulthood (Spergel and Paller, 2003). About 70% of adult patients suffer from the extrinsic form of AD, which is defined by an elevated level of IgE and / or specific sensitizations against allergens.

AD patients may be sensitized against multiple allergens including microbial antigens such as enterotoxins of *Staphylococcus aureus* (*S. aureus*), *Malassezia sympodialis* (*M. sympodialis*), *Candida albicans* or *Aspergillus fumigatus* (Novak et al., 2003; Reefer et al., 2007).

The clinical features of AD change during lifetime from typical involvement of the cheeks in infancy and flexural eczema in childhood to a variable clinical picture in adulthood, which includes minimal forms of AD such as hand- or lid eczema. Beyond, severe disseminated forms exist, which are very difficult to treat.

In some AD patients, especially in those suffering from severe adult forms, no clear connection between the symptoms and exposure to environmental allergens exists. Since scratching due to intense pruritus represents a characteristic feature of AD patients and human proteins might be released through scratching-related tissue damage, it was hypothesized that reactivity to self proteins could represent a trigger factor, which contributes to the chronification of the disease (Valenta et al., 1996).

Definition

Autoreactivity is defined as antigen-antibody response to self-antigens (Zeller et al., 2008). In contrast to autoimmunity, which results from the production of autoantibodies against self-antigens, autoreactivity is caused by structural similarities between environmental antigens and IgE-binding self antigens as kind of a molecular mimicry (Zeller et al., 2008).

Sensitivity of human beings to human dander was first described a long time ago (Keller, 1924; Hampton and Crooke, 1941). After many years, methods were developed which made it possible to gain more detailed insights into the molecular background of this phenomenon, including isolation of cDNAs of IgE-binding proteins or the production of recombinant self antigens. Consequently, more than 50 years later, cross reactivity between birch profilin and human profilin as well as a plethora of other IgE reactive self antigens were detected (Valenta et al., 1991).

Molecular background of IgE autoreactivity

The analysis of the molecular structure of allergens revealed remarkable similarities between environmental allergens and human proteins (Valenta et al., 1991). For example, birch pollen allergen Bet v 2 was demonstrated to share significant sequence homology with human profilins (Valenta et al., 1991). The phenomenon of IgE autoreactivity has been partially identified with the help of a complementary DNA (cDNA) library which had been screened with serum IgE from a patient sensitized to birch pollen (Valenta et al., 1991).

Since skin test challenges with human profilins performed in individuals sensitized to Bet v 2 did not induce any allergic reactions, it has been speculated that the affinity of cross reactive IgE against Bet v 2 to bind to IgE receptors on the surface of effector cells might not be high enough to provoke a type 1 reaction.

Conversely, there are other self antigens such as Manganese Superoxide Dismutase (MnSOD) with striking structural similarities to exoallergens, which have been shown to induce positive reactions in skin test challenges (Zeller et al., 2008). This might mirror distinct affinity of IgE antibodies to autoallergens and environmental allergens. Recent data from research work revealing the crystal structure and the immunological functions of allergens and related self antigens show that the phenomenon of autoreactivity may be mainly caused by a molecular mimicry between shared B cell epitopes (Zeller et al., 2008 88; Fluckiger et al., 2002; Glaser et al., 2006). This B cell cross reactivity depends on similarities and characteristics of the conformation of B cell epitopes (Natter et al., 1998). The structure of B cell epitopes is extremely complex and can only be revealed by the use of antigen-antibody complexes, followed by co-crystallisation of the complex and analysis of its x-ray structure (Limacher et al., 2007). To date, it is possible to reveal the 3-dimensonal structure of many allergens, which allows the comparison of the structural composition of allergens and related human proteins. Nevertheless, structural similarities between environmental allergens and self antigens are far from being completely elucidated.

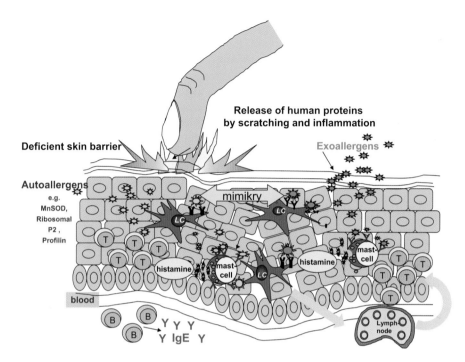

Fig. 1. Mechanisms which might lead to IgE-autoreactivity in AD: Deficient skin barrier as well as release of human proteins by scratching or other triggers and a molecular mimicry between exoallergens and human proteins leads to the development of IgE autreactivity. Later on, cross linking of FceRI on effector cells and antigen presenting cells might occur, leading to the release of mediators and chronification of skin inflammation. Abbreviations: LC=Langerhans cell; B=B cell; T=T cell.

Sensitization to self antigens in AD patients is already detectable in early infancy

Screening of sera from adult AD patients revealed that about 23% of patients with moderate to severe forms of AD display IgE reactivity to human proteins. Conversely, healthy controls and patients with other inflammatory skin diseases such as psoriasis, did not show any autoreactivity to atopy related autoantigens (Mothes et al., 2005).

The most intensive IgE reactivity to human proteins was observed in patients suffering from severe AD (Valenta et al., 1996). Beyond, an increased level of IgE autoantibodies was demonstrated during flare-ups or seasonal allergen exposure (Natter et al., 1998). Autoreactivitiy occurs mainly in patients with the extrinsic form of AD, which goes along with elevated serum IgE and / or high number of specific sensitizations to aeroallergens. However, autoreactivity has also been shown in some patients with the non-allergic (intrinsic) form of AD (Mothes et al., 2005).

Very severe xerosis, ichthyosis and dishydrosis of the skin were other features of AD patients with IgE autoreactivity, furthermore, those patients suffered much more often from
recurrent bacterial and viral infections and had an early onset of the disease (Mothes et al.,
2005). Systematic screening of sera from children with AD younger than 1 year for autoreactive IgE showed that already about 15% of the infants display autoreactivity. Most of
those children had sensitizations against food allergens. Autoreactivity was furthermore
detectable in 80% of children older than 2 years with total serum IgE levels $> 1000\,kU\,/\,l$
IgE. Thus, it has been supposed, that the mechanism of sensitization against self antigens
may already start at very early time points of life together with the onset of first sensitizations to exogenous allergens (Mothes et al., 2005).

Self antigens in AD

Screening of sera from individuals with allergic diseases and healthy controls for IgE reactivity to a human epithelial cell line (A431) derived from an epidermoid mammary carcinoma by western blotting revealed IgE reactivity to several human proteins in AD patients
(Valenta et al., 1996).

Some antigens expressed in the skin (e. g. ara KER) might be released in response to inflammation and scratching of the skin lesions (Natter et al., 1998).

Conversely, other autoantigens expressed in various tissues (e. g. ara NAC) are supposed
to be transported as antigen-antibody complexes to cells expressing the high affinity receptor for IgE (FcεRI) (Natter et al., 1998). In this context, it has been assumed, that complexes
of IgE antibodies and autoantigens, which bind to effector cells such as mast cells, basophils and eosinophils, induce mediator release (Natter et al., 1998). Moreover, IgE autoantibodies may also play a role during delayed type skin reactions which are characteristic for
AD. IgE autoantibodies might be presented to T cells by antigen presenting cells such as
dendritic cells (Natter et al., 1998).

Recently, it could be demonstrated that serum IgE autoantibodies target cells of the respiratory epithelia and epidermal keratinocytes and might cause tissue damage by induction of interferon (IFN)-γ release of these cells (Mittermann et al., 2008) Figure 1.

About 140 IgE-binding self antigens have been identified so far, which seem to be associated with AD (Zeller et al., 2009). Below, the most important self antigens and their potential relevance in AD are described.

Hom s 2

Hom s 2 is the α-chain of the nascent polypeptide-associated complex (α-NAC), an evolu-
tionary conserved protein, which has been attributed to play a role in the transport of polypeptides from the ribosome to appropriate cellular locations.

Recent data show, that recombinant Hom s 2 was able to release IFN-γ from cultured blood mononuclear cells of atopic and non-atopic individuals (Mittermann et al., 2008). This might be of particular immunologic importance in view of the capability of IFN-γ to promote tissue damage and keratinocyte apoptosis, which might influence the course and severity of AD.

Hom s 4

Hom s 4 is an IgE-reactive autoantigen belonging to a subfamily of calcium binding proteins. It is cross reactive to calcium binding allergens from plants and fish such as Phl p 7 and Cryp c 1. Whereas Hom s 4 could induce only a weak histamine release from the patients' basophils, it is capable of inducing Th1-autoreactivity by the release of IFN-γ, which may contribute to the chronification of skin inflammation in AD patients.

Human Acid Ribosomal P2 Protein (P2-protein)

Aspergillus fumigatus (*A. fumigatus*) is an ubiquitous mould which acts as an agent for a broad spectrum of bronchopulmonary diseases. Its major allergen Asp f 1 is a ribotoxin.

IgE-cross reactivity between P2 protein from *A. fumigatus* and human and aspergillus MnSOD could be shown *in vitro* by ELISA and Western blot experiments. Moreover, it was demonstrated *in vivo,* that the protein is able to provoke positive skin test reactions (Crameri et al., 1996; Mayer et al., 1999).

Malassezia sympodialis and "Head and Neck Dermatitis"

The lipophilic yeast *Malassezia sympodialis* (M. sympodialis) colonizes the seborrhoic areas of the head, breast and shoulders after puberty. Sensitizations against M. sympodialis are frequent in AD patients, especially in those showing an accentuation of eczema in the head and neck area, the so called "head and neck dermatitis".

Several allergens of M. sympodialis have been identified to contribute to cross reactivity between human M. sympodialis and human proteins. Genes coding for M. sympodialis allergens (Mala s 1 and Mala s 5–13) have been cloned and sequenced (Schmid-Grendelmeier et al., 2006).

Interestingly, cross reactivity between human MnSOD and MnSOD from M. sympodialis are caused most likely by sequence similarities between the enzyme form M. sympodialis (Mala s 11) (Schmid-Grendelmeier et al., 2006) and human MnSOD.

MnSOD is an essential enzyme which is inducible by UV-radiation, mechanical trauma, and chronic inflammation (Hirose et al., 1993). It has been shown to be upregulated in eczematous areas (Schmid-Grendelmeier et al., 2006) and a high rate of specific sensitizations against human MnSOD could be demonstrated in AD patients. Consequently, patients sensitized to M. sympodialis show frequently positive atopy-patch-test reactions to M. sympodialis. Furthermore, human MnSOD expression is frequently upregulated in eczematous skin lesions of AD patients, which underlines the clinical relevance of this self antigen to aggravate eczema (Schmid-Grendelmeier et al., 2006). Moreover, other allergens of M. sympodialis have been shown to crossreact with human proteins:

Mala s 6 belongs to the cyclophilin pan-allergen family (Glaser et al., 2006). Cyclophilins are cytosolic proteins important for protein folding through enzymatic catalysis. After revealing the 3D structure of Mala s 6 and comparing it to the structure of human cyclophilin, a high grade of similarity between the two structures was discovered, which may explain their cross reactivity detected by Western blot analysis and inhibition ELISAs (Glaser et al., 2006).

Thioredoxins (Trx) from M. sympodialis (Mala s 13) and Aspergillus fumigatus are small redox proteins which are located in all living cells. They have been revealed to be cross reactive structures to human thioredoxins and have been shown to be able to provoke type I-reactions (Limacher et al., 2007).

As a clinical consequence of these findings, a reduction of the colonization with M. sympodialis by topical or systemic antifungal treatment can lead to an improvement of eczema in patients with "Head an Neck Dermatitis" and sensitizations to M. sympodialis (Darabi et al., 2009).

Summary

A subgroup of AD patients characterized by a severe form of the disease, high serum IgE levels and an early age of onset, displays IgE reactivity to self antigens, which share structural similarities with environmental allergens. This process of autosensitization appears to start in early infancy together with the development of first skin lesions and first allergic reactions of the children. Sensitization to self antigens is supposed to be facilitated by chronic tissue damage caused by permanent scratching and skin inflammation, although the exact pathophysiologic mechanisms are largely unclear.

Autoreactivity might explain the severe courses in some of the patients suffering from nearly constant flares of the disease independently of exposition to environmental trigger factors. However, autoreactivity is still a controversial issue because cross reactivity between environmental allergens and self antigens is never complete and ELISA and western blot analysis are not sensitive enough to show the grade of the antigen-anibody binding affinity.

Taken together, autoreactivity in AD patients remains a field, in which much more research work is required to characterize more potential self antigens in AD and prove their assumed function in the pathogenesis of AD.

16

References

Crameri R, Faith A, Hemmann S, Jaussi R, Ismail C, Menz G, Blaser K (1996) Humoral and cell-mediated autoimmunity in allergy to Aspergillus fumigatus. J Exp Med:184:265–70

Darabi K, Hostetler SG, Bechtel MA, Zirwas M (2009). The role of Malassezia in atopic dermatitis affecting the head and neck of adults. J Am Acad Dermatol January;60:125–36

Fluckiger S, Scapozza L, Mayer C, Blaser K, Folkers G, Crameri R (2002) Immunological and structural analysis of IgE-mediated cross-reactivity between manganese superoxide dismutases. Int Arch Allergy Immunol:128:292–303

Glaser AG, Limacher A, Fluckiger S, Scheynius A, Scapozza L, Crameri R (2006) Analysis of the cross-reactivity and of the 1.5 A crystal structure of the Malassezia sympodialis Mala s 6 allergen, a member of the cyclophilin pan-allergen family. Biochem J:396:41–9

Hampton SF, Cooke RA (1941) The sensitivity of man to human dander, with particular reference to eczema (allergic dermatitis) J Allergy:13:63–76

Hirose K, Longo DL, Oppenheim JJ, Matsushima K (1993) Overexpression of mitochondrial manganese superoxide dismutase promotes the survival of tumor cells exposed to interleukin-1, tumor necrosis factor, selected anticancer drugs, and ionizing radiation. FASEB J :7(2):361–8

Keller P (1924) Beitrag zu den Beziehungen von Asthma und Ekzem. Arch Derm Syph Berl:148:82–91

Limacher A, Glaser AG, Meier C, Schmid-Grendelmeier P, Zeller S, Scapozza L, Crameri R (2007) Cross-reactivity and 1.4-A crystal structure of Malassezia sympodialis thioredoxin (Mala s 13), a member of a new pan-allergen family. J Immunol:1;178:389–96

Mayer C, Appenzeller U, Seelbach H, Achatz G, Oberkofler H, Breitenbach M, Blaser K, Crameri R (1999). Humoral and cell-mediated autoimmune reactions to human acidic ribosomal P2 protein in individuals sensitized to Aspergillus fumigatus P2 protein. J Exp Med:189:1507–12

Mittermann I, Reininger R, Zimmermann M, Gangl K, Reisinger J, Aichberger KJ, Greisenegger EK, Niederberger V, Seipelt J, Bohle B, Kopp T, Akdis CA, Spitzauer S, Valent P, Valenta R (2008) The IgE-reactive autoantigen Hom s 2 induces damage of respiratory epithelial cells and keratinocytes via induction of IFN-gamma. J Invest Dermatol;128:1451–9

Mothes N, Niggemann B, Jenneck C, Hagemann T, Weidinger S, Bieber T, Valenta R, Novak N (2005) The cradle of IgE autoreactivity in atopic eczema lies in early infancy. J Allergy Clin Immunol;116:706–9

Natter S, Seiberler S, Hufnagl P, Binder BR, Hirschl AM, Ring J, Abeck D, Schmidt T, Valent P, Valenta R (1998) Isolation of cDNA clones coding for IgE autoantigens with serum IgE from atopic dermatitis patients. FASEB J:12:1559–69

Novak N, Allam JP, Bieber T (2003) Allergic hyperreactivity to microbial components: a trigger factor of "intrinsic" atopic dermatitis? J Allergy Clin Immunol:112:215–6

Reefer AJ, Satinover SM, Wilson BB, Woodfolk JA 2007) The relevance of microbial allergens to the IgE antibody repertoire in atopic and nonatopic eczema. J Allergy Clin Immunol:120:156–63

Sampson HA (2004) Update on food allergy. J Allergy Clin Immunol:113:805–19

Schmid-Grendelmeier P, Scheynius A, Crameri R (2006) The role of sensitization to Malassezia sympodialis in atopic eczema. Chem Immunol Allergy:91:98–109

Schmid-Grendelmeier P, Fluckiger S, Disch R, Trautmann A, Wuthrich B, Blaser K, Scheynius A, Crameri R (2005) IgE-mediated and T cell-mediated autoimmunity against manganese superoxide dismutase in atopic dermatitis. J Allergy Clin Immunol May;115:1068–75

Spergel JM, Paller AS (2003) Atopic dermatitis and the atopic march. J Allergy Clin Immunol:112:S118–S127

Valenta R, Duchene M, Pettenburger K, Sillaber C, Valent P, Bettelheim P, Breitenbach M, Rumpold H, Kraft D, Scheiner O (1991) Identification of profilin as a novel pollen allergen; IgE autoreactivity in sensitized individuals. Science August 2;253:557–60

Valenta R, Maurer D, Steiner R, Seiberler S, Sperr WR, Valent P, Spitzauer S, Kapiotis S, Smolen J, Stingl G (1996) Immunoglobulin E response to human proteins in atopic patients. J Invest Dermatol;107:203–8

Zeller S, Glaser AG, Vilhelmsson M, Rhyner C, Crameri R (2008) Immunoglobulin-E-mediated reactivity to self antigens: a controversial issue. Int Arch Allergy Immunol:145:87–93

Zeller S, Rhyner C, Meyer N, Schmid-Grendelmeier P, Akdis CA, Crameri R (2009) Exploring the repertoire of IgE-binding self-antigens associated with atopic eczema. J Allergy Clin Immunol:124:278–85

Dagmar Simon and Hans-Uwe Simon

Eosinophils under physiologic conditions

Under physiologic conditions, the distribution of eosinophils is restricted to few organs: the hematopoietic and lymphatic organs such as the bone marrow, spleen, lymph nodes and thymus (Rothenberg, Hogan, 2006) and in the gastrointestinal tract with the exception of the esophagus (Straumann, Simon, 2004). Recent studies reported the essential role of eosinophils in mammary gland branch formation (Guon-Evans et al., 2000) and maturation of the pubertal uterus in mice (Guon-Evans et al., 2001). The baseline tissue levels of eosinophils are controlled by eotaxin-1 (Matthews et al., 1998).

Eosinophils are generated and differentiate in the bone marrow, from where they are released into the circulation. In the peripheral blood, they represent 1% to 5% of the leukocytes (Osgood et al., 1939). Eosinophil numbers and activation are under control of eosinophil hematopoietins, such as interleukin (IL)-3, IL-5, and GM-CSF. For eosinophilia, IL-5 particularly plays a critical role by regulating the production, differentiation, activation, trafficking, and survival of eosinophils (Sanderson, 1992).

Eosinophil infiltration in autoimmune bullous diseases

Eosinophil infiltration is found in a broad spectrum of skin disorders. It is a characteristic feature of allergic diseases and parasitic infestations, but it is also observed in auto-immune diseases, hematologic diseases, as well as in association with tumors, and bacterial or viral infections (Simon, Simon, 2007). The presence or absence of eosinophils in skin specimens is often taken as a criterion for differential diagnoses by dermatopathologists. For instance, for the diagnosis of early lesions of bullous pemphigoid (BP), the presence of eosinophils in the upper dermis might be a hint even in the absence of blisters. In addition to BP, eosinophils have also been observed in other autoimmune bullous diseases including cicatricial pemphigoid (Heiligenhaus et al., 1998), pemphigoid gestationis (Borrego et al.,

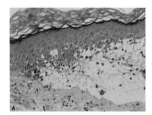 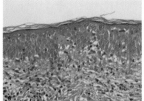 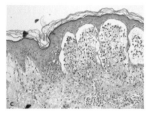

Fig. 1. Eosinophis in autoimmune bullous diseases. (A) Eosinophils in the dermis and blister of bullous pemphigois. (B) Eosinophil spongiosis in pemphigus foliaceus. (C) Eosinophils and Neutrophils in the papillary dermis of dermatitis herpetiformis.

1999), pemphigus vulgaris (Emmerson, Wilson-Jones, 1968), pemphigus foliaceus (Osteen et al., 1976), pemphigus vegetans (Pearson et al., 1980), dermatitis herpetiformis (Blenkinsopp et al., 1983), linear IgA disease (Caproni et al., 1999), and epidermolysis bullosa aquisita (Ward et al., 1992) (Fig. 1). With regard to the spectrum of autoimmune diseases, eosinophilia is a striking feature in eosinophilic fasciitis, but has also been reported in systemic sclerosis and localized scleroderma (Falanga et al., 1987). Furthermore, in morphea profunda and lupus panniculitis, eosinophils may be present in the tissue (Peters, Su, 1991). Graft versus host reactions containing eosinophils may histologically mimic drug hypersensitivity (Marra et al., 2004). In chronic urticaria, including autoimmune variants, the inflammatory infiltrates of the wheals contain eosinophils (Sabroe et al., 1999).

In hematoxylin & eosin (H&E) stained skin specimens, eosinophils are remarkable as round shaped cells stuffed with coarse eosinophil granules. Disrupted oval shaped eosinophils may also be found, and have been reported in subacute and chronic eczematous lesions. Extracellular granular proteins can be detected in varying amounts either as separate deposits or as a thin coating on collagen bundles. The latter are called flame figures. Both phenomena have been observed in BP (Borrego et al., 1996, Beer et al., 1994, Watanabe et al., 1998). Immunofluorescence staining using antibodies directed against eosinophilic cationic protein (ECP) or major basic protein (MBP) allows a more sensitive detection of eosinophils and extracellular granular protein depositions than H&E staining.

17

Eosinophil activation and mediator release

Eosinophils that are primed by IL-5 or IFN-γ and activated by lipopolysaccharide from gram-negative bacteria were reported to release mitochondrial DNA in a catapult-like manner (Yousefi et al., 2008). Granule proteins, such as ECP and MBP, were shown to colocalize with the extracellular DNA structures, indicating that eosinophils are involved in acute defence mechanisms against pathogens. In contrast to DNA, the release of granule proteins occurs through exocytosis or piecemeal degranulation (Logan et al., 2003, Scepek et al., 1994). In classical exocytosis, single secretory granules are extruded to the cell exterior, whereas in compound exocytosis the fusion of intracellular granules precedes their release through a single fusion pore (Logan et al., 2003). Piecemeal degranulation has been identified as mechanism by which cytoplasmic secretory vesicles containing cytoplasmic crystalloid granules with core components are released from eosinophils (Scepek et al., 2004). In addition to the classical eosinophil hematopoietins IL-3, IL-5 and GM-CSF, eosinophils can be activated by complement, eotaxin, IL-13, pro-inflammatory cytokines, such as TNF-α and IFN-γ, immunoglobulines (Schmid-Grendelmeier et al., 2001; Hogan et al., 2008, Yousefi et al., 2008), as well as bacteria or viruses via Toll-like receptors (TLR) (Plötz et al., 2001; Mansson, Cardell, 2009).

The distinct functions of eosinophils

The primary function of eosinophils has been related to the protection against helminth parasites (Klion, Nutman, 2004). Recently, a novel mechanism of eosinophil function in innate immunity has been reported. By releasing mitochondrial DNA and granule proteins, eosinophils form extracellular structures, which are able to bind and kill bacteria invading the gastrointestinal tract (Yousefi et al., 2008). Furthermore, eosinophils are accused to cause tissue damage (Frigas et al., 1991; Klion, Nutman, 2004). In addition, eosinophils play an important role in repair and remodelling processes as well as in immunomodulation (Jacobsson et al., 2007; Straumann et al., 2010). The role of eosinophils under pathological conditions has mostly been studied in parasitic infections and in bronchial asthma. However, in skin diseases, eosinophils are much less investigated.

The cytoplasmic granules, which are belived to be important for tissue damage, are composed of four distinct populations that can be identified under electron microscopy: primary and secondary granules, small granules and lipid bodies (Kariyawasam, Robinson, 2006). The cytotoxic cationic proteins are stored in the secondary granules that are formed by a core containing major basic protein (MBP) and a matrix composed of eosinophil cationic protein (ECP), eosinophil peroxidase (EPO) and eosinophil derived neurotoxin (EDN) (Peters et al., 1986). MBP is highly cytotoxic (Gleich et al., 1979). Because of its cationic nature, it affects the charge of surface membranes resulting in disturbed permeability, disruption and injuring of cell membranes (Kroegel et al., 1987). ECP damages target cell membranes through the formation of pores or transmembrane channels (Young et al., 1986). ECP and EDN have been identified as ribonucleases (Gleich et al., 1986) and possess antiviral activity (Rosenberg, Domachowske, 2001). Eosinophils store abundant amounts of ECP and may release it upon repetitive stimulation with the same agonist, implying that mature eosinophils do not require a significant ECP resynthesis (Simon et al., 2000).

Eosinophils exhibit immunoregulatory functions by producing a large number of cytokines that modulate the activation and function of leukocytes, such as dendritic cells, macrophages, lymphocytes, mast cells and neutrophils, and of resident tissue cells, including epithelial cells, endothelial cells and fibroblasts (Jacobson et al., 2007). Depending on the tissue and inflammatory response, eosinophils modulate and / or sustain either T helper 1

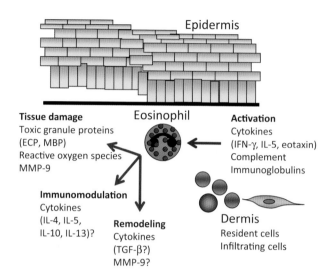

Fig. 2. Potential roles of eosinophils in autoimmune bullous diseases

(by releasing e. g. IL-2, IL-12, IL-18, IFN-γ) or T helper 2 (by production of IL-4, IL-5, IL-13, IL-25) immune responses (Lamkhioued et al., 1996; Ohno et al., 1996; Schmid-Grendelmeier et al., 2002; Lampinen et al., 2004; Jacobson et al., 2007; Wang et al., 2009). On the other hand, eosinophils may promote acute inflammation (TNF-α) or might also be involved in the regulation of T regulatory cells (Casale et al., 1996; Spencer et al., 2009). Moreover, eosinophils produce tumor growth factor (TGF)-β, which is involved in Th17 cell differentiation, a newly identified T helper subtype producing IL-17 and IL-22 (Deenik, Tangye, 2007).

Eosinophils express a number mediators that are implicated in remodelling including fibroblast growth factor (FGF)-2, IL-4, IL-6, IL-11, IL-13, IL-17, IL-25, TGF-β, nerve growth factor (NGF), matrix metalloproteinase (MMP)-9 and vascular endothelial growth factor (VEGF) (Kay et al., 2004; Foley et al., 2007). TGF-β by autocrine-paracrine actions may stimulate eosinophils to generate IL-11, another cytokine with fibrogenic potential (Foley et al., 2007). Furthermore, eotaxin (CCL11) was shown to exhibit a direct profibrogenic effect on fibroblasts (Puxeddu et al., 2006). Eotaxin is secreted by a various resident and inflammatory cells, e. g. epithelial cells, to recruit eosinophils into the tissues, but it is also released by eosinophils (Rothenberg, 1999). Moreover, MBP interacts with IL-1 and TGF-β and thus stimulates lung fibroblasts (Rochester et al., 1996). EPO products that are generated by infiltrating eosinophils may affect endothelial cells and thus promote the thrombotic diathesis characteristic of the hypereosinophilic syndrome (Wang et al., 2006). By secreting metalloproteinases, especially MMP-9, eosinophils may also directly affect remodelling (Wiehler et al., 2004).

Eosinophils in bullous pemphigoid

The histopathology of BP reveals eosinophil infiltration in and below blisters and along the basement membrane (Blenkinsopp et al., 1983). Moreover, eosinophils are found in non-blistering, urticarial or eczematous lesions of BP (Strohal et al., 1993). Eosinophils migrate through the basement membrane and can be detected in newly formed blisters after 12 to 24 hour (Iryo et al., 1992). Peripheral blood eosinophilia has been observed in 50% of BP patients ranging between 5% and 43% (Bushkell et al., 1983).

BP is associated with T cell activation reflected by the production of both Th1 (IFN-γ) and Th2 cytokines (IL-4, IL-5 and IL-13) (Ameglio et al., 1998; Rico et al., 1999). Patients with active BP exhibit increased IL-5 levels and eosinophil numbers in the blood compared with patients in clinical remission and healthy controls (Engineer et al., 2001). Furthermore, serum eotaxin levels are increased in BP patients correlating with disease activity (Frezzolini et al., 2002; Nakashima et al., 2007). IL-5 as well as eotaxin are abundantly found in blister fluids. The production of IL-5 is associated with blood eosinophilia and significant eosinophil infiltration in the skin of BP patients as well as disease intensity (Ameglio et al., 1998; Wakugawa et al., 2000). Upon exposure of eosinophils to blister fluids from BP lesions an increased survival has been observed that was inhibited by blocking IL-5 and IL-3 (Borrego et al., 1996). IL-5, eotaxin and eotaxin receptor CCR3 are expressed by skin infiltrating cells (Frezzoloini et al., 2002). Eosinophil priming with IL-5 and subsequent stimulation with immunue complexes of the IgG, IgA or IgE types resulted in an increased production of the Th2 chemokines eotaxin and MCP-4 (Abdelilah et al., 2006).

In addition to IL-5 and eotaxin, which are essential for the recruitment, activation and survival of eosinophils at the inflammatory tissue, immunoglobulins as well as complement are able to activate eosinophils. Whether BP180 and/or BP230 autoantibodies of the IgG or IgE types are able to directly activate eosinophil has not been investigated so far. Eosinophils exhibit CD16, the Fc gamma receptor, and degranulate upon stimulation with IgG immune complexes (Davoine et al., 2004). The presence of Fc epsilon RI-positive eosinophils has also been suggested (Kasahara et al., 2001). Furthermore, IL-5 primed eosinophils release granule proteins upon stimulation with complement C5a (Simon et al., 2000).

Already in the 1980ies, it has been hypothesized that in the presence of complement, eosinophils release enzymes and reactive oxygen onto the basement membrane causing tissue destruction and blister formation in BP (Sams, Gammon, 1982). Eosinophil granule protein depositions have been observed in both blistering and evolving lesions (Borrego et al., 1996). Analogous to BP, eosinophils and extracellular MBP deposition have been found in pemphigoid gestationis (Scheman et al., 1989). ECP can be detected in blister fluid (Czech et al., 1993). Serum ECP levels are elevated in BP patients compared with controls (Caproni et al., 1995). MMP-9 has been reported to be expressed by eosinophils in lesional skin as well as in the blister fluids of BP (Stahle-Bäckdahl et al., 1994). Moreover, MMP-9 cleaves the extracellular, collagenous domain of BP180 autoantigen in vitro (Stahle-Bäckdahl et al., 1994). Taken together, eosinophils are thought to be critically implicated in blister formation by releasing toxic granule proteins (ECP, MBP) and proteolytic enzymes (Stahle-Bäckdahl et al., 1994; Caproni et al., 1995; Wakugawa et al., 2000).

It should be noted, that, although there is strong evidence that eosinophils are important players in the pathogenesis of BP, their direct contribution and the molecular mechanisms are not fully understood (Fig. 2). Recently, it has been demonstrated in SCID mice that IgE basement membrane zone antibodies induce BP like lesions with eosinophil infiltration and blister formation (Zone et al., 2007). However, other established mouse models were not suitable for studying the role of eosinophils in BP (Leighty et al., 2007).

Eosinophils in other autoimmune bullous diseases

Compared to BP, in other autoimmune bullous diseases, eosinophils have less been studied. Eosinophilic spongiosis can be observed in early pemphigus including pemphigus foliaceus (Brodersen et al., 1978). Although eosinophils are a common feature in cutaneous drug reactions, the presence of eosinophil spongiosis may not discriminate drug-induced pemphigus from pemphigus vulgaris (Landau, Brenner, 1997). The presence of eosinophils may be due to IL-5 as part of the mixed Th1 / Th2 cytokine profile that has been found in pemphigus vulgaris (Rico et al., 1999). Complement fixing antibodies were shown to induce eosinophil infiltration in pemphigus (Iwatsuki et al., 1983). Charcot-Leyden crystals that are derived from eosinophil granule proteins have been observed in pemphigus vegetans (Kanitakis, 1987).

Although neutrophils and leukocytoklasis are typical for dermatitis herpetiformis, occasionally undermingled eosinophils can be seen in the papillary dermis (Blenkinsopp et al., 1983). Furthermore, both neutrophils and eosinophils are the predominant infiltrating cells in linear IgA bullous dermatosis (Caproni et al., 1999). Epidermolysis bullosa aquisita following GM-CSF therapy has been related to eosinophil infiltration and deposition of EPO and MBP at the dermal-epidermal junction (Ward et al., 1992).

Eosinophils as therapeutic targets

Corticosteroids that are widely used for the treatment of autoimmune bullous diseases affect most cells that contribute to inflammation and blister formation. They inhibit cytokine and chemokine release of infiltrating immune cells, in particular T cells, as well as resident cells and thus decrease the production, activation and survival of eosinophils. Moreover, corticosteroids exhibit direct effects on eosinophils, i.e. by causing apoptosis (Meagher et al., 1996). However, long-term corticosteroid therapy is accompanied by a number of side effects, which might be relevant in particular in elderly patients. Therefore, specific targeting of cells and / or cytokines relevant in the pathogenesis of autoimmune bullous diseases is a promising approach.

Since the eosinophilopoietin IL-5 critically regulates eosinophil numbers and activation, antagonizing IL-5 or its receptor by specific antibodies is thought to be useful in treating eosinophilic diseases. Anti-IL-5 antibody therapy has been shown to be effective in eosinophilic diseases such as hypereosinophilic syndrome, eosinophilic esophagitis, and bronchial asthma (Plötz et al., 2003; Rothenberg et al., 2008; Stein et al., 2006; Haldar et al., 2009; Nair et al., 2009). It drastically decreases eosinophil numbers in the peripheral blood and to some extent in the tissues (Plötz et al., 2003, Straumann et al., 2010). In HES and in bronchial asthma, anti-IL-5 therapy had a significant steroid-sparing effect (Rothenberg et al., 2008, Nair et al., 2009). Moreover, it was shown to reduce remodelling in bronchial asthma (Phipps et al., 2004) and eosinophilic esophagitis (Straumann et al., 2010). Clinical trials investigating an anti-IL-5 receptor antibody in asthma have just started. So far, studies evaluating anti-IL-5 therapy in autoimmune bullous diseases such as BP have not been performed yet.

Blocking chemokines and its receptors represents another approach to downregulate eosinophil inflammatory responses. Eotaxins are chemokines that are involved in eosinophil recruitment into the tissue and remodeling. Blocking eotaxins by a monoclonal antibody and inhibiting the receptor for eotaxins, CCR3, are current strategies to treat eosinophilic diseases.

Summary

Eosinophils may be present in most of the autoimmune bullous diseases, in particular in BP. In BP, the number of eosinophils as well the levels of eosinophil derived products in the peripheral blood correlate with disease severity. However, the exact mechanisms how eosinophils are recruited and activated as well as their pathogenic role is not fully understood. The detectable eosinophil granule proteins and cytokines point to the possibility that eosinophils play a role in tissue damage, immunomodulation and / or remodeling. It should be noted, however, that the pathogenic role of eosinophils in autoimmune bullous diseases remains unclear. Clinical trials with novel drugs that specifically target eosinophils, cytokines or their receptors may provide new insights into the pathogenesis of these diseases, besides the analysis of clinical efficacy.

References

Abdelilah SG, Weilemans V, Agouli M, Guenounou M, Hamid Q, Beck LA, Lamkhioued B (2006) Increased expression of Th2-associated cytokines in bullous pemphigoid diesease. Role of eosinophils in the production and release of these cytokines. Clin Immunol 120:220–231
Ameglio F, D'Auria L, Bonifati C, Ferrano C, Mastroianni A, Giacalone B (1998) Cytokine pattern in blister fluid and serum of patients with bullous pemphigoid: relationships with disease intensity. Br J Dermatol 138:611–614
Beer TW, Langtry JA, Phillips WG, Wojnarowska F (1994) Flame figures in bullous pemphigoid. Dermatology 188:310–312

Blenkinsopp WK, Haffenden GP, Fry L, Leonard JN (1983) Histology of linear IgA disease, dermatitis herpetiformis, and bullous pemphigoid. Am J Dermatopathol 5:547–554

Borrego L, Maynard B, Peterson EA, George T, Iglesias L, Peters MS, Newman W, Gleich GJ, Leiferman KM (1996) Deposition of eosinophil granule proteins precedes blister formation in bullous pemphigoid. Comparison with neutrophil and mast cell granule proteins. Am J Pathol 148:897–909

Borrego L, Peterson EA, Diez LI, de Pablo Martin P, Wagner JM, Gleich GJ, Leiferman KM (1999) Polymorphic eruption of pregnancy and herpes gestationis: comparison of granulated cell proteins in tissue and serum. Clin Exp Dermatol 24:213–225

Brodersen I, Frentz G, Thomsen K (1978) Eosinophilic spongiosis in early pemphigus foliaceus. Acta Derm Venereol 58:368–369

Bushkell LL, Jordon RE (1983) Bullous pemphigoid: a cause of peripheral blood eosinophilia. J Am Acad Dermatol 8:648–651

Caproni M, Palleschi GM, Falcos D, D'Agata A, Cappelli G, Fabbri P (1995) Serum eosinophil cationic protein (ECP) in bullous pemphigoid. Int J Dermatol 34:177–180

Caproni M, Rolfo S, Bernacchi E, Bianchi B, Brazzini B, Fabbri P (1999) The role of lymphocytes, granulocytes, mast cells and their related cytokines in lesional skin of linear IgA bullous dermatosis. Br J Dermatol 140:1072–1078

Casale TB, Costa JJ, Galli SJ (1996) TNF alpha is important in human lung allergic reactions. Am J Respir Cell Mol Biol 15:35–44

Czech W, Schaller J, Schöpf E, Kapp A (1993) Granulocyte activation in bullous diseases: release of granular proteins in bullous pemphigoid and pemphigus vulgaris. J Am Acad Dermatol 29:210–215

Davoine F, Labonte I, Ferland C, Mazer B, Chakir J, Laviolette M (2004) Role and modulation of CD16 expression on eosinophils by cytokines and immune complexes. Int Arch Allergy Immunol 134:165–172

Deenick EK, Tangye SG (2007) IL-21: a new player in Th17-cell differentiation. Immunol Cell Biol 85:503–505

Emmerson RW, Wilson-Jones E (1968) Eosinophilic spongiosis in pemphigus. A report of an unusual hitological change in pemphigus. Arch Dermatol 97:252–257

Engineer L, Bhol K, Kumari S, Razzaque Ahmed A (2001) Bullous pemphigoid: interaction of interleukin5, anti-basement membrane zone antibodies and eosinophils. A preliminary observation. Cytokine 2001;13:32–38

Falanga V, Medsger TA (1987) Frequency, levels, and significance of blood eosinophilia in systemic sclerosis, localized scleroderma, and eosinophilic fasciitis. J Am Acad Dermatol 17:6486–56

Foley SC, Prefontaine D, Hamid Q (2007) Role of eosinophils in airway remodeling. J Allergy Clin Immunol 119:1563–1566

Frezzolini A, Teofoli P, Cianchini G, Barduagni S, Ruffelli M, Ferranti G, Puddu P, Pita OD (2002) Increased expression of eotaxin and its specific receptor CCR3 in bullous pemphigoid. Eur J Dermatol 12:27–31

Frigas E, Motojima S, Gleich GJ (1991) The eosinophilic injury to the mucosa of the airways in the pathogenesis of bronchial asthma. Eur Respir J 13:S123-S135

Gleich GJ, Frigas E, Loegering DA, Wassom DL, Steinmuller D (1979) Cytotoxic properties of the eosinophil major basic protein. J Immunol 123:2925–2927

Gleich GJ, Loegering DA, Bell MP, Checkel JL, Ackerman SJ, McKean DJ (1986) Biochemical and functional similarities between human eosinophil-derived neurotoxin and eosinophil cationic protein: homology with ribonucleases. Proc Natl Acad Sci USA 83:3146–3150

Gouon-Evans V, Rothenberg ME, Pollard JW (2000) Postnatal mammary gland development requires macrophages and eosinophils. Development 127:2269–2282

Gouon-Evans V, Pollard JW (2001) Eotaxin is required for eosinophil homing into the stroma of the pubertal and cycling uterus. Endocrinology 142:4515–4521

17

Haldar P, Brightling CE, Hargadon B, Gupta S, Monteiro W, Sousa A, Marshall RP, Bradding P, Green RH, Wardlaw AJ, Pavord ID. (2009) Mepolizumab and exacerbations of refractory eosinophilic asthma. N Engl J Med 360:973–984

Heiligenhaus A, Schaller J, Mauss S, Engelbrecht S, Dutt JE, Foster CS, Steuhl KP (1998) Eosinophil granule proteins expressed in ocular cicatricial pemphigoid. Br J Ophthalmol 82:312–317

Hogan SP, Rosenberg HF, Moqbel R, Phipps S, Foster PS, Lacy P, Kay AB, Rothenberg ME (2008) Eosinophils: Biological properties and role in health and disease. Clin Exp Allergy 38:709–750

Iryo K, Tsuda S, Sasai (1992) Ultrastructural aspects of infiltrated eosinophils in bullous pemphigoid. J Dermatol 19:393–399

Iwatsuki K, Tagami H, Yamada M (1983) Pemphigus antibodies mediate the development of an inflammatory change in the epidermis. A possible mechanism underlying the feature of eosinophilic spongiosis. Acta Derm Venereol 63:495–500

Jacobsen EA, Taranova AG, Lee NA, Lee JJ (2007) Eosinophils: singularly destructive effector cells or purveyors of immunoregulation. J Allergy Clin Immunol 119:1313–1320

Kanitakis J. Charcot-Leyden crystals in pemphigus vegetans (1987) J Cutan Pathol 14:127

Kariyawasam HH, Robinson DS (2006) The eosinophil: the cell and its weapons, the cytokines, its locations. Semin Respir Crit Care Med 27:117–127

Kasahara-Imamura M, Hosokawa H, Maekawa N, Horio T (2001) Activation of Fc epsilon RI-positive eosinophils in bullous pemphigoid. Int J Mol Med 7:249–253

Kay AB, Phipps S, Robinson DS (2004) A role for eosinophils in airway remodelling in asthma. Trends Immunol 25:477–482

Klion AD, Nutman TB (2004) The role of eosinophils in host defense against helminth parasites. J Allergy Clin Immunol 113:30–37

Kroegel C, Costabel U, Matthys H (1987) Mechanism of membrane damage mediated by eosinophil major basic protein. Lancet 1:1380–1381

Lamkhioued B, Gounni AS, Aldebert D, Delaporte E, Prin L, Capron A, Capron M (1996) Synthesis of type 1 (IFN gamma) and type 2 (IL-4, IL-5, and IL-10) cytokines by human eosinophils. Ann N Y Acad Sci 796:203–208

Lampinen M, Carlson M, Håkansson LD, Venge P (2004) Cytokine-regulated accumulation of eosinophils in inflammatory disease. Allergy 59:793–805

Landau M, Brenner S (1997) Histopathologic findings in drug-induced pemphigus. Am J Dermatopathol 19:411–414

Leighty L, Li N, Diaz LA, Liu Z (2007) Experimental models of autoimmune and inflammatory blistering disease, bullous pemphigoid. Arch Dermatol 299:417–422

Logan MR, Odemuyiwa SO, Moqbel R (2003) Understanding exocytosis in immune and inflammatory cells: the molecular basis of mediator secretion. J Allergy Clin Immunol 111:923–932

Meagher LC, Cousin JM, Seckl JR, Haslett C (1996) Opposing effects of glucocorticoids on the rate of apoptosis in neutrophilic and eosinophilic granulocytes. J Immunol 156:4422–4428

Månsson A, Cardell LO (2009) Role of atopic status in Toll-like receptor (TLR) 7- and TLR9-mediated activation of human eosinophils. J Leukoc Biol 85:719–727

Marra DE, McKee PH, Nghiem P (2004) Tissue eosinophils and the perils of using skin biopsy specimens to distinguish between drug hypersensitivity and cutaneous graft-versus-host disease. J Am Acad Dermatol 51:543–546

Matthews AN, Friend DS, Zimmermann N, Sarafi MN, Luster AD, Pearlman E, Wert SE, Rothenberg ME (1998) Eotaxin is required for the baseline level of tissue eosinophils. Proc Natl Acad Sci USA 95:6273–6278

Nair P, Pizzichini MM, Kjarsgaard M, Inman MD, Efthimiadis A, Pizzichini E, Hargreave FE, O'Byrne PM (2009) Mepolizumab for prednisone-dependent asthma with sputum eosinophilia. N Engl J Med 360:985–993

Nakashima H, Fujimoto M, Asashima N, Watanabe R, Kuwano Y, Yazawa N, Maruyama N, Okochi H, Kumanogoh A, Tamaki K (2007) Serum chemokine profile in patients with bullous pemphigoid. Br J Dermatol 156:454–459

Ohno I, Nitta Y, Yamauchi K, Hoshi H, Honma M, Woolley K, O'Byrne P, Tamura G, Jordana M, Shirato K (1996) Transforming growth factor beta 1 (TGF beta 1) gene expression by eosinophils in asthmatic airway inflammation. Am J Respir Cell Mol Biol 15:404–409

Osgood EE, Brownlee IE, Osgood MW, Ellis DM, Cohen W (1939) Total differential and absolute leukocyte counts and sedimentation rates. Arch Int Med 64:105–120

Osteen FB, Wheeler CE Jr, Briggaman RA, Puritz EM (1976) Pemphigus foliaceus. Early clinical appearance as dermatitis herpetiformis with eosinophilic spongiosis. Arch Dermatol 112:1148–1152

Pearson RW, O'Donoghue M, Kaplan SJ (1980) Pemphigus vegetans: its relationship to eosinophilic spongiosis and favorable response to dapsone. Arch Dermatol 116:65–68

Peters MS, Rodriguez M, Gleich GJ (1986) Localization of human eosinophil granule major basic protein, eosinophil cationic protein, and eosinophil-derived neurotoxin by immunoelectron microscopy. Lab Invest 54:656–662

Peters MS, Su WP (1991) Eosinophild in lupus panniculitis and morphea profunda. J Cut Pathol 18:189–192

Phipps S, Flood-Page P, Menzies-Gow A, Ong YE, Kay AB (2004) Intravenous anti-IL-5 monoclonal antibody reduces eosinophils and tenascin deposition in allergen-challenged human atopic skin. J Invest Dermatol 122:1406–1412

Plötz SG, Lentschat A, Behrendt H, Plötz W, Hamann L, Ring J, Rietschel ET, Flad HD, Ulmer AJ (2001) The interaction of human peripheral blood eosinophils with bacterial lipopolysaccharide is CD14 dependent. Blood 97:235–241

Plötz SG, Simon HU, Darsow U, Simon D, Vassina E, Yousefi S, Hein R, Smith T, Behrendt H, Ring J (2003) Use of an anti-interleukin-5 antibody in the hypereosinophilic syndrome with eosinophilic dermatitis. N Engl J Med 349:2334–2339

Puxeddu I, Bader R, Piliponsky AM, Reich R, Levi-Schaffer F, Berkman N (2006) The CC chemokine eotaxin/CCL11 has a selective profibrogenic effect on lung fibroblasts. J Allergy Clin Immunol 117:103–110

Rico MJ, Benning C, Weingart ES, Streilein RD, Hall RP (1999) Characterization of skin cytokines in bullous pemphigoid and pemphigus vulgaris. Br J Dermatol 140:1079–1086

Rochester CL, Ackerman SJ, Zheng T, Elias JA (1996) Eosinophil-fibroblast interactions. Granule major basic protein interacts with IL-1 and transforming growth factor-beta in the stimulation of lung fibroblast IL-6-type cytokine production. J Immunol 156:4449–4456

Rosenberg HF, Domachowske JB (2001) Eosinophils, eosinophil ribonucleases, and their role in host defence against respiratory virus pathogens. J Leukoc Biol 70:691–698

Rothenberg ME (1999) Eotaxin: an essential mediator of eosinophil trafficking into mucosal tissues. Am J Respir Cell Mol Biol 21:291–295

Rothenberg ME, Hogan SP (2006) The eosinophil. Annu Rev Immunol 24:147–174

Rothenberg ME, Klion AD, Roufosse FE, Kahn JE, Weller PF, Simon HU, Schwartz LB, Rosenwasser LJ, Ring J, Griffin EF, Haig AE, Frewer PI, Parkin JM, Gleich GJ; Mepolizumab HES Study Group (2008) Treatment of patients with the hypereosinophilic syndrome with mepolizumab. N Engl J Med 358:1215–1228

Sabroe RA, Poon E, Orchard GE, Lane D, Francis DM, Barr RM, Black MM, Black AK, Greaves MW (1999) Cutaneous inflammatory cell infiltrate in chronic idiopathic urticaria: comparison of patients with and without anti-FcepsilonRI or anti-IgE autoantibodies. J Allergy Clin Immunol 103:484–493

Sams WM Jr, Gammon WR (1982) Mechanism of lesion production in pemphigus and pemphigoid. J Am Acad Dermatol 6:431–452

Sanderson CJ (1992) Interleukin-5, eosinophils, and disease. Blood 79:3101–3109

Scepek S, Moqbel R, Lindau M (1994) Compound exocytosis and cumulative degranulation by eosinophils and its role in parasite killing. Parasitol Today 10:276–278

Scheman AJ, Hordinsky MD, Groth DW, Vercellotti GM, Leiferman KM (1989) Evidence for eosinophil degranulation in the pathogenesis of herpes gestationis. Arch Dermatol 125:1079–1083

17

Schmid-Grendelmeier P, Altznauer F, Fischer B, Bizer C, Straumann A, Menz G, Blaser K, Wüthrich B, Simon HU (2002) Eosinophils express functional IL-13 in eosinophilic inflammatory diseases. J Immunol 169:1021–1027

Simon D, Simon HU (2007) Eosinophilic disorders. J Allergy Clin Immunol 119:1291–1300

Simon HU, Weber M, Becker E, Zilberman Y, Blaser K, Levi-Schaffer F (2000) Eosinophils maintain their capacity to signal and release eosinophil cationic protein upon repetitive stimulation with the same agonist. J Immunol 165:4069–4075

Spencer LA, Szela CT, Perez SA, Kirchhoffer CL, Neves JS, Radke AL, Weller PF (2009) Human eosinophils constitutively express multiple Th1, Th2, and immunoregulatory cytokines that are secreted rapidly and differentially. J Leukoc Biol 85:117–23

Ståhle-Bäckdahl M, Inoue M, Guidice GJ, Parks WC (1994) 92-kD gelatinase is produced by eosinophils at the site of blister formation in bullous pemphigoid and cleaves the extracellular domain of recombinant 180-kD bullous pemphigoid autoantigen. J Clin Invest 93:2022–2030

Stein ML, Collins MH, Villanueva JM, Kushner JP, Putnam PE, Buckmeier BK, Filipovich AH, Assa'ad AH, Rothenberg ME (2006) Anti-IL-5 (mepolizumab) therapy for eosinophilic esophagitis. J Allergy Clin Immunol 118:1312–1319

Straumann A, Simon HU (2004) The physiological and pathophysiological roles of eosinophils in the gastrointestinal tract. Allergy 59:15–25

Straumann A, Conus S, Gronzka P, Kita H, Kephart G, Bussmann C, Beglinger C, Patel J, Byrne M, Simon HU (2010) Anti-interleukin-5 antibody treatment (mepolizumab) in active eosinophilic esophagitis: A Randomized, Placebo-Controlled, Double-Blind Trial. Gut 59:21–30

Strohal R, Rappersberger K, Pehamberger H, Wolff K (1993) Nonbullous pemphigoid: prodrome of bullous pemphigoid or a distinct pemphigoid variant? J Am Acad Dermatol 29:293–2999

Wakugawa M, Nakamura K, Hino H, Toyama K, Hattori N, Okochi H, Yamada H, Hirai K, Tamaki K, Furue M (2000) Elevated levels of eotaxin and interleukin-5 in blister fluid of bullous pemphigoid: correlation with tissue eosinophilia. Br J Dermatol 143:112–116

Wang JG, Mahmud SA, Thompson JA, Geng JG, Key NS, Slungaard A (2006) The principal eosinophil peroxidase product, HOSNC, is a uniquely potent phagocyte oxidant inducer of endothelial cell tissue factor activity: a potential mechanism for thrombosis in eosinophilic inflammatory states. Blood 107:558–565

Wang YH, Liu YJ (2009) Thymic stromal lymphopoietin, OX40-ligand, and interleukin-25 in allergic responses. Clin Exp Allergy 39:798–806

Ward JC, Gitlin JB, Garry DJ, Jatoi A, Luikart SD, Zelickson BD, Dahl MV, Skubitz KM (1992) Epidermolysis bullosa acquisita induced by GM-CSF: a role for eosinophils in treatment-related toxicity. Br J Haematol 81:27–32

Watanabe H, Sueki H, Kitami A, Kakuchi C, Ikeda Y, Nagata S, Hashimoto T, Iijima M (1998) Flame figures associated with bullous pemphigoid. J Dermatol 25:632–636

Wiehler S, Cuvelier SL, Chakrabarti S, Patel KD (2004) p38 MAP kinase regulates rapid matrix metalloproteinase-9 releases from eosinophils. Biochem Biophys Res Commun 315:463–467

Young JD, Peterson CG, Venge P, Cohn ZA (1986) Mechanism of membrane damage mediated by human eosinophil cationic protein. Nature 321:613–616

Yousefi S, Gold JA, Andina N, Lee JJ, Kelly AM, Kozlowski E, Schmid I, Straumann A, Reichenbach J, Gleich GJ, Simon HU (2008) Catapult-like release of mitochondrial DNA by eosinophils contributes to antibacterial defense. Nat Med 14:949–953

Zone JJ, Taylor T, Hull C, Schmidt L, Meyer L (2007) IgE basement membrane zone antibodies induce eosinophil infiltration and histological blisters in engrafted human skin on SCID mice. J Invest Dermatol. 127:1167–1174

Paraneoplastic Syndromes of the Skin

18

Peter Fritsch

What are paraneoplasias?

Paraneoplasias (paraneoplastic signs, syndromes or diseases) are accessory expressions of malignancies which are neither caused directly by the primary tumor itself nor by metastases, but represent distant effects of the neoplastic process. They are thought to be caused by the production of biologically active mediators (hormones, peptides, cytokines), tumor-related immune reactions or metabolic disturbances, or other as yet unidentified mechanisms. Paraneoplasias are a time-honored concept which were first put forward by the neurologist Denny-Brown (Denny-Brown, 1948) and readily accepted by dermatology. Paraneoplasias attracted attention not only because of their potential to provide insight into tumor biology but also because they might make possible the earlier detection of malignant tumors. Paraneoplastic syndromes have been recognized in many fields of medicine, prominently in neurology, hematology, nephrology and endocrinology; in dermatology alone, more than 50 skin signs / diseases have been labeled as paraneoplasias (Callen, 2008; DeWitt et al., 2008; Nguyen et al., 2008).

Fuzziness of the term "paraneoplasia". In the past decades, we have witnessed an enthusiasm in dermatology to unveil new paraneoplasias which led to an undue expansion of this disease group and to a blurring of the concept. Several developments have contributed to confusion:

1. Cause and effects are not always held apart. By definition, the malignancy is the cause of paraneoplasias, and it is not reasonable to use this term for diseases in which malignant tumors may arise due to the disease proper or to common underlying pathomechanisms. So, dermatitis herpetiformis is not a paraneoplasia even if lymphomas of the bowels may arise in the setting of gluten sensitivity. Similarly, systemic scleroderma is not, even if lung cancer may rarely arise in fibrotic lungs, and erythropoietic protoporphyria is not, although hepatic carcinoma may develop.
2. Skin neoplasias should not be called themselves paraneoplasias. So, Bowen´s disease is not, although it may be accompanied by internal malignancies – it is not caused by

these. Paget´s disease of the nipple is not, because it represents the cutaneous extension of an underlying mammary duct carcinoma.

3. Simple signs, particularly if nonspecific, are not good candidates for the paraneoplasias, though they are clearly a valuable help for being aware of internal cancer in the management of skin patients. So, pseudoichthyosis is associated with many diseases leading to malnutrition, including some neoplasms. In others, skin signs may be a direct and expectable effect of the tumor's hormonal activity, such as the flush symptom in carcinoid syndrome, and diffuse hyperpigmentation associated with ACTH-secreting neoplasms (e. g. small cell carcinoma of the lung). Interestingly, hirsutism accompanying ovarian carcinoma has never been included in the paraneoplasia group.

4. Associations which lack a certain degree of statistical likelihood should not be called paraneoplasias. Bullous pemphigoid and herpes zoster are examples in kind, and so is the paraneoplastic subacute cutaneous lupus erythematosus which has been described in very few instances as compared to the general incidence of SCLE.

5. Skin signs which per se may be found both in malignant and non-malignant disease pose the problem of specificity. So, it is often stated in reviews that hypertrichosis lanuginosa acquisita is a paraneoplasia in close to 100% although up to 10 non-malignant conditions are often listed in which excessive hair growth may occur as well.

Criteria for the classification of skin signs as "paraneoplastic". For paraneoplasias, it is obviously the core problem to distinguish between causal relationship vs. by chance coincidence of (internal) neoplasms and skin signs. Helen O. Curth (Curth, 1971) was hitherto the only author to suggest criteria for this distinction: concurrent onset (the neoplasm is detected at the same time as the skin sign or shortly thereafter), parallel course (remissions and recurrences of neoplasm and skin sign occur at approximately the same time), uniform type or site of the causative neoplasm, statistical association and genetic linkage. Curth's criteria are still cited in most reviews; however, only the statistical association and the temporal linkage of paraneoplasias and neoplasms have remained as meaningful and useful parameters. These purely clinical parameters are, of course, flexible and provided for a good deal of ambiguity.

General features of skin paraneoplasias. Most skin paraneoplasias (SP) are rare or very rare conditions which cover a wide spectrum of clinical appearances. Epidemiological data are fragmentary or not existent for most SP; it is evident, though, that most malignancies are not accompanied by SP, making SP rare even for their respective neoplasms. SP may be strongly (up to close to 100%) or weakly linked to malignancies – which led to the distinction of "obligatory" vs. "facultative" SP. In most SP, we know very little on the pathogenesis. SP are often resistant to standard therapeutic measures.

What would be an "ideal" SP? This should be a conspicuous and unmistakable sign, preferably not found otherwise in clinical dermatology – a sign specific for individual tumors or groups of tumors which arises early in the neoplastic process thus allowing timely diagnosis and treatment. This is the case in some instances, but in general the clinical reality differs from this idealized model:

Concurrent onset. Logic dictates that the cause (malignancy) precede the effect (SP). Still, the malignancy may become clinically apparent only months or even years after the emergence of the SP. Conversely, the SP may develop late in the course of the associated neoplasm (e. g. acquired ichthyosis in lymphomas).

Parallel course. It is a cardinal feature of SP that clinical symptoms recede when a remission of the malignancy is accomplished, and recur when the latter relapses. While this is true often enough, it is not invariably the case. Some SP stay on while the neoplasm regresses (e. g. Leser-Trélat, hypertrichosis lanuginosa), or improvement sets in with delay (necrolytic migratory erythema) or remains incomplete (acanthosis nigricans). For SP associated with monoclonal gammopathy, the question of therapeutic intervention does not apply.

Uniqueness of the clinical appearance of SP. The clinical picture of many SP is indeed unambiguous. Nevertheless, the evaluation may be complicated by the fact that these are easy diagnoses but may also arise as non-paraneoplasias. This is best illustrated by acanthosis nigricans which is not linked to malignancy in 80% but to up to 50 different non-malignant conditions, most often insulin resistance and obesity. In obese females suffering from e. g. uterine carcinoma, it may thus be imposible to decide if their acanthosis nigricans is due to obesity or the malignancy. This dilemma has provoked the establishment of categories like "pseudoacanthosis nigricans" or "benign and malignant acanthosis nigricans" but most authors agree that the SP and non-SP variants are fairly indistinguishable, except that, as an SP, acanthosis nigricans tends to develop more rapidly and extensively. Similar quantitative differences exist between SP- and non-SP variants of dermatomyositis, and erythema gyratum repens: this figurate erythema differs from ordinary variants only by the number, extent and migratory rapidity of lesions. The same may be true for the Leser-Trélat sign which is not accepted as a SP by all: it differs from ordinary eruptive seborrheic keratoses only by the enormous amount of lesions and inflammation. In a few instances, an SP may closely resemble other, related entities which are not SP but can be differentiated by laboratory tests: the SP anti-epiligrin pemphigoid is clinically equivalent to other kinds of mucous membrane pemphigoid (but features autoantibodies against epiligrin / laminin-332); paraneoplastic pemphigus resembles severe pemphigus vulgaris (but displays a different autoantibody profile).

"Paraneoplasia without malignancy". For probably all clinical entities, non-SP variants exist parallel to SP variants, even in those SP with an almost 100% association with malignancies (e. g. Bazex syndrome, tripe palms, necrolytic migratory erythema). It is thus tempting to postulate that none of the SP is characterized by completely independent clinical lesions which are not found otherwise (Bazex syndrome may be an exception) – but they are often distinct because of the number and extent of their lesions. Moreover, there is no SP which does not ever arise in the absence of a malignancy.

Specificity of SP for individual malignancies. In very few instances, a specific SP is linked to a specific malignancy (e. g. glucagon producing pancreatic carcinoma and necrolytic migratory erythema); in many, there is a predilection for a distinct group of malignancies, but in others SP can be found linked to many malignancies with little predilection.

Clinical entities

The purpose of this text book is to present the autoimmune diseases of the skin. Only very few of the SP are definite autoimmune dermatoses, the vast majority is not or is linked to ill-defined inflammatory processes which may, of course, include immune mechanisms.

1. "Hyperkeratotic" SP.

This group comprises non-inflammatory SP which are characterized by epidermal hyperplasia. They are thought to be caused by the effects of growth factors.

Acanthosis nigricans (AN) (Fig. 1) is a prototypical SP: it was the first to be described (see 5) and is probably the best known and best documented SP of all. AN is much more often (80:20) associated with nonmalignant conditions (hereditary diseases, endocrinopathies – particularly insulin resistant diabetes, obesity) than with malignancies. As a SP, AN has been found associated with a wide spectrum of tumors, but gastrointestinal, especially gastric adenocarcinomas are the most common (ca 90%): in the latter, AN is found in approximately 1/35 cases compared to only 1/6000 cases in the general cancer population (DeWitt et al., 2008).

AN is a generally non-pruritic symmetric eruption which occupies the large body folds and the neck but may be more widespread in more advanced stages, including face, palms

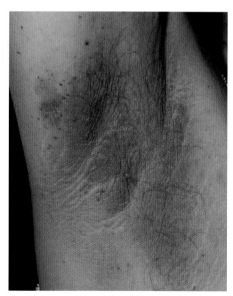

Fig. 1. Acanthosis nigricans: hyperpigmentation, velvety surface and multiple acrochorda of the axillary fold.

18

and soles and even the lips and oral mucosa. The presenting sign is an ill-defined hyper-pigmentation ("dirty neck") in which gradually small and then larger papillomas arise, resulting in a velvety and then irregular texture. Acrochordons and wart-like lesions may develop. Histopathology shows acanthosis, papillomatosis and hyperkeratosis and (at times) increased epidermal melanin. There is no inflammation except in lesions of the oral mucosa and in association with scratching.

The pathogenesis is still unresolved. In "benign" AN, elevated insulin levels are held responsible, in the "malignant" type hypotheses first centered on insulin like growth factors, later on dysregulation of the transforming growth factor α-epidermal growth factor receptor-axis. More recently, activation of epidermal fibroblast growth factor receptor 3 has been put forward – in mice, activating mutations of this receptor result in an AN-like clinical picture.

Removal of the malignancy results in improvement or even resolution of AN. Topical therapies are only moderately effective.

SP related to acanthosis nigricans. "**Tripe palms**" represent an extremely rare SP which coincides in 75% with AN and is considered an analogous process modified by the anatomical individuality of palms and soles. It is characterized by a diffuse thickening of palmar skin with a prominent rugged surface texture due to disproportionately hypertrophic dermatoglyphics (tripe – a simile to the corrugated mucosa of the bovine stomach). As an isolated SP, tripe palms are highly associated with pulmonary carcinoma.

Leser-Trélat sign. This sign is defined as the sudden and massive development of seborrheic keratoses which are often inflamed and pruritic. Excessive numbers of seborrheic keratoses are a commonplace finding in elderly persons, and since large series of patients did not reveal a significant increase in malignancies, the qualification as SP is uncertain. Arguments in favor are a sometimes observed overlap with AN as well as the occurrence in young adults with internal malignancies (mostly of the gastrointestinal tract). The lesions of Leser-Trélat do not readily regress when the malignancy is removed.

Acquired ichthyosis is a not uncommon finding characterized by generalized hyperkeratosis and scaling resembling ichthyosis vulgaris. It occurs most often in malnourished patients in whom dryness of the skin, catabolism due to consuming infectious (HIV!) or other systemic disease, and nutritional and / or hygienic neglect interact. It is no surprise that internal malignancies are among the chief causes of this sign. Acquired ichthyosis can be associated with many types of malignancies, but there is a high predilection for lymphomas, especially Hodgkin's lymphoma. This is again not surprising because Hodgkin's lymphoma often displays dryness of the skin and pruritus sine materia even in its early stages. Acquired ichthyosis arises often late in the disease, but remission can be observed when the malignancy is successfully treated.

Bazex syndrome (acrokeratosis neoplastica, BS) (Fig. 2) is a very rare condition which is possibly the only SP with a unique clinical profile not duplicated by other dermatoses – although it may be confused with psoriasis in its initial stages. BS is both a hyperkeratotic

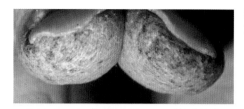

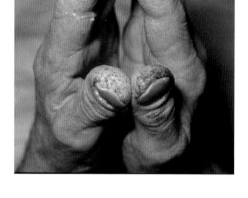

Fig. 2. Acrokeratosis neoplastica Bazex: Hyperkeratotic plaques at the finger tips.

and an inflammatory disorder. It develops typically in men over 50 years and is associated in close to 100% to malignancies, mostly squamous cell carcinomas of the oropharynx or (less common) lung and esophagus.

BS is an erythemato-papulosquamous eruption which symmetrically affects the acral regions (fingers / toes but also nose and ears – clinical hallmark!) and progresses to involve hand and feet (typically sparing the central parts), nails (paronychia, onychodystrophy, onycholysis, ridging) and later the extensor surfaces of the extremities, face and trunk. Lesions are initially erythematous, later hyperkeratotic and scaling and may become erosive and crusted. Bullae arise infrequently (hand and feet). Differential diagnoses include psoriasis, dermatophyte infection and eczema. Histopathology exhibits psoriasiform features, but also epidermal vacuolar degeneration and dyskeratosis, and superficial lymphohistiocytic inflammation.

The pathogenesis is unclear. Hypotheses put forward include immune reactions against epidermal or basement membrane antigens which may cross react with tumor antigens, or a dysbalance of growth factors.

BS tends to arise in the early stages of the underlying malignancy and to regress upon successful removal. Attempts at symptomatic treatment of BS are largely ineffective.

Hypertrichosis lanuginosa acquisita is not a hyperkeratotic SP but it similarly represents a growth stimulus on lanugo hair follicles caused by as not yet identified growth factors. Clinically it is characterized by the sudden appearance of excessively long, fine nonpigmented lanugo hairs, particularly in the face. It has to be distinguished from acquired hypertrichosis in the context of systemic disease (e.g. HIV infection, porphyria cutanea tarda) and from hypertrichosis caused by drugs (e.g. phenytoin, minoxidil, cyclosporine).

18

As a SP, it tends to arise late in the course of the neoplasm (most often of the lungs and colon, but a variety of other tumors have been recorded).

2. Inflammatory paraneoplasias of the skin

Erythema gyratum repens (EGR) (Fig. 3) is a "classic" SP which formally belongs to the group of figurate erythemas. Its hallmark are thus polycyclic macular and urticarial lesions which enlarge (migrate) and may display scaling on their inner slopes. It is not the morphology of the lesions, however, which sets EGR apart from all other types of figurate erythemas but their enormous number and their relatively quick concentric migration (ca 1 cm / day). There results a distinctive picture of parallel serpiginous lines and bands ("wood grain design") which may cover most of the body except the acral areas and face. EGR may be very pruritic. Histopathology is nonspecific.

The appearance of EGR is striking and distinct, but localized as well as atypical forms have been described in which the characteristic array of lesions is absent. In such cases, differential diagnosis from other types of e. g. erythroderma, erythema anulare centrifugum, pityriasis rubra pilaris, subacute cutaneous lupus erythematosus and others may be difficult. It is therefore surprising that EGR is said to be associated with internal malignancies in 80% – most commonly lung cancer, but many other types of malignancy have been recorded as well. EGR should thus qualify as an "obligatory" SP, but many instances have been reported where no malignancy was found, or where it was linked to "benign diseases", such as tuberculosis, pregnancy and bullous dermatoses. As a SP, EGR tends to develop months before the malignancy becomes manifest. It occurs predominantly in persons over 60 years and in males (2:1). It improves with removal of the tumor, but is resistant to symptomatic therapy.

The pathogenesis of EGR is unclear. IgG and C3 deposits have been detected by immunofluorescence and electron microscopy at the epidermal basement membrane in instances (Letko et al., 2007), but the significance of these findings remains to be elucidated.

Necrolytic migratory erythema (Glucagonoma syndrome, NME) (Fig. 4). NME is an exceptional SP because it is characterized by a highly typical clinical and histopathological appearance and by a typical profile of laboratory values, is highly specifically associated

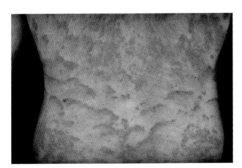

Fig. 3. Erythema gyratum repens: Figurate erythemas of the trunk with concentric migration pattern.

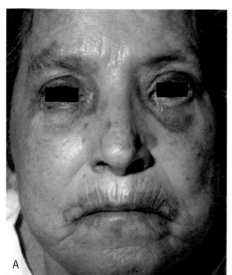

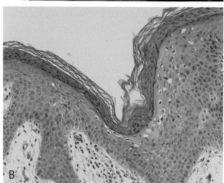

Fig. 4. A. Necrolytic migratory erythema in glucagonoma syndrome: erythematous and erosive lesions of the periorbital and perioral regions. **B.** Necrolytic migratory erythema (chronic lesion): vacuolization and dyskeratotic keratinocytes of the upper spinous layer, parakeratosis.

with glucagon producing pancreatic islet tumors, and its pathogenesis is fairly well understood.

NME is a very rare SP, occurs in persons well in their second half of life and has no gender predilection. It is a systemic disease which usually presents with weight loss, malaise, weakness, neuropsychiatric disturbances, diabetes and diarrhea. Skin signs include tender dermatitis-like erythematous patches with occasional blistering, erosions and crusts which appear in the groins, anogenital areas (where painful fissures may arise) and buttocks, in the distant extremities and in the face with a predilection for the perioral region. The lesions tend to expand to large areas with pronounced circinate borders. Oral lesions include stomatitis, atrophic glossitis and angular cheilitis. Histopathology displays dyskeratosis and necrosis in the upper Malpighian layers, neutrophilic infiltration and a psoriasiform reaction of the epidermis (parakeratosis, loss of the granular layer). Prominent laboratory signs include hyperglycemia, often excessively high glucagon serum levels, normochromic anemia, abnormal liver function tests and low levels of serum amino acids, total protein, and often zinc deficiency.

The pathogenesis appears to be predominantly due to metabolic disturbances (Dewitt, 2008). Glucagon has been shown to use up tissue pools of amino acids (histidine, tryptophan) by stimulating gluconeogenesis and amino acid oxidation. Epidermal protein deficiency develops and in turn leads to necrosis of the upper stratum spinosum, producing eroded erythematous lesions. Diarrhea and malabsorption often result in deficiencies of vitamins (B2, B3, B6), zinc, and essential fatty acids. The resulting clinical image is a composite of the complex nutritional dysregulation. A number of other entities may mimic the dermatological and systemic symptoms of NME in the absence of an islet cell tumor ("pseudoglucagonoma syndrome"): pancreatitis, acquired zinc deficiency syndrome, inflammatory bowel disease, pellagra and others. These entities must be considered in the differential diagnosis; the glucagonoma must be verified or ruled out by imaging techniques. The dermatological differential diagnosis is particularly important because NME in its early stages may be easily mistaken as intertrigo, seborrheic dermatitis or candidiasis.

Complete removal of the glucagonoma results in remission of NME. Although NME often arises in late stages, surgical reduction of the tumor load may still lead to improvement. In contrast to many other SP, conservative treatment of NME may lead to amelioration (correction of nutritional deficiencies, administration of the glucagon antagonist somatostatin).

3. Collagen vascular diseases

Dermatomyositis is a classic complex disease entity which is covered extensively in Chapter 6. It is also a classic SP in adult patients – its risk of association with internal malignancies is estimated at 25–30%, most often with breast and ovarian cancer in females, and colonic and pulmonary cancer in males – but a host of other underlying neoplasms have been reported. Females are involved more often and succumb to the disease more frequently than males. The signs of dermatomyositis are usually the presenting complaints; neoplasms already may be detectable in about 20% but may also become manifest years later. Regular cancer screening is therefore recommended for several years. Following removal of the malignancy, dermatomyositis remits but relapses when metastatic disease develops.

Considerable pains have been taken to better identify the subgroups most prone for association with cancer. It is generally agreed that the adult but not the juvenile type of dermatomyositis qualifies as a SP. Similarly, polymyositis and amyopathic dermatomyositis are not significantly linked to neoplastic disease. Clinical symptomatology and laboratory profile of dermatomyositis is the same for both SP and non-SP varieties, except that the former may be more severe and progress more rapidly.

It is unclear by which mechanisms malignancies trigger the symptoms of dermatomyositis.

Lupus erythematosus and systemic scleroderma. Both disease entities are not generally considered as SP although anecdotal reports exist to suggest such association.

Several cases of subacute cutaneous LE (but not of systemic or chronic discoid LE) have been described in association with internal malignancies (Trüeb et al., 1999). In all, the courses of LE and of the tumor (most often pulmonary carcinomas) were parallel.

There appears to exist a certain tendency in advanced systemic scleroderma with respiratory tract involvement to develop lung cancer and cancer of the tongue. Such statistical association is not supported by large series, and is very low at any rate (3%) but may be significant for cancer of the tongue. There is nothing to suggest, though, that the scleroderma is caused by these cancers as the definition of a SP would require.

Paraneoplastic vasculitis. Necrotizing cutaneous vasculitis as a SP is an old paradigm which is referred to in many reviews. The incidence appears to be very low (less than 2%) and is supported by anecdotal evidence mainly. It is most often encountered in patients with paraproteinemia (multiple myeloma) or lympho / myeloproliferative disorders (e. g. hairy cell leukemia), occasionally with a variety of solid tumors. The relationship between neoplasms and the putative SP is tenuous in many instances; the mechanisms operative are immune complex formation and deposition.

Paraneoplastic vasculitis should be differentiated from paraneoplastic Raynaud syndrome and paraneoplastic acral vascular syndrome (Poszepczynska-Guine et al., 2002).

4. Autoimmune bullous diseases

Paraneoplastic pemphigus (PNP) is fully covered in Chapter 3.1. PNP appears to be a truly "obligatory" paraneoplasia which is linked to just a small number of lymphoproliferative neoplasms: NHL, chronic lymphocytic leukemia, thymoma and, most notably, to Castleman disease (16% of PNP – particularly in pediatric cases). Association with solid tumors is exceptionally rare. Interestingly, the courses of PNP and of the underlying malignancy are not well correlated. PNP may arise prior to or following the emergence of the malignancy. Treatment of the latter does not always or markedly improve the skin symptoms, and pulmonary involvement (see below) may persist despite tumor eradication. One exception is apparently the Castleman tumor which is found most often in young patients: if of the solitary type, the chances of complete elimination are high, and a complete remission of PNP does ensue.

PNP is considerably rarer than pemphigus vulgaris, but its actual incidence is not known. Clinical hallmark is a severely inflammatory and extensive involvement of the oral mucosa which does not respond well to conventional treatment. The clinical appearance is more polymorphous than that of pemphigus vulgaris: blisters, multiforme-like erythemas and lichenoid lesions are found. Histopathology mirrors this polymorphous character by exhibiting acantholysis, lichenoid and interphase changes.

PNP is caused by pathogenic IgG autoantibodies against desmogleins 1 and 3. In addition, antibodies are found against proteins of the plakin family (such as desmoplakin and others). Direct immunofluorescence shows intercellular IgG and complement deposits, and complement deposits at the junction zone. As a unique feature, the antibodies do not bind to epidermal antigens only but also to simple columnar or transitional epithelia (such as in the rat bladder which is used as a diagnostic substrate). The pathogenesis is not fully elucidated. In addition to autoantibodies, cellular immune reactions are likely to be

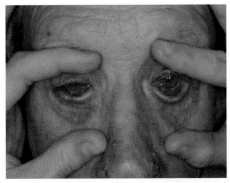

Fig. 5. Mucous membrane pemphigoid: Different stages of progressive conjuctival involvement with end stage symblepharon

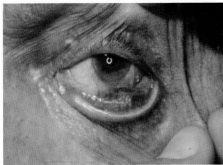

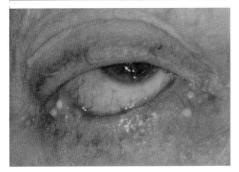

involved in the formation of lichenoid and multiforme-like lesions. In the newborn mouse model, injection of antibody produces only acantholysis. Recently, dysregulated secretion of IL-6 (which is known for its capacity to drive immunoglobulin production) has been considered as a main causative factor. Serum IL-6 is highly elevated in PNP; Castleman tumors and some subsets of CLL and NHL have been shown to produce high amounts of this cytokine.

PNP is in 40% complicated by pulmonary involvement (bronchiolitis obliterans) which may be a cause of death. As a skin disease, PNP is very resistant to traditional therapeutic regimens, and the patients are troubled and incapacitated by the painful PNP lesions.

Antiepiligrin cicatricial pemphigoid (AECP) (Fig. 5) is a relatively rare but distinct subset of mucous membrane pemphigoid which is defined by tissue specific pathogenic autoantibodies against laminin 332 (formerly laminin 5). An increased risk of internal cancer (RR 6,8) (Egan et al., 2001) has been determined which is not shared by the other subtypes of mucous membrane pemphigoid caused by autoantibodies against the ß4integrin subunit (Letko et al., 2007).The malignancies involved are predominantly solid tumors of the respiratory and digestive tract, occasionally lymphoproliferative disorders. AECP tends to arise only shortly before the neoplasm is detected, and the courses of SP and tumor prove largely parallel.

Patient sera contain circulating IgG antibodies which are bound to the dermal side of NaCl split human skin; in immunoblot, they prove reactive with the α subunit of laminin 332. AECP is clinically indistinguishable from other types of cicatricial pemphigoid except for a higher tendency for skin involvement.

Laminin 332, previously termed epiligrin or laminin 5, is a major adhesive component of the epidermal basement membrane. It is localized to the border between the lamina lucida and lamina densa and has been shown by immunoelectron microscopy to form a link between anchoring filaments and the lamina densa and the anchoring fibrils beneath. Laminin 332 and/or its subunits are highly expressed in a variety of human cancers and appear to play a relevant role in cancer biology. Tumor cells are capable of regulating the activity of laminin 332 by proteolytic processing; cleavage of laminin 332 down-regulates their adhesive activities but up-regulates cell locomotion (Sadler et al., 2007).

5. Neutrophilic dermatoses

Sweet syndrome (SS) is a not infrequent classical acute, relapsing dermatosis which is characterized by acute fever, blood neutrophilia, distinct (papular, erythematous, vesicle-like) skin lesions and variable involvement of internal organs. Histologically, SS exhibits a dense diffuse neutrophilic infiltrate of the upper dermis and massive edema. The classical type of SS is triggered by a variety of infections; the malignancy-associated type (approximately 20% of cases) is most often found with acute myelocytic leukemia, less often with myelodysplastic syndrome, other types of leukemias and lymphomas (Buck et al., 2008). An association with solid tumors is exceptional. Clinical features of the malignancy-associated SS do not differ clearly from those of the classic type; there is no female preponderance, however, and the frequency of relapses may be increased. The pathophysiology is not well understood, a disturbance of cytokine regulation (particularly of GMCSF) has been considered (Cohen et al., 2007).

Pyoderma gangrenosum (PG) is likewise a not infrequent classical dermatosis featuring dense neutrophilic infiltrates of the skin which, however, lead to the necrotic breakdown of the affected tissue. The resulting ulcers are excessively painful and tend to enlarge rapidly. PG is associated with other systemic diseases in more than half of the cases, including arthritis, inflammatory bowel disease, monoclonal gammopathy (IgA, up to 20%) and various, predominantly hematologic malignancies (10–20%, acute myeloid leukemia, multiple myeloma). Interestingly, malignancy-associated PG often becomes manifest as "atypical", i.e. bullous PG, the most acute clinical subset of PG. The pathophysiology of PG is unclear. It appears to be a candidate for the newly established disease category of "autoinflammatory syndromes".

6. Paraneoplasias associated with plasma cell dyscrasia and monoclonal gammopathy

POEMS syndrome (PS) (Fig. 6) is a uncommon complex multisystem disorder with prominent skin involvement. It represents a monoclonal plasma cell proliferative disorder (most often IgG κ light chain), is in close to 100% linked to osteosclerotic myeloma and often (10–20%) associated with Castleman disease. It differs from monoclonal gam-

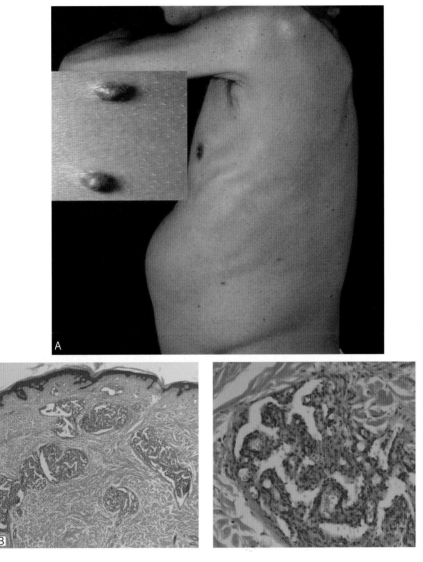

Fig. 6. **A**. POEMS syndrome: hyperpigmentation, ascites and glomeruloid hemangiomas (inset). **B**. Glomeruloid hemangiomas: vascular channels resembling the architecture of renal glomeruli.

mopathy of unknown significance (MGUS), one of its main differential diagnoses, by the nature of the paraprotein (IgG λ light chain in MGUS) and its clinical expression: MGUS is asymptomatic for long periods of time, whereas PS displays prominent end organ damage. POEMS is an acronym for the main clinical features (P – polyneuropathy, O – organomegaly, E – endocrinopathy, M – monoclonal gammopathy, S – skin changes); to this list, however, a number of other important symptoms must be added: edema (pleural effusion, ascites), pulmonary hypertension and restrictive lung disease, arthralgias, cardiomyopathy, thrombocytosis and thrombotic diathesis, polycythemia and others. Elevated levels of VEGF, TNFα, IL-1 and IL-6 are regularly found, the levels correlating with disease activity (Dispenzieri, 2005).

Skin changes are seen in 50–90% of patients: diffuse hyperpigmentation, hypertrichosis, skin thickening and formation of "glomeruloid" hemangiomas – a type of capillary angioma which clinically resembles senile angiomas, but differs histologically with vascular channels resembling renal glomeruli. Glomeruloid hemangiomas are considered diagnostic for PS; not surprisingly, they may also occur at times in healthy individuals and those with unrelated conditions (Lee et al., 2008).

VEGF is thought to play a major role in the pathogenesis of PS. It could at least explain some of the skin changes, organomegaly and edema formation, possibly also neuropathy (myelin edema and non-compacted myelin lamellae are a characteristic abnormality in POEMS) (Vallat et al., 2008).

PS sets in usually around 50 years of age. Presenting signs are most often a peripheral sensory / motor polyneuropathy and endocrine dysfunction (diabetes, hypothyroidism, erectile dysfunction). PS is a chronic disease but can less often take a fulminant course. The median survival time in a large series has been found 13.8 years (Dipenzieri et al., 2003). Main causes of death are cardiorespiratory failure, infection, capillary leak syndrome and inanition, but interestingly not progression to multiple myeloma. Treatment focuses on radiation therapy to eliminate Castleman disease and osteosclerotic myeloma; medical treatment rests on chemotherapy (cyclophosphamide, melphalan, corticosteroids). Recently, autologous hematopoietic stem cell transplantation and the anti-VEGF monoclonal antibody bevacizumab have proved highly effective (Dipenzieri et al., 2003).

Schnitzler syndrome (SchS) is a relatively new acquisition (Schnitzler L, 1972) to the realm of paraneoplasias which appears to be fairly rare with around 100 published cases. SchS is characterized by two major criteria (chronic urticaria with often daily eruptions, and monoclonal gammopathy, most frequently IgM κ), and a number of minor criteria (intermittent fever, arthralgias and bone pain, hepato / splenomegaly, lymphadenopathy, radiologically demonstrable bone densities, leuko- and thrombocytosis) (DeKoning et al., 2007; Claes K et al., 2008). Bence Jones protein is found in up to 30% of cases. SchS markedly affects the quality of life due to pruritus (which may be mild at the beginning), bone pains, fever, fatigue and weakness, but the life expectancy is not significantly reduced when compared with the general population (DeKoning et al., 2007). In the course of SchS, however, lymphoproliferative diseases may develop with an estimated 10 years risk of 15% (or possibly more, most often Waldenström macroglobulinemia, more rarely IgM myeloma or B cell lymphomas). The risk for amyloidosis A is increased (DeKoning et al., 2007; Claes K et al., 2008).

The diagnosis of SchS is principally one of exclusion (for differential diagnoses see DeKoning et al., 2007). The urticarial lesions do not differ much from those of plain urticaria (though they may persist somewhat longer, are mainly located on the trunk and are not accompanied by angioedema); histopathology is non-contributory. Immunofluorescence revealed paraprotein deposits at the dermoepidermal junction zone and in dermal capillaries in a subset of cases (but such deposits are found in Waldenström disease as well where no wheals are formed). Circulating IL-6 levels and IL-1 secretion from PBMC were found increased. Although various autoantibodies were discovered, an autoimmune basis for the disease is not evident.

The pathogenesis of SchS was enigmatic for long time and is still not fully elucidated. Some features, however, are parallel to some of the hereditary periodic fever syndromes, now included in the so called autoinflammatory diseases group (Masters et al., 2009). This disease category is characterized by generalized inflammation (e. g. fever, skin rashes, arthritis) without evidence of infection, high-titer autoantibodies or autoreactive T cells. They are thus considered not a dysregulation of the adaptive but of the innate immune system, caused by mutations in various relevant genes, e. g. the TNF-αR gene or the NLRP3 gene which encodes NALP3 (cryopyrin) – an intracellular pattern recognition receptor mediating monocyte and macrophage IL-1ß secretion. SchS is a disease of advanced age, getting manifest at average at 50 years, whereas the fever syndromes are of neonatal onset. SchS was therefore hypothesized to be an (acquired?) autoinflammatory disease, with IL-1ß playing a major pathophysiological role (DeKoning et al., 2007; Eiling et al., 2007a). Recently, a gain-of-function mutation in the NLRP3 gene was described in one patient with SchS and in 4 asymptomatic first degree relatives, suggesting an hereditary basis for SchS as well – possibly representing a genetic predisposition which needs a second factor to trigger disease manifestation (Loock et al., 2010).

Previous efforts to treat SchS with traditional methods, including corticosteroids, interferon, colchicine and many others, were disappointing. In contrast, the IL-1 receptor blocker anakinra results in rapid and complete symptom relief, just as in the cryopyrin-associated periodic fever syndromes (Schuster et al., 2009; Eiling et al., 2007b).

Scleromyxedema (Fig. 7) is the systemic form of lichen myxedematosus, a rare syndrome characterized by mucin deposits in the skin leading to a scleroderma-like induration (face, upper extremities); deposits are less marked in internal organs (coronary vessels, kidneys, peripheral nerves and others). It is a slowly progressive incapacitating disorder which is associated with a monoclonal gammopathy (IgG λ light chain) in up to 80%. Myeloma (or much more rarely other lymphoproliferative diseases) develop in less than 10%. The pathophysiology of the disease is unclear.

Normolipemic diffuse plane xanthoma is a rare non-Langerhans cell histiocytosis characterized by flat yellow plaques predominantly of the face. It is frequently (but not always) associated with monoclonal gammopathies (IgG) and has been reported in myeloma and other lymphoproliferative disorders. It is believed that paraproteins and lipoproteins form complexes which are taken up by the histiocytes.

Necrobiotic xanthogranuloma is likewise a rare instance of a non-Langerhans cell histiocytosis which is characterized by papulonodular lesions predominantly of the face (espe-

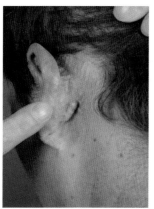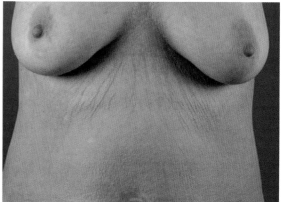

Fig. 7. Scleromyxedema: pearl-like arrangement of indurated opaque papules retroauricularly and on the abdomen.

cially periorbital region) with a tendency to become atrophic and/or ulcerated. Histopathology shows a granulomatous infiltration of inflammatory cells, foam cells and Touton giant cells, with sharply delineated necrotic areas. It is associated in 80% with a monoclonal gammopathy (most often IgG κ). Myeloma arises in 10% of patients, less often Hodgkin or non-Hodgkin lymphomas. The pathogenesis is unclear.

Amyloidosis L (AL) is a classic systemic disease in which amyloid chains are formed from monoclonal immunoglobulin light chains (VL domain). AL is thus linked to plasma cell dyscrasias and can occur in any of them. The incidence is highest in subjects with MGUS (80%); in myeloma, amyloid L deposits occur in about 15%.

Cryoglobulinemia type I is characterized by the presence of a single monoclonal immunoglobulin (IgM or IgG) with the properties of cryoglobulins, i.e. precipitation in cold temperatures. It is almost always associated with hematologic malignancies, in particular with multiple myeloma or B-cell lymphomas. Dermatological expressions, if any, are Raynaud syndrome, acrocyanosis, and a noninflammatory occlusive arteriopathy leading to purpura, necroses and at times gangrene, most often of the lower leg. In contrast, type II mixed cryoglobulinemia typically presents as cutaneous necrotizing vasculitis; it may be associated with a number of systemic disorders (connective tissue and hepatic diseases, infections), among these lymphoproliferative diseases.

7. Miscellaneous

Acquired C1 esterase inhibitor dysfunction has been described in a few instances of systemic lymphoproliferative disease, monoclonal gammopathy and lupus erythematosus.

Multicentric reticulohistiocytosis (MRH) is an uncommon member of the non-Langerhans cell histiocytoses group. It is characterized by mucocutaneous papulonodular lesions, predominantly of the fingers and hands, more rarely of the face, arms and legs, by severe arthritis (hands or, more infrequently, the large joints) and variable involvement of internal organs (muscles, cardiopulmonary and respiratory systems, eyes and thyroid gland). Presenting sign is often severe polyarthritis, accompanied by systemic symptoms (fever, weight loss, weakness). The cutaneous lesions of MRH may remit spontaneously; joint involvement may become stable but leads to progressive destruction in up to 50%. MRH may be associated with autoimmune diseases and chronic infections. It is also associated in up to 30% with internal malignancies of various kinds (often pulmonary and breast carcinomas). MRH would thus certainly qualify as a paraneoplasia, but surprisingly, there is no indication for a parallel course with the given malignancy.

Thrombophlebitis migrans (Trousseau syndrome, TS) was the first paraneoplasia to be described (Trousseau et al., 1865) and still is, at the same time, one of the most relevant and practically important associations of internal malignancies. Unfortunately, there is some blurring of terminology (Varki, 2007): clinical hallmark of the syndrome is the recurring nature of superficial and deep phlebothrombosis (often complicated by pulmonary embolism), which leads to the impression of a migratory process. Later, it was recognized that TS often encompasses the features of chronic disseminated intravascular coagulation, including platelet-rich microthrombi, microangiopathic hemolytic anemia, verrucous endocarditis and thromboembolic events (Sacket al., 1977). Today, the term is often used as a synonym for malignancy-associated hypercoagulability in general. It should be reserved, however, for thromboses emerging while the neoplasm is still occult – because in more advanced stages, multiple additional factors appear which may promote blood coagulation (infections, chemotherapy, dehydration, mechanical factors and others).

Venous thromboembolic events (VTE) are the second leading cause of death in malignant disease. There is an overall 7x increased relative risk for VTE across all types of malignant neoplasms (Sack et al., 1977). It is higher for specific malignancies (gastrointestinal, pancreatic, pulmonary, renal, ovarian, and brain) and runs as high as 28x for hematological disorders. The risk is markedly increased around the time of detection of the neoplasm and in metastatic disease, and it is additionally considerably higher in patients undergoing surgery, chemotherapy, antiangiogenetic and hormonal therapy.

Multiple mechanisms may be (and usually are) involved in creating a thrombophilic milieu in cancer patients, and many of them are operative well before the neoplasm is detected, as e. g. shown by the elevation of coagulation activity markers (fibrinopeptides, D-dimer and others) (Noble and Pasi, 2010). The mechanisms overlap and may specifically shape the risk profile and clinical course in individual neoplasms. Many originate from the phenotypic changes of the tumor cells proper, consequent to oncogene (ras, EGFR, C-MET, HER-2) or tumor suppressor gene mutations (p53, PTEN) (Rak et al., 2006). Cancer cells produce substances with procoagulant, antifibrinolytic (plasminogen activator inhibitor) and profibrinolytic as well as proaggregating activities; they release proinflammatory (TNFα) and pro-angiogenic cytokines (VEGF), and they interact with the host vascular cells and blood cells via adhesion molecules.

One of the most important and probably longest known procoagulant mediators produced by cancer cells is tissue factor (TF), the initiator of the extrinsic coagulation pathway. TF is constitutively expressed by cancer cells; in addition to its local action, it may be released from cancer cells as TF-laden vesicles. Other relevant cancer cell activities are: the expression of the tumor coagulant – a cysteine protease only expressed in malignant tissue which directly activates factor X; deficient activity of von Willebrand factor cleaving proteases; down-regulation of thrombomodulin and thrombospondin.

Importantly, VTE and tumor progression are linked in a two-way association – the procoagulant milieu enhances tumor growth and metastasis formation (promotion of tumor angiogenesis, mitogenesis, migration, "sealing off" of tumors etc). Several mechanisms have been detected, the most relevant being linked to TF expression.

Treatment of TS is directed at the management of the VTE and the elimination of the malignancy. For the former, anticoagulation therapy with unfractionated heparin is recommended (Varki, 2007) in view of its broad biological activities which may be more suited in dealing with a multifaceted coagulation disturbance than low molecular weight heparins. Screening for occult neoplasms is mandatory in any event of spontaneous ("unprovoked") VTE. Not surprisingly, the likelihood to detect undiagnosed malignancies is higher the more extensive the screening is (Carrier et al., 2008) – which does not answer the question up to which point of diagnostic endeavors the criteria of improvement of quality of life and / or cost-effectiveness are met.

Summary

Cutaneous paraneoplasias include a number of dermatoses which are associated in a variable degree with internal malignancies. They are a very heterogenous group of diseases, differing greatly in their clinical appearance and pathogenesis (which is not well understood in most of them). Most of the paraneoplasias are very rare. Some of the more recently described entities promise a better insight in the mechanisms of cancer pathophysiology. Dermatology has taken a keen interest in the paraneoplasias, particularly because of the expectation that they may lead to earlier detection of malignancies at a time when they are more likely to be curable.

References

Buck T, González LM, Lambert C, Schwartz RA (2008) Sweet's syndrome with hematologic disorders: a review and reappraisal. Int J Dermatol 47:775–782

Callen JP (2008) Dermatologic manifestations in patients with systemic disease. In: Bolognia JL, Jorizzo JL, Rapini RP (eds): Dermatology, 2nd Edition, Elsevier, 675–692

Carrier M, Le Gal G, Wells PS, Ferguson D, Ramsay T, Rodger MA (2008) Systematic review: the Trousseau syndrome revisited: should we screen extensively for cancer in patients with venous thromboembolism? Ann Intern Med 149:323–333

Caux F, Ebbe C, Thomine E, Benyahia B, Flageul B, Joly P, Rybojad M, Morel P (1994) Erythema gyratum repens. A case studied with immunofluorescence, immunoelectron microscopy and immunohistochemistry. Br J Dermatol 131:102–107

Claes K, Bammens B, Delforge M, Evenepoel P, Kuypers D, Vanrenterghem Y (2008) Another devastating complication of the Schnitzler syndrome: AA amyloidosis. Brit J Dermatol 158:182–184

Cohen PR (2007) Sweet´s syndrome – a comprehensive review of an acute febrile neutrophilic dermatosis. Orphanet J Rare Dis 2:34–68

Curth HO (1971) Cutaneous manifestations associated with malignant internal diseases. In: Fitzpatrick TB, Arndt KA, Clark WH Jr, Eisen AZ, Van Scott EJ, Vaughan JH (eds): Dermatology in General Medicine 1st Edition (McGraw-Hill, New York), 1561–81

De Koning HD, Bodar EJ, can der Meer JWM, Simon A (2007): Schnitzler syndrome: beyond the case reports: review and follow-up of 94 patients with an emphysis on prognosis and treatment. Semin Arthritis Rheum 37, 137–148

Denny-Brown DE (1948) Primary sensory neuropathy with muscular changes associated with carcinoma. J Neurol, Neurosurg and Psych, 11:73–87

DeWitt CA, Buescher LS, Stone SP (2008) Cutaneous manifestations of internal malignant disease: cutaneous paraneoplastic syndromes. In: Wolff K, Goldsmith LA, Gilchrest BA, Paller AS, Leffell DJ (eds): Fitzpatrick's Dermatology in General Medicine, 7th Edition, McGrawHill, 1493–1507

Dispenzieri A, Kyle RA, Lacy MQ (2003) POEMS syndrome: definitions and long-term outcome. Blood 101:2496–2506

Dispenzieri A, Moreno-Aspitia A, Suarez GA, Lacy MQ, Colon-Otero G, Tefferi A, Litzow MR, Roy V, Hogan W, Kyle RA, Gertz MA (2004): Peripheral blood stem cell transplantationin 16 patients with POEMS syndrome, and a review of the literature. Blood 104:3400–3407

Dispenzieri A (2005) POEMS syndrome. Hematology 2005:360–367

Egan CA, Lazarova E, Darling TN, Yee C, Coté T, Yancey KB (2001) Anti-epiligrin cicatricial pemphigoid and relative risk for cancer. Lancet 357:1850–1851

Eiling E, Möller M, Kreiselmaier I, Brasch J, Schwarz T (2007) Schnitzler syndrome: treatment failure to rituximab but response to anakinra. J Am Acad Dermatol 57:361–364

Lee H, Meier FH, Ma CK, Ormsby AH, Lee MW (2008) Eosinophilic globules in 3 cases of glomeruloid hemangioma of the head and neck: a characteristic offering more evidence for thanatosomes with or without POEMS. Am J Dermatopathol 30:539–544

Letko E, Gürcan HM, Papaliodis GN, Christen W, Foster CS, Ahmed AR (2007): Relative risk for cancer in mucous membrane pempohigoid associated with antibodies to the ß4 integrin subunit. Clin Exp Dermatol 32:637–641

Lipsker D, Veran Y, Grunenberger F, Cribier B, Heid E, Grosshans E (2001): The Schnitzler syndrome: four new cases and review of the literature. Medicine 80:37–44

Loock J, Lamprecht P, Timmann C, Mrowietz U, Csermak E, Gross WL (2010): Genetic predisposition (NLRP3 V198M mutation) for IL-1 mediated inflammation in a patient with Schnitzler syndrome. J Allergy Clin Immunol 125:500–502

Masters SL, Simon A, Aksentijevich I, Kastner DL (2009) Horror autoinflammaticus: the molecular pathophysiology of autoinflammatorty disease Ann Rev Immunol 27:621–668

Nguyen VQ, Levin WJ, Raugi GJ (2008) Paraneoplastic diseases. E Medicine Dermatology, Internal Medicine

Noble S, Pasi J (2010) Epidemiology and pathophysiology of cancer-associated thrombosis. Br J Cancer 102: S2–S9

Poszepczynska-Guiné E, Viguier M, Chosido O, Orcel B, Emmerich J, Dubertret L (2002) Paraneoplastic acral vascular syndrome: epidemiologic features, clinical manifestations, and disease sequelae. J Am Acad Dermatol 47:47–52

Rak J, Yu JL, Luyendyk J, Mackman N (2006) Oncogenes, Trousseau syndrome, and cancer-related changes in the coagulome of mice and humans. Cancer Res 66:10643–10646

Sack GH, Levin J, Bell WR Trousseau's syndrome and other manifestations of chronic disseminated coagulopathy in patients with neoplasms: cilinical, pathophysiologic, and therapeutic features (1977). Medicine 56:1–37

Sadler E, Lazarova Z, Sarasombath, Yancey KB (2007): A widening perspective regarding the relationship between anti-epiligrin cicatricial pemphigoid and cancer. J Dermatol Science 47:1–7

Schnitzler L (1972): Lésions urticarienne chroniques permanentes (érythéme pétaloide?). Case clinique n. 46B. Journée Dermatologique d'Angers 1972, Oct. 28 (abstr. 46)

Schuster C, Kränke B, Aberer E, Arbab E, Sturm G, Aberer W (2009): Schnitzler syndrome: response to anakinra in two cases and a review of the literature. Internat J Dermatol 48:1190–1194

Trousseau, A (1865) Phlegmasia alba dolens. Lectures in clinical medicine, delivered at the Hotel-Dieu, Paris 5:381–232

Trüeb RF, Trüeb RM (1999) Paraneoplastic subacute cutaneous lupus erythematosus: example of cutaneous paraneoplasias as an immunologic phenomenon. Praxis 88:1803–1810

Vallat JM, Magy L. Richard L, Sturtz F, Couratier P (2008) Contribution of electron microscopy to the study of neuropathies associated with an IgG monoclonal paraproteinemia. Micron 39:61–70

Varki A (2007) Trousseau's syndrome: multiple definitions and multiple mechanisms. Blood 110:1723–1729

Targeted Therapies in Autoimmune and Inflammatory Skin Disorders

Rüdiger Eming and Ingo H. Tarner

Introduction

Autoimmune diseases represent the clinical manifestation of a complex dysregulation of immune mechanisms and regulatory networks finally resulting in loss of self-tolerance. In recent years the principal insight into underlying immune processes has greatly advanced. Novel therapeutic strategies in autoimmunity aim at specifically targeting defined cellular and humoral components of the immune system, thus trying to reduce severe side effects and comorbidity which currently arise from broad unspecific high-dose immunosuppressive therapies. Due to a more defined understanding of basic immune mechanisms shaping the complex network of chronic inflammation and autoimmunity, these diseases have attracted a plethora of promising therapies targeting a variety of cell surface molecules, soluble mediators and intracellular proteins that are of importance for the function of immune cells. Monoclonal antibodies directed against defined receptors on the surface mostly of B-lymphocytes and to a lesser extent of T-lymphocytes as well as soluble receptor fusion proteins interfering with important inflammatory mediators, such as tumor necrosis factor alpha, have been the dominant tools recently applied in various autoimmune and chronic inflammatory disorders. Moreover, stem cell therapy and small molecule inhibitors are being validated in clinical trials for the treatment of different autoimmune disease. This chapter aims at providing a concise review of the most recent developments and their corresponding clinical translation in dermatological diseases and closely related rheumatic autoimmune disorders.

Antigen Specific Approaches for the Therapy of Autoimmune Diseases

The majority of therapies approved for autoimmune diseases involve global immunosuppressive and immunoregulatory strategies, respectively, inhibiting inflammatory (auto)immune processes. Although partly effective in controlling autoimmune dysregulation, these drugs harbour numerous side effects leading to severe comorbidity and thus continous immunosuppressive therapy is mostly not feasible. So far, none of the currently applied therapies in autoimmunity has been able to induce long-term, drug-free remission in any auto-immune disease. In this context, over the past decades great emphasis has been placed on therapeutical efforts to restore immune tolerance in autoimmune disorders. A highly de-sired alternative approach is the attempted induction of antigen-specific tolerance to the respective autoantigen. However, precise knowledge about the molecular and cellular tar-gets of the autoimmune response are mandatory to design new and more specific strategies in a given autoimmune disorder. However, recent studies revealed that here are numer-ous pitfalls and limitations to the translation of preclinical findings to the clinic (Luo et al., 2010). The following section will focus on the clinically most advanced strategies, that have recently concentrated on autoimmune diabetes mellitus (type 1 DM) and multiple sclero-sis (MS) (St Clair, 2009).

Therapy by Autoantigen Administration

In type 1DM, glutamic acid decarboxylase (GAD) and insulin have been identified as ma-jor autoantigens (Miller et al., 2007). The Diabetes Prevention Trial demonstrated that in relatives of patients with type 1DM who are at high risk of developing type 1DM, neither treatment with oral insulin nor subcutaneous insulin injection prevented a delayed the on-set of diabetes compared with controls (Diabetes Prevention Trial-Type 1 Diabetes Study Group, 2002; Skyler et al., 2005). The authors discussed several reasons for the lack of ef-fect in these two prevention studies, such as different dosing schemes and therapy regi-mens (Diabetes Prevention Trial-Type 1 Diabetes Study Group, 2002; Skyler et al., 2005). Thrower et al. conducted a first-in-man phase I safety study using an HLA-DR4-restricted proinsulin epitope for intradermal administration in a total of 36 type 1 DM patients (Thrower et al., 2008). The peptide was injected at two different doses (30 µg vs 300 µg; $n = 18$ each group) at 0, 1 and 2 months. This randomized, open-label study assessed two aspects: the dosing regimen was well tolerated and study patients did not show signs of sys-temic hypersensitivity, and secondly peptide administration did not induce or reactivate proinsulin-specific proinflammatory T cells, and proinsulin-specific IgG antibodies were not detected (Thrower et al., 2009). Interestingly, four of 18 patients from the low-dose group demonstrated peptide-specific, IL10-positive T cells. Promising results were demon-strated in a recent placebo-controlled randomized trial including 70 young type 1 diabet-ics of recent onset treated with two subcutaneous injections of a GAD alum vaccine (Lud-vigsson et al., 2008). While insulin secretion gradually decreased in both study groups, fasting C-peptide levels declined from baseline levels significantly less over 30 months in the GAD-alum group compared to the placebo group (Ludvigsson et al., 2008). Within the GAD-alum treated group, peripheral blood mononuclear cells (PBMC) demonstrated se-cretion of IL-5, IL-10, IL-13 and IL-17 as well as Foxp3 and TGFß-expression upon GAD stimulation at month 15 compared to baseline (Ludvigsson et al., 2008). Although GAD-alum treatment did not change the insulin requirement, this vaccine treatment might con-tribute to the preservation of residual insulin secretion in patients with recent-onset type 1 diabetes. Recently, a dose escalation phase I/II trial showed preservation of ß-cell func-tion (as measured by stable C-peptide levels) in type I DM patients, using a DNA plasmid encoding a full-length human proinsulin (BHT-3021) (Steinman, 2010a). 12 weekly intramuscular injections of this vaccine improved glycemic control for up to 12 months whereas insulin secretion decreased in the placebo group as expected (Steinman, 2010a). A very similar approach was taken in a phase I/II randomized double-blind placebo-controlled trial including 30 patients with relapsing-remitting multiple sclerosis (RRMS), applying a tolerizing DNA vaccine (BHT-3009) encoding full human myelin basic protein (MBP) (Bar-Or et al., 2007). BHT-3009 treatment was safe and well tolerated. Compared to the placebo group, the vaccine induced beneficial antigen-specific immune changes including a marked decrease in IFNγ+, MBP-reactive CD4+ T cells from peripheral blood and myelin-specific autoantibodies from spinal fluid. Clinically, BHT-3009 treatment provided favorable trends on brain MRI (Bar-Or et al., 2007). The MBP peptide MBP8298 (dirucotide) is of potential therapeutic interest, as it contains both an HLA-DR2 restricted T cell epitope and an immunodominant B cell epitope defined by residues aa85-96 in MBP. In a phase II placebo-controlled trial MBP8298 was given intravenously to 32 MS patients (Warren et al., 2006). Although no difference in clinical outcome was apparent, there was a significant reduction in MBP-specific autoantibodies in cerebrospinal fluid in most of the MBP8298-treated patients (Warren et al., 2006). Two phase III trials (MAESTRO-01 and -03) of MBP8298 for secondary progressive MS are ongoing, but preliminary results of MAESTRO-01 indicate that the MBP-peptide did not meet its primary endpoint in delaying disease progression (St Clair, 2009). So far, the results of antigen-specific immunotherapies in different autoimmune disorders have demonstrated variable clinical success. However, currently ongoing and future studies have to clarify the ideal route of administration, i. e. soluble peptide injection, orally or nasally applied peptides or DNA vaccination. Moreover, the timing of immunotherapy in autoimmune diseases seems to be another crucial, most likely disease-related, aspect. Up to now, the different clinical studies suggest that antigen-specific therapies seem to be safe and well tolerated. Among the very promising methods of inducing tolerance for the prevention and treatment of autoimmune diseases, is intravenous treatment with antigen-coupled, ethylene carbodiimide (ECDI)-fixed splenocytes (Miller et al., 2007). In various studies it has been shown that antigen-coupled cells can induce anergy in vitro and peripheral tolerance in vivo (Miller et al., 2007). Especially in the EAE mouse model, antigen-coupled cells have been successfully applied both in preventive experimental settings and for ameliorating the progression of established disease (Smith and Miller, 2006; Sriram et al., 1983; Vandenbark et al., 1996). Based on these encouraging preclinical data, future clinical investigations have to evaluate the safety and effectiveness of this therapeutic approach in autoimmune patients.

Targeting cellular components of the immune system

B cell targeted strategies

B cells fulfill a variety of important functions which in the context of autoimmunity initiate and perpetuate inflammatory immune mechanisms, respectively (Shlomchik, 2009). For a long time, autoantibody secretion and resulting immune complexes have been considered the main pathogenic contribution of B cells in autoimmune diseases. Now, it has become obvious that B cells exert different (auto) antibody-independent mechanisms that are crucial in chronic inflammation, including antigen presentation to T cells, especially in situations when antigen is limited (Lanzavecchia, 1990) and the release of cytokines and chemokines (Martin and Chan, 2006). Recently, a new subset of B cells (CD19+, CD24hi, CD38hi) exhibiting regulatory capacity has been identified (Blair et al., 2010). In this study, CD19+, CD24hi, CD38hi B cells have been shown to suppress the differentiation of T helper 1 cells partially by the secretion of IL-10 (Blair et al., 2010). There is evidence that in SLE patients, these regulatory B cells might be impaired in their suppressive function (Blair et al., 2010). Moreover, Yang et al. demonstrated that BAFF increased the number of IL-10-secreting B cells in vitro and in vivo (Yang et al., 2010). In mice, BAFF-induced IL-10+ B cells showed a distinct CD1dhi, CD5+ phenotype mainly derived from marginal zone B cells (Yang et al., 2010). Due to their central role, B cell targeted therapies have been applied in various autoimmune disorders (Levesque, 2009). Several B cell targeting strategies are currently being investigated and clinically applied, respectively. In general, these approaches include either direct B cell killing using depleting antibodies, or agents interfering with B cell survival or differentiation factors. Furthermore, abrogation of B cell receptor and co-stimulatory signaling and alteration of lymphoid microarchitecture (ectopic lymphoid neogenesis) might be promising targets of B cell therapy in autoimmune diseases (Sanz and Lee, 2010).

Anti-CD20 antibody therapy

The chimeric IgG1 anti-CD20 antibody, rituximab, is by now the best studied B cell directed antibody in autoimmunity and in addition to its use in B cell lymphomas, it has been approved for the treatment of active rheumatoid arthritis (RA) refractory to therapy with anti-tumor necrosis factor (TNF) by the FDA in 2007. CD20 is a transmembrane phosphoprotein expressed on most B cells from late stage pre-B cell until terminal plasma cell differentiation (Cragg et al., 2005). The CD20 molecule is a particularly suitable target for immunotherapy, as it is neither shed from the surface of CD20+ B cells after antibody binding nor internalized or downregulated (Press et al., 1987). Several mechanisms have been identified to explain the B cell depleting properties of anti-CD20 antibodies, including complement dependent cytotoxicity, direct induction of apoptosis and, most importantly, antibody dependent cell mediated cytotoxicity (Clark and Ledbetter, 2005). The success of B cell depleting strategies provided the impetus for further investigations of this approach in other autoimmune diseases, such as systemic lupus erythematodes (SLE), idiopathic thrombocytopenic purpura (ITP), primary Sjorgen's Syndrome (pSS), systemic sclerosis (SSc), vasculitides and blistering autoimmune diseases of the skin, mostly pemphigus (Nagel et al., 2009a). Two large, randomized, placebo-controlled phase II/III trials of rituximab in moderate-to-severe nonrenal lupus and lupus nephritis failed to meet the superiority endpoints (Merrill et al., 2010b). In these investigations, rituximab was compared to placebo in an adjuvant setting combined with conventional immunosuppressive therapy. In the EXPLORER study a benefit in clinical response was noticed at 1 year in African American and Hispanic SLE patients and improved platelet counts in patients with baseline thrombocytopenia (Merrill et al., 2010b). Although inducing profound depletion of circulating B cells, several studies demonstrated that rituximab does not significantly reduce levels of total IgM, IgA and IgG in RA, SLE and Wegener's granulomatosis (Cambridge et al., 2003; Vallerskog et al., 2007; Ferraro et al., 2008). Moreover, after anti-CD20 antibody treatment, there is no statistically significant decline in antibodies to common pathogens (CMV, EBV) or recall antigens such as tetanus toxoid (Ferraro et al., 2008). A recent study by Nagel et al. showed even an increase in anti-VZV-IgG and anti-EBV-IgG in 11 pemphigus patients treated with rituximab (Nagel et al., 2009b). A very interesting aspect of B cell directed therapies in autoimmune disorders is the correlation of autoantibody titers and clinical response. While in systemic autoimmunity such as RA and SLE, the relationship between B cell depletion, clinical response and autoantibody titers are inconsistent (Cambridge et al., 2006; Cohen, 2006), in organ specific disorders like pemphigus, the rituximab induced decline in autoantibodies correlates well with clinical responses (Ahmed et al., 2006; Joly et al., 2007; Eming et al., 2008). Within the group of blistering skin disorders, pemphigus has been mostly treated with anti-CD20 antibodies. To date, the data of rituximab in pemphigus is primarily based on numerous case reports and smaller cohort studies (Schmidt et al., 2009). A phase III trial comparing rituximab with standard oral corticosteroids is currently ongoing at the University Hospital of Rouen, France. One evident rationale for applying rituximab in pemphigus is the removal of precursors of autoantibody-secreting plasma cells. Studies by different groups provided evidence for the important role of autoreactive CD4+ T cells in the initiation of the autoimmune response in pemphigus (Wucherpfennig et al., 1995; Lin et al., 1997; Tsunoda et al., 2002; Hertl et al., 2006). Based on these matching in vitro and in vivo findings, the depletion of autoreactive B cells as antigen presenting cells might exert an indirect effect on autoreactive, desmoglein 3-specific CD4+ T cells. A recent study demonstrated a statistically significant decrease in desmoglein 3-reactive CD4+ T cells in peripheral blood of pemphigus patients on rituximab treatment (Eming et al., 2008). In a cohort of 11 pemphigus vulgaris patients treated with rituximab ($4 \times 375 \, \text{mg} / \text{m}^2$), the frequency of desmoglein 3- reactive, peripheral Th1 (interferon-γ+) and Th2 (IL-4+) cells were determined over a period of 12 months after rituximab treatment (Eming et al., 2008). The frequencies of total CD3+CD4+ T helper cells remained unaffected by rituximab, whereas the frequencies of autoreactive Th1 and Th2 cells decreased significantly over 6 and 12 months after rituximab therapy, respectively. Moreover, the frequencies of interferon-γ+ tetanus toxoid-reactive Th1 cells were not affected by rituximab, suggesting that desmoglein 3-specific CD4+ T cells strongly depend on autoreactive B cells as antigen presenting cells (Eming et al., 2008). In autoimmune blistering diseases, rituximab has been mostly applied to treat pemphigus vulgaris and pemphigus foliaceus. The excellent clinical efficacy of rituximab treatment in refractory and severe pemphigus has been documented in several, mostly monocenter, smaller cohort studies. A multicenter study using a single cycle of rituximab in 14 pemphigus vulgaris and 7 pemphigus foliaceus patients who previously did not respond to immunosuppressive therapy showed that 18 of 21 patients experienced complete remission within 3 months after rituximab ($4 \times 375 \, \text{mg} / \text{m}^2$) therapy (Joly et al., 2007). During follow-up, 9 pemphigus patients relapsed after a mean of 19 months in this study (Joly et al., 2007). Ahmed et al. combined rituximab with high-dose intravenous immunoglobulin (IVIG) treatment in 11 pemphigus vulgaris patients previously showing an inadequate response to immunosuppression and IVIG alone (Ahmed et al., 2006). During the first 2 months patients received three weekly infusions of rituximab ($375 \, \text{mg} / \text{m}^2$) followed by

IVIG (2 g / kg) in the fourth week while in months 3–6, rituximab was administered once per month plus a single infusion of IVIG (2 g / kg). Nine of 11 patients experienced a complete remission within 7–9 weeks after the first rituximab infusion, lasting 22 to 37 months, whereas 2 patients showed a relapse 12 months after beginning of the study (Ahmed et al., 2006). Recently, Schmidt et al. summerized the clinical experience with rituximab in pemphigus (Schmidt et al., 2009). Of 103 published pepmphigus vulgaris patients treated with rituximab, 79 patients (77%) showed either a complete remission (defined as clinical remission and no further medication required) or a clinical remission (healing of all clinical lesions on immunosuppression), while 21 patients at least showed a partial clinical response, i. e. healing of > 50% of initial lesions at baseline) (Schmidt et al., 2009). The results of 20 pemphigus foliaceus patients included in this review were very similar to the ones obtained in pemphigus vulgaris. In about 10% of the pemphigus patients severe infections were reported; 3% of these were fatal events whereas infusion-related adverse events were rarely reported (Schmidt et al., 2009).

Second generation anti-CD20 monoclonal antibodies and small modular immunopharmaceutical proteins

Rituximab is a chimeric antibody carrying murine Fab fragments that might induce the development of human anti-chimeric antibodies (HACAT) potentially limiting its efficacy and habouring the risk of allergic reactions in form of infusion-related adverse events. Moreover, complement dependent cytotoxicity (CDC) has been shown to be one mechanism of B cell depletion by rituximab. The activation of the complement system is another potential risk of infusion-related adverse events. Based on these findings, new humanized and fully human anti-CD20 monoclonal antibodies have been developed and are currently in clinical evaluation. Finally, other anti-CD20 antibodies are likely to recognize different epitopes of the CD20 molecule, theoretically accompanied by more effective B cell depletion. Ocrelizumab is a humanized anti-CD20 monoclonal antibody recognizing the same epitope as rituximab. It is being applied in different phase I/II studies for the treatment of RA, MS and lupus nephritis in SLE (Tarner, 2009). Genovese et al. published results of a phase I/II trial in moderate to severe RA (Genovese et al., 2008). Although CDC was expected to be reduced, infusion related reactions appeared more often compared to the placebo group (Genovese et al., 2008). However, in this study patients initially did not receive steroid-based premedication. In addition to MTX, patients received 200 mg and 1000 mg ocrelizumab, respectively, and demonstrated a ACR 20, 50 and 70 response of 50, 20 and 8% (for 200 mg) and 50, 28 and 18% (1000 mg) versus 22, 7 and 2% in the placebo group (Genovese et al., 2008). Severe adverse events including infections were not significantly increased compared to placebo. Similar results of a European study applying ocrelizumab in RA were reported at the EULAR congress in 2008 (Tak et al., 2008). Based on the currently available data, ocrelizumab seems to induce clinical responses in RA similar to rituximab (Tarner, 2009). Veltuzumab is a humanized anti-CD20 antibody with complementarity determining regions (CDR) indentical to rituximab except for the replacement of asparagine with aspartic acid at position 101. In vitro studies revealed that veltuzumab exhibits higher binding affinities to CD20 compared with rituximab and CDC activity by veltuzumab ap-

19

pears to be enhanced (Milani, Costillo, 2009). Preclinical studies for the treatment of RA are being conducted. Ofatumumab is a fully human anti-CD20 monoclonal antibody. So far, abstracts on preliminary results of phase I and II studies in refractory RA patients, most of them receiving MTX with or without prednisone, have been recently reported (Østergaard, 2008b). In the phase II study, 226 RA patients received 2 infusions of ofatuzumab in three different dosing categories (300, 700 and 1000 mg). 24 weeks after start of treatment all dosing groups of the intention to treat population demonstrated statistically significant clinical efficacy by ACR 20 rates. These positive results were confirmed at 48 weeks, suggesting that compared to placebo, ofatumumab induced a sustained clinical response in RA (Østergaard, 2008a). This promising clinical outcome prompted the initiation of ongoing phase III clinical investigations. In contrast to the above mentioned monoclonal antibodies, TRU-015 and SBI-087 are CD20-specific single chain variable fragments (scFv), also known as small modular immunopharmaceutical proteins (SMIP). Due to their small molecular weight these constructs are thought to have an improved tissue penetration compared to complete antibodies. TRU-015 binds to CD20 on pre- to mature B cells. A recent phase I, open label, dose-escalation trial in RA demonstrated dose-dependent B cell depletion, no dose-limiting toxicity and an acceptable tolerability profile (Burge et al., 2008). Up to date, there is only limited data on the clinical efficacy of TRU-015 in RA available, due to the small number of patients included in the current studies. Preliminary results show that ACR 20 rates seem to be comparable with the other anti-CD20 agents tested in RA. Studies are being conducted to asses the long-term efficacy and safety in the treatment of RA and lymphoma. Currently, phase I studies in RA and SLE are ongoing to evaluate the other SMIP SBI-087. In summary, these new anti-CD20 agents have been generally well tolerated in clinical studies with infusion reactions the most commonly reported adverse events. As expected with huanized and fully human antibodies, they have been associated with less immunogenicity and compared with rituximab with fewer infusion reactions (Burge, 2008; Hutas G, 2008; Castillo, Milani, 2009).

Anti-CD22 antibody (epratuzumab)

CD22 is a lektin-like type I transmembrane glycoprotein (135kDa) expressed on immature B cells and at higher levels on mature circulating (IgD+, IgM+) B cells until the transitional stage whereas differentiated plasma cells lack CD22 expression (Tedder et al., 2005). Consisting of 7 immunoglobulin-like domains, CD22 mediates adhesion of B cells to oligosaccharides bearing 2.6-linked sialic acid residues present on most leucocytes (Engel et al., 1995). In addition to its function as a homing receptor for recirculating B cells, CD22 might attenuate B cell receptor signaling by cytoplasmatic inhibitory domains (O'Keefe et al., 1996). CD22-deficient mice exhibit a reduced number of mature B cells, hyperreactivity to B cell receptor signaling and an increased risk for developing a lupus-like disease (Samardzic et al., 2002; Jellusova et al., 2010). Epratuzumab is a humanized monoclonal IgG1 anti-CD22 antibody preferentially depleting naïve and transitional B cells, leading to a reduction of 35–50% of peripheral B cell counts (Carnahan et al., 2007). In contrast to rituximab, anti-CD22 treatment does not induce apoptosis and CDC (Carnahan et al., 2007). Epratuzumab has been applied in phase I/II trials for the treatment of

Sjögren's syndrome and SLE, respectively. In a study with 16 Sjögren's syndrome patients, epratuzumab led to at least a 20% improvement in at least two parameters including lacrimal fluid, salivary flow, fatigue and IgG levels in 53% of the patients at 6 weeks. A 50% improvement in at least 2 of the above mentioned symptoms were recorded in 45% of the patients at week 32 (Steinfeld et al., 2006). Circulating B cell counts were moderately decreased by 39–54% and epratuzumab was given in four infusions of $360\,mg/m^2$ every other week (Steinfeld et al., 2006). Dörner et al., assessed the efficacy and safety of epratuzumab in 14 SLE patients reporting a modest decline in circulating B cell numbers and at least a 50% improvement of clinical activity (as quantified by BILAG score) in all the patients (Dörner et al., 2006). Preliminary results of interrupted phase III trials in SLE demonstrated a clinically relevant response, a steroid sparing effect and an improvement in life quality, indicated by a 2.5–3-fold increase in SF-36 quality of life assessment at week 48 compared to the placebo group. (Petri, 2008). So far, epratuzumab demonstrated a promising clinical efficacy and safety profile in these clinical conditions, prompting larger phase III trials in the future.

Anti-CD19 antibody

Except for the early stages of B cell development, CD19 is expressed by all B cells and at low levels on antibody secreting plasma cells (Levesque and St Clair, 2008). The anti-CD19 antibody MDX-1342 results in B cell depletion and elimination and is currently in phase I trials for RA. Currently, it remains unclear whether anti-CD19 antibody treatment will lead to more profound B cell depletion than anti-CD20 therapy (Levesque, 2009).

Inhibitors of B cell survival and signaling factors

In various autoimmune disorders there is growing evidence that the release of cytokines and growth factors by inflamed nonlymphoid target tissues, such as the synovium in RA or the kidneys in lupus nephritis, and infiltrating cells are important mediators of B cell activation (Groom and Mackay, 2008). In the context of autoimmune disorders, B cell tolerance and homeostasis are of major interest and thus, factors influencing B cell maturation have been thoroughly investigated in various autoimmune diseases (Daridon et al., 2009). The B cell activating factor from the tumor necrosis family (BAFF) or B lymphocyte stimulator (BlyS) has been identified to influence B cell differentiation and survival. Its complex function for B cell tolerance is not completely defined, yet (Mackay and Ambrose, 2003; Schneider, 2005). However, BAFF drives the maturation of B cells mainly at early transitional stages and has been suggested to interfere with humoral tolerance by rescuing autoreactive B cells from apoptosis (Mackay et al., 2003). BAFF is able to transduce signaling on B cells by three different receptors, B cell maturation antigen (BCMA), transmembrane activator and calcium modulator and cyclophilin ligand interactor (TACI) and BAFF receptor (BAFF-R) (Zhang et al., 2005). Another ligand of the TNF family, a proliferation-inducing ligand (APRIL), is closely related to BAFF and shares binding to BCMA and TACI. Depending on their maturation status, B cells express BAFF-R, BCMA and TACI in different

19

intensities, whereas BAFF-R is also expressed by activate and regulatory T cells. BCMA has been identified on plasma blasts and plasma cells (Bossen et al., 2008). Furthermore, there is evidence that BAFF-BAFF-R interaction mainly triggers the generation and maintenance of mature B cells, whereas BAFF induces T cell independent B cell activation, immunoglobulin switching and B cell homeostasis by binding to TACI (Sasaki et al., 2004). BAFF and APRIL can form biologically active heterotrimers that are significantly increased in systemic autoimmune diseases, probably due to an overexpression. However, the functional relevance of these heterotrimers is currently not completely understood (Roschke et al., 2002). Transgenic mice overexpressing BAFF develop a lupus-like autoimmune disorder including the production of anti-DNA autoantibodies, autoimmune nephritis and glandular infiltrations by B cells resulting in Sjögren-like disease (Groom et al., 2002). Moreover, BAFF overexpression resulted in hypergammaglobulinemia and dysregulation of B cell subsets with increased marginal zone B cells, mature and transitional type 2 B cells (Mackay et al., 1999). In SLE, RA and Sjögren's syndrome, various studies have found substantially increased levels of BAFF, APRIL and BAFF / APRIL heterotrimers in serum and target tissues, further enhancing the pathogenic relevance of raised BAFF and APRIL in systemic autoimmunity (Pers et al., 2005; Seyler et al., 2005). Some investigations demonstrated a positive correlation of elevated BAFF / APRIL serum levels and autoantibody titers and clinical activity, respectively (Jonsson et al., 2005; Zhang et al., 2005). In Sjögren's syndrome it has been shown that the level of circulating BAFF in the serum before B cell depleting therapy influences the duration of mature B cell depletion (Pers et al., 2007) and moreover, BAFF is dramatically enhanced during B cell depletion probably supporting re-emerging B cell differentiation (Edwards and Cambridge, 2006). The concept that impaired BAFF expression and dysregulation of the BAFF / APRIL system enforce the maturation of autoreactive B cell clones, provides the rationale for therapeutically targeting this system.

Therapeutic approaches targeting BAFF and APRIL

Two different strategies have been developed to target BAFF either by applying an anti-BAFF antibody or using a BAFF-R fusion protein, respectively. Belimumab (Lympho Stat B) is a fully human IgG1 anti BAFF monoclonal antibody targeting soluble BAFF with high affinity thus preventing binding of BAFF to its receptors (Baker et al., 2003). Briobacept (BR3-Fc) is a recombinant BAFF-R-Ig fusion protein, uniquely blocking soluble and membrane bound BAFF, as it does not bind to APRIL. So far, briobacept has been applied in two phase I trials for the treatment of RA, providing pharmacodynamic and pharmacokinetic data, but lacking an assessment of its clinical efficacy, yet (Fleischmann, 2006; Shaw, 2007; Shaw M, 2007). Briobacept was well tolerated with minor local reactions at the injection sites. Immunological effects included a 50–70% decrease in naïve CD19+CD27- B cells, a 10% reduction of total immunoglobulin levels and a doubling of CD19+CD27+ memory B cells (Shaw, 2007). Belimumab is currently assessed in seven active NIH trials, including different phase II/III studies in SLE and one phase II trial in RA (Tarner, 2009). With respect to tolerability and safety, all studies including around 800 patients demonstrate a favorable safety profile of belimumab without increased incidence of severe infections and malignancies, respectively. Belimumab treatment led to a significant reduction in circulating B cells and immunoglobulin levels including disease-related autoantibody titers decreased. However, the clinical responses to belimumab in SLE and RA demonstrated modest efficacy. The phase I trial in SLE did not show meaningful clinical responses irrespective of the dosing regimen. Furthermore, in the randomized, double-blind placebo-controlled phase II study in SLE, the primary endpoint at week 52 was not achieved (Chatham, 2008). A subgroup analysis revealed that autoantibody positive patients demonstrated a higher incidence of clinical responses, as measured by "SLE responder index" (Furie, 2008). Results of a two year open-label extension study showed that belimumab at a dose of 10 mg / kg every four weeks led to a significant stabilization of disease activity and reduced flare rates (Furie, 2008). Atacicept, a decoy receptor TACI-Ig prevents binding of BAFF and APRIL to the TACI receptor on B cells and has been studied in a phase I trial in RA and a phase Ib trial in RA and SLE (Tak et al., 2008). Atacicept induced a marked reduction of immunoglobulins, especially of IgM, and in RA there was a decrease in rheumatoid factor and anti-CCP-antibodies, while pathogen specific, protective antibodies, such as anti-tetanus toxoid antibodies, in 11 RA patients remained unchanged (Dall'Era et al., 2007). By flow cytometry analysis, atacicept induced a reduction in all B cell subsets, with the most prominent reduction was noticed in naïve B cells. As seen in SLE, atacicept induced a brief initial increase in memory B cells in RA, with no effect on T cells and monocytes (Tak et al., 2008). Both in SLE and RA, clinical benefits were moderate and no serious infections were noted (Dall'Era et al., 2007; Tak et al., 2008). Although there are promising results of the above mentioned clinical trails using different strategies of interfering with B cell activation, maturation and differentiation in autoimmune diseases, the field still lacks precise knowledge of the relative functions of BAFF and APRIL and their receptors. The indirect effect on plasma cells by BAFF inhibition and theoretically synergistic effects with B cell depleting strategies are required to be evaluated in the future.

Strategies of blocking T-B cell interactions and germinal center reactions

For autoantibody-mediated autoimmune diseases, T cell help is thought to be crucially linked to B cell memory and plasma cell induction concentrated in the germinal center. Therefore, blockade of T cell help and targeting pathways of the germinal center reaction are possible objects of selective cellular therapy. This strategy is clinically already available by the recombinant fusion protein CTLA-4 Ig (abatacept) consisting of the extracellular domain of CTLA-4 linked to the Fc portion of IgG1. Abatacept was approved in 2005 for the treatment of refractory RA showing inadequate response to previous anti-TNF treatment. Currently, abatacept is being evaluated in various phase II trials for the treatment in SLE, vasculitis syndromes, systemic sclerosis and ankylosing spondylitis. Recently, Merrill et al. reported results of a 12-month exploratory phase II trial to evaluate abatacept in non-life-threatening SLE (Merrill et al., 2010a). In this study, SLE patients received abatacept (approx. 10 mg / kg) or placebo combined with prednisone (30 mg / d) for one month and then tapered. Abatacept did not show a meaningful clinical effect, since primary and secondary endpoints were not met. Compared with placebo, abatacept led to significantly higher severe adverse events that require further assessment. Blocking the CD40/CD40L (CD154) interaction in SLE using the humanized antibody ruplizumab (BG9588) resulted in good clinical responses, a decreasing anti-dsDNA autoantibodies, a 50% improvement of proteinuria in lupus nephritis and led to reduced plasmablasts (Boumpas et al., 2003). However, thromboembolic events occurring during the early trial phase resulted in its early termination, probably related to CD154 expression on activated platelets (Mirabet et al., 2008). IDEC-131 is another humanized anti-CD154 antibody that was well tolerated and safe in a phase I trial in SLE, but failed to demonstrate clinical benefits in a SLE phase II-trail (Kalunian et al., 2002). Lymphotoxin is essential as survival factor for stromal cells providing the cellular basis for secondary lymphoid organs. A decoy receptor, lymphotoxin-ß receptor – IgG1 (baminercept, BG9924) is able to inhibt binding of lymphotoxin on activated T and B cells and has been investigated in randomized phase II trials in RA patients showing an inadequate response to MTX (Genovese, 2009). Baminercept was dosed with 1 and 3 mg/kg leading to best improvements of ACR score at day 77. Up to 30% of the patients experienced flu-like symptoms after the first dose representing the most frequent side effect. The clinical value of strategies targeting the germinal center reaction will be determined in future studies.

T cell targeted strategies

Alemtuzumab (Campath-1H) is a humanized monoclonal antibody directed against CD52, a glycoprotein present on all T- and B lymphocytes, monocytes and eosinophils, but it is not expressed by hematopoietic precursors (Gilleece and Dexter, 1993). The exact function of this abundantly expressed protein remains unclear. Alemtuzumab rapidly induces a profound lymphopenia with CD4+ T cells being particularly slow to recover, taking 5 years to reach pre-treatment levels (Coles et al., 2008). Anti-CD52 antibody treatment is licensed for the treatment of chronic lymphocytic leukemia (CLL), but has been applied in various autoimmune diseases, in renal transplantation and non-myeloablative conditioning prior to stem cell transplantation (Jones and Coles, 2009). Since the early 1990s alemtuzumab has been studied for the treatment of relapsing-remitting MS (RRMS). CAMMS-223 was a multicenter, randomized, single-blind phase II trial designed to compare alemtuzumab with interferon beta 1a in early active MS. 334 patients with active MS were randomized either to interferon beta-1b subcutaneously three times a week or alemtuzumab at one of two doses (12 or 24 mg daily i.v.) on five consecutive days. Alemtuzumab was shown to reduce the risk of relapse and the risk of sustained accumulation of disability by more than 70% compared with interferon (Coles et al., 2008). These clinical observations were paralleled by changes in brain volume as measured by MRI. Between 12 and 36 months post-alemtuzumab an increased brain volume was noticed suggesting a restoration of brain structure (Coles et al., 2008). The CAMMS-223 trial revealed more infectious events in the alemtuzumab group than in the interferon beta I treated patients, largely due to mild-to-moderate respiratory tract infections, whereas malignancies were not statistically more frequent after alemtuzumab therapy. However, the principal adverse event of alemtuzumab is the occurrence of novel autoimmunity arising months to years after treatment. Typically, 20–30% of these patients develop some kind of thyroid autoimmunity, mostly Graves' disease and in the CAMMS-223 trial 2.8% of the patients developed ITP (Coles et al., 2008). One obvious explanation for its efficacy in the treatment of MS is the ability of anti-CD52 antibody

Table 1. Strategies for therapeutic targeting of B cells, T cells and plasma cells in autoimmune diseases

Molecular target	Effect on cellular targets			Agent	Reference
	T cell	B cell	Plasma cell*		
T cell targets					
T cell receptor complex	induces T cell apoptosis/anergy; induces Treg			anti-CD3 mAb otelixizumab tepilizumab	Bisikirska et al., 2005; Chatenoud and Bluestone, 2007; Keymeulen et al., 2005
Co-stimulatory receptors					
CD154 / CD40L	blocks T – B cell interaction	inhibits early B cell activation; GC formation	probably inhibits the generation	anti-CD154 mAb ruplizumab toralizumab	Davis et al., 2001; Kalunian et al., 2002
CTLA-4	blocks costimulation; CD28-CD80/86 interaction	blocks costimulation; CD28-CD80/86 interaction		CTLA-4-Ig abatacept	Emery et al., 2010; Maxwell and Singh, 2009; Merrill et al., 2010a
CD2	prevents T cell (CD2) – APC (LFA-3) interaction			LFA3-Ig alefacept	Kraan et al., 2002; Krueger et al., 2002; Roberts et al., 2010
Other T cell targets					
CD25	inhibits T cell activation/expansion; blocks IL-2 receptor binding			anti-CD25 mAb basiliximab daclizumab	Bielekova et al., 2009; Bielekova et al., 2004
B cell depletion					
CD20	reduces activation	depletion	depletes precursors	anti-CD 20 mAb rituximab ocrelizumab ofatumumab veltuzumab Tru-015 SBI-087	Edwards and Cambridge, 2006; Levesque and St Clair, 2008; Merrill et al., 2010b
CD19		depletion	depletes precursors; plasma blasts and some PC	anti-CD19 mAb MDX-1342	Tedder, 2009

19

Table 1. (continued) Strategies for therapeutic targeting of B cells, T cells and plasma cells in autoiummue diseases

Molecular target	Effect on cellular targets			Agent	Reference
	T cell	B cell	Plasma cell*		
Proteasome		kills activated B cells / GC cells	kills PC	bortezumib	Neubert et al., 2008
CD22		depletes / inhibits proliferation	depletes precursors / inhibits differentiation	anti-CD22 mAb epratuzumab	Carnahan et al., 2007; Dorner et al., 2006; Steinfeld et al., 2006; Tedder et al., 2005
B cell survival / differentiation					
BAFF		reduces survival of naive and transitional cells; reduced GC survival	depletes some precursors	anti-BAFF mAb belimumab; BAFF-R-Ig (BR3-Fc) briobacept	Chatham, 2008; Furie, 2008 Fleischmann, 2006; Shaw, 2007
BAFF & APRIL		reduces survival of naive and transitional cells; reduced GC survival	reduces BM PC; depletes short / long lived PC	TACI-Ig atacicept	Dall'Era et al., 2007; Tak et al., 2008
GC reaction / homing					
Lymphotoxin-ß		disrupts GC reaction, ectopic lymphogenesis		LT-ßR-Ig baminercept	Genovese, 2009
CD154 / CD40L	see above				
CTLA-4	see above				
T & B cell targets					
CD52	depletion	depletion		anti-CD52 mAb alemtuzumab	Gilleece and Dexter, 1993; Jones and Coles, 2009

Mechanisms range from preclinical studies to phase III clinical trials. The described biologic effects are mainly derived from animal models and human studies if available.

* The effects on plasma cells are rather deducted from effects of the respective intervention on the (auto) antibody levels than from direct experimental evidence.

Animal modles of SLE; preclinical data;
APC: antigen presenting cell; BM PC: bone marrow-derived plasma cells; BAFF: B cell activating factor; Ig: immunoglobulin; IL-2: interleukin-2; GC: germinal center; LT-ß: lymphotoxin-beta; mAb: monoclonal antibody; PC: plasma cell; TACI: transmembrane activator and calcium-modulating and cyclophilin ligand interactor; Treg: regulatory T cell

treatment to induce a long-lasting lymphopenia. However, the occurrence of autoimmunity after alemtuzumab treatment and the lack of severe infectious events suggests that the patients are not profoundly immunocompromised. There is recent evidence that one putative effect of alemtuzumab is the homeostatic reponse it induces. Cox et al. showed that the circulating lymphocyte pool is dramatically altered by alemtuzumab (Cox et al., 2005). Especially, while memory T cells are reduced, there is a predominance of regulatory T cells (CD4+CD25hiFoxp3+), possibly providing a "tolerogenic environment" for newly generated lymphocytes. This latter finding somewhat contradicts the novel development of autoimmunity after alemtuzumab (Jones and Coles, 2009). Another T cell directed therapeutic strategy includes Fc receptor non-binding (FcR)-non-binding anti-CD3 antibodies that have been shown to minimally deplete T cells but might induce a tolerogenic state of the T cells by altering TCR-signaling (Chatenoud and Bluestone, 2007). Anti-CD3 antibodies modulate the TCR-CD3 complex resulting in the T cells becoming "blind" (also referred to as antigenic modulation). In type I DM, FcR-non-binding CD3-specific antibodies are thought to induce remission by two mechanisms, first induction of T cell apoptosis and anergy and secondly induction of adaptive regulatory T cells secreting transforming growth factor beta (Chatenoud and Bluestone, 2007). The early results of anti-CD3 antibody treatment in Type I DM have been promising. Keymeulen et al. demonstrated that otelixizumab, an anti-CD3-antibody, maintained ß-islet cell function better than placebo in a randomized, placebo controlled trial including 80 new-onset type I diabetics (Keymeulen et al., 2005). More recently, it was shown that tepilizumab (hOKT3γ1), another anti-CD3 antibody, preserved pancreatic ß-cell function associated with activation of CD8+CD25+ regulatory T cells in peripheral blood (Bisikirska et al., 2005). Based on these promising findings, phase III clinical trials are ongoing to confirm these results in a larger cohort of type I DM patients. In this context, a very interesting report by Ilan et al. showed that oral administration of OKT3 antibody in humans exerts a dose-dependent immunologic effect in T cells and dendritic cells (Ilan et al., 2010). For 5 days, healthy volunteers (three per group) received orally administered OKT3 antibody in a dose range of 0.2 to 5.0 mg daily and immune parameters were measured thereafter on days 5, 10 and 30 (Ilan et al., 2010). In this observational study, no severe side effects were reported and the development of human anti-mouse antibodies was not noticed. There were interesting immunologic changes including enhanced T cell proliferation, increased TGF-ß/L-10 secretion, decrease in Th1 and Th17 reponses and lower IL-23/IL-6 expression by dendritic cells (Ilan et al., 2010).

Cellular therapies

Hematopoietic stem cell transplantation

As detailed above, autoimmunity results from failure of the immune system to discriminate "immunologic self", e.g. own organ structures from "non-self", such as pathogens. This complex dysregulation of the immune system includes both cellular and humoral factors of the innate immune system as well as the tightly regulated adaptive immune response.

For systemic autoimmune diseases, such as SLE, the multilayered interaction of autoreactive B- and T cells has become increasingly evident (Shlomchik, 2009). Thus, the approach of correcting the autoaggressive immune aberrations by resetting the immune system appears very attractive. Moreover, there is evidence that autoreactive long-lived plasma cells could maintain chronic inflammation and autoimmune processes by persistent autoantibody secretion (Manz et al., 2006). Several studies demonstrate that plasma cells are resistant to immunosuppression, irradiation and anti-CD20 antibody treatment (Anolik et al., 2004; Radbruch et al., 2006). Thus, the depletion of autoreactive long-lived plasma cells by immunoablation followed by autologous hematopoietic stem cell transplantation might be a key-point for the success of sustained control of disease activity at least in some autoimmune diseases, such as SLE. The results of pioneering animal experiments using various autoimmune models suggested that stem cell therapy might be beneficial for patients with severe refractory autoimmune diseases. Animal models of collagen-induced arthritis (CIA) and experimental autoimmune encephalomyelitis (EAE) demonstrated that hematopoetic cell transplantation (HCT) can ameliorate autoimmune diseases and induce tolerance, respectively (Ikehara et al., 1985). Moreover, appreciation of the potential cure of autoimmune diseases was fostered by illustrative case reports of patients with coincident autoimmune disease and hematologic malignancy who remained in long-term remission of both diseases after allogeneic transplantation (Marmont, 2004). Since 1996, especially the European League Against Rheumatism (EULAR) and the European Group of Blood and Marrow Transplantation (EBMT) have encouraged the exploration of hematopoetic stem cell transplantation (HSCT) in severe autoimmune diseases (Sullivan et al., 2010). Since then, more than 1500 autoimmune patients have received an HCST (Tyndall and Gratwohl, 2009). The clinical experience with HCST in autoimmunity is further supplemented by three large multinational randomized trials for systemic sclerosis (ASTIS), multiple sclerosis (ASTIMS) and Crohn's disease (ASTIC study). Currently, randomized phase III studies are recruiting patients in the USA with these three autoimmune conditions (Sullivan et al., 2010). The ultimate goal of this therapy is to induce durable medication-free remission by correcting the autoreactive immune aberration.

Clinical experience with HSCT in autoimmune diseases

A recent analysis of the EBMT / EULAR database included nearly 1000 patients who underwent an HSCT for the indication of autoimmune diseases (Tyndall and Gratwohl, 2009). The leading indications for autologous HSCT comprised MS in 353 patients, SSc in 176, RA in 86, SLE in 85, vasculitis in 29 patients and other autoimmune disorders in fewer patients including inflammatory bowel disease and neurological disorders (Tyndall and Gratwohl, 2009). A recent retrospective analysis of more than 400 MS patients demonstrated that 60–70% of MS patients having received HSCT showed a 3-year progression-free survival and treatment-related mortality (TRM) was reported in 1–2% (Mancardi and Saccardi, 2008). In SSc, recent reports demonstrated that HSCT seems to be able to reverse fibrosis (Fleming et al., 2008; Nash et al., 2007) and to improve microvascularization (Aschwanden et al., 2008). In a series of 26 patients transplanted for SSc, 81% demonstrated a beneficial response (Vonk et al., 2008). TRM with HSCT has decreased over time from 17% in a cohort of 41 patients to 9% in a subsequent analysis of 65 patients (Nash

Table 2. Indications for hematopoietic stem cell transplantation in autoimmune diseases

Autoimmune disease	Number of patients
Multiple sclerosis	352
Connective tissue diseases	
• Systemic sclerosis	176
• Systemic lupus erythematodes	85
• Polymyositis / dermatomyositis	11
• Sjögren's syndrome	3
Arthritis	
• Rheumatoid Arthritis	86
• Systemic juvenile idiopathic arthritis	40
• Psoriatic arthritis	3
Inflammatory bowel disease	
• Crohn's disease	15
Vasculitis	
• Wegener's granulomatosis	7
• Behcet's disease	6
• Microscopic polyangiitis	2
• Churg-Strauss syndrome	2
• Classical polyarteritis nodosa	1

Until March 2008, nearly 1000 patients were registered in the The European League Against Rheumatism (EULAR) / The European Group for Blood and Marrow Transplantation (EBMT) database as having received an HSCT for the indication of autoimmune disorders. Shown are selected indications of the complete database; modified from (Tyndall and Gratwohl, 2009)

et al., 2007). Two prospective multicenter randomized trials of HSCT for SSc are currently ongoing in Europe and the US (van Laar et al., 2008). In one of these studies event-free survival, defined as survival without mortality, relapse or progression of SSc, was 64.3% at 5 years and 57.1% at 7 years (Vonk et al., 2008). A retrospective analysis of 53 SLE patients treated with HSCT, recorded in the EBMT / EULAR database, was previously reported (Jayne et al., 2004). Survival at 48 weeks was 62% and 50% of the patients achieved a 5-year disease free survival and TRM was 12% (Jayne et al., 2004). Additional results of phase I and II studies have been reported in Europe and the USA (Tyndall and Gratwohl, 2009). HSCT treatment for vasculitic disorders included, among others, cryoglobulinemia, Wegner's granulomatosis and Behcet's disease (Daikeler et al., 2007). Farge et al. performed a retrospective observational study on all first autologous HSCT for autoimmune diseases refractory to approved therapies that were reported to the EBMT registry between 1996–2007 (Farge et al., 2010). 900 patients were analyzed and the primary end-points for analysis were overall survival, progression-free survival and TRM at 100 days post transplantation (Farge et al., 2010). Among all patients, the 5-year survival was 85% and the progression-free survival 43%, although these results varied depending on the type of autoimmune disease. The 100-day TRM was significantly associated with the experience of the transplant center and the type of autoimmune disorder, but there was no significant correlation with the transplant technique (Farge et al., 2010). Progression-free survival was significantly correlated with age less than 35 years, the diagnosis and whether transplantation was performed after the year 2000 (Farge et al., 2010). The authors conclude that this largest cohort studied worldwide proves autologous HSCT to induce sustained remission for more than 5 years in patients with severe autoimmune diseases refractory to conventional therapies. The most relevant determinant of outcome was the type of autoimmune disease rather than the transplant technique (Farge et al., 2010).

Evidence for immune resetting by HSCT in autoimmunity

The rationale for applying HSCT in autoimmune diseases is to regenerate a new and self-tolerant repertoire of immune cells. A study by Roland Martin's group demonstrated in 7 MS patients who had been treated with autologous HSCT the regeneration of a new, naïve T cell repertoire emerging from the thymus (Muraro et al., 2005). Compared with pretherapy, analysis of the T cell receptor repertoire showed an overall broader clonal diversity and renewal of clonal specificities (Muraro et al., 2005). A more recent study by Alexander et al. in 7 SLE patients treated with autologous HSCT demonstrated that clinical remission correlated well with the depletion of autoreactive immunologic memory (Alexander et al., 2009). Anti-dsDNA autoantibodies and protective pathogen-specific antibodies disappeared after autologous HSCT treatment in these patients, whereas recent thymic emigrants (CD31+CD45RA+CD4+ T cells) reoccurred with a doubling in absolute numbers compared with age-matched healthy controls at 3-year follow-up. Morever, the authors noticed an increase in CD4+CD25bright Foxp3+ T cells from 2 to 7 years after HSCT, suggesting a restoration of impaired immune regulation seen in active SLE patients (Alexander et al., 2009).

Future aspects of autologous HSCT in autoimmune disorders

The data of patients registered in the EBMT / EULAR database suggest a reduction in TRM most likely due to more precise patient selection (Sullivan et al., 2010). The focus in the field is to initiate planned and to complete ongoing prospective randomized clinical trials to validate the effectiveness and toxicity of HSCT in autoimmune diseases.

Mesenchymal stem cells for autoimmune diseases

Within the past years there has been substantial interest in mesenchymal stem cells (MSC) for the treatment of chronic inflammatory and autoimmune diseases. MSC have been applied as vehicles for gene therapy, as anti-inflammatory and immunomodulatory cells and

Table 3. Proposed mechanisms for immune modulation by mesenchymal stem cells

Immunomodulatory properties	Proposed mechanism	Reference
Immunosuppressive effect on T cell proliferation and cytokine release (enhanced after proinflammatory stimuli, i. e. TNFα, IFNγ, IL-6)	Soluble factors: TGF-ß; hepatocyte growth factor (HGF); HLA-G; indoleamine 2.3 dioxygenase (IDO); nitric oxide	(Di Nicola et al., 2002; Krampera et al., 2003)
Induction of T cell anergy / unresponsiveness	Partially reversible by IL-2; also shown: divison arrest anergy	(Glennie et al., 2005; Zappia et al., 2005)
Immunosuppressive effects on macrophages and attenuating sepsis	Release of prostaglandins, i. e. PGE₂, PGE₁, PGE₃, PGI₂; PGE2 induces IL-10 secretion by macrophages	(Nemeth et al., 2009)
Antigen presentation	Upregulation of MHC class I / II under inflammatpry conditions; antigen cross-presentation to CD8+ T cells	(Chan et al., 2008; Francois et al., 2009)
Secretion of proinflammatory cytokines; chemotaxis	Upon IFNγ-stimulation: secretion of IL-6, CXCL10, CCL2, CCL8, sICAM-1	(Hoogduijn et al., 2010)
Inhibition of generation and maturation of dendritic cells	Various soluble factors; dose-dependent inhibition of both CD34+ and monocyte-derived dendritic cells	(Nauta et al., 2006)
Inhibition of antibody secretionby B cells	Third party MSC suppress alloantigen-specific antibody production in mixed lymphocyte cultures; cell-cell contact independent mechanism, but cell-cell contact enhances inhibitory function of MSC	(Comoli et al., 2008)
Induction of CD4+CD25+ T cells with regulatory function	Unknown mechanism	(Maccario et al., 2005)

Mesenchymal stem cells (MSC) have been shown to exert various immunomodulatory functions in vitro and in vivo. The most prominent effects of MSC are listed in this table. CXCL10: chemokine (C-X-C motif) ligand 10; CCL2: chemokine (C-C motif) ligand 2; IFN-γ: interferon-gamma; TNFα: tumor necrosis factor-alpha; IL-2: interleukin-2; IL-6: interleukin-6; TGF-ß: transforming growth factor-beta; HLA-G: human leucocyte antigen-G; PGE: prostaglandin E; MHC: major histocompatibility complex

19

to support the engraftment of hematopoietic stem cells (Passweg and Tyndall, 2007). Both in vitro and in vivo MSC are able of differentiating to various cell lineages including muscle, bone and myelosupportive stroma (Horwitz et al., 2005). MSC can be isolated from different organs including adipose tissue, skeletal muscle, bone marrow, cord blood and placental products (Tyndall and Gratwohl, 2009). MSC are defined by the expression profile of certain cell surface markers and functional properties, as they lack unique cell surface markers (Pittenger et al., 2002). MSC express surface markers such as CD13, CD29, CD44, CD73, CD90 and CD166 but they are negative for CD34, CD45, CD80, CD86, HLA class II and HLA class I[low] separating them from hematopoietic stem cells which are CD13, CD34 and CD45 positive (Hoogduijn et al., 2010; Tolar et al., 2010). This expression profile suggests that MSC are of low immunogenic-genicity. MSC demonstrate a robust proliferation potential in vitro and they can clonally regenerate. Especially their immunomodulatory, antiproliferative capacities make MSC an interesting therapeutic candidate in the treatment of autoimmune diseases and acute graft versus host disease (GvHD) (Tyndall et al., 2007; Dazzi and Marelli-Berg, 2008). The exact immunosuppressive effect of MSC remains to be completely understood. However, clinical effectiveness of MSC may not require engraftment of large cell numbers or further differentiation into clinically affected or specific tissues. There is evidence suggesting that therapeutical benefit might be achieved by local release of antiproliferative and immunomodulatory factors (Tyndall and Gratwohl, 2009). Human MSC suppress T and B cell proliferation in mixed lymphocyte reactions in a dose-dependent, MHC-independent manner which does not require cell-cell contact (Aggarwal and Pittenger, 2005). Depending on the experimental setting, multiple mechanisms of immunosuppression have been described including transforming growth factor-beta (TGF-ß) (Di Nicola et al., 2002) IL-1 receptor antagonism (Ortiz et al., 2007), HLA class I G (HLA-G) and recently MSC have been shown to express Toll-like receptors (TLR) which might contribute to the anti-inflammatory effects on macrophages (Nemeth et al., 2009).

Mesenchymal stem cells in animal models and clinical experiences

In EAE models, MSC treatment demonstrated both histological and clinical improvement. Early treatment with MSC showed better results which were reversed by IL-2 treatment, suggesting rather an anergy inducing effect of MSC in these models (Zappia et al., 2005). In murine arthritis models, MSC application showed mixed outcomes in collagen induced arthritis models (Augello et al., 2007; Djouad et al., 2005). Recent results of a phase II study in acute, steroid-resistant GvHD showed favorable clinical results without immediate toxicity. Thirty of 55 patients had a complete response, with reduced TRM at 12 months and higher overall 2-year survival (Le Blanc et al., 2008). MSC in SSc patients were normal in respect to proliferation and specific differentiation (Larghero et al., 2008). Several ongoing phase I / II trials of MSC treatment in MS, SLE, type I diabetes and Chrohn's disease aim at exploring their effectiveness in these autoimmune diseases (Tyndall and Gratwohl, 2009).

Targeting the fibrotic pathway in systemic sclerosis

With regard to its therapeutic management, SSc continues to be one of the most complex systemic autoimmune diseases. In addition to autoimmune inflammation and vasculopathy, extensive fibrosis is considered a fundamental etiopathogenic factor (Gabrielli et al.,

2009). Thus, selective therapies interfering with fibrotic pathways are considered among the most promising novel therapeutic strategies in SSc (Ramos-Casals et al., 2010). A variety of potential molecular targets have been identified including Abelson kinase (c-abl), platelet derived growth factor (PDGF), connective tissue growth factor (CCN2) and TGF-ß (Denton et al., 2005). Surprisingly, a pilot phase I/II study of a human monoclonal antibody against TGF-ß1 (CAT-192) in SSc failed to meet the efficacy outcomes (Denton et al., 2007). Pathological activation of tyrosine kinases (TK) might enhance carcinogenesis, vascular remodeling and fibrogenesis (Beyer et al., 2010). Recently, TK inhibitors have been explored for the treatment of SSc (Distler and Distler, 2009). Imatinib mesylate is a small molecule TK inhibitor effectively blocking the activity of c-abl by binding to its ATP-pocket (Distler and Distler, 2010). Moreover, imatinib mesylate interferes with PDGF signaling by blocking the TK activity of its receptor (Savage and Antman, 2002). By simultaneously targeting two important proliferative pathways activated in SSc, imatinib mesylate represents an interesting small molecule for the treatment of this autoimmune disease. Several preclinical studies using various experimental animal models of dermal, renal and lung fibrosis provided in vivo evidence that imatinib might reduce even established fibrosis (Akhmetshina et al., 2009). Two pilot studies in refractory chronic GvHD reported an antifibrotic effect of imatinib (Magro et al., 2008; Olivieri et al., 2009). Furthermore, several case reports demonstrated beneficial effects of imatinib mesylate in refractory SSc (Beyer et al., 2010). Based on these promising results of imatinib mesylate in SSc, clinical trials have been initiated (Ong and Denton, 2010). An interim analysis of a phase II open-label study including 30 patients with SSc showed that imatinib led to an improved skin score at 12 months, associated with corresponding histological improvement (Akhmetshina et al., 2009). Previous clinical trials in CML patients showed that imatinib is well tolerated with discontinuation of the treatment in < 1% of patients due to severe side effects (Distler and Distler, 2009). So far, in SSc the most common, but often self-limited, adverse events included edema (80%), nausea (73%), myalgia (60%) and fatigue (53%) (Ong and Denton, 2010). To evaluate the safety and toxicity of imatinib in SSc, larger clinical studies are manfatory. Currently, several clinical trials of imatinib for the treatment of fibrosis in SSc are ongoing. Dasatinib and nilotinib, two novel inhibitors of c–abl and PDGFR, represent interesting alternatives to imatinib in the anti-fibrotic treatment in SSc (Distler and Distler, 2010). Additionally, there is recent evidence that nilotinib might exert positive effects on the proliferative vasculopathy (Akhmetshina et al., 2008). Furthermore, the inhibition of Src kinases that regulate the activation of c-abl, might be an additional therapeutic effect of dasatinib (Skhirtladze et al., 2008).

Targeting cytokines and cytokine receptors

The identification of new cytokines and other soluble mediators affecting immune responses is probably among the most dynamic area of biomedical research. Translational research projects aim at exploring newly identified immune mediators for their potential therapeutic benefit. In the category of immunomodulating therapies targeting cytokines, monoclonal antibodies against the IL-6 receptor (IL-6R) and the IL-12/23 p40 receptor subunit, rank as the most exciting of these recent developments.

Anti-Il-6 receptor antibody (tocilizumab)

Tocilizumab is a humanized monoclonal antibody against the alpha chain of the IL-6R preventing binding of IL-6 to both membrane-bound and soluble IL-6R and finally preventing its biological activity (Nishimoto and Kishimoto, 2008). IL-6 is a multifunctional cytokine involved in the acute immune response, in the regulation of hematopoiesis, in the production of acute phase proteins in the liver and in B cell proliferation and differentiation (Kishimoto, 2005). Interestingly, IL-6 together with TGF-ß is also involved in the differentiation of Th17 cells, whereas TGF-ß in the absence of IL-6 has been reported to promote differentiation of CD4+CD25brightFoxp3+ regulatory T cells (Sakaguchi, 2004). High levels of IL-6 have been found in synovial fluid from inflamed joints of acute RA patients, causing angiogenesis by the induction of vascular endothelial growth factor (VEGF) (Ushiyama et al., 2003). Multiple phase III studies demonstrated that tocilizumab rapidly reduced RA disease activity and improved the functional status (Genovese et al., 2008). Furthermore, tocilizumab slows radiographic progression with improvement in bone and cartilage turnover markers (Hashimoto et al., 2010). Tocilizumab has first been approved in 2005 in Japan for the treatment of Castleman's disease and in 2008 the approval was extended to the treatment of RA, juvenile arthritis and Still's syndrome. Since the beginning of 2010, tocilizumab is approved by the FDA for the treatment of RA patients who did not respond to anti-TNF treatment. In murine models of lupus, IL-6 and IL-6R expression has been shown to be associated with disease activity (Nagafuchi et al., 1993; Ryffel et al., 1994). Moreover, lupus patients demonstrate elevated IL-6 serum levels correlating with disease activity and with anti-dsDNA autoantibodies in some studies (Richards et al., 1998). In lupus nephritis, an increased urinary excretion of IL-6 in acute patients has been shown (Peterson et al., 1996). Taken together, there are increasing preclinical models and clinical observations that IL-6 plays an important role in lupus. A recent open-label phase I, dosage-escalation study assessed the safety of IL-6R inhibition by tocilizumab and presented preliminary results on clinical and immunological efficacy in SLE (Illei et al., 2010). In this study, 16 SLE patients with mild to moderate disease activity received tocilizumab given intravenously every other week for 12 weeks, followed by a 8-week follow-up period. Three dosing groups included 2 mg / kg, 4 mg / kg and 8 mg / kg. Overall-tocilizumab was well tolerated, but it induced dose-dependent decrease in neutrophil counts. One patient was withdrawn due to neutropenia. In 8 of 15 patients there was a significant decrease of > 4 points in the disease activity index. Moreover, arthritis improved in all affected patients and anti-dsDNA autoantibodies decreased by a median of 47% (Illei et al., 2010). Together with a 7.8% decrease in total IgG levels, the frequency of circulating plasma cells decreased significantly, suggesting a specific effect of anti-IL6R treatment on autoantibody-secreting plasma cells (Illei et al., 2010). This pilot study demonstrates improved clinical and serological markers of lupus activity and encourages further studies to establish treatment regimens, safety and efficacy in SLE. Finally, other clinical applications of anti-IL-6R treatment are currently being investigated such as vasculitis syndromes (Nishimoto and Kishimoto, 2008).

Anti-IL-12/23 monoclonal antibody (ustekinumab)

The differentiation of naïve CD4+ T cells into distinct lineages with different effector functions has been limited to Th1 and Th2 subsets for many years. Recently, the diversification of CD4+ T effector cells has been enlarged by the discovery of new functional subsets, including Th9, Th17 and Th22 cells, facilitated by the identification of new cytokines and differentiation factors (Zhou et al., 2009). In the context of autoimmunity, the characterization of IL-17-secreting CD4+ T cells (Th17 cells) was of particular interest. The identification of Th17 cells as a distinct CD4+ T cell subset was mainly achieved in murine models of autoimmunity, such as EAE, CIA and inflammatory bowel diseases. The initial concept that these inflammatory autoimmune disorders were principally Th1-driven, IFNγ-mediated diseases, has been challenged by the finding that IFNγ- and IFNγ-receptor-deficient mice, respectively, were not resistant but even more susceptible to auto-immune reactions in the central nervous system (Krakowski and Owens, 1996). Furthermore, Il-23, a IL-12 family member, shares the p40 subunit with IL-12 and its receptor is composed of the IL-12ß1 and IL-23R chains (Oppmann et al., 2000). These findings led to studies demonstrating that IL-23 is critically linked to autoimmunity in these models (Cua et al., 2003; Murphy et al., 2003). Investigations in humans demonstrated that Th17 cells express CCR6, CCR4, RORC and IL23R and they secrete IL17A, IL-17F, IL-22 and IL-26 and the chemokine CCL20 (Acosta-Rodriguez et al., 2007; Annunziato et al., 2007). A proportion of human Th17 cells produce IFNγ in addition to IL-17A, therefore these cells were described as Th17/Th1 cells (Boniface et al., 2008). Thus far, modulation of Th17 cell function has largely proceeded using monoclonal antibodies to the p40 subunit of IL-12 (heterodimer of p35 and p40) and IL-23 (heterodimer of p19 and p40), targeting both IL-12 dependent Th1 and IL-23-promoted Th17 cells (Steinman, 2010b). Two completely humanized anti-IL12/23 p40 antibodies, ustekinumab (IgG1κ) and briakinumab /ABT-874 , were successfully applied in psoriasis (Kimball et al., 2008; Krueger et al., 2007). Two large multicenter, randomized, placebo-controlled clinical trials (PHOENIX 1 and 2) demonstrated an excellent clinical response with 67% of patients achieving a PASI 75 response at week 12 to ustekinumab treatment (that is, an improvement of the Psoriasis Area and Severity Index of at least 75% relative to baseline) (Leonardi et al., 2008; Papp et al., 2008). Patients who were randomized to ustekinumab received 45 mg or 90 mg doses subcutaneously at weeks 0 and 4, followed by the same dose every 12 weeks. A recent randomized, placebo-controlled phase II study demonstrated very similar clinical results using briakinumab/ABT-874 in moderate to severe chronic plaque psoriasis in five different dosing and frequency combinations versus placebo for 12 weeks (Kimball et al., 2008). At week 12, PASI 75 results were achieved depending on the treatment ranging from 63% (200 mg single dose) up to 93% (200 mg weekly for 12 weeks). ABT-874 was well tolerated and the most common adverse event was injection-site reaction, whereas the most common infectious event were upper respiratory tract infection (Kimball et al., 2008). For both antibod-

19

ies, ustekinumab and briakinumab, clinical responses were very similar to those seen with anti-TNF treatment that has been approved for psoriasis for several years. In Crohn's disease several lines of evidence support an important role of IL-23, including IL-23R polymorphisms strongly associated with susceptibility to Crohn's disease (Duerr et al., 2006). In addition, elevated transcripts encoding IL-17A and IL-6 are detected in biopsies from patients with active Crohn's disease (Holtta et al., 2008) and different groups succeeded in cloning Th17/Th1 cells from the lamina propria of Crohn's patients (Annunziato et al., 2007; Pene et al., 2008). Based on these results, studies were conducted evaluating the clinical effectiveness of anti-IL12/23 antibody treatment in Crohn's disease. Mannon et al. included 79 patients with active Crohn's disease in a multicenter, randomized, placebo-controlled phase II study, applying the anti-IL12/23 antibody briakinumab in different dosing groups (Mannon et al., 2004). Briakinumab treatment achieved the primary and secondary endpoints versus placebo in Crohn's disease activity index after seven weekly injections. The clinical remission correlated with a decrease of IL-12, IFN-γ and TNFα secretion by mononuclear cells of the colonic lamina propria (Mannon et al., 2004). Interestingly, in the second study, the use of ustekinumab in 104 patients with moderate to severe Crohn's disease, induced a clinical response especially in patients previously treated with anti-TNF antibodies (infliximab) (Sandborn et al., 2008). In both trials there were no significant toxicities reported. In contrast to the promising results of anti-IL12/23 antibody treatment in psoriasis and Crohn's disease, ustekinumab did not induce a significant clinical response in a phase II trial treating relapsing-remitting multiple sclerosis (Segal et al., 2008). In this investigation, the primary endpoint, the reduction of new gadolinium positive lesions, was not achieved compared to placebo treated patients (Segal et al., 2008). These clinical results in MS patients are in contrast to impressive preclinical data on the influence of blocking the IL-12 p40 family in EAE models (Cua et al., 2003).

Summary and Conclusions

The character of treatment for autoimmune diseases is dramatically changing due to the constant identification of new targets and the subsequent development of corresponding agents. The enormous efforts in identifying new target structures are based on a substantially refined understanding of the underlying autoimmune disorder. B cells symbolize this recent development, since they attract a lot of attention as key players in the dysregulation of autoimmune mechanisms. It has been appreciated that B cells are not restricted to (auto) antibody dependent functions, but they demonstrate various effects contributing to the complex procedures finally resulting in clinical symptoms of autoimmunity. Consequently, new targets directly affecting B cell function and interfering with (auto) antibody release, respectively, are being developed and evaluated for their clinical benefit. High clinical need for better therapeutic outcomes still exists for many autoimmune disorders, although major progress since the initial introduction of the biologic agents, at least for treatment of diseases such as rheumatoid arthritis, psoriasis or pemphigus, has been made. It can be expected that additional monoclonal antibodies and fusion proteins directed against newly identified targets as well as pharmacologically improved compounds directed against existing targets will be brought to the clinic. Translational research and the decision for some therapeutic agents to move to clinical application has mainly been based on preclinical, and that means animal, studies. It has been a disappointing experience that in some cases results from animal studies poorly predicted successful application in humans. Thus, factors that need to be considered in the future include deeper knowledge of the pathogenic mechanisms, the identification of valuable biomarkers assessing efficacy and safety and finally the more defined characterization of optimum treatment paradigms and most appropriate patient populations for the use of new therapeutic agents.

References

Acosta-Rodriguez, E. V., Rivino, L., Geginat, J., Jarrossay, D., Gattorno, M., Lanzavecchia, A., Sallusto, F., and Napolitani, G. (2007). Surface phenotype and antigenic specificity of human interleukin 17-producing T helper memory cells. Nat Immunol 8, 639–646

Aggarwal, S., and Pittenger, M. F. (2005). Human mesenchymal stem cells modulate allogeneic immune cell responses. Blood 105, 1815–1822

Ahmed, A. R., Spigelman, Z., Cavacini, L. A., and Posner, M. R. (2006). Treatment of pemphigus vulgaris with rituximab and intravenous immune globulin. N Engl J Med 355, 1772–1779

Akhmetshina, A., Dees, C., Pileckyte, M., Maurer, B., Axmann, R., Jungel, A., Zwerina, J., Gay, S., Schett, G., Distler, O., and Distler, J. H. (2008). Dual inhibition of c-abl and PDGF receptor signaling by dasatinib and nilotinib for the treatment of dermal fibrosis. Faseb J 22, 2214–2222

Akhmetshina, A., Venalis, P., Dees, C., Busch, N., Zwerina, J., Schett, G., Distler, O., and Distler, J. H. (2009). Treatment with imatinib prevents fibrosis in different preclinical models of systemic sclerosis and induces regression of established fibrosis. Arthritis Rheum 60, 219–224

Alexander, C. M., Puchalski, J., Klos, K. S., Badders, N., Ailles, L., Kim, C. F., Dirks, P., and Smalley, M. J. (2009). Separating stem cells by flow cytometry: reducing variability for solid tissues. Cell Stem Cell 5, 579–583

Annunziato, F., Cosmi, L., Santarlasci, V., Maggi, L., Liotta, F., Mazzinghi, B., Parente, E., Fili, L., Ferri, S., Frosali, F., et al. (2007). Phenotypic and functional features of human Th17 cells. J Exp Med 204, 1849–1861

Anolik, J. H., Barnard, J., Cappione, A., Pugh-Bernard, A. E., Felgar, R. E., Looney, R. J., and Sanz, I. (2004). Rituximab improves peripheral B cell abnormalities in human systemic lupus erythematosus. Arthritis Rheum 50, 3580–3590

Aschwanden, M., Daikeler, T., Jaeger, K. A., Thalhammer, C., Gratwohl, A., Matucci-Cerinic, M., and Tyndall, A. (2008). Rapid improvement of nailfold capillaroscopy after intense immunosuppression for systemic sclerosis and mixed connective tissue disease. Ann Rheum Dis 67, 1057–1059

Augello, A., Tasso, R., Negrini, S. M., Cancedda, R., and Pennesi, G. (2007). Cell therapy using allogeneic bone marrow mesenchymal stem cells prevents tissue damage in collagen-induced arthritis. Arthritis Rheum 56, 1175–1186

Baker, K. P., Edwards, B. M., Main, S. H., Choi, G. H., Wager, R. E., Halpern, W. G., Lappin, P. B., Riccobene, T., Abramian, D., Sekut, L., et al. (2003). Generation and characterization of LymphoStat-B, a human monoclonal antibody that antagonizes the bioactivities of B lymphocyte stimulator. Arthritis Rheum 48, 3253–3265

19

Bar-Or, A., Vollmer, T., Antel, J., Arnold, D. L., Bodner, C. A., Campagnolo, D., Gianettoni, J., Jalili, F., Kachuck, N., Lapierre, Y., et al. (2007). Induction of antigen-specific tolerance in multiple sclerosis after immunization with DNA encoding myelin basic protein in a randomized, placebo-controlled phase 1/2 trial. Arch Neurol 64, 1407–1415

Beyer, C., Distler, J. H., and Distler, O. (2010). Are tyrosine kinase inhibitors promising for the treatment of systemic sclerosis and other fibrotic diseases? Swiss Med Wkly

Bielekova, B., Richert, N., Howard, T., Blevins, G., Markovic-Plese, S., McCartin, J., Frank, J. A., Wurfel, J., Ohayon, J., Waldmann, T. A., et al. (2004). Humanized anti-CD25 (daclizumab) inhibits disease activity in multiple sclerosis patients failing to respond to interferon beta. Proc Natl Acad Sci U S A 101, 8705–8708

Bielekova, B., Howard, T., Packer, A. N., Richert, N., Blevins, G., Ohayon, J., Waldmann, T. A., McFarland, H. F., and Martin, R. (2009). Effect of anti-CD25 antibody daclizumab in the inhibition of inflammation and stabilization of disease progression in multiple sclerosis. Arch Neurol 66, 483–489

Bisikirska, B., Colgan, J., Luban, J., Bluestone, J. A., and Herold, K. C. (2005). TCR stimulation with modified anti-CD3 mAb expands CD8+ T cell population and induces CD8+CD25+ Tregs. J Clin Invest 115, 2904–2913

Blair, P. A., Norena, L. Y., Flores-Borja, F., Rawlings, D. J., Isenberg, D. A., Ehrenstein, M. R., and Mauri, C. (2010). CD19(+)CD24(hi)CD38(hi) B cells exhibit regulatory capacity in healthy individuals but are functionally impaired in systemic Lupus Erythematosus patients. Immunity 32, 129–140

Boniface, K., Blom, B., Liu, Y. J., and de Waal Malefyt, R. (2008). From interleukin-23 to T-helper 17 cells: human T-helper cell differentiation revisited. Immunol Rev 226, 132–146

Bossen, C., Cachero, T. G., Tardivel, A., Ingold, K., Willen, L., Dobles, M., Scott, M. L., Maquelin, A., Belnoue, E., Siegrist, C. A., et al. (2008). TACI, unlike BAFF-R, is solely activated by oligomeric BAFF and APRIL to support survival of activated B cells and plasmablasts. Blood 111, 1004–1012

Boumpas, D. T., Furie, R., Manzi, S., Illei, G. G., Wallace, D. J., Balow, J. E., and Vaishnaw, A. (2003). A short course of BG9588 (anti-CD40 ligand antibody) improves serologic activity and decreases hematuria in patients with proliferative lupus glomerulonephritis. Arthritis Rheum 48, 719–727

Cambridge, G., Leandro, M. J., Edwards, J. C., Ehrenstein, M. R., Salden, M., Bodman-Smith, M., and Webster, A. D. (2003). Serologic changes following B lymphocyte depletion therapy for rheumatoid arthritis. Arthritis Rheum 48, 2146–2154

Cambridge, G., Stohl, W., Leandro, M. J., Migone, T. S., Hilbert, D. M., and Edwards, J. C. (2006). Circulating levels of B lymphocyte stimulator in patients with rheumatoid arthritis following rituximab treatment: relationships with B cell depletion, circulating antibodies, and clinical relapse. Arthritis Rheum 54, 723–732

Carnahan, J., Stein, R., Qu, Z., Hess, K., Cesano, A., Hansen, H. J., and Goldenberg, D. M. (2007). Epratuzumab, a CD22-targeting recombinant humanized antibody with a different mode of action from rituximab. Mol Immunol 44, 1331–1341

Chan, W. K., Lau, A. S., Li, J. C., Law, H. K., Lau, Y. L., and Chan, G. C. (2008). MHC expression kinetics and immunogenicity of mesenchymal stromal cells after short-term IFN-gamma challenge. Exp Hematol 36, 1545–1555

Chatenoud, L. and Bluestone, J. A. (2007). CD3-specific antibodies: a portal to the treatment of autoimmunity. Nat Rev Immunol 7, 622–632

Chatham, A. C., Furie R (2008). Progressive normalization of autoantibody, immunoglobulin, and complement levels over 3 years of belimumab (fully human monoclonal antibody to BlyS) therapy in systemic lupus erythematosus (SLE) patients. Ann Rheum Dis 67, 217

Clark, E. A. and Ledbetter, J. A. (2005). How does B cell depletion therapy work, and how can it be improved? Ann Rheum Dis 64 Suppl 4, iv77–80

Cohen, S. B. (2006). Updates from B Cell Trials: Efficacy. J Rheumatol Suppl 77, 12–17

Coles, A. J., Compston, D. A., Selmaj, K. W., Lake, S. L., Moran, S., Margolin, D. H., Norris, K., and Tandon, P. K. (2008). Alemtuzumab vs. interferon beta-1a in early multiple sclerosis. N Engl J Med 359, 1786–1801

Comoli, P., Ginevri, F., Maccario, R., Avanzini, M. A., Marconi, M., Groff, A., Cometa, A., Cioni, M., Porretti, L., Barberi, W., et al. (2008). Human mesenchymal stem cells inhibit antibody production induced in vitro by allostimulation. Nephrol Dial Transplant 23, 1196–1202

Cox, A. L., Thompson, S. A., Jones, J. L., Robertson, V. H., Hale, G., Waldmann, H., Compston, D. A., and Coles, A. J. (2005). Lymphocyte homeostasis following therapeutic lymphocyte depletion in multiple sclerosis. Eur J Immunol 35, 3332–3342

Cragg, M. S., Walshe, C. A., Ivanov, A. O., and Glennie, M. J. (2005). The biology of CD20 and its potential as a target for mAb therapy. Curr Dir Autoimmun 8, 140–174

Cua, D. J., Sherlock, J., Chen, Y., Murphy, C. A., Joyce, B., Seymour, B., Lucian, L., To, W., Kwan, S., Churakova, T., et al. (2003). Interleukin-23 rather than interleukin-12 is the critical cytokine for autoimmune inflammation of the brain. Nature 421, 744–748

Daikeler, T., Kotter, I., Bocelli Tyndall, C., Apperley, J., Attarbaschi, A., Guardiola, P., Gratwohl, A., Jantunen, E., Marmont, A., Porretto, F., et al. (2007). Haematopoietic stem cell transplantation for vasculitis including Behcet's disease and polychondritis: a retrospective analysis of patients recorded in the European Bone Marrow Transplantation and European League Against Rheumatism databases and a review of the literature. Ann Rheum Dis 66, 202–207

Dall'Era, M., Chakravarty, E., Wallace, D., Genovese, M., Weisman, M., Kavanaugh, A., Kalunian, K., Dhar, P., Vincent, E., Pena-Rossi, C., and Wofsy, D. (2007). Reduced B lymphocyte and immunoglobulin levels after atacicept treatment in patients with systemic lupus erythematosus: results of a multicenter, phase Ib, double-blind, placebo-controlled, dose-escalating trial. Arthritis Rheum 56, 4142–4150

Daridon, C., Burmester, G. R., and Dorner, T. (2009). Anticytokine therapy impacting on B cells in autoimmune diseases. Curr Opin Rheumatol 21, 205–210

Davis, J. C., Jr., Totoritis, M. C., Rosenberg, J., Sklenar, T. A., and Wofsy, D. (2001). Phase I clinical trial of a monoclonal antibody against CD40-ligand (IDEC-131) in patients with systemic lupus erythematosus. J Rheumatol 28, 95–101

Dazzi, F. and Marelli-Berg, F. M. (2008). Mesenchymal stem cells for graft-versus-host disease: close encounters with T cells. Eur J Immunol 38, 1479–1482

Denton, C. P., Lindahl, G. E., Khan, K., Shiwen, X., Ong, V. H., Gaspar, N. J., Lazaridis, K., Edwards, D. R., Leask, A., Eastwood, M., et al. (2005). Activation of key profibrotic mechanisms in transgenic fibroblasts expressing kinase-deficient type II Transforming growth factor-{beta} receptor (T{beta}RII{delta}k). J Biol Chem 280, 16053–16065

Denton, C. P., Merkel, P. A., Furst, D. E., Khanna, D., Emery, P., Hsu, V. M., Silliman, N., Streisand, J., Powell, J., Akesson, A., et al. (2007). Recombinant human anti-transforming growth factor beta1 antibody therapy in systemic sclerosis: a multicenter, randomized, placebo-controlled phase I/II trial of CAT-192. Arthritis Rheum 56, 323–333

Di Nicola, M., Carlo-Stella, C., Magni, M., Milanesi, M., Longoni, P. D., Matteucci, P., Grisanti, S., and Gianni, A. M. (2002). Human bone marrow stromal cells suppress T-lymphocyte proliferation induced by cellular or nonspecific mitogenic stimuli. Blood 99, 3838–3843

Diabetes Prevention Trial-Type 1 Diabetes Study Group (2002). Effects of insulin in relatives of patients with type 1 diabetes mellitus. N Engl J Med 346, 1685–1691

Distler, J. H. and Distler, O. (2009). Imatinib as a novel therapeutic approach for fibrotic disorders. Rheumatology (Oxford) 48, 2–4

Distler, J. H. and Distler, O. (2010). Tyrosine kinase inhibitors for the treatment of fibrotic diseases such as systemic sclerosis: towards molecular targeted therapies. Ann Rheum Dis 69 Suppl 1, i48–51

19

Djouad, F., Fritz, V., Apparailly, F., Louis-Plence, P., Bony, C., Sany, J., Jorgensen, C., and Noel, D. (2005). Reversal of the immunosuppressive properties of mesenchymal stem cells by tumor necrosis factor alpha in collagen-induced arthritis. Arthritis Rheum 52, 1595–1603

Dorner, T., Kaufmann, J., Wegener, W. A., Teoh, N., Goldenberg, D. M., and Burmester, G. R. (2006). Initial clinical trial of epratuzumab (humanized anti-CD22 antibody) for immunotherapy of systemic lupus erythematosus. Arthritis Res Ther 8, R74

Duerr, R. H., Taylor, K. D., Brant, S. R., Rioux, J. D., Silverberg, M. S., Daly, M. J., Steinhart, A. H., Abraham, C., Regueiro, M., Griffiths, A., et al. (2006). A genome-wide association study identifies IL23R as an inflammatory bowel disease gene. Science 314, 1461–1463

Edwards, J. C. and Cambridge, G. (2006). B-cell targeting in rheumatoid arthritis and other autoimmune diseases. Nat Rev Immunol 6, 394–403

Emery, P., Durez, P., Dougados, M., Legerton, C. W., Becker, J. C., Vratsanos, G., Genant, H. K., Peterfy, C., Mitra, P., Overfield, S., et al. (2010). Impact of T-cell costimulation modulation in patients with undifferentiated inflammatory arthritis or very early rheumatoid arthritis: a clinical and imaging study of abatacept (the ADJUST trial). Ann Rheum Dis 69, 510–516

Eming, R., Nagel, A., Wolff-Franke, S., Podstawa, E., Debus, D., and Hertl, M. (2008). Rituximab exerts a dual effect in pemphigus vulgaris. J Invest Dermatol 128, 2850–2858

Engel, P., Wagner, N., Miller, A. S., and Tedder, T. F. (1995). Identification of the ligand-binding domains of CD22, a member of the immunoglobulin superfamily that uniquely binds a sialic acid-dependent ligand. J Exp Med 181, 1581–1586

Farge, D., Labopin, M., Tyndall, A., Fassas, A., Mancardi, G. L., Van Laar, J., Ouyang, J., Kozak, T., Moore, J., Kotter, I., et al. (2010). Autologous hematopoietic stem cell transplantation for autoimmune diseases: an observational study on 12 years' experience from the European Group for Blood and Marrow Transplantation Working Party on Autoimmune Diseases. Haematologica 95, 284–292

Ferraro, A. J., Drayson, M. T., Savage, C. O., and MacLennan, I. C. (2008). Levels of autoantibodies, unlike antibodies to all extrinsic antigen groups, fall following B cell depletion with Rituximab. Eur J Immunol 38, 292–298

Fleischmann, W. N., Shaw M (2006). BR3-Fc phase I study: Safety, pharmacokinetics (PK) and pharmacodynamic (PD) effects of a novel BR3-Fc fusion protein in patients with rheumatoid arthritis. Arthritis Rheum 54, S229–S230

Fleming, J. N., Nash, R. A., McLeod, D. O., Fiorentino, D. F., Shulman, H. M., Connolly, M. K., Molitor, J. A., Henstorf, G., Lafyatis, R., Pritchard, D. K., et al. (2008). Capillary regeneration in scleroderma: stem cell therapy reverses phenotype? PLoS One 3, e1452

Francois, M., Romieu-Mourez, R., Stock-Martineau, S., Boivin, M. N., Bramson, J. L., and Galipeau, J. (2009). Mesenchymal stromal cells cross-present soluble exogenous antigens as part of their antigen-presenting cell properties. Blood 114, 2632–2638

Furie, P. M., Weisman MH (2008). Belimumab (fully human monoclonal antibody to BlyS) improved or stabilized systemic lupus erythematosus (SLE) disease activity and reduced flare rate during 3 years of therapy. Ann Rheum Dis 67, 53

Gabrielli, A., Avvedimento, E. V., and Krieg, T. (2009). Scleroderma. N Engl J Med 360, 1989–2003

Genovese, M. C., McKay, J. D., Nasonov, E. L., Mysler, E. F., da Silva, N. A., Alecock, E., Woodworth, T., and Gomez-Reino, J. J. (2008). Interleukin-6 receptor inhibition with tocilizumab reduces disease activity in rheumatoid arthritis with inadequate response to disease-modifying antirheumatic drugs: the tocilizumab in combination with traditional disease-modifying antirheumatic drug therapy study. Arthritis Rheum 58, 2968–2980

Genovese, M. C., Greenwald, M. W., Alloway, J. A., Baldassare, A. R., Chase, W., Newman, C. (2009). Efficacy and Safety of Baminercept in the Treatment of Rheumatoid Arthritis (RA) Results of the Phase 2B Study in the TNF-IR Population. Arthritis Rheum 60, Suppl 10:417

Gilleece, M. H. and Dexter, T. M. (1993). Effect of Campath-1H antibody on human hematopoietic progenitors in vitro. Blood 82, 807–812

Glennie, S., Soeiro, I., Dyson, P. J., Lam, E. W., and Dazzi, F. (2005). Bone marrow mesenchymal stem cells induce division arrest anergy of activated T cells. Blood 105, 2821–2827

Groom, J. and Mackay, F. (2008). B cells flying solo. Immunol Cell Biol 86, 40–46

Groom, J., Kalled, S. L., Cutler, A. H., Olson, C., Woodcock, S. A., Schneider, P., Tschopp, J., Cachero, T. G., Batten, M., Wheway, J., et al. (2002). Association of BAFF/BLyS overexpression and altered B cell differentiation with Sjogren's syndrome. J Clin Invest 109, 59–68

Hashimoto, J., Garnero, P., van der Heijde, D., Miyasaka, N., Yamamoto, K., Kawai, S., Takeuchi, T., Yoshikawa, H., and Nishimoto, N. (2010). Humanized anti-interleukin-6-receptor antibody (tocilizumab) monotherapy is more effective in slowing radiographic progression in patients with rheumatoid arthritis at high baseline risk for structural damage evaluated with levels of biomarkers, radiography, and BMI: data from the SAMURAI study. Mod Rheumatol

Hertl, M., Eming, R., and Veldman, C. (2006). T cell control in autoimmune bullous skin disorders. J Clin Invest 116, 1159–1166

Holtta, V., Klemetti, P., Sipponen, T., Westerholm-Ormio, M., Kociubinski, G., Salo, H., Rasanen, L., Kolho, K. L., Farkkila, M., Savilahti, E., and Vaarala, O. (2008). IL-23/IL-17 immunity as a hallmark of Crohn's disease. Inflamm Bowel Dis 14, 1175–1184

Hoogduijn, M. J., Popp, F., Verbeek, R., Masoodi, M., Nicolaou, A., Baan, C., and Dahlke, M. H. (2010). The immunomodulatory properties of mesenchymal stem cells and their use for immunotherapy. Int Immunopharmacol

Horwitz, E. M., Le Blanc, K., Dominici, M., Mueller, I., Slaper-Cortenbach, I., Marini, F. C., Deans, R. J., Krause, D. S., and Keating, A. (2005). Clarification of the nomenclature for MSC: The International Society for Cellular Therapy position statement. Cytotherapy 7, 393–395

Ikehara, S., Ohtsuki, H., Good, R. A., Asamoto, H., Nakamura, T., Sekita, K., Muso, E., Tochino, Y., Ida, T., Kuzuya, H., and et al. (1985). Prevention of type I diabetes in nonobese diabetic mice by allogenic bone marrow transplantation. Proc Natl Acad Sci U S A 82, 7743–7747

Ilan, Y., Zigmond, E., Lalazar, G., Dembinsky, A., Ben Ya'acov, A., Hemed, N., Kasis, I., Axelrod, E., Zolotarov, L., Klein, A., et al. (2010). Oral administration of OKT3 monoclonal antibody to human subjects induces a dose-dependent immunologic effect in T cells and dendritic cells. J Clin Immunol 30, 167–177

Illei, G. G., Shirota, Y., Yarboro, C. H., Daruwalla, J., Tackey, E., Takada, K., Fleisher, T., Balow, J. E., and Lipsky, P. E. (2010). Tocilizumab in systemic lupus erythematosus: data on safety, preliminary efficacy, and impact on circulating plasma cells from an open-label phase I dosage-escalation study. Arthritis Rheum 62, 542–552

Jayne, D., Passweg, J., Marmont, A., Farge, D., Zhao, X., Arnold, R., Hiepe, F., Lisukov, I., Musso, M., Ou-Yang, J., et al. (2004). Autologous stem cell transplantation for systemic lupus erythematosus. Lupus 13, 168–176

Jellusova, J., Wellmann, U., Amann, K., Winkler, T. H., and Nitschke, L. (2010). CD22 x Siglec-G double-deficient mice have massively increased B1 cell numbers and develop systemic autoimmunity. J Immunol 184, 3618–3627

Joly, P., Mouquet, H., Roujeau, J. C., D'Incan, M., Gilbert, D., Jacquot, S., Gougeon, M. L., Bedane, C., Muller, R., Dreno, B., et al. (2007). A single cycle of rituximab for the treatment of severe pemphigus. N Engl J Med 357, 545–552

Jones, J. L. and Coles, A. J. (2009). Spotlight on alemtuzumab. Int MS J 16, 77–81

Jonsson, M. V., Szodoray, P., Jellestad, S., Jonsson, R., and Skarstein, K. (2005). Association between circulating levels of the novel TNF family members APRIL and BAFF and lymphoid organization in primary Sjogren's syndrome. J Clin Immunol 25, 189–201

Kalunian, K. C., Davis, J. C., Jr., Merrill, J. T., Totoritis, M. C., and Wofsy, D. (2002). Treatment of systemic lupus erythematosus by inhibition of T cell costimulation with anti-CD154: a randomized, double-blind, placebo-controlled trial. Arthritis Rheum 46, 3251–3258

19

Keymeulen, B., Vandemeulebroucke, E., Ziegler, A. G., Mathieu, C., Kaufman, L., Hale, G., Gorus, F., Goldman, M., Walter, M., Candon, S., et al. (2005). Insulin needs after CD3-antibody therapy in new-onset type 1 diabetes. N Engl J Med 352, 2598–2608

Kimball, A. B., Gordon, K. B., Langley, R. G., Menter, A., Chartash, E. K., and Valdes, J. (2008). Safety and efficacy of ABT-874, a fully human interleukin 12/23 monoclonal antibody, in the treatment of moderate to severe chronic plaque psoriasis: results of a randomized, placebo-controlled, phase 2 trial. Arch Dermatol 144, 200–207

Kishimoto, T. (2005). Interleukin-6: from basic science to medicine – 40 years in immunology. Annu Rev Immunol 23, 1–21

Kraan, M. C., van Kuijk, A. W., Dinant, H. J., Goedkoop, A. Y., Smeets, T. J., de Rie, M. A., Dijkmans, B. A., Vaishnaw, A. K., Bos, J. D., and Tak, P. P. (2002). Alefacept treatment in psoriatic arthritis: reduction of the effector T cell population in peripheral blood and synovial tissue is associated with improvement of clinical signs of arthritis. Arthritis Rheum 46, 2776–2784

Krakowski, M. and Owens, T. (1996). Interferon-gamma confers resistance to experimental allergic encephalomyelitis. Eur J Immunol 26, 1641–1646

Krampera, M., Glennie, S., Dyson, J., Scott, D., Laylor, R., Simpson, E., and Dazzi, F. (2003). Bone marrow mesenchymal stem cells inhibit the response of naive and memory antigen-specific T cells to their cognate peptide. Blood 101, 3722–3729

Krueger, G. G., Langley, R. G., Leonardi, C., Yeilding, N., Guzzo, C., Wang, Y., Dooley, L. T., and Lebwohl, M. (2007). A human interleukin-12/23 monoclonal antibody for the treatment of psoriasis. N Engl J Med 356, 580–592

Krueger, G. G., Papp, K. A., Stough, D. B., Loven, K. H., Gulliver, W. P., and Ellis, C. N. (2002). A randomized, double-blind, placebo-controlled phase III study evaluating efficacy and tolerability of 2 courses of alefacept in patients with chronic plaque psoriasis. J Am Acad Dermatol 47, 821–833

Lanzavecchia, A. (1990). Receptor-mediated antigen uptake and its effect on antigen presentation to class II-restricted T lymphocytes. Annu Rev Immunol 8, 773–793

Larghero, J., Farge, D., Braccini, A., Lecourt, S., Scherberich, A., Fois, E., Verrecchia, F., Daikeler, T., Gluckman, E., Tyndall, A., and Bocelli-Tyndall, C. (2008). Phenotypical and functional characteristics of in vitro expanded bone marrow mesenchymal stem cells from patients with systemic sclerosis. Ann Rheum Dis 67, 443–449

Le Blanc, K., Frassoni, F., Ball, L., Locatelli, F., Roelofs, H., Lewis, I., Lanino, E., Sundberg, B., Bernardo, M. E., Remberger, M., et al. (2008). Mesenchymal stem cells for treatment of steroid-resistant, severe, acute graft-versus-host disease: a phase II study. Lancet 371, 1579–1586

Leonardi, C. L., Kimball, A. B., Papp, K. A., Yeilding, N., Guzzo, C., Wang, Y., Li, S., Dooley, L. T., and Gordon, K. B. (2008). Efficacy and safety of ustekinumab, a human interleukin-12/23 monoclonal antibody, in patients with psoriasis:76-week results from a randomised, double-blind, placebo-controlled trial (PHOENIX 1). Lancet 371, 1665–1674

Levesque, M. C. (2009). Translational Mini-Review Series on B Cell-Directed Therapies: Recent advances in B cell-directed biological therapies for autoimmune disorders. Clin Exp Immunol 157, 198–208

Levesque, M. C. and St Clair, E. W. (2008). B cell-directed therapies for autoimmune disease and correlates of disease response and relapse. J Allergy Clin Immunol 121, 13-21; quiz 22–13

Lin, M. S., Swartz, S. J., Lopez, A., Ding, X., Fernandez-Vina, M. A., Stastny, P., Fairley, J. A., and Diaz, L. A. (1997). Development and characterization of desmoglein-3 specific T cells from patients with pemphigus vulgaris. J Clin Invest 99, 31–40

Ludvigsson, J., Faresjo, M., Hjorth, M., Axelsson, S., Cheramy, M., Pihl, M., Vaarala, O., Forsander, G., Ivarsson, S., Johansson, C., et al. (2008). GAD treatment and insulin secretion in recent-onset type 1 diabetes. N Engl J Med 359, 1909–1920

Luo, X., Herold, K. C., and Miller, S. D. (2010). Immunotherapy of type 1 diabetes: where are we and where should we be going? Immunity 32, 488–499

Maccario, R., Podesta, M., Moretta, A., Cometa, A., Comoli, P., Montagna, D., Daudt, L., Ibatici, A., Piaggio, G., Pozzi, S., et al. (2005). Interaction of human mesenchymal stem cells with cells involved in alloantigen-specific immune response favors the differentiation of CD4+ T-cell subsets expressing a regulatory/suppressive phenotype. Haematologica 90, 516–525

Mackay, F. and Ambrose, C. (2003). The TNF family members BAFF and APRIL: the growing complexity. Cytokine Growth Factor Rev 14, 311–324

Mackay, F., Schneider, P., Rennert, P., and Browning, J. (2003). BAFF AND APRIL: a tutorial on B cell survival. Annu Rev Immunol 21, 231–264

Mackay, F., Woodcock, S. A., Lawton, P., Ambrose, C., Baetscher, M., Schneider, P., Tschopp, J., and Browning, J. L. (1999). Mice transgenic for BAFF develop lymphocytic disorders along with autoimmune manifestations. J Exp Med 190, 1697–1710

Magro, L., Catteau, B., Coiteux, V., Bruno, B., Jouet, J. P., and Yakoub-Agha, I. (2008). Efficacy of imatinib mesylate in the treatment of refractory sclerodermatous chronic GVHD. Bone Marrow Transplant 42, 757–760

Mancardi, G. and Saccardi, R. (2008). Autologous haematopoietic stem-cell transplantation in multiple sclerosis. Lancet Neurol 7, 626–636

Mannon, P. J., Fuss, I. J., Mayer, L., Elson, C. O., Sandborn, W. J., Present, D., Dolin, B., Goodman, N., Groden, C., Hornung, R. L., et al. (2004). Anti-interleukin-12 antibody for active Crohn's disease. N Engl J Med 351, 2069–2079

Manz, R. A., Moser, K., Burmester, G. R., Radbruch, A., and Hiepe, F. (2006). Immunological memory stabilizing autoreactivity. Curr Top Microbiol Immunol 305, 241–257

Marmont, A. M. (2004). Stem cell transplantation for autoimmune disorders. Coincidental autoimmune disease in patients transplanted for conventional indications. Best Pract Res Clin Haematol 17, 223–232

Martin, F. and Chan, A. C. (2006). B cell immunobiology in disease: evolving concepts from the clinic. Annu Rev Immunol 24, 467–496

Maxwell, L. and Singh, J. A. (2009). Abatacept for rheumatoid arthritis. Cochrane Database Syst Rev, CD007277

Merrill, J. T., Burgos-Vargas, R., Westhovens, R., Chalmers, A., D'Cruz, D., Wallace, D. J., Bae, S. C., Sigal, L., Becker, J. C., Kelly, S., et al. (2010a). The efficacy and safety of abatacept in patients with non-life-threatening manifestations of SLE: Results of A 12-month exploratory study. Arthritis Rheum

Merrill, J. T., Neuwelt, C. M., Wallace, D. J., Shanahan, J. C., Latinis, K. M., Oates, J. C., Utset, T. O., Gordon, C., Isenberg, D. A., Hsieh, H. J., et al. (2010b). Efficacy and safety of rituximab in moderately-to-severely active systemic lupus erythematosus: the randomized, double-blind, phase II/III systemic lupus erythematosus evaluation of rituximab trial. Arthritis Rheum 62, 222–233

Miller, S. D., Turley, D. M., and Podojil, J. R. (2007). Antigen-specific tolerance strategies for the prevention and treatment of autoimmune disease. Nat Rev Immunol 7, 665–677

Mirabet, M., Barrabes, J. A., Quiroga, A., and Garcia-Dorado, D. (2008). Platelet pro-aggregatory effects of CD40L monoclonal antibody. Mol Immunol 45, 937–944

Muraro, P. A., Douek, D. C., Packer, A., Chung, K., Guenaga, F. J., Cassiani-Ingoni, R., Campbell, C., Memon, S., Nagle, J. W., Hakim, F. T., et al. (2005). Thymic output generates a new and diverse TCR repertoire after autologous stem cell transplantation in multiple sclerosis patients. J Exp Med 201, 805–816

Murphy, C. A., Langrish, C. L., Chen, Y., Blumenschein, W., McClanahan, T., Kastelein, R. A., Sedgwick, J. D., and Cua, D. J. (2003). Divergent pro- and antiinflammatory roles for IL-23 and IL-12 in joint autoimmune inflammation. J Exp Med 198, 1951–1957

Nagafuchi, H., Suzuki, N., Mizushima, Y., and Sakane, T. (1993). Constitutive expression of IL-6 receptors and their role in the excessive B cell function in patients with systemic lupus erythematosus. J Immunol 151, 6525–6534

19

Nagel, A., Hertl, M., and Eming, R. (2009a). B-cell-directed therapy for inflammatory skin diseases. J Invest Dermatol 129, 289–301

Nagel, A., Podstawa, E., Eickmann, M., Muller, H. H., Hertl, M., and Eming, R. (2009b). Rituximab mediates a strong elevation of B-cell-activating factor associated with increased pathogen-specific IgG but not autoantibodies in pemphigus vulgaris. J Invest Dermatol 129, 2202–2210

Nash, R. A., McSweeney, P. A., Crofford, L. J., Abidi, M., Chen, C. S., Godwin, J. D., Gooley, T. A., Holmberg, L., Henstorf, G., LeMaistre, C. F., et al. (2007). High-dose immunosuppressive therapy and autologous hematopoietic cell transplantation for severe systemic sclerosis: long-term follow-up of the US multicenter pilot study. Blood 110, 1388–1396

Nauta, A. J., Kruisselbrink, A. B., Lurvink, E., Willemze, R., and Fibbe, W. E. (2006). Mesenchymal stem cells inhibit generation and function of both CD34+-derived and monocyte-derived dendritic cells. J Immunol 177, 2080–2087

Nemeth, K., Leelahavanichkul, A., Yuen, P. S., Mayer, B., Parmelee, A., Doi, K., Robey, P. G., Leelahavanichkul, K., Koller, B. H., Brown, J. M., et al. (2009). Bone marrow stromal cells attenuate sepsis via prostaglandin E(2)-dependent reprogramming of host macrophages to increase their interleukin-10 production. Nat Med 15, 42–49

Neubert, K., Meister, S., Moser, K., Weisel, F., Maseda, D., Amann, K., Wiethe, C., Winkler, T. H., Kalden, J. R., Manz, R. A., and Voll, R. E. (2008). The proteasome inhibitor bortezomib depletes plasma cells and protects mice with lupus-like disease from nephritis. Nat Med 14, 748–755

Nishimoto, N. and Kishimoto, T. (2008). Humanized antihuman IL-6 receptor antibody, tocilizumab. Handb Exp Pharmacol, 151–160

O'Keefe, T. L., Williams, G. T., Davies, S. L., and Neuberger, M. S. (1996). Hyperresponsive B cells in CD22-deficient mice. Science 274, 798–801

Olivieri, A., Locatelli, F., Zecca, M., Sanna, A., Cimminiello, M., Raimondi, R., Gini, G., Mordini, N., Balduzzi, A., Leoni, P., et al. (2009). Imatinib for refractory chronic graft-versus-host disease with fibrotic features. Blood 114, 709–718

Ong, V. H. and Denton, C. P. (2010). Innovative therapies for systemic sclerosis. Curr Opin Rheumatol 22, 264–272

Oppmann, B., Lesley, R., Blom, B., Timans, J. C., Xu, Y., Hunte, B., Vega, F., Yu, N., Wang, J., Singh, K., et al. (2000). Novel p19 protein engages IL-12p40 to form a cytokine, IL-23, with biological activities similar as well as distinct from IL-12. Immunity 13, 715–725

Ortiz, L. A., Dutreil, M., Fattman, C., Pandey, A. C., Torres, G., Go, K., and Phinney, D. G. (2007). Interleukin 1 receptor antagonist mediates the antiinflammatory and antifibrotic effect of mesenchymal stem cells during lung injury. Proc Natl Acad Sci U S A 104, 11002–11007

Østergaard, B. B., Rigby W et al. (2008a). Efficacy of ofatumumab in rheumatoid arthritis (RA) patients with inadequate response to one or more DMARDs:48 weeks follow up. Arthritis Rheum 58, S306

Østergaard, B. B., Rigby W, et al. (2008b). Ofatuzumab, a human CD20 monoclonal antibody, in th etreatment of rheumatoid arthritis (RA): Subgroup analysis at week 24 from a phase I/II clinical trial. . Arthritis Rheum 58, S305

Papp, K. A., Langley, R. G., Lebwohl, M., Krueger, G. G., Szapary, P., Yeilding, N., Guzzo, C., Hsu, M. C., Wang, Y., Li, S., et al. (2008). Efficacy and safety of ustekinumab, a human interleukin-12/23 monoclonal antibody, in patients with psoriasis:52-week results from a randomised, double-blind, placebo-controlled trial (PHOENIX 2). Lancet 371, 1675–1684

Passweg, J. and Tyndall, A. (2007). Autologous stem cell transplantation in autoimmune diseases. Semin Hematol 44, 278–285

Pene, J., Chevalier, S., Preisser, L., Venereau, E., Guilleux, M. H., Ghannam, S., Moles, J. P., Danger, Y., Ravon, E., Lesaux, S., et al. (2008). Chronically inflamed human tissues are infiltrated by highly differentiated Th17 lymphocytes. J Immunol 180, 7423–7430

Pers, J. O., Daridon, C., Devauchelle, V., Jousse, S., Saraux, A., Jamin, C., and Youinou, P. (2005). BAFF overexpression is associated with autoantibody production in autoimmune diseases. Ann N Y Acad Sci 1050, 34–39

Pers, J. O., Devauchelle, V., Daridon, C., Bendaoud, B., Le Berre, R., Bordron, A., Hutin, P., Renaudineau, Y., Dueymes, M., Loisel, S., et al. (2007). BAFF-modulated repopulation of B lymphocytes in the blood and salivary glands of rituximab-treated patients with Sjogren's syndrome. Arthritis Rheum 56, 1464–1477

Peterson, E., Robertson, A. D., and Emlen, W. (1996). Serum and urinary interleukin-6 in systemic lupus erythematosus. Lupus 5, 571–575

Petri, H. K., Gordon C (2008). Clinically meaningful improvements with Epratuzumab (anti-CD22 mAb targeting B-cells) in patients (Pts) with moderate/severe SLE flares: results from 2 randomized controlled trials. Arthritis Rheum 58, S571

Petri M, H. K., Gordon C (2008). Clinically meaningful improvements with Epratuzumab (anti-CD22 mAb targeting B-cells) in patients (Pts) with moderate/severe SLE flares: results from 2 randomized controlled trials. Arthritis Rheumatism 58, S571

Pittenger, M., Vanguri, P., Simonetti, D., and Young, R. (2002). Adult mesenchymal stem cells: potential for muscle and tendon regeneration and use in gene therapy. J Musculoskelet Neuronal Interact 2, 309–320

Press, O. W., Appelbaum, F., Ledbetter, J. A., Martin, P. J., Zarling, J., Kidd, P., and Thomas, E. D. (1987). Monoclonal antibody 1F5 (anti-CD20) serotherapy of human B cell lymphomas. Blood 69, 584–591

Radbruch, A., Muehlinghaus, G., Luger, E. O., Inamine, A., Smith, K. G., Dorner, T., and Hiepe, F. (2006). Competence and competition: the challenge of becoming a long-lived plasma cell. Nat Rev Immunol 6, 741–750

Ramos-Casals, M., Fonollosa-Pla, V., Brito-Zeron, P., and Siso-Almirall, A. (2010). Targeted therapy for systemic sclerosis: how close are we? Nat Rev Rheumatol 6, 269–278

Richards, H. B., Satoh, M., Shaw, M., Libert, C., Poli, V., and Reeves, W. H. (1998). Interleukin 6 dependence of anti-DNA antibody production: evidence for two pathways of autoantibody formation in pristane-induced lupus. J Exp Med 188, 985–990

Roberts, J. L., Ortonne, J. P., Tan, J. K., Jaracz, E., and Frankel, E. (2010). The safety profile and sustained remission associated with response to multiple courses of intramuscular alefacept for treatment of chronic plaque psoriasis. J Am Acad Dermatol 62, 968–978

Roschke, V., Sosnovtseva, S., Ward, C. D., Hong, J. S., Smith, R., Albert, V., Stohl, W., Baker, K. P., Ullrich, S., Nardelli, B., et al. (2002). BLyS and APRIL form biologically active heterotrimers that are expressed in patients with systemic immune-based rheumatic diseases. J Immunol 169, 4314–4321

Ryffel, B., Car, B. D., Gunn, H., Roman, D., Hiestand, P., and Mihatsch, M. J. (1994). Interleukin-6 exacerbates glomerulonephritis in (NZB x NZW)F1 mice. Am J Pathol 144, 927–937

Sakaguchi, S. (2004). Naturally arising CD4+ regulatory t cells for immunologic self-tolerance and negative control of immune responses. Annu Rev Immunol 22, 531–562

Samardzic, T., Marinkovic, D., Danzer, C. P., Gerlach, J., Nitschke, L., and Wirth, T. (2002). Reduction of marginal zone B cells in CD22-deficient mice. Eur J Immunol 32, 561–567

Sandborn, W. J., Feagan, B. G., Fedorak, R. N., Scherl, E., Fleisher, M. R., Katz, S., Johanns, J., Blank, M., and Rutgeerts, P. (2008). A randomized trial of Ustekinumab, a human interleukin-12/23 monoclonal antibody, in patients with moderate-to-severe Crohn's disease. Gastroenterology 135, 1130–1141

Sanz, I. and Lee, F. E. (2010). B cells as therapeutic targets in SLE. Nat Rev Rheumatol 6, 326–337

Sasaki, Y., Casola, S., Kutok, J. L., Rajewsky, K., and Schmidt-Supprian, M. (2004). TNF family member B cell-activating factor (BAFF) receptor-dependent and -independent roles for BAFF in B cell physiology. J Immunol 173, 2245–2252

Savage, D. G. and Antman, K. H. (2002). Imatinib mesylate – a new oral targeted therapy. N Engl J Med 346, 683–693

Schmidt, E., Goebeler, M., and Zillikens, D. (2009). Rituximab in severe pemphigus. Ann N Y Acad Sci 1173, 683–691

19

Schneider, P. (2005). The role of APRIL and BAFF in lymphocyte activation. Curr Opin Immunol 17, 282–289

Segal, B. M., Constantinescu, C. S., Raychaudhuri, A., Kim, L., Fidelus-Gort, R., and Kasper, L. H. (2008). Repeated subcutaneous injections of IL12/23 p40 neutralising antibody, ustekinumab, in patients with relapsing-remitting multiple sclerosis: a phase II, double-blind, placebo-controlled, randomised, dose-ranging study. Lancet Neurol 7, 796–804

Seyler, T. M., Park, Y. W., Takemura, S., Bram, R. J., Kurtin, P. J., Goronzy, J. J., and Weyand, C. M. (2005). BLyS and APRIL in rheumatoid arthritis. J Clin Invest 115, 3083–3092

Shaw, D. G. J., Trapp R (2007). The safety, pharmacokinetics (PK) and pharmacodynamic (PD) effects of repeated doses of BR3-Fc in patients with rheumatoid arthritis (RA). Arthritis Rheum 56, S568–569

Shaw M, D. G. J., Trapp R (2007). The safety, pharmacokinetics (PK) and pharmacodynamic (PD) effects of repeated doses of BR3-Fc in patients with rheumatoid arthritis (RA). Arthritis Rheum 56, S568–569

Shlomchik, M. J. (2009). Activating systemic autoimmunity: B's, T's, and tolls. Curr Opin Immunol 21, 626–633

Skhirtladze, C., Distler, O., Dees, C., Akhmetshina, A., Busch, N., Venalis, P., Zwerina, J., Spriewald, B., Pileckyte, M., Schett, G., and Distler, J. H. (2008). Src kinases in systemic sclerosis: central roles in fibroblast activation and in skin fibrosis. Arthritis Rheum 58, 1475–1484

Skyler, J. S., Krischer, J. P., Wolfsdorf, J., Cowie, C., Palmer, J. P., Greenbaum, C., Cuthbertson, D., Rafkin-Mervis, L. E., Chase, H. P., and Leschek, E. (2005). Effects of oral insulin in relatives of patients with type 1 diabetes: The Diabetes Prevention Trial – Type 1. Diabetes Care 28, 1068–1076

Smith, C. E. and Miller, S. D. (2006). Multi-peptide coupled-cell tolerance ameliorates ongoing relapsing EAE associated with multiple pathogenic autoreactivities. J Autoimmun 27, 218–231

Sriram, S., Schwartz, G., and Steinman, L. (1983). Administration of myelin basic protein-coupled spleen cells prevents experimental allergic encephalitis. Cell Immunol 75, 378–382

St Clair, E. W. (2009). Novel targeted therapies for autoimmunity. Curr Opin Immunol 21, 648–657

Steinfeld, S. D., Tant, L., Burmester, G. R., Teoh, N. K., Wegener, W. A., Goldenberg, D. M., and Pradier, O. (2006). Epratuzumab (humanised anti-CD22 antibody) in primary Sjogren's syndrome: an open-label phase I/II study. Arthritis Res Ther 8, R129

Steinman, L. (2010a). Inverse vaccination, the opposite of Jenner's concept, for therapy of autoimmunity. J Intern Med 267, 441–451

Steinman, L. (2010b). Mixed results with modulation of TH-17 cells in human autoimmune diseases. Nat Immunol 11, 41–44

Sullivan, K. M., Muraro, P., and Tyndall, A. (2010). Hematopoietic cell transplantation for autoimmune disease: updates from Europe and the United States. Biol Blood Marrow Transplant 16, S48–56

Tak, P. P., Thurlings, R. M., Rossier, C., Nestorov, I., Dimic, A., Mircetic, V., Rischmueller, M., Nasonov, E., Shmidt, E., Emery, P., and Munafo, A. (2008). Atacicept in patients with rheumatoid arthritis: results of a multicenter, phase Ib, double-blind, placebo-controlled, dose-escalating, single- and repeated-dose study. Arthritis Rheum 58, 61–72

Tarner, I. H. (2009). [Novel B-cell directed strategies for the treatment of rheumatic diseases]. Z Rheumatol 68, 380–389

Tedder, T. F. (2009). CD19: a promising B cell target for rheumatoid arthritis. Nat Rev Rheumatol 5, 572–577

Tedder, T. F., Poe, J. C., and Haas, K. M. (2005). CD22: a multifunctional receptor that regulates B lymphocyte survival and signal transduction. Adv Immunol 88, 1–50

Thrower, S. L., James, L., Hall, W., Green, K. M., Arif, S., Allen, J. S., Van-Krinks, C., Lozanoska-Ochser, B., Marquesini, L., Brown, S., et al. (2009). Proinsulin peptide immunotherapy in type 1 diabetes: report of a first-in-man Phase I safety study. Clin Exp Immunol 155, 156–165

Tolar, J., Le Blanc, K., Keating, A., and Blazar, B. R. (2010). Hitting the Right Spot with Mesenchymal Stromal Cells (MSCs). Stem Cells

Tsunoda, K., Ota, T., Suzuki, H., Ohyama, M., Nagai, T., Nishikawa, T., Amagai, M., and Koyasu, S. (2002). Pathogenic autoantibody production requires loss of tolerance against desmoglein 3 in both T and B cells in experimental pemphigus vulgaris. Eur J Immunol 32, 627–633

Tyndall, A., Walker, U. A., Cope, A., Dazzi, F., De Bari, C., Fibbe, W., Guiducci, S., Jones, S., Jorgensen, C., Le Blanc, K., et al. (2007). Immunomodulatory properties of mesenchymal stem cells: a review based on an interdisciplinary meeting held at the Kennedy Institute of Rheumatology Division, London, UK, 31 October 2005. Arthritis Res Ther 9, 301

Tyndall, A. and Gratwohl, A. (2009). Adult stem cell transplantation in autoimmune disease. Curr Opin Hematol 16, 285–291

Ushiyama, T., Chano, T., Inoue, K., and Matsusue, Y. (2003). Cytokine production in the infrapatellar fat pad: another source of cytokines in knee synovial fluids. Ann Rheum Dis 62, 108–112

Vallerskog, T., Gunnarsson, I., Widhe, M., Risselada, A., Klareskog, L., van Vollenhoven, R., Malmstrom, V., and Trollmo, C. (2007). Treatment with rituximab affects both the cellular and the humoral arm of the immune system in patients with SLE. Clin Immunol 122, 62–74

van Laar, J. M., Farge, D., and Tyndall, A. (2008). Stem cell transplantation: a treatment option for severe systemic sclerosis? Ann Rheum Dis 67 Suppl 3, iii35–38

Vandenbark, A. A., Vainiene, M., Ariail, K., Miller, S. D., and Offner, H. (1996). Prevention and treatment of relapsing autoimmune encephalomyelitis with myelin peptide-coupled splenocytes. J Neurosci Res 45, 430–438

Vonk, M. C., Marjanovic, Z., van den Hoogen, F. H., Zohar, S., Schattenberg, A. V., Fibbe, W. E., Larghero, J., Gluckman, E., Preijers, F. W., van Dijk, A. P., et al. (2008). Long-term follow-up results after autologous haematopoietic stem cell transplantation for severe systemic sclerosis. Ann Rheum Dis 67, 98–104

Warren, K. G., Catz, I., Ferenczi, L. Z., and Krantz, M. J. (2006). Intravenous synthetic peptide MBP8298 delayed disease progression in an HLA Class II-defined cohort of patients with progressive multiple sclerosis: results of a 24-month double-blind placebo-controlled clinical trial and 5 years of follow-up treatment. Eur J Neurol 13, 887–895

Wucherpfennig, K. W., Yu, B., Bhol, K., Monos, D. S., Argyris, E., Karr, R. W., Ahmed, A. R., and Strominger, J. L. (1995). Structural basis for major histocompatibility complex (MHC)-linked susceptibility to autoimmunity: charged residues of a single MHC binding pocket confer selective presentation of self-peptides in pemphigus vulgaris. Proc Natl Acad Sci U S A 92, 11935–11939

Yang, M., Sun, L., Wang, S., Ko, K. H., Xu, H., Zheng, B. J., Cao, X., and Lu, L. (2010). Novel function of B cell-activating factor in the induction of IL-10-producing regulatory B cells. J Immunol 184, 3321–3325

Zappia, E., Casazza, S., Pedemonte, E., Benvenuto, F., Bonanni, I., Gerdoni, E., Giunti, D., Ceravolo, A., Cazzanti, F., Frassoni, F., et al. (2005). Mesenchymal stem cells ameliorate experimental autoimmune encephalomyelitis inducing T-cell anergy. Blood 106, 1755–1761

Zhang, M., Ko, K. H., Lam, Q. L., Lo, C. K., Srivastava, G., Zheng, B., Lau, Y. L., and Lu, L. (2005). Expression and function of TNF family member B cell-activating factor in the development of autoimmune arthritis. Int Immunol 17, 1081–1092

Zhou, L., Chong, M. M., and Littman, D. R. (2009). Plasticity of CD4+ T cell lineage differentiation. Immunity 30, 646–655

19

Subject Index